Clinics in Developmental Medicine No.162
SHAKING AND OTHER NON-ACCIDENTAL
HEAD INJURIES IN CHILDREN

© 2005 Mac Keith Press
High Holborn House, 30 Furnival Street, London EC4A 1JQ

Editor: Hilary M Hart
Managing Editor: Michael Pountney

First published in this edition 2005

Reprinted March 2006

British Library Cataloguing-in-Publication data:
A catalogue record for this book is available from the British Library

ISSN: 0069 4835
ISBN: 1 898683 35 2

Printed by The Lavenham Press Ltd, Water Street, Lavenham, Suffolk
Mac Keith Press is supported by Scope

Clinics in Developmental Medicine No. 162

Shaking and Other Non-accidental Head Injuries in Children

Edited by

ROBERT A MINNS
J KEITH BROWN

University of Edinburgh, *and*
Royal Hospital for Sick Children
Edinburgh, Scotland

2005
Mac Keith Press

Distributed by 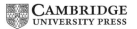 **CAMBRIDGE**
UNIVERSITY PRESS

This book is
dedicated to

A Norman Guthkelch

CONTENTS

AUTHORS' APPOINTMENTS

Karen M Barlow — Assistant Professor, Division of Neurology, University of Calgary, Alberta Children's Hospital, Canada; *formerly* Research Fellow, Neurology Department, Royal Hospital for Sick Children, Edinburgh, Scotland

Jeanne E Bell — Professor of Neuropathology, University of Edinburgh; *and* Honorary Consultant Neuropathologist, Western General Hospital, Edinburgh, Scotland

J Keith Brown — Consultant Paediatric Neurologist, Royal Hospital for Sick Children, Edinburgh; *and* Part-time Senior Lecturer, Section of Child Life and Health, University of Edinburgh, Scotland

Anne-Marie Childs — Consultant Paediatric Neurologist, Neonatal Unit, Leeds General Infirmary, Leeds, England

Cathy Cobley — Senior Lecturer in Law, Cardiff Law School, Cardiff University, Wales

Robert Doran — Consultant Ophthalmologist, Department of Ophthalmology, Leeds General Infirmary, Leeds, England

Elaine Ennis — Training and Development Consultant, Outcomes UK Ltd, Winchester; *formerly* Lecturer in Social Work, Centre for Child Care and Protection Studies, Department of Social Work, University of Dundee, Scotland

Tim Jaspan — Consultant Paediatric Radiologist, Queen's Medical Centre, Nottingham, England

Patricia A Jones — Research Fellow, Child Life and Health, University of Edinburgh, Scotland

John H Livingston — Consultant Paediatric Neurologist, Neurology Department, The General Infirmary, Leeds, England

TY Milly Lo — Research Fellow, Paediatric Neurosciences, Child Life and Health, University of Edinburgh, Scotland

Stephanie Mackenzie — Consultant Paediatric Radiologist, Royal Hospital for Sick Children, Edinburgh, Scotland

Kristina May — Specialist Registrar in Ophthalmology, Department of Ophthalmology, Royal Hallamshire Hospital, Sheffield, England

Maeve McPhillips — Consultant Paediatric Radiologist, Royal Hospital for Sick Children, Edinburgh, Scotland

Caroline Millar — Research Nurse, Child Life and Health, University of Edinburgh, Scotland

Fiona C Minns — Senior House Officer, Western General Hospital, Edinburgh, Scotland

Robert A Minns — Professor of Paediatric Neurology, University of Edinburgh; Academic Head, University of Edinburgh, Section of Child Life and Health; Honorary Consultant Paediatric Neurologist, Royal Hospital for Sick Children, Edinburgh, Scotland

Jacqueline Mok — Consultant Paediatrician, Community Child Health Services, Edinburgh, Scotland

Chris N Morison — Research and Development Engineer, Postgraduate, University of Birmingham, England

M Andrew Parsons — Director, Ophthalmic Sciences Unit, Royal Hallamshire Hospital; and Senior Lecturer in Ophthalmic Pathology, University of Sheffield, England

Jonathan Punt — Consultant Paediatric Neurosurgeon, Nottingham, England

Nina Punt — Independent Researcher, Nottingham, England

K Kamath Tallur — Specialist Paediatric Registrar, Royal Hospital for Sick Children, Edinburgh, Scotland

Philip Wheeler — Detective Chief Inspector, Metropolitan Police, New Scotland Yard, London, England

FOREWORD

The last few years have seen an intense spotlight on non-accidental injury in children. The tragic case in London of Victoria Climbié, who was systematically abused and then murdered by her carers, highlighted the difficulties encountered when abuse was eventually clear for all to see. The more subtle forms of child abuse have also come under media scrutiny. Three high-profile cases involving sudden infant death where mothers were either released from a life sentence for murder, or not convicted, because of disputed medical evidence, has left the public and professionals understandably confused.

Child abuse in all its myriad forms is one of the most challenging areas of medical practice. The cornerstone of all medical practice is the initial consultation with a person who is ill or perceives themselves to be so. In paediatric practice this is, of necessity, a triadic consultation with a parent or carer speaking for the child. An accurate history followed by examination and necessary investigation gives the best chance of arriving at a correct diagnosis, which is then followed by a management and treatment plan.

Head injury can be a difficult area. Skull fractures, and retinal and subdural haemorrhages, are all conditions that may occur both accidentally and non accidentally. Occasionally we do get an accurate history either because an event has been witnessed or a 'perpetrator' confesses.

This volume of *Clinics in Developmental Medicine* is edited, and indeed substantially authored, by leading experts Bob Minns and Keith Brown from Edinburgh. They have undertaken a great deal of original research and drawn this together with other contemporary work into a single source of reference for all those involved in this difficult area. Medical practitioners should find it invaluable and the legal profession will be able to use it as an authoritative source of the 'state of the art'.

This, along with experimental work in the laboratory, is helping us to understand the true meaning of clinical and pathological findings. However, the area remains controversial and it is timely for a review of the evidence.

Alan Craft
President
Royal College of Paediatrics and Child Health

ACKNOWLEDGEMENTS

We are greatly indebted to Mr Andrew S Muirhead FCIBS MBA, Chief Executive of Lloyds TSB Foundation for Scotland, and successive Chairpersons, Mr Charles McGregor (Hon Sec), Sir Andrew Bruce, Earl of Elgin and Kincardine KT JP DL, Hon. Dame Mary Corsar DBE, Mr JDM Robertson CBE, Mr J George Mathieson CBE TD DL, Mr Archie Robb Dip SW CQSW ACIS Hon D Litt, Mr Norman Drummond, and former Chief Executive of Lloyds TSB Scotland, Mr Alistair Dempster, for generous financial support for research into non-accidental head injury at the Royal Hospital for Sick Children, Edinburgh, and the University of Edinburgh.

We are similarly grateful to Mr RK Austin and the trustees of the RS Macdonald Charitable Trust and to the Morton Stewart Bequest.

We have had support and encouragement from Dr Andrew Fraser (Deputy Chief Medical Officer, Scotland) and the Hon. Catherine Stihler (MEP Dunfermline), and fruitful discussion with Professor Aubrey Manning, OBE BSc DPhil FIBiol FRSE FRZSS, Emeritus Professor of Natural History, University of Edinburgh.

Our special thanks are reserved for Mrs Patricia Jones who has not only contributed to the content of this volume but has laboured tirelessly over much of the presentation, revisions and corrections in various chapters.

Much of the scholarship and research would not have been possible without the support of our colleagues in Paediatric Neurosciences in Edinburgh, Mr James Steers, Miss Lynn Myles, Dr Paul Eunson, Dr Ailsa McLellan, Charge Nurse Joan Saunders and our paediatric colleagues at the Royal Hospital for Sick Children in Edinburgh, consultant colleagues in South East Scotland and to those throughout Scotland in the 'Non-Accidental Head Injury Interest Group' who have contributed cases and illustrations to the Scottish database.

We are indebted to colleagues in various specialties: (Pathology and Neuropathology) Professor Jeanne Bell, Dr Colin Smith, Dr Jean Keeling; (Forensic Medicine) Professor Anthony Busuttil; (Neuropsychology) Dr David Johnson; (Radiology) Dr Maeve McPhillips, Dr Rod Gibson, Dr Graham Wilkinson, Dr Mike Hendry, Dr Stephanie MacKenzie; (Child Protection Consultants) Dr Jacqui Mok, Dr Helen Hammond; (Social Work colleagues) Mr Kenny Dickson, the late Mr John McBride; (Child Protection Coordinator Lothian) Mr Martin Henry and (University of St Andrews Social Work) Elaine Ennis; (Secretarial support) Kim Motion, Elaine Forbes, Angela Smith; (Establishing and maintaining the Scottish database) Dr Karen Barlow, Mrs Frances Wright, Dr Milly Lo, Ms Caroline Miller, Ms Gillian Lawson, Dr Fiona Minns, Mrs Eleanor Kerr; (Statisticians) Ms Gillian Taylor and Ms Mandy Lee; (Medical Physics and Physiology) Dr Harry Brash, Ms Karne McBride, Mr Bill Duval and in particular the late Dr Geoffrey Walsh; (Photography) Mr Len Cumming; (Ophthalmologists) Dr Brian Fleck, Dr Alan Mulvihill; (Forensic Statistics, Edinburgh) Professor CGG Aitken: (Librarian RHSC Edinburgh) Ms Anne Donnelly.

We are particularly indebted to our national and international colleagues for their intellectual and other support, in particular Professor Tina Duhaime, Professor Susan Margulies, Ms Marilyn Sandberg, Professor Ronald Barr, Professor Randal Alexander, Professor Tim David and Detective Chief Inspector Phil Wheeler, and ex-University of Edinburgh medical students who undertook studies on inflicted head injury in children as part of their studies – Dr Francesca Clough, Dr Rachel Cooke and Dr Isabel Boyd.

We are grateful to those publishers who have kindly allowed us to reproduce figures and illustrations from their publications.

Finally, we thank the staff at Mac Keith Press for their perseverance in what has been a very protracted exercise, often changing or being modified in the light of new thinking or research findings in this very complex subject.

RAM
JKB

PREFACE

This book is written in the hope that it will be of value to all paediatricians, both hospital and community, and to child protection teams including legal, police and social work personnel who have to deal with the always very difficult cases of inflicted head injuries to young infants and the vexatious arguments that surround them.

There are people with entrenched and extreme views on both sides of the arguments surrounding non-accidental head injury (NAHI) and shaken baby syndrome (SBS), with some denying that adults ever cause inflicted brain trauma to children. Others argue that shaking does not cause brain injury to infants, still others maintain that SBS is not an entity and cannot be diagnosed, and that the child's clinical findings are explicable from other causes such as minor falls, hypoxia, or earlier from birth, or that it does not occur in particular cultures. While it is inevitable that the child presenting with a subdural haemorrhage (SDH) or retinal haemorrhage, or combinations of features, will and should trigger thoughts about the possibility of abuse, there are those at the other extreme who report large series of NAHI/SBS, some cases of which might not stand up to current exhaustive scrutiny. In the current medico-legal climate the easiest approach would be to sit on the fence and look in both directions. However, decisions have got to be made using the best possible information and knowledge available at the time when faced with an infant who is suffering a life threatening injury.

The book attempts a uniform hypothesis involving different mechanisms of brain injury and how rotational injury (shaking) fits into these. It also outlines an approach to the diagnosis of NAHI made from the history, examination and contributory social risk factors, leading to a diagnosis of 'suspected' NAHI (after thorough investigations about the circumstances of the injury, and exclusion of potential differential diagnoses). This diagnosis is made with varying levels of certainty (definite, probable/presumptive, possible/not certain, or not NAHI). Separately, comment is offered about whether the mechanism/s of the injury is/are consistent with impact, rotational injury, rotational and impact deceleration, whiplashing, compression, etc. There may be many cases, however, where the physician is unsure and cannot make a diagnosis of NAHI or attempt to offer a mechanism of injuring, for example chronic SDH, and it is vital that the paediatrician does not try to force the signs and symptoms into a preconceived diagnosis. Although courts of law demand absolute proof, one cannot expect to provide a greater level of proof with the best possible clinical judgement than is available in other fields of medicine. It is clear, however, that there is no single pathognomonic feature which is positive proof of NAHI. The book attempts to produce an evidence base from the current medical literature, from our own clinical experience, and from our own research findings in NAHI at the Department of Child Life and Health in the University of Edinburgh, and from a database of suspected NAHI cases in Scotland.

The book comprises a number of specialist chapters concerned with retinopathy, epidemiology, SDH, outcome, etc., with a substantial initial overview chapter that attempts to tie together the various facets of this multidimensional injury of infants.

Recent topical controversies, such as the 'short fall' controversy, the hypothesis that SDHs and retinal haemorrhages are due to hypoxia, the arguments concerning the role of re-bleeding of SDHs, the aetiology of posterior fossa SDHs, and the question of whether perinatal SDHs mimic infant-inflicted injuries, are all raised and discussed.

This publication does not attempt to be a text on the whole of head injury in childhood but does include other types of head injury that illustrate a pathology or pathophysiology, or produce a similar clinical syndrome to NAHI (such as neonatal compression head injury, boxing injuries, accidental traumatic acceleration–deceleration injuries, rotational injury in adults subjected to shaking injury, and similar patterns of damage associated with conflict blast injury and the use of body armour helmets). It does not cover other types of NAHI, e.g. gunshots wounds to the head, which may be common in other cultures but are rarely encountered by paediatricians working in the United Kingdom.

Associated with media attention there may have been some confusion in the public perception of the relationship between cot death and NAHI. This work does not attempt to be a treatise on cot death, but it is recognized that although some cot deaths may rarely be a result of non-accidental suffocation, NAHI is not a feature of the pathology of cot death at autopsy. Double pathology may occur, for example in an adult suffocating a child to stop them crying after having caused a NAHI. Such situations require much pathological expertise in differentiating this from the pathology of hypoxic–ischaemic injury consequent on cervicomedullary junction injury associated with shaking.

In an ideal world paediatricians would be without bias or preconceptions, but because of their close contact with the child, they may be the only person in the court who has seen a reported previously normal child change to a blind, cognitively and motor-impaired infant. Traditionally paediatricians have always considered themselves as advocates for the child, and while this still remains largely true, they cannot fail to be aware of the consequences of their diagnosis for the child divorced from his/her family. This is one of the few unenviable situations where paediatricians may find themselves trying to protect the child and possibly siblings from further injury, and acting against the parents.

Paediatricians should not regard conviction/acquittal in court as success or failure, or as their responsibility. However, a question arises as to whether the existing legal processes are the most appropriate way for dealing with 'disciplinary' or 'frustration' type injuries when the perpetrator is without the intent to injure, loses control and has subsequent remorse, when a system of intense family support may be a more appropriate option than breaking up the family with a custodial sentence. The existing legal processes may be theoretically very appropriate for 'malicious type injuries' where the intent is to injure and no remorse is shown (although one could question whether the punitive sanctions for this latter group are sufficient), but actually in existing legal systems, criminal charges are laid in approximately 26% of cases and only 7% are convicted.

The illustrations in this text are of actual cases, and accordingly we have removed all identifying features and have actively sought to conceal identity by altering age, sex, etc., while maintaining the points pertinent in the illustration.

We are particularly indebted to the chapter authors who have provided an up-to-date review of current knowledge and we readily recognize that further research will undoubtedly refine the diagnostic and pathophysiological understanding of NAHI in infants.

Robert A Minns
J Keith Brown

1

NEUROLOGICAL PERSPECTIVES OF NON-ACCIDENTAL HEAD INJURY AND WHIPLASH/SHAKEN BABY SYNDROME: AN OVERVIEW

Robert A Minns and J Keith Brown

Child abuse may take the form of physical, emotional or sexual abuse, or neglect (Fig. 1.1). The American National Center for Injury Prevention and Control (NCIPC) in Atlanta, Georgia defines child abuse as "an act or failure to act by a parent, caretaker, or other person . . . that results in physical abuse, neglect including medical neglect, sexual abuse, emotional abuse, or an imminent risk of serious harm to a child."

Four types of maltreatment may be identified:

- *Physical abuse* is infliction of physical injury by punching, beating, kicking, biting, burning, shaking, or otherwise harming a child.
- *Neglect* is failure to provide for a child's basic needs. Neglect can be physical, educational, or emotional. It includes withholding of medically indicated treatment.
- *Sexual abuse* includes fondling a child's genitals, intercourse, rape, sodomy, exhibition-ism, and commercial exploitation through prostitution or the production of pornographic materials.
- *Emotional abuse* (psychological/verbal abuse, mental injury) involves acts or failures to act by parents or other caregivers that have caused or could cause serious behavioural, cognitive, emotional, or mental disorders.

In 2002 a total of 1900 children in Scotland (and 25,000 in England and Wales) were recorded by government statistics as abused. Physical abuse constitutes about 33% of all cases of child abuse in Scotland (Fig. 1.1); in England, where there is a separate group of mixed abuse, the figure is 16%. Of these 16%, only about 2% are head injuries in infants under 1 year of age. In the USA in the year 2002, an estimated 896,000 children experienced or were at risk for child abuse and/or neglect: 60.5% suffered neglect; 18.6% were physically abused; 9.9% were sexually abused; and 6.5% were emotionally maltreated (National Clearinghouse on Child Abuse and Neglect Information 2004). An estimated 1400 children (1.8/100,000) died from such maltreatment, 38% from neglect, 30% from physical abuse, and 30% from multiple types of maltreatment.

The prevalence of non-accidental head injury in infants is 25/100,000 infants under 1 year (Barlow et al. 2000), which for an annual birth rate of 50,000 in Scotland and 500,000 in England and Wales provides an estimated 12 cases per year in Scotland and 125 cases

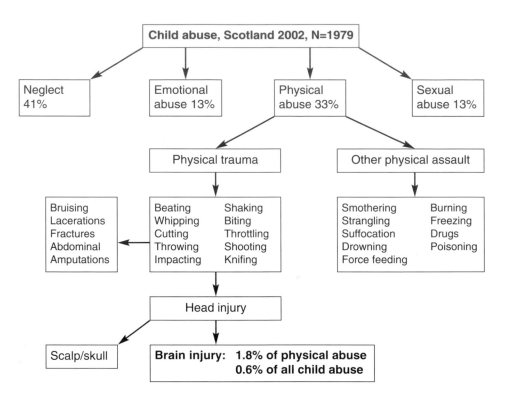

Fig 1.1. Non-accidental brain injury as a percentage of all child (and physical) abuse in Scotland in 2002.

per year in England and Wales. Extrapolating from the above, only about 0.5% of all cases of child abuse therefore have a non-accidental head injury.

Although non-accidental head injury forms only a very small part of the total picture of child abuse there is an added tragedy in the case of head injury, of brain damage causing learning difficulties, motor disability, blindness, epilepsy and organic behavioural problems. As a direct result of shaking, in a Canadian study of 364 children, 69 children (19%) died and, of those who survived, 162 (55%) had ongoing neurological injury and 192 (65%) had visual impairment. Only 65 (22%) of those who survived were considered to show no signs of health or developmental impairment at the time of discharge (King et al. 2003).

Abusive head trauma accounts for the overwhelming number of fatal or life-threatening injuries attributed to physical abuse under one year of age. Accidental intracranial traumatic injury is rare in children aged less than 1 year. Death is more likely to result from neglect and head injury than other injuries and so the clinician becomes involved in protracted legal proceedings. The increasing rate of fatalities compared to earlier years is hypothesized to be largely attributable to improved reporting.

The youngest children are the most vulnerable. Children under 1 year of age accounted for 41% of child fatalities, and 88% of child fatalities were in children under 6 years of age (Fig. 1.2).

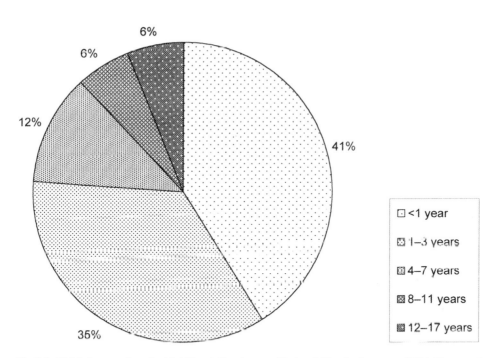

Fig 1.2. Child abuse and neglect fatality victims by age (National Clearinghouse on Child Abuse and Neglect Information 2004).

The young infant is probably less protected by society now than in the past, with recent failed court battles, expert witness disagreement, reluctance to imprison women and in particular mothers, and prosecuting authorities' reluctance to risk an unsuccessful prosecution in court. There now appears to be not only disagreement with what constitutes non-accidental head injury (NAHI) but also confusion of NAHI with cot death and Munchausen syndrome by proxy. There is also the added difficulty for the paediatrician of the disabled child requiring long-term medical support and treatment when the legal proceedings may have alienated the whole family against the paediatrician.

Definitions
Non-accidental head injury may refer to trauma to the scalp, skull or brain. *Non-accidental brain injury* refers to inflicted traumatic brain injury (traumatic encephalopathy), usually by an adult, to infants and young children, sustained as a result of deliberate impact (acceleration or deceleration), head compression, penetrating head injury, repetitive rotational injury (shaken baby syndrome), rotation and impact (shaken impact syndrome) or whiplash (cervico-medullary syndrome). Any one mechanism or combination of mechanisms may be present in the individual child. Child maltreatment through blunt trauma to the head or violent shaking is a leading cause of head injury among infants and young children (American Academy of Pediatrics Committee on Child Abuse and Neglect 2001).

The term 'shaken baby syndrome' is often used as a generic term for non-accidental (inflicted or abusive) head injury and this has caused confusion in court proceedings as it implies shaking as the cause of all non-accidental head injuries. The term 'non-accidental head injury' is to be preferred as no mechanism of injury is inferred. This is not to deny that shaking can cause brain injury and that shaken baby syndrome does exist with a certain constellation of clinical and investigative findings. However, a diagnosis of shaken baby syndrome requires confession or corroboration of the mechanism of the injury. Each component of the syndrome has other potential mechanisms of causation.

Some of the different definitions of abusive head trauma offered in the literature include the following:

- Caffey (1946) drew attention to the association of (a) intracranial and intraocular haemorrhages in the absence of signs of external trauma to the head or fractures of the calvarium, and (b) traction lesions of the periosteum of the long bones in the absence of fractures and traumatic changes in the overlying skin of the extremities.
- Caffey (1974) defined "shaken baby syndrome" (SBS) as an association in infants of multiple fractures in the long bones together with chronic subdural haemorrhage.
- Frank et al. (1985) drew attention to the importance of retinal haemorrhages (which they regarded as a cardinal sign of abusive head injury) in conjunction with an encephalopathy and without other necessary "classical" signs of trauma such as skull and limb fractures.
- Ewing-Cobbs et al. (1998a) defined SBS as a clinical syndrome of infants with subdural haemorrhage, subarachnoid haemorrhage, retinal haemorrhage and associated long bone changes.
- Gilles and Nelson (1998) defined NAHI as head injury caused by acts of commission by a caregiver, which required sufficient force to cause craniospinal injury. It encompassed rotation, translation, biomechanical forces and other contributing factors such as smothering, strangulation or cardiac arrest occurring at the time of injury.
- King et al. (2003) defined cases of NAHI as those with intracranial haemorrhage, intraocular haemorrhage or cervical spine injury, resulting from substantiated or suspected shaking with or without impact in children under the age of 5.
- Reece (2002) divided inflicted traumatic brain injury for research purposes into three categories: (1) shaking injuries, (2) shaken impact syndrome, and (3) the "battered child" with inflicted brain injury.

Shaking is a mechanism of injury and not a syndrome and should be considered in the context of other mechanisms of NAHI. Restricting the definition to the classic descriptions of Caffey excludes deliberate head compression, stamping, squeezing, shooting, impact, and whiplash cervico-medullary syndrome as non-accidental head injuries.

Presenting history

The typical case presents in the first 6 months of life, with a peak around 8 weeks of age. Presentation may be of bruising, fractures, burns, knife cuts or obvious trauma or some history of trauma may be given even if not the true mechanism. In many cases the presentation is of a nonspecific acute encephalopathy and the true nature may not at first be obvious when meningitis, metabolic disease, poisoning, encephalitis or status epilepticus are suspected.

In the large Canadian study (King et al. 2003) the median age of subjects was 4.6 months (range 7 days to 58 months), and 56% were boys. Presenting complaints for the 364 children identified as having SBS were nonspecific (seizure-like episodes in 45%, decreased level of consciousness in 43%, and respiratory difficulty in 34%), though bruising was noted on examination in 46%. A history and/or clinical evidence of previous maltreatment was noted in 220 children (60%), and 80 families (22%) had had previous involvement with child welfare authorities.

In the following sections, the frequencies of various points of history, symptoms and signs (shown in brackets) at presentation were taken from a database of 98 Scottish cases held by the Department of Child Life & Health in the University of Edinburgh, described in Chapter 4.

HISTORY OF TRAUMA

A history of preceding events is taken at several levels, e.g. at the Accident & Emergency department, by the house officer or registrar, and by the ITU consultant or neuropaediatrician, and the consistency of these multiple interviews is an important sign.

A history of a traumatic event or a potentially traumatic event was given by the parent or guardian to the medical enquirers at the time of presentation in 25% of cases, thus at least pointing the thinking to a possible traumatic encephalopathy.

This was thought to be a significant trauma in 16% and a minor traumatic explanation in 9%. Even when the traumatic origin of the child's condition eventually became obvious no explanation for the trauma was offered by the caregiver in 23% of cases and an inappropriate history was offered in 44% of cases. This included many improbable explanations (see below) and in approximately half of these (20%) multiple possible explanations were serially offered.

SKELETAL INJURY

Skull fractures were seen in 26% of cases, and overall some evidence of impact was seen in a total of 53% of cases. In a further 5% of cases it was not possible to clinically confirm impact, for example in cases with scalp bruising and alopecia.

It is vital that any signs of impact, particularly to the head, are carefully sought. This indicates trauma, and since infants of less than 5 months of age are not able to injure themselves accidentally, signs of impact may be a strong indicator of intent.

Clinical evidence of impact may comprise: (i) cutaneous or subcutaneous bruising, (ii) subgaleal haemorrhage, (iii) skull fracture, (iv) extradural haemorrhage, (v) focal subdural haemorrhage, (vi) focal cerebral contusion, and/or (vii) contra coup injury.

Some 53% of cases had no fracture on skeletal survey. Rib fractures were noted in 31% of cases, fracture of the long bones was seen in 24%, and fracture of the clavicles in 2.5%. The most frequent combination of fractures was that of rib and long bone fractures (12%). Skull and rib fractures occurred together in only 1%, and skull, rib and long bone fractures also in 1%.

EXTERNAL EVIDENCE OF TRAUMA

Bruising and oedema of the scalp, periorbital bruising or Battle's sign (bruising over the

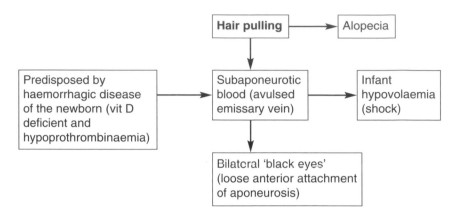

```
              ┌─────────────┐        ┌──────────┐
              │ Hair pulling ├───────►│ Alopecia │
              └──────┬──────┘        └──────────┘
                     │
                     ▼
┌──────────────────┐   ┌──────────────┐   ┌──────────────┐
│ Predisposed by   │   │ Subaponeurotic│   │ Infant       │
│ haemorrhagic     ├──►│ blood (avulsed├──►│ hypovolaemia │
│ disease          │   │ emissary vein)│   │ (shock)      │
│ of the newborn   │   └──────┬───────┘   └──────────────┘
│ (vit D           │          │
│ deficient and    │          ▼
│ hypoprothrombin- │   ┌──────────────────────┐
│ aemia)           │   │ Bilateral 'black eyes'│
└──────────────────┘   │ (loose anterior       │
                       │ attachment            │
                       │ of aponeurosis)       │
                       └──────────────────────┘
```

Fig. 1.3. Mechanisms of scalp injury from hair pulling.

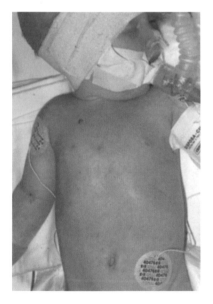

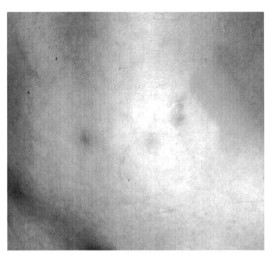

Fig. 1.4. Bruising over the anterior chest wall from thumb pressure.

mastoid, indicating a fracture of the base of the skull) indicates an impact injury, but absence of these signs does not preclude impact, especially in NAHI. Some bruising and superficial abrasion was evident in 41% of cases and this included "new bruises" in 24% and scalp haematomas in 7%. There were additionally abrasions, scratches, lacerations, hair loss, subconjunctival haemorrhages and bleeding from the ears and mouth in a further 8% of cases. Evidence of "old bleeding" was seen in 2%.

In order to shake a child a firm grip is necessary, so careful examination should be made of the chest wall and upper arms and the pattern of bruises documented graphically and

TABLE 1.1
History at presentation, in cases of NAHI*

Irritability and crying − 41%
Bruising and superficial injury − 41%
Vomiting and anorexia − 38%
Apnoea and respiratory symptomatology − 38%
Extensor stiffness (due to seizure, hypoxic rigidity or raised intracranial pressure) − 34%
Probable seizures − 21%
Pallor or cyanosis − 29%
'Potential traumatic event' − 26%
Depressed consciousness state − 21%

*Scottish National Database data.

photographically. This may reflect the way the child has been grasped. *Methods of grasping the child include:*
• by the hair (Fig. 1.3)
• by the chest – thumb marks at the side of the nipples (Fig. 1.4), fractured ribs and retinopathy
• by the arms – spiral fracture of the humerus
• by the legs – 'bucket handle' metaphyseal fracture
• by the throat – carotid trauma (unilateral or ipsilateral infarction, loss of venous pulsation in the retina, contralateral hemiplegia, facial and retinal petechiae)
• by the abdomen – finger bruising, retroperitoneal haemorrhages and bowel bruising
• by the shoulders – finger and thumb bruises.

Bruising around the mouth suggests possible suffocation to prevent the infant screaming. Thumb marks should be carefully sought under the mandible. Tears of the frenulum, often desribed as a hallmark of child abuse due to a direct blow, or forcing an object into the child's mouth must be differentiated from congenital tags of the frenulum.

PRESENTING SYMPTOMS (Table 1.1)
Symptoms prior to hospital admission were irritability, crying, inconsolability, unsettled behaviour, and being distressed or unwell in 41% of presentations. A "high-pitched" cerebral cry was reported in only two cases. Vomiting and/or deterioration in feeding were reported in 38% of cases. Haematemesis was reported in one case. Three per cent presented because of pyrexia and 2% because of hypothermia.

NEUROLOGICAL PRESENTATIONS OF CHILD ABUSE
The whiplash element of SBS was originally highlighted by Guthkelch (1971) and Caffey (1972). The more obvious supratentorial rotational injuries, e.g. subdural haematoma, have been easier to see and therefore have dominated the clinician's description.
    Classifications of NAHI may be based on:
(1) the type of injury (confirmed by imaging)
(2) the mechanism of injury, i.e. contact or inertial (in the contact injury the head strikes an object, while in the inertial the brain is in movement; most injuries involve both mechanical elements, with both translational and angular forces)

7

TABLE 1.2
Temporal classification of neurological presentations*

1. Hyperacute cervico-medullary syndrome (whiplash shaking injury – 6%)
2. Acute encephalopathy (classical SBS) with rotation plus or minus impact (seizures, coma, decerebration and central apnoea – ventilation) – 53%
3. Subacute non-encephalopathic presentation (subdural haemorrhage, haemorrhagic retinopathy, fractures, bruising) – 19%
4. Recurrent encephalopathy (none recorded in this series)
5. Chronic extracerebral non-encephalopathic (isolated subdural haemorrhage) – 22%

*Data from Scottish National Database.

(3) the severity of injury, as measured by either the Glasgow Coma Score (GCS) or the more interrater reliable 'Infant Face Scale' (Durham 2000)
(4) the timing of injury, based on the neurological presentation (Table 1.2).

Hyperacute cervico-medullary syndrome

The hyperacute presentation results from severe flexion/extension whiplash shaking forces and the infants suffer the equivalent of a 'broken neck' or more correctly a 'broken brainstem'. Geddes et al. (2001b) found localized axonal damage at the cranio-cervical junction, in the corticospinal tracts in the lower brainstem, and in the cervical cord roots, and additionally there is the possibility of traumatic thrombosis of the vertebral arteries as they wind through the foramina of the cervical vertebrae. Damage to these areas presumably results from hyperflexion and hyperextension movements, and as such these cases would truly reflect a 'whiplash' shaking stem injury. These cases are infrequently seen by the clinician (6%) and are either dead on arrival at hospital or die shortly thereafter, and are the groups most likely seen by pathologists. The infants in the Geddes et al. (2001b) study survived a median of 1 day after injury, and the children over 1 year of age survived a median of 0.7 days. Young infants at 2–3 months of age present with apnoea as part of this cervico-medullary syndrome with only 'trivial' subdural bleeding. The apnoea gives rise to severe secondary hypoxic brain injury with cerebral oedema but little in the way of axonal shearing. Subdural haematomas seen in this hyperacute presentation are small both on imaging and at autopsy. This may be a result of the acute cerebral oedema compressing the subdural space and the fact that the bleed is still 100% blood with a high haematocrit (since haemodilution has not yet occurred), and it may not become more evident until 2–3 days later.

Combined sequential MRI and CT has given a much more dynamic picture of pathology than autopsy, which occurs often after a period of reanimation and secondary insult or acutely before classical findings appear. The subdural haemorrhage in most cases, not just the hyperacute ones, is very unimpressive in the first 24 hours but has dramatically increased in size on imaging 7 days later. This presentation with death with a thin subdural haemorrhage or prior to the development of a combined subdural haematoma and effusion (low haematocrit) does not negate the shaking mechanism; that is, the presentation of this hyperacute pattern is a respiratory one with apnoea, acute respiratory failure and death with severe hypoxic–ischaemic damage found at autopsy.

Acute encephalopathic presentation

This is characterized by seizures, coma, decerebration, homeostatic derangements, bilateral large subdural haematomas and widespread haemorrhagic retinopathy. There may be additional skeletal fractures such as rib or metaphyseal 'corner' or 'chip' fractures or other evidence of non-accidental injuries such as bruising, cuts, cigarette burns, etc. This type of presentation is the commonest pattern seen by hospital paediatricians and has frequently been referred to by clinicians as the classical 'shaken baby syndrome'. Depending on whether there are additional signs of impact, the syndrome could then be more accurately referred to as 'shaken impact syndrome'.

In a typical case the young infant is irritable and resents handling, s/he may suddenly quieten, which is a bad sign, feeding becomes difficult and there is vomiting. Pallor with severe anaemia at presentation is likely due to haemodilution following acute blood loss in the head (subdural, subgaleal, skin, extradural, fracture sites, retinal, etc.). The degree of anaemia (compared to the normal haemoglobin for age) may reflect the time interval between the injury and presentation. Intravascular expansion, however, will alter this possible relationship. In addition to the hypovolaemic shock there may be a central vasoparalytic shock with marked loss of vasomotor tone, tachycardia and an expanded vascular volume rather than a low circulating blood volume. Young infants will produce an initial tachycardia before blood pressure drops [unless there is an inherent myocardial contractility problem or, very rarely, ventricular fibrillation resulting from blunt chest trauma ("commotio cordis" – Zangwill and Strasburger 2004)], although the antecedent tachycardia may not always be recognized. The newborn, particularly preterm, infant may not be able to increase their already fast heart rate without impairing venous return. Failure of peripheral circulation causes the cold extremities, decreased capillary return and low blood pressure, and these are serious signs as they may further interfere with cerebral perfusion pressure. Although the babies feel cold due to the shock, core hypothermia is rarely present. A depressed conscious state with unresponsiveness, floppiness and reduced movements is a common finding.

• *Respiratory symptomatology*. This appears as the intracranial pressure rises but may also, as in the hyperacute presentation, represent direct medullary trauma or vertebral artery trauma due to the whiplashing or due to fits or chest injury. Abnormal breathing such as apnoea and respiratory arrest, grunting respirations, shallow respirations or choking, featured in approximately 40% of cases. Pallor or cyanosis was recorded in approximately a third. A history of previous respiratory symptoms, which may have required medical attention or antibiotics in the weeks prior to presentation, may represent an earlier traumatic episode and old fractures of ribs should be carefully sought. Cardiorespiratory arrest occurred in the accident and emergency department in only 3% but cardiopulmonary resuscitation or mouth to mouth resuscitation was attempted in at least 10% of the children prior to arrival at hospital. Forty-two per cent required subsequent ventilation.

• *Epileptic seizures*. Seizures prior to presentation were described in 20% of children, and decerebrate posturing due to the tonic phase of the seizure, hypoxic rigidity, or raised intra-

9

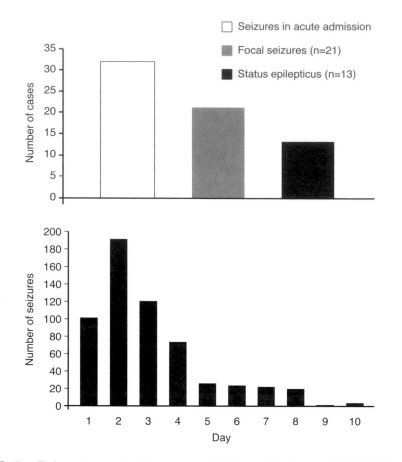

Fig. 1.5. *(Top)* Early post-traumatic seizures occurred in 32 out of 43 of cases of NAHI. Of these, focal seizures were present in 21/32, and 13/32 had one or more episodes of status epilepticus. *(Bottom)* The greatest frequency of seizures occurred in the second 24-hour period after admission, and all seizures had resolved after day 10. (Redrawn by permission from Barlow et al. 2000.)

cranial pressure was evident from the history in a third of cases. Following admission to hospital two thirds of children developed seizures, a much higher incidence than that occurring following accidental traumatic brain injury. Seizures are often severe and drug resistant, reaching a climax at 24–48 hours but usually decreasing and ceasing by the fifth day. EEG recordings often show more discharges than those witnessed clinically. Seizures cause a rise in intracranial pressure every time there is a clinical and electrical discharge.

Since this is an age when epileptic fits are relatively uncommon, their high frequency does suggest that there have been diffuse cortical insults, either primary or secondary, and Barlow et al. (2000) have shown a significant relationship between the early post-traumatic seizures and outcome in NAHI (Fig. 1.5). It is therefore likely that the fits are an epiphenomenon reflecting the extensive brain injury.

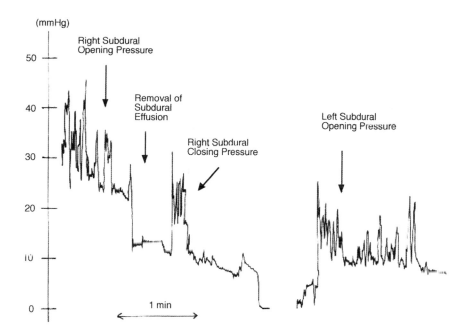

Fig. 1.6. Intracranial pressure measurement obtained during bilateral subdural taps via the fontanelle showing an opening pressure of 22.5 mmHg on the right and 10 mmHg on the left. A total of 20 ml of fluid was removed to normalize the pressure.

• *Raised intracranial pressure (ICP)*. Evidence of raised ICP, including increased head circumference, tense non-pulsatile anterior fontanelle, and distended scalp veins, was present in 22% of cases. Pupillary changes are not helpful and only 3% showed pupil abnormalities. Fixed dilated pupils are more likely to indicate brain death and are not reliable as an early warning of raised ICP. Cerebral oedema was evident on brain imaging in 23% of children at first imaging after admission.

On admission more than two-thirds of children had documented raised ICP, which was objectively measured (Fig. 1.6). The average of the mean opening pressures was 31 mmHg (SD 25 mmHg), approximately seven times the expected pressure for age. In cases where the ICP was measured, raised ICP did not show a direct relationship with outcome. The increased ICP, together with shock and hypotension, further reduces the cerebral perfusion pressure (CPP) and increases the risk of secondary ischaemic brain damage. The low CPP correlates with long-term disability (Fig. 1.7; Barlow and Minns 1999). The reason for this apparent disparity is that the CPP is dependent on the mean arterial pressure (which is regulated via the brainstem in the Cushing response), cerebral vasoreactivity control, and peripheral vasomotor tone with resultant defective cerebrovascular autoregulation in addition to the raised ICP.

Almost half of the children require admission to an intensive care unit. The aim of intensive care management in traumatic brain injury is to reduce the risk of death or aggravated brain

11

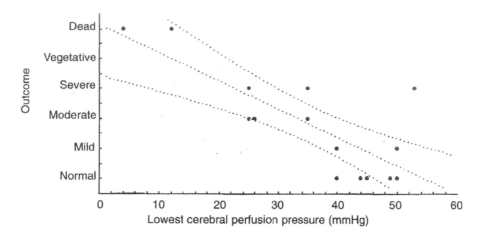

Fig. 1.7. Scatter plot demonstrating that cerebral perfusion pressure is highly significantly related to outcome ($\tau = -0.544$; $p=0.0047$). Dotted lines show 95% confidence limits. (Reproduced by permission from Barlow and Minns 1999.)

damage and resultant disability from the secondary injury. The primary injury in shaking appears to cause more irreversible brain damage than the contusional injury of a single impact. The response to the treatment of seizures, brain swelling and the maintenance of cerebral perfusion is often more disappointing than in accidental injuries. Duhaime et al. (1996) found that in infants presenting with coma and bilateral or unilateral diffuse hypodensities the outcome was independent of aggressive management. Ten per cent of cases died in this series, but the rate can be double that.

• *Subdural haemorrhage (SDH)*. Bleeding from torn bridging veins into the subdural space is the hallmark of non-accidental shaking injury in the first year of life. Eighty-nine per cent of cases from our series suffered a SDH. This was in addition to a subarachnoid haemorrhage in 19% of cases. The SDH was bilateral in approximately 78% of all cases. A unilateral SDH does not negate the diagnosis of NAHI and was seen in 14% of confirmed cases.

The subdural bleeding, although usually most obvious over the surface convexity of the cerebral hemispheres, also occurs in the interhemispheric fissure, and Zimmerman et al. (1979) regarded this as diagnostic of NAHI. They may also be seen in the subtemporal and less often in the suboccipital or posterior fossa providing MRI is available.

The presentation of anaemia, shock, tense fontanelle and an expanded head circumference does not differentiate cerebral oedema from bilateral SDH under pressure. It is therefore mandatory that the child is examined immediately with ultrasound or CT, which are the imaging modalities most likely to be available on an emergency basis. This must be followed up with MRI if one is later to discuss mechanisms, prognosis and pathophysiology in court.

Intraparenchymal haemorrhage was noted in 10%, while other haemorrhages such as extradural and intraventricular were infrequently noted (3%). Fewer than 5% of cases had no

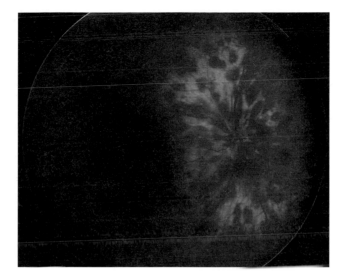

Fig. 1.8. Extensive multi-layer retinal haemorrhages including retinal folds, extending to the ora serrata in a 5-month-old child presenting with shock, encephalopathy, skull fracture, subdural haemorrhages and retinal haemorrhages.

reported haemorrhages. A chronic bilateral subdural haematoma was noted in one case and subgaleal haemorrhages were infrequently noted. Cortical tears were reported in one case.

• *Retinal haemorrhage (RH).* In the series reported by Duhaime et al. (1992) nine out of 10 children with RH had non-accidental injuries, the other case being a fatal high speed impact injury in a car. Retinopathy can occur without SDH or cerebral oedema. Tomasi and Rosman (1975) described two children with classical retinal angiopathy who presented with isolated seizures and no intracranial haemorrhage, which emphasizes the need to examine the fundi in any child under 3 years with an acute neurological disorder. Conversely, however, retinopathy is seen in 50–70% of cases with subdural haematomas. RHs alone can be due to many causes; when combined with SDH, cerebral oedema and fractured ribs the syndromic combination becomes reliable as a pointer to non-accidental injury.

Inflicted head injuries are associated with a high incidence of RH (70% in our series). In 11% of cases the RH was unilateral. In a review of 20 cases of SBS, bilateral RHs were reported to occur in 16, and four were unilateral (Ludwig and Warman 1984). Levin (2000) found that 84% of RHs were associated with NAHI. There appears to be a correlation between the severity of the RHs and the degree of brain injury, suggesting a possible common mechanism of causation, i.e. a rotational shearing injury.

In a typical haemorrhagic retinopathy the haemorrhages are not around the optic disc or flame shaped, but tend to be paravenous, occurring throughout the retina usually bilaterally and extending to the periphery, although one eye may be much more seriously affected than the other. The RHs are severe and extensive throughout the retina and predominantly involve sub-, intra- and pre-retinal layers and extend to the ora serrata (Fig. 1.8). Traumatic

13

retinoschisis and retinal folds were thought to be the most pathognomonic type of retinal injury, being a shearing type injury, but rarely can be due to accidental causes (Lantz et al. 2004).

Bleeding can extend into the vitreous or backwards (sub-retinal) to cause retinal detachment. The red cells and plasma may separate out or exudates appear and the lens can dislocate. If one adds to this the optic atrophy from raised ICP, optic nerve trauma, optic nerve ischaemia and trans-synaptic degeneration as well as calcarine infarction of the visual area from tentorial herniation compressing the posterior cerebral arteries, it is not surprising that severe visual defect is common in survivors. Mushin (1971) found that 12 of 19 physically abused babies had some form of residual visual defect. Sixty-five per cent of the 364 infants in the Canadian study had some visual deficiency (King et al. 2003).

RHs may also be caused by *accidental head injury*, but in many published studies the reported incidences have usually been less than 3%. They are often small posterior pole haemorrhages. Up to 16% of children injured in motor vehicle accidents have RHs, particularly if there is associated chest injury.

Duhaime et al. (1992) found one out of three cases of motor vehicle accident had RHs but failed to find any in 69 other children with traumatic brain injury. Elder et al. (1991) reported no cases of RH in serious accidental traumatic brain injury. This view has recently been challenged by Plunkett (2001) who described an older group of children with playground injuries that were witnessed and noted that RHs were seen in 4 out of 6 children who had ophthalmological examinations. RHs following accidental head injury are more likely to occur following high velocity road traffic accidents involving side impact. They are exceptionally rare after cardiopulmonary resuscitation (CPR). We accept that RHs are not all that rare after accidental injury, and when detailed RETCAM examinations were performed in the acute phase we found (in an ongoing study) that 3 out of 9 children had RHs (personal observations, unpublished). There is nothing pathognomonic about the RHs from shaking or other NAHI. Any injury in which the mechanism involves rotation and shearing, e.g. boxing, side impact vehicular accidents or wing mirror injuries, may produce intracranial damage and RH.

RHs are not an homogenous entity, and may be due to several factors.

Purtscher's retinopathy is a retinal angiopathy with paravenous haemorrhages secondary to sudden thoracic compression in adults (Kaur and Taylor 1992). Purtscher's retinopathy, petechial paravenous RHs with white patches due to chest compression, occurs infrequently in the infant with inflicted head injury. Fifty per cent of neonates show RHs following chest compression during vaginal delivery (Kivlin 2001), but RHs are rare after elective caesarean section (Sezen 1970). Schenker and Gombos (1966) reported no cases after caesarean section, 8% following breech extraction, and 31% when delay in delivery required forceps.

Supportive evidence for chest compression as a cause of RH comes not only from the very frequent association with fractured ribs (adults with sudden chest compression or following a Valsava manoeuvre get blurred vision from a haemorrhagic retinopathy – Duane 1973), but also from the occurrence of RHs following compression injuries caused by 'over the shoulder' type seat belts. Mothers squeezing their children tightly in an accident have also caused RHs, as have prolonged coughing in pertussis, struggling during gastric lavage, smothering with struggling, and accidental traumatic asphyxia due to chest compression in road traffic accidents.

In *Terson syndrome* (intracranial haemorrhage including SAH, and RH), haemorrhage tracts through the optic nerve sheath, but this mechanism does not occur in NAHI and must be differentiated from the optic nerve sheath tears and haemorrhages and injury and/or bruising found at autopsy in NAHI. It is seen as peridiscal flame-shaped bleeding.

The most favoured explanation for the aetiology of RHs in shaking injury is that of *vitreous traction*. The firmer vitreous and its stronger adhesion to the retina in the young infant could cause bleeding from acceleration–deceleration injuries to the retina itself without chest compression. The vitreous is attached to the retina at its periphery and this is the site where shearing forces will tear the vitreous attachments from the retina (or ora serrata) and cause disruption of ocular and orbital blood vessel integrity. The eyeball may be shaken in its socket like a marble in a cup and this may also bruise the optic nerve, cause optic sheath haemorrhage or dislocate the lens from its suspensory ligament. The mechanism is therefore similar to the shearing forces causing subdural bleeding and cortical tears. The shearing affects multiple layers of the retina, and macular retinoschisis and paramacular folds occur in approximately one-third of cases from the vitreous shaking.

Raised ICP can certainly be associated with RHs but usually when associated with papilloedema, which is present in less than 10% of cases of inflicted head trauma. No study has been undertaken to establish a relationship between RHs and the level of ICP in shaking injury cases. Retinal venous occlusion from optic nerve trauma would cause severe RHs. There is no relationship between the side of the RH and the side of the SDH. Convulsions are extremely common in shaking injury but there is no evidence that these raise central venous pressure sufficient to cause asphyxial haemorrhages (Sandramouli et al. 1997). Hypertension can occur as the Cushing response to raised ICP and this can occasionally cause RHs to appear at very high blood pressures, e.g. 200/140 (Eden and Brown 1977). Severe hypertension has not been documented in NAHI, and shock, anaemia and hypotension are more common. The most common mechanism of RH production claimed by the defence in court is by chest compression during CPR, and although RH may be seen very rarely after prolonged attempts at reanimation most studies have failed to show CPR as a cause of retinal haemorrhages (Kanter 1986, Gilliland and Luckenbach 1993, Odom et al. 1997). Experimentally, CPR in young piglets also failed to produce RHs (Fackler et al. 1992).

Other causes of RH not associated with trauma (e.g. meningococcal meningitis) are discussed in Chapter 6.

In summary, retinal damage can be due to venous rupture from very high central venous pressure in chest compression (i.e. a Purtscher retinopathy) but it is also part of the same rotational shearing injury that causes subdural and subcortical tears. This suggests a unified pathophysiology for the main components of shaking injury. A multi-layer extensive RH can only be due to such shearing mechanisms as occur in SBS.

Subacute non-encephalopathic presentation
In this group the acute brain injury is less intense, i.e. no acute swelling or diffuse cerebral hypodensities and no accompanying encephalopathic features (seizures, coma, decerebration,

15

etc.). However, the presentation is with SDHs, RHs, rib and other skeletal fractures, and bruising. The outcome in this group is better than in those with an acute encephalopathic presentation, although timing of the injury may be more problematic.

Recurrent encephalopathy
The child may present with a recurrent encephalopathy when encephalitis or a metabolic cause is suspected, rather than repeated poisoning, suffocation or shaking (Rogers et al. 1976). Fabrication of symptoms, especially seizures (fictitious epilepsy), is a form of child abuse in 'Munchausen syndrome by proxy' (Meadow 1984). The child may present with an isolated fit from shaking or with status epilepticus. Odd turns or fits, apnoeic attacks, cyanotic attacks, rigidity or coma may be due to repeated attempts to suffocate the child. Video recordings have shown that a parent may carry a rolled up item of clothing in order to put over the child's mouth and they will do this even in hospital or in the intensive care unit (Meadow 1987, Southall et al. 1987). Polygraphic studies with ambulatory monitoring indicate the child struggling as shown by EMG activity, apnoea and bradycardia, until the EEG flattens from hypoxaemia but without epileptic spikes. The difficulty in separating the rare child who presents as a cot death from a non-accidental suffocation has been the subject of much media speculation (Berger 1979, Emery 1983, Rosen et al. 1983, Roberts et al. 1984).

Chronic extracerebral (non-encephalopathic) isolated subdural haemorrhage
This is the late presenting SDH (weeks or months after the injury) in a child with an expanding head circumference, vomiting, failure to thrive, hypotonicity and mild developmental delay. There is no RH, no encephalopathy, and no accompanying fractures or bruising, and the SDH has occurred weeks prior to presentation. These children are at risk of the effects of raised ICP and visual compromise, but the prognosis with recognition and appropriate treatment is good. This group is the most problematic from the point of view of determining the timing of the injury, the mechanism, and who was the caregiver at that time. The differential diagnosis for chronic subdural space expansion encompasses a wide variety of conditions and these must be excluded by appropriate investigation. Although cases may be due to late presentation of NAHI, the possibility of some other cause, including the nebulous 'idiopathic spontaneous SDH', means that there is not sufficient evidence to start legal proceedings. One cannot state the timing, who was looking after the child, the certainty of trauma, or a possible mechanism. Suspicion may be strong in the mind of the paediatrician and social worker but sometimes proof depends on further injury to the child or death of a sibling.

Diagnosis of non-accidental head injury
The diagnosis is considered under three headings: (1) History, (2) Syndromic Combination, (3) Social Pathology.

HISTORY
The history at presentation is usually unreliable and inconsistent, changing with each

16

interviewer, and there may be a delay in seeking treatment. It is also inadequate to explain the clinical findings. This is at variance with the classical teaching in medicine that the history contributes to or makes the diagnosis in about 80% of cases. In some cases no attempt is made by the caregiver to explain the clinical findings. A history of acknowledging or admitting to injuring the child is obtained in some 23% of cases. A history of trauma should be deliberately enquired about, and a denial documented, as the story may change as the clinical course evolves. A history of 'no trauma' is important and not the same as 'no history of trauma'. If trauma is admitted, then the exact circumstances must be documented and whether it is significant trauma (i.e. a fall down stairs in a baby walker, etc.) or minor trauma (i.e. a short fall of less than 1 metre or so).

SYNDROMIC COMBINATION
Shaking injury is a syndromic diagnosis that is dependent on the total picture of clinical, ophthalmological, radiological and brain imaging features, all of which are individually compatible with an injury of non-accidental origin and lead to a presumptive diagnosis of 'suspected NAHI'.

With the above guidelines this syndromic diagnosis is as secure as any other syndromic diagnosis in medicine. The individual components must be compatible with a non-accidental aetiology. The American Academy of Pediatrics Committee on Child Abuse and Neglect (2001) state that "the shaken baby syndrome is a clearly definable medical condition. The syndrome is reproducible in males and females, and in all races, and is seen in nearly every country in the world as a consistent constellation of signs and symptoms."

This syndromic concept has been likened in court to the 'Duck test' – i.e. a bird, that waddles, swims on water, has webbed feet, has a flat bill, and quacks, where increasing combinations of these descriptors secure identification as a duck. One item, i.e. 'quacks' secures the identification beyond reasonable doubt; others, e.g. 'webbed feet', arouse suspicion; whilst 'a bird' or 'swims' are too insecure to warrant calling it a duck. The above are not all independent variables and some components carry more weight than others. In a similar fashion *we can expand the basic syndrome of SBS to the expanded syndrome of NAHI* (Table 1.3).

The more components there are, the more secure the diagnosis, and while a single component, e.g. subdural haematoma or isolated haemorrhagic retinopathy in a young infant, is still most likely (on a balance of probability) to be due to non-accidental injury, it may be due to other causes. Whilst individual components may have multiple causes and features that are more characteristic of non-accidental injury, the diagnosis becomes more statistically secure (i.e. beyond reasonable doubt) only when the several component parts are taken in combination. The most secure diagnosis of NAHI is when there has been confession on the part of the perpetrator, or the abuse has been witnessed, or when the head injury is seen in combination with evidence of other malicious injury (multiple fractures of different ages, malicious cutting, cigarette burns, multiple beatings, etc.).

A young infant presenting with a head injury plus a combination of any two of the following three factors – (1) inconsistent history/physical examination, (2) retinal haemorrhages, (3) parental risk factors (alcohol or drug abuse, previous social service intervention

TABLE 1.3
**Expanded syndromic components of non-accidental
head injury**

- Acute encephalopathy
- Subdural haematoma
- Age usually less than 1 year
- Acute cervico-medullary injury
- Haemorrhagic retinopathy
- Bruising and subgaleal haemorrhage
- Skull fracture
- Rib or limb fracture
- Evidence of malicious injury (bites, cuts, cigarette burns, whip marks, etc.)
- A history that is incompatible or inconsistent
- Acute cerebral oedema or diffuse cerebral hypodensities
- Early cerebral atrophy
- Poor long-term prognosis

within the family, past history of child abuse or neglect) – is especially consistent with NAHI. Such dual combinations are highly predictive of inflicted head injury (p<0.001, Goldstein et al. 1993).

There are no clinical ocular findings that in isolation are pathognomonic for SBS, although extensive multi-layer RHs are most unlikely to be due to anything else (one is highly unlikely to shear the retina in isolation). It is important to recognize that when the above factors are taken into consideration and after full investigation of all potential differential diagnoses, then the diagnosis is made of 'suspected NAHI' with varying *degrees of certainty* (Thomas et al. 1991).

A diagnosis of 'suspected NAHI' will be arrived at on the basis of the initial clinical assessment. This will then be confirmed or rebutted based upon subsequent investigation, and social work/police enquiry. The degree of suspicion will then be qualified by a degree of certainty:

1. Definite (i.e. beyond reasonable doubt)
2. Probable (most likely, on a balance of probability)
3. Possible/questionable (legally not provable at the time)
4. Not non-accidental (suspicion not sustained).

There is no formal statistical definition for the level of proof. A 'balance of probabilities' should indicate a greater than 50% chance (p≤0.5), whereas 'beyond reasonable doubt' has been variously equated with statistical levels of p<0.01 to p<0.001. As described above, Goldstein et al. (1993) showed that syndromic combinations could achieve this degree (p<0.001) of certainty.

Kivlin et al. (2000) state that: "The mere presence of any retinal hemorrhage is adequate to raise the concern of SBS. The extent or type of the hemorrhage is less clinically important."

The SDH is more likely to be non-accidental in origin if it is convex and bilateral, interhemispheric, associated with cerebral tears, and with ruptured bridging veins visible

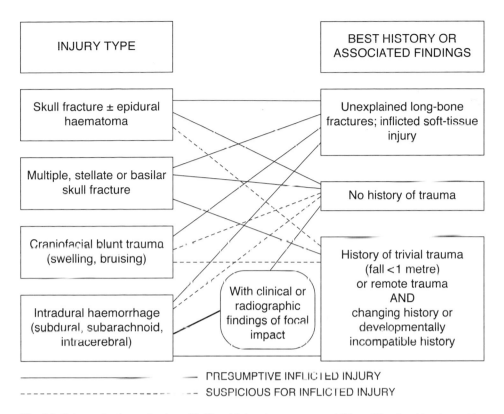

Fig. 1.9. Scheme for determination of inflicted injury in very young children. The algorithm is used by finding the patient's injury type in the left-hand column, then matching it with the appropriate best history or associated findings in the right-hand column. If the columns are connected by a solid line, the injury is classified as 'presumed inflicted injury'. If the columns are connected by a broken line, the injury is suspicious for inflicted injury but does not meet criteria for a presumption of inflicted injury. Note that concussive injuries are assigned to a category in the left-hand column according to their associated objective clinical or radiographic findings, such as bruising, fracture or haemorrhage. (Adapted by permission from Duhaime et al. 1992.)

on imaging. The original description of SBS was of SDH in combination with long bone fractures (Guthkelch 1971, Caffey 1972). 'Definite' combinations would be the type of SDH (as described above) combined with an extensive multi-layer haemorrhagic retinopathy, bruising and fractures of different ages.

There is nothing characteristic about the presentation of the traumatic encephalopathy in NAHI to distinguish it from other causes. For the purpose of definition, encephalopathy here refers to a new acute presentation of fits, coma, decerebration, central apnoea and homeostatic disturbance. It is again the total environment in which it is seen. Ewing Cobbs et al. (1998) reported that early post-traumatic seizures occur very much more frequently in inflicted than in non-inflicted head injury, and disappear by the fifth day. Rao et al. (1999) concluded that hypoxic–ischaemic encephalopathy (HIE) plus interhemispheric SDH was highly specific for the diagnosis of NAHI, occurring in 89% of cases. Zimmerman et al. (1978) suggested that interhemispheric SDH may be specific for NAHI (61% of cases).

Duhaime et al. (1992) developed an algorithm for determining the probability that an injury was inflicted (Fig. 1.9). It results in a diagnosis of presumptive inflicted injury or suspicious for inflicted injury. There was a 95% agreement between the categorization of the injury and that concluded by the child protection team. Adaptations of this algorithm were developed by Ewing-Cobbs et al. (1998b) and Dashti et al. (1999).

There is clearly a spectrum of possible combinations from the 'full house' in which there are: metaphyseal and rib fractures; skull fracture; multi-layer RHs with retinoschisis; bilateral SDHs with interhemispheric extension and acute encephalopathy with seizures; cortical tears on MRI with cerebral oedema and rapidly expanding subdural spaces; ventricular dilatation and white matter shrinkage within 10 days, with cerebral atrophy; inconsistent history; delay in presentation; and a background of social pathology.

At the other end of the spectrum there may be children who present with only one or two components of the full syndrome, e.g. hypoxic–ischaemic brain swelling, or an isolated SDH, or a fit with RHs. In any of these presentations there is a strong clinical suspicion of abuse, but proof would need to come from investigative or other supportive evidence.

In previous studies (Barlow and Minns 2000) we have used the entry criteria of an acute encephalopathy plus two of the following: (i) skeletal fractures (rib, long bone, metaphyseal), (ii) inconsistent history, (iii) SDH without skull fracture, (iv) RHs, (v) other malicious injury (burns, bite marks, etc.). The presence of any one of these individual features in a child must raise concerns or suspicion about the possibility of abuse and be an indication for investigation by the child abuse team and police. However, only the syndromic combinations allow a diagnosis of suspected child abuse to be made by the paediatrician. Where the mechanism of the NAHI is not purely shaking the diagnosis may be difficult, e.g. with compression head injury or other impact head injures where interpretation of the injury is not as specific as the syndromic diagnosis of SBS.

The two main problems concern firstly making a diagnosis that an injury is non-accidental in origin (Fig. 1.10) and secondly attributing a mechanism to the particular clinical pattern of injuries where these have occurred in private. It is therefore paramount that the diagnosis of 'suspected NAHI' is made with various degrees of certainty, and separately, that an opinion is offered that the mechanism of the injury is consistent with either rotation/deceleration, or other mechanism as on the flow diagram.

SOCIAL PATHOLOGY

In our experience it is rare for non-accidental injury to occur in a 'clear blue sky' without any adverse social factors or pathology. The 'perpetrator type' will vary from country to country depending on the social structure of childcare.

Just as there is a 'full house' for the medical syndromic features, there is an equally extreme social picture, e.g. the non-biological father, unemployed, drug abusing, having been abused himself in the past, known to social workers and police, and with a previous history of child abuse. However, we have also seen cases with very supportive extended family structure and equally seen professional people as perpetrators in very supported

20

extended family situations. From our database (see Chapter 4) we have identified the following social factors in the NAHI population:

- *Marital status.* Forty-four per cent of the children's parents were married, 11% were single, and 45% were cohabiting.
- *Age of parents.* The mean age of mothers was 22 years (SD 5.0 years), and that of the biological father or partner was 26 years (SD 5.8 years).
- *Past history of child abuse.* There was a previous history of abuse to children in 41% of cases. A past history of abuse to the parent as a child was noted in 2.5% of cases. This latter figure is smaller than would be expected in other forms of abuse (such as sexual abuse).
- *Drug or alcohol abuse.* Major drug or alcohol abuse was found in 25% of cases: 9% had a history predominantly of alcohol abuse and 16% predominantly of drug abuse.
- *Domestic abuse.* The injury occurred in an abusive context, i.e. there was a reported history of violence within the family, in 25% of cases, emphasizing the seamless nature of violence.
- *Mental health history.* A background of psychiatric illness was found in 32% of cases (27% in the mother and 5% in the father or partner).
- *Preterm birth.* Twenty-nine per cent of cases were born at less than 37 weeks gestation; 65% were born at term and 6% beyond 42 weeks gestation.
- *Twins.* Eight sets of twins (9%) were identified in 92 cases of NAHI. In some cases both twins were abused and in others one was singled out for abuse.
- *Recurrent medical consultations and hospital admissions.* Forty-six per cent of children were noted to have had recurrent consultations with the GP or hospital, and in two thirds of these the consultation was for 'suspicious' events that could have had an abusive aetiology. In one third of cases the recurrent consultations were for likely unrelated medical reasons.
- *Past history of social work enquiry or involvement.* This was found in 34% of cases from the Edinburgh cohort.

These social factors support the expectations that such children are frequently low birthweight and born preterm, with twins overly represented, and living with unmarried parents in an abusive environment (previous child abuse, drug and alcohol abuse, domestic abuse) where many have had previous contact with medical and social workers.

MISSED CASES OF ABUSIVE HEAD TRAUMA

Missed cases of abusive head trauma from families where there were no risk factors were investigated by Jenny et al. (1999) in a retrospective study of 173 children, younger than 3 years with head injuries caused by abuse. Almost one third had been seen by physicians after abusive head trauma and the diagnosis was not recognized until a mean of 7 days later (range 0–189 days). The diagnosis was more likely to be missed in very young white children from intact families, and in children without respiratory compromise or seizures. The errors resulted from a misinterpretation of the radiology in 7 cases. Twenty-eight per cent were re-injured, 41% experienced medical complications from the delay, and four of five deaths within the group might have been prevented by earlier recognition of the abuse.

21

Approach to the Diagnosis of Non-Accidental Head Injury

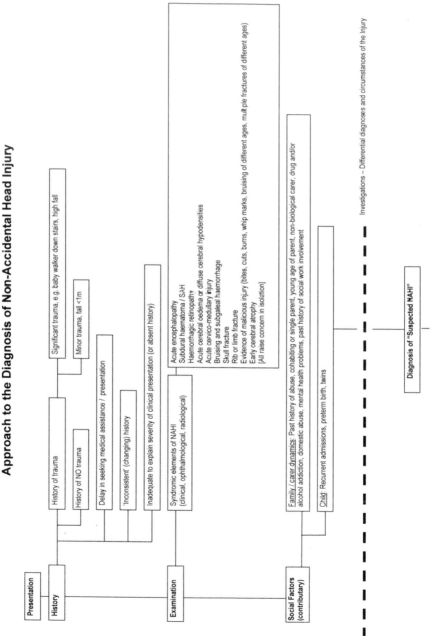

Presentation

History

History of trauma
- Significant trauma, e.g. baby walker down stairs, high fall
- Minor trauma, fall <1m

History of NO trauma

Delay in seeking medical assistance / presentation

'Inconsistent' (changing) history

Inadequate to explain severity of clinical presentation (or absent history)

Examination

Syndromic elements of NAHI
(clinical, ophthalmological, radiological)
- Acute encephalopathy
- Subdural haematoma / SAH
- Haemorrhagic retinopathy
- Acute cerebral oedema or diffuse cerebral hypodensities
- Acute cervico-medullary injury
- Bruising and subgaleal haemorrhage
- Skull fracture
- Rib or limb fracture
- Evidence of malicious injury (bites, cuts, burns, whip marks, bruising of different ages, multiple fractures of different ages)
- Early cerebral atrophy
- [All raise concern in isolation]

Social Factors (contributary)

Family / carer dynamics: Past history of abuse, cohabiting or single parent, young age of parent, non-biological carer, drug and/or alcohol addiction, domestic abuse, mental health problems, past history of social work involvement

Child: Recurrent admissions, preterm birth, twins

Investigations – Differential diagnoses and circumstances of the Injury

Diagnosis of "Suspected NAHI"

22

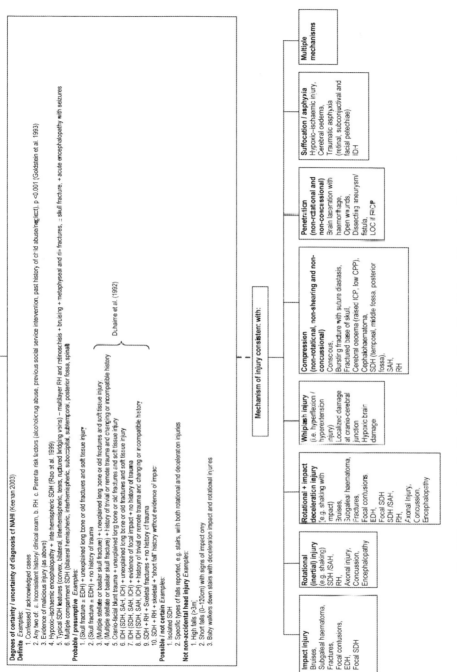
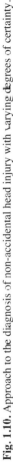

Fig. 1.10. Approach to the diagnosis of non-accidental head injury with varying degrees of certainty.

Re-injury may occur not only from missed diagnosis by medical staff and social workers, but also from failure of child protection investigations and failed legal actions. In one study, of 49 babies with suspected abuse returned home, 31% were re-abused (Ellaway et al. 2004).

MEDICO-SOCIAL ASPECTS OF PHYSICAL ABUSE
The physically abused child can be of either sex, any social class, race, colour and religion, able bodied or disabled, and living with his or her natural mother, a foster mother or in residential care. However, suspected physical abuse was reported in 23% of white children but in twice as many (53%) of other races (Lane et al. 2002). The child may be abused by any member of the family – father, mother, partner, grandparent, uncle or sibling, or by a lodger, babysitter, housemaid, nanny, child minder, or other care staff. Copeland (1985) identified the mother as the abuser in 28% of cases; the father, stepfather or boyfriend in 42%; and a babysitter in 10%. The figures vary in different places and different countries, but a common factor is that no person or group is above suspicion. Males tend to outnumber females as perpetrators of physical abuse and in the case of NAHI from the Edinburgh database with known prime perpetrators, 38/48 were male (and 34 of these were the biological father), but 5 of the cases involved the mother as a secondary perpetrator. In 10 cases the biological mother was the prime perpetrator (with 3 cases involving the biological father as well). In the USA in 2001, of *all types of child abuse*, 59.3% of perpetrators were women and 40.7% were men. The median age of female perpetrators was 31 years, and of male perpetrators was 34 years. Eighty-four per cent of victims were abused by one or both parents. Almost half (41%) were maltreated by just their mother, and one-fifth (19%) by both their mother and father (US Department of Health & Human Services 2001).

Malicious injury
This type of injury is premeditated, with the intent to injure, and the perpetrator cannot be in any doubt about the consequences of their actions. They do not show any remorse and if they get away with their actions in court, it is seen as a triumph in a game. The perpetrator may have a long history of violence and sadistic behaviour (e.g. hanging a child upside down over a deep stairwell and getting pleasure out of the child's terror). Many previous contacts with the police and courts (e.g. 26 in one case) may be discovered after the court proceedings. Such examples as burning the child with a lighted cigarette, cutting the genitalia with a knife, breaking the fingers, swinging the child by the legs against a wall or repeatedly hitting the child's head against a hard surface have all been seen in our practice. The psychopath has no feelings for the baby who cries, or will not take feeds, or who interferes with sex, and they may inflict the most horrendous injuries without any remorse. The type of injury may be such that no normal adult could fail to recognize that what they were doing to the child would cause injury. The child's screams and cries of pain leave them unmoved and may actually cause pleasure. Both the perceived intent and the absence of any remorse are important in the subsequent legal proceedings. When there is evidence of malicious intent accompanying the child's brain damage this is prima facie evidence of NAHI.

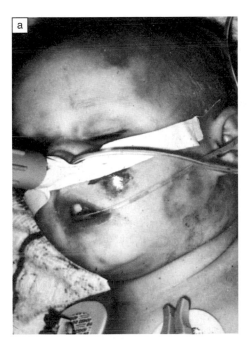

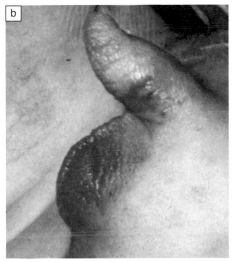

Fig. 1.11. (a) Multiple bruising and abrasions about the head and neck in an infant who did not survive a malicious assault. (b) Cuts to the genitalia and cigarettes burns to the same infant.

Clinical findings in malicious injury

Malicious intent can be reasonably inferred if there is:

- external evidence of *multiple bruising injuries* in multiple sites with bruising of different ages and patterns (Fig. 1.11a)
- *multiple fractures of different ages*, indicating a pattern of repeated abuse
- specific types of injury, as from biting, cutting, burning, strapping, etc. (Fig. 1.11b).

Repeated medical contact and recurrent admissions with physical injuries are suggestive of inflicted injury; recurrent admissions (i.e. more than two) were experienced in 27% of our cases.

Disciplinary and frustration injuries

A *disciplinary injury* is an injury that results from an attempt to correct a perceived abnormal behaviour (e.g. screaming, uncontrollable crying or food refusal); a *frustration injury* is an injury that results from the inability of the parent/carer to tolerate such behaviour. Parents may have no knowledge of child development and feel that normal crying and tantrums represent naughty behaviour that has to be corrected. It is thought by the abuser that the forbidden behaviour is maliciously thought out, deliberately provocative, and antisocial, even at 5 months of age. Disciplinary injuries are easy to recognize if there is finger bruising from slapping or strap marks on the bottom (Fig. 1.12), and the parent may admit to them. If annoyed by a child continuously crying there is an almost instinctive reaction to want to slap the child, shake the child or grab a limb and twist it. One only needs to see how a mother cat or primate in the zoo deals with an unruly youngster. There may be no intention of actually

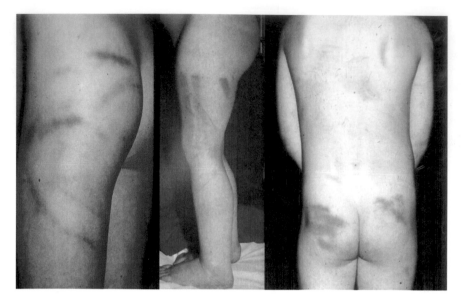

Fig. 1.12. Patterned bruising from belts, hands and buckles.

harming the child. It is sometimes felt that a shake is less harmful than a smacked bottom when the converse is very definitely the case (Guthkelch 1971).

True disciplinary/frustration injuries are not premeditated, nor sadistic, and the parent is very distressed at their occurrence. Thus in disciplinary injuries there is no intent to injure and there is remorse which is different from the malicious injury where there is every intention to injure and no remorse. The high morbidity and mortality from a shaking injury means that a parent who truly did not know the danger of shaking an infant as a means of supposedly disciplining them, will spend the rest of their life grief stricken at the damage they have done.

Normal parents tell of having to leave the house, or lock themselves in a bathroom or even a garden shed, when they feel they can stand no more from a crying or irritable child, because they recognize that there is a risk of them doing an injury to the child. When annoyed, all of us have a threshold beyond which we have an uncontrolled rage reaction (fight as opposed to flight). If these thresholds are lowered or the stimulus is sufficiently marked, persistent, or recurrent, we lose our self-control. This threshold for rage or panic is lower if we are anxious and tired from lack of sleep due to a crying infant, or if we are overworked and have several children below school age and no social life. Frontal lobe brain damage with epilepsy or cognitive deficits following traumatic brain injury (such as from motor vehicle accidents) may result in a lowered flight threshold and abuse to the child.

An area that is unresearched and newly recognized is attention deficit–hyperactivity disorder (ADHD) persisting into adult life, with its associated poor impulse control and cataclysmic rage reactions. It may be difficult to separate such individuals with poor school performance, truanting and low achievement from true psychopathic personalities. Just as alcohol and drugs, in the same group of people, may lower the threshold for aggression, so may hormones, as in the premenstrual syndrome or puerperal depression. Everyone is more irritable when anxious, for example when they have been made redundant with loss of self esteem. Although one may be sympathetic and acknowledge the extenuating circumstances, if the child has been abused, then when the stress is repeated so the abuse may reoccur. The environment may be more amenable to social manipulation and alleviation of stress factors than trying to train or change a personality disorder but in the meantime the child still needs protection and a place of safety.

Extenuating circumstances in the child
One child in the family may be selected out for abuse. Many cases occur where parental bonding has been weak, for instance when the child resulted from an unwanted pregnancy or the parents were not in a committed relationship. It is suggested that the strongest test of parental love is the 'suicide test': would you risk your life for the child? The greatest protection that the child has is that of parental love. The child plays a part in the interaction of this dyad and must cuddle in, smile, greet, show eye contact and console when the parent cuddles the child. If the child is irritable, does not smile, will not console, constantly rejects attention, arches away rather than cuddles in, will not accept food as a gift and cries every time a particular person picks them up, then the attachment and bonding, and therefore protection, is lessened. It is claimed that this is why the preterm infant is more likely to be abused. Similarly the child with cerebral palsy and learning disability is slower in achieving social skills and appropriate responses to the carers, while at the same time the parents may have gone through a mourning reaction and covertly rejected the child who is then left emotionally unprotected and at risk of abuse (Bax 1983, Cohen and Warren 1987).

MUNCHAUSEN SYNDROME BY PROXY
In this syndrome the perpetrator fabricates symptoms in which the intent is to satisfy an internal need for dependence or reassurance of the absence of a serious illness. This is a form of abuse, which involves other parts of the spectrum of child maltreatment, and while physical abuse with head injury may occur, it more commonly presents with an enceph-alopathy due to suffocation, administration of medication such as barbiturates or insulin, salt poisoning, etc., where there is a consequential brain injury. This appears to arise from impulsion on the part of the parent, as a result of a phobic anxiety state, which requires constant attention, reassurance, or investigation of the child's fabricated symptoms.

PUERPERAL PSYCHOSIS
There is no conscious or volitional intent here to cause harm but rather an organic depressive psychosis that commonly results in infanticide and also in many cases suicide. Where a shaking injury has occurred between 2 and 6 months of age, and the perpetrator is the mother, the question arises as to whether this is due to a puerperal depressive illness.

MERCY KILLING (EUTHANASIA)
This is most often seen when the child has a pre-existing medical or neurological abnormality with associated brain damage or a progressive or degenerative disease, and by definition

27

there is the intent to kill but without malice and with the intention of compassion (compassion aforethought).

PSYCHOSIS
Although rare, one does occasionally see a child suffering an inflicted injury from a parent with a known psychotic schizophrenic diagnosis. Delusional thought processes, such as voices in schizophrenia, or severe depression with suicide pacts, etc., are without normal intent.

DYSCONTROL
The threshold for fight and flight is altered by acute or chronic intoxication with drugs or alcohol, i.e. during the acute toxic delirium, during the withdrawal phase or due to long-term effects of drugs. All these situations are associated with increased aggression, and there are theoretically other drugs than recreational drugs, such as anabolic steroids, which may have a similar effect. Although drugs and alcohol will lower the tolerance to frustration and increase aggression, this explains the actions and intent, it does not excuse them, as the person remains responsible for their actions unlike with psychotic states as outlined above.

Mechanism of injury offered by parents/caregiver
Changing stories, different reasons for the injury given by each parent, or a mechanism of injury inconsistent with the physical finding are all pointers to non-accidental injury. The reasons submitted are varied and sometimes fanciful, but falls from short distances are particularly blamed and a source of disagreement in court. Some explanations seem reasonable but are thought up after initial denial of any injury, or are not substantiated by the other caregiver who may give an alternative explanation, or the story is changed as the seriousness of the child's injuries becomes apparent. The timing may be inconsistent with injury weeks before the acute presentation. Some such explanations that we have heard include:
- The child had difficulty getting his breath and mother held him upside down to help.
- The child was left in the care of the babysitter who rocked the baby on her knee and noticed him turn blue.
- Two boys kicked a ball into the child's pram where the child was lying and 12 hours later the child became drowsy.
- Four days previously the child slipped from the parent's hands into the bath and bruised her buttocks.
- A 2-year-old sibling had thrown a bag at the baby the previous day.
- The child was dropped on his head at delivery.

An inappropriate or changed history was recorded in the acute admission in 65% of cases. A recent immunization was blamed for the injury in 3% of cases; however, no scientific support for a causal relationship between DTP immunization and long-term neurological injury has been found (Aldershlade et al. 1981, Griffin et al. 1990). Accusations against other people such as siblings, grandparents, hospital staff in the A&E department or intensive care, ambulance personnel, maternity staff and other unrelated children were made in 12% of cases. In view of the varied histories obtained it can be appreciated how important it is to describe the pattern and timing of the injuries and whether the claimed mechanism for this unwitnessed event could have been responsible for the injury. Histories where 'short falls' were part of the proffered explanation were given in 18% of cases, and mild shaking to revive the child was offered in 5% of cases; these, along with the effects of subsequent cardiopulmonary resuscitation, are often the most contentious issues.

ACCIDENTAL SHORT FALLS

Some parents have learned, or been advised, that to deny any knowledge of how the injury occurred is a good defence, and this occurred in 60% of cases. Others will blame a fall from a low level in a domestic setting, e.g. from a settee or bed, from a changing table, or from the carer's knee. Accidental falls are divided arbitrarily into 'short falls', variously considered as <120–150 cm or <200 cm (<3–4 ft or <6 ft), and 'high falls', generally >300–450 cm (>10–15 ft). Short falls are often cited as an explanation or defence in shaken baby cases.

Toddler falls

A prospective observational study by an Edinburgh medical student of more than 700 child hours of 1- to 2-year-olds in a nursery setting showed that toddlers fall short distances frequently (0.53 falls per hour), but only 13% of these falls involved hitting the head and rarely (1%) caused minor injury (cuts). Boy toddlers fell twice as often as girls (0.65 vs 0.35 falls per hour). All the falls were short (<100 cm), and there were no fractures or serious injuries (Isabel Boyd and RA Minns, personal data, unpublished). Joffe and Diamond (1990), however, reported that toddlers fell only 3–5 times per week. Falls in infants who are not yet weight-bearing are initiated in most instances by an adult or by equipment failure and only rarely by the infant. Nevertheless, falls out of incubator portholes, papooses and front-carrying harnesses, baby bouncers and baby walkers can all undoubtedly cause true accidental impact head injuries to infants.

Fatalities due to falls from a low height do occur but are exceptionally rare. Hall et al. (1989) estimated an annual rate for short fall deaths of 0.14–0.22 per 100,000 children between birth and 4 years of age. Death from extradural haemorrhage can occur from being swung in a baby bouncer (Claydon 1996). In a prospective study of 65 infants who 'fell down stairs' in an infant walker, 29% had serious injuries, and there was one fatality associated with SDH and cervical and skull fractures. Falls from the top bunk and from a rocking chair have also been noted to result in SDHs and death in two children (Reiber 1993). What is clear from most short fall reports is that they cause predominantly typical impact injuries with bruising, fractures, contusions and extradural haemorrhages but without encephalopathy.

Plunkett (2001) reviewed the US Consumer Products Safety Commission database for the period 1/1/88 to 30/6/99 and found 18 fall-related head injury fatalities. He reviewed the primary source data, i.e. the hospital and emergency medical service records, law enforcement reports, and coroner or medical examiner records. The children in this report were from 12 months to 13 years old, they all had a witnessed impact deceleration injury from playground equipment, the falls were from 2 to 10 feet (60–300 cm), and two thirds were independently witnessed and had a lucid interval. Four of the six children whose fundoscopy examination was documented had bilateral RHs, and the author concluded that an infant or child may suffer a fatal head injury from a fall of less than 10 ft (300 cm). There were no infants amongst this group, and in no case is it reported that the paediatrician who saw the child suspected an injury of non-accidental origin. The report needs to be seen in the context of more than 75,000 reports of injuries related to playground falls in young children. Maxeiner (2001) reported injuries over a 20 year period in Berlin, documenting a total of 80 traumatic or violent deaths from a population of 440,000 infants. However, not a single death with SDH from a minor fall was recorded in that series.

The infrequency of serious injury after low falls has been reported by several authors (Crabit 1969, Helfer et al. 1977, Garrettson and Gallagher 1985, Nimitjongskul and Anderson 1987, Williams 1991, Lyons and Oates 1993, Rivara et al. 1993, Di Scala et al. 2000). Four of these studies (Crabit 1969, Helfer et al. 1977, Nimitjongskul and Anderson 1987, Lyons and Oates 1993) cumulatively yield a total of 839 short falls in children, including many publicly observed, with only three fractures and one SDH recorded. The overwhelming balance of evidence is that fatalities and serious injuries are rare in young children with short falls, although falls associated with a high angular velocity are potentially more dangerous (Ommaya and Hirsch 1971). Despite the rarity of such injuries, however, it is apparent that there is an imprecise relationship between the severity of the head injury and the appearance of haematomas or parenchymal injury. With extremely short falls the possibility of achieving significant angular velocity is particularly small unless that fall is associated with lateral rotation such as a fall from a swing. The presence of a subdural haematoma usually indicates a rotational injury; the critical rotational velocity for an infant for concussion is 100 radians per second and for SDH is higher. The impact times during falls or in situations where the child is thrown are typically 5–10 ms, and for very short falls, the short impact time would be associated with a low terminal velocity. In summary, short falls can be fatal, and a distinction must be made between 'benign falls' and 'short falls'.

In general, impact injuries arising from linear acceleration or deceleration result in fractures, extradural haemorrhage, etc., but importantly there is usually an absence of concussion, SDHs and RHs. By contrast, rotational injuries result in a concussive syndrome with SDHs, RHs and shearing.

Can we prove the syndrome really is due to abuse?

One cannot experimentally shake a series of babies under controlled conditions, so absolute proof will never be possible. Ultimately, proof that the combination of encephalopathy, SDHs and retinopathy is due to shaking must come from indirect evidence. Proof that the syndromic SBS features (encephalopathy, SDHs, retinopathy, etc.) are due to abuse requires evidence in three parts:

   1. Are these syndromic features a result of trauma? Evidence:

   (a) The pathology of shearing in such widely spaced areas (retina, cortical veins, corpus callosum, cerebellar peduncle, grey–white matter interface) can be produced only by *rotational shearing type injury*.

   (b) The evidence for trauma as a cause is supported by the fact that an *identical neurological syndrome* occurs when there is unambiguous evidence of trauma, when it is accompanied by fractured skull, fractured ribs, fractured limbs, bruising or internal haemorrhage.

(c) The other scenarios that include SDH, RH, cervicospinal injury and encephalopathy include *boxing, side-impact and wing-mirror injuries*. Birth trauma may also produce a similar clinical picture when traction and distortion occur due to the readily moulded newborn head. All of these mechanisms have a clear traumatic aetiology.

(d) *Closed circuit television evidence* of cases proving absolutely that in those particular cases, the trauma of shaking was the mechanism of injuring the child.

(e) From our database, the features of those acknowledged or *confessed cases of traumatic inflicted head injury are not significantly different* from the 'unconfessed' cases.

2. *Can shaking damage the infant's brain? Evidence:*

(a) Many clinical studies in the *medical literature* report cases of bilateral SDH, intra-ocular haemorrhage, and multiple traction changes in the long bones, without evidence of external head trauma and/or strong testimony, suggesting approximately 33% could only have been from shaking.

(b) *Perpetrator acknowledged/confessed cases.* Of the 23% of children in the Scottish Database where the perpetrator acknowledged or confessed to injuring the child, only 14% had a skull fracture. The relatively small proportion with skull or skeletal fractures, bruising and external injuries is consistent with a pure 'shaking' aetiology. The reliability of a confession may be questioned, and there are reasons why an accused may admit to an unwitnessed episode of injuring, but there is no reason to believe that any of the above were anything but uncoerced confessions.

(c) *A single carefully documented case* can establish the principle that shaking alone may result in such head injury. A case was documented (Minns 2005) where the perpetrator admitted angrily shaking a 4-month-old child "in the air" (without impacting on any hard or soft surface) for 5–10 seconds, as a response to protracted crying, verifying that adults can and do shake infants resulting in encephalopathy, SDH and RH, and that impaction need not be necessary for these to occur.

(d) *Experimental animal models.* An 'inflicted injury' model is difficult because the acceleration, duration, direction, and presence or absence of impact are unknown and cannot be accurately factored into an experiment, which should ideally utilize immature animals. Ommaya et al. (1968) and Gennarelli and Thibault (1982), however, proved that impact was not necessary to cause acute SDH in primates subjected to experimental whiplash injuries.

(e) *Biomechanical models.* Duhaime (1987) established with doll models that impact produced peak accelerations up to 50 times those caused by shaking alone. They predicted, after scaled comparison, no injury for shaking alone, but injury for all, even soft, impacts. Edinburgh studies show lower peak values for angular acceleration. De San Lazaro et al. (2003) recorded peak acceleration values of 3G for "normal" and 7G for "violent" shaking. Different mannequin designs of the infant neck hinder extrapolation to the live infant and are not strictly comparable.

(f) *Computer or finite element modelling.* Zhou et al. (1996), using a 3D model of the human head loaded with an impulsive angular acceleration, found bridging vein stretch ratios of 1.383 during sagittal rotation. A 3D model of SBS that included representation of the CSF (Morison 2002) showed that shaking at a frequency of 4 Hz and an amplitude of ±60° can produce increased stretch ratios, confirming that SDH is a possible result of manually shaking a baby.

(g) *Pathology from neuroimaging of non-impact NAHI cases.* Barlow et al. (1999) reported the MRI findings in a subgroup of 7 infants without evidence of impact, and showed that all had SDHs in various sites, with tearing of the surface veins in 2/7.

(h) Shaking injury has been described rarely in adults (shaken adult syndrome) where extreme violence by shaking has been the mechanism of injury (Pounder 1997, Carrigan et al. 2000).

   3. If presented with the clinical features of encephalopathy, SDH, RH, etc., can we diagnose a 'shaking' or other mechanism of abuse? Evidence:

The presence of focal (contact or translational) or diffuse (inertial) injuries should allow the clinician to report that the injury *may be consistent* with an impact, rotational, rotational plus impact deceleration, whiplash, compression or penetration injury, suffocation/ asphyxia, or any combination of the above mechanisms. While a fracture is evidence of a contact injury, an SDH (after eliminating the other differential diagnoses such as coagulation problems) usually results from (i) an inertial injury with sheared bridging veins, but may be (ii) focal from impact (e.g. from a short fall), or (iii) a true focal subarachnoid haemorrhage that rapidly disappears, or (iv) a benign external hydrocephalus that very uncommonly could predispose to bleeding, particularly after major trauma, or (v) a venous-origin epidural haematoma from bleeding between the ends of the bony fracture. As the injury to the child is almost always unwitnessed, and there is an imperfect relationship between the clinical features and mechanism of injuring, it is important that the clinician is careful about attributing an unequivocal injury mechanism in a particular case, and should therefore diagnose, with varying degreees of certainty (Fig. 1.9), an inflicted or non-accidental injury rather than SBS (although the injury may be consistent with a shaking mechanism).

Bony injuries
The principle features of non-accidental skeletal injury are summarized in Table 1.4.

Skull Fractures
Skull fractures are a common accompaniment of non-accidental as well as accidental injuries, occurring in about a quarter of cases. The skull in the neonate consists of poorly mineralized membranous bone, which can easily be cut at autopsy with a pair of scissors. Linear fractures due to birth trauma occur but are rare in the compressive head injuries of birth unless post-term. This is because mineralization is switched on very rapidly at 40 weeks and within a few weeks the bone is well mineralized and cracks under pressure, needing to be sawed at autopsy. Obviously the poorly mineralized skull bends and may indent, causing the 'ping-pong ball' or Pond fracture. Under these circumstances it offers little protection to the underlying brain, which is easily compressed. Severe local bruising and haemorrhage into the brain is then seen with a minimal fracture. Splintering, i.e. a cerebral green stick fracture, may be seen under a cephalohaematoma. In a so-called Hemsath fracture, indentation of the occipital bone (which arises from eight ossification centres) by

TABLE 1.4
The principle features of non-accidental skeletal injury

- Multiple sites of fracture
- Multiple ages of fracture
- 'Bucket handle' and 'corner' fractures of the metaphysis
- Radiolucent metaphyseal lines (extensions of the growth plate into metaphysis in healing fractures)
- Spiral fractures in a non-mobile child
- Non-supracondylar humeral fractures
- Rib fractures
- Multiple metacarpal fractures (stamping injury)
- Unusual fractures – bilateral clavicle, scapula, sternum
- Exuberant callus (non-immobilized fracture or refracture)

the maternal pubis, especially in breech extraction, causes osteodiastasis, and little may be seen on the X-ray, splintering may be seen at autopsy, but severe cerebellar haemorrhage can result (Pape and Wigglesworth 1979).

Skull fractures do not heal by callus formation and so dating of an injury is difficult; if the edges are round and smooth it is more than 2 weeks old. At autopsy the margins are heaped, smooth and discoloured with haemosiderin. A skull fracture normally heals in 2–3 months and has disappeared on X-ray by 6 months (Milhorat 1978). In small infants the fracture site may not heal but form a growing skull fracture as described below. There may be no bruising at all over the skull, even with a severe impact fracture, although bruising of the aponeurosis may be very evident at autopsy or operation. Equally, fractures may not be seen on X-ray so that a simple disciplinary shaking injury is suspected when again at autopsy or surgery well defined fractures may be seen suggesting a more severe impact injury. A study of skull fractures in 100 consecutive children under 2 years of age revealed that 27 were linear, 8 depressed, 3 multiple, 1 stellate, 3 bilateral and 4 basal (Duhaime et al. 1992).

Biomechanics of skull fracture
- *Force.* The force with which the skull impacts the surface in deceleration injuries, or when a moving object hits the head in acceleration injuries, depends upon the mass of either the child (and the head in particular) or the moving object, and also the velocity (force = mass × acceleration). If the child is dropped then the force depends upon the weight of the child and the height dropped. As the height increases so does the terminal velocity, to a maximum of 67 m/s, and therefore the force is a vector quantity with magnitude and direction. The initial linear velocity will be zero if associated with a fall but a positive value if the child is thrown or pushed.

The force required to cause multiple fractures is not necessarily a great deal more than that needed to cause a simple linear fracture. In experiments on isolated adult heads of known weight dropped from a known height onto a solid steel plate (unforgiving surface), Gurdjian et al. (1949) showed that a 10 lb (4.5 kg) head dropped only 3.5 ft (108 cm), i.e. a force of 35 ft-lb (SI 47 Nm), could cause a linear fracture of the skull. The extra force to cause

33

multiple fractures was not great (40 ft-lb, 54 Nm), but skulls that were thicker and with more hair did not produce any fracture at 90 ft-lb (122 Nm).

Duhaime et al. (1992) point out that the height the child falls is judged by the distance through which the child's head moves, whether sitting, lying in an adult's arms, or from a bed. Falls from beds onto carpets, often given as a reason for NAHI, do not often cause fractures in the elastic infant skull. Helfer et al. (1977) reviewed 246 children who fell less than 3 ft (1 m) out of bed: there were three skull fractures, all unilateral and none more than 1 mm wide, and no single child was seriously injured. Duhaime et al. (1992) found that linear skull fractures could occur from falls of less than 4 ft (120 cm) but that all basal, depressed or stellate fractures were due to accidental falls of more than 4 ft (120 cm) or falls down stairs. A similar study of 22 infants who fell out of baby walkers found that there were no deaths or severe brain injuries and only one parietal fracture (Fazen and Felizberto 1982). Acute cerebral contusions, cerebral oedema, cortical tears, diffuse axonal injury, intracranial haematomas or permanent brain damage from falls like these are therefore extremely unlikely but can rarely occur.

• *Skull protection*. The amount of hair, the presence of temporalis and occipitalis muscle, the thickness of the skull, and the wearing of any protective head gear, all help to dissipate force. The thicker the skull the more the energy is widely dissipated. Cycle helmets in older children have already proved their worth in skull protection.

• *Skull elasticity*. The elastic, partially ossified membranous bone of the young infant will bend and recoil without fracture but with less brain protection than a thick, fully ossified skull. At the site of impact the skull in-bends and flattens. At a distance from the edge of the blow the skull out-bends. Fractures are most likely at the point between the in-bending and out-bending, as when breaking a stick.

The inner table will stretch more than the outer table, especially if the bone is very thick, so the resulting fracture is more likely to start in the inner table. The viscoelastic properties of bone are functions of its water content (Sasaki and Enyo 1995) and the infant's skull with less calcium and more water shows a greater elasticity than that of the adult and can deform without fracture as shown by gross deformation of some infant's heads at birth (Margulies and Thibault 2000). Elderly people may fracture their skull from a fall from a standing position. A skull fracture indicates an impact injury, but it may be accompanying either a translational or linear acceleration or a rotational force. The extent of fracture depends upon the amount of force that has been used. A fracture therefore indicates that a force has been applied to the head but does not indicate whether it is rotational or linear. Weber (1984, 1985) dropped infant cadavers on their head from a height of 32 ins (82 cm) onto different surfaces at unspecified times after death, and caused fractures. These craniums would have had reduced elasticity due to reduced water content after death, and it is not known if any measures were taken to maintain normal bone hydration.

• *Area of impact*. This is important in that if the impact is over a very small area, penetration of the skull, as with a bullet, dart, scissors or knife blade, is likely. The greater the area of impact the more the force will be dissipated and the less likely is a fracture, e.g. a slap with an open hand dissipates the same force more than a clenched fist.

• *Forgiveness of the surface.* According to Newton's third law of motion both the child and the surface experience the same force, but if there is elastic deformation of both skull and surface then deceleration occurs more gradually over the same distance. Forgiving surfaces such as sand, forest bark, grass, carpet with underlay or a trampoline lead to a more prolonged 'impact time'. Impact times above 10 ms are associated with a low force; 5 ms is a quick deceleration and associated with a high force. Concrete does not 'give', i.e. is unforgiving. The force of deceleration injury can then be more devastating, and severe injury can be sustained from a fall from a lower height. One very effective way to dissipate force in physical systems is to impart bounce or skid. The protective effect of bounce is made use of when jumping from buildings onto a fireman's trampoline. Babies and young children are more elastic than old people who have lost much of the elasticity in their skin, vertebral discs and skull, and therefore babies are more likely to bounce than older people.

• *Site of impact.* Another important parameter is the site of impact. Skull fractures tend to occur along the lines of least reinforcement, e.g. squamous temporal and parietal regions. A skull fracture tends to extend from suture to suture, buttress to buttress, or suture to buttress (Milhorat 1978). Fracture lines pass to the sides of bony buttresses such as the petrous temporal bone and zygoma. Most simple fractures are parietal. A low frontal impact causes the fracture to go through the orbital plate of the frontal bone and ethmoids. A high frontal impact tends to fracture towards the temporal fossae. A similar situation arises in the occipital region where low impact causes the fracture line to pass through the foramen magnum and impact higher up the posterior skull causes the fracture to pass towards the temporal fossa (Hooper 1969). These general principles are not absolute and exceptions do occur. In the small infant, the compressibility of the skull may cause a so-called 'bursting fracture' when the suture lines rupture, and this is not easily recognized clinically or radiologically. Side to side compression of the infant's head may cause the base and not the vertex to fracture (see compression injury, pp. 43–47)

Characteristics of non-accidental skull fractures
Certain characteristics of a skull fracture suggest that it is more likely to be non-accidental than accidental in origin. Most accidental fractures are simple linear fractures, and are usually parietal and over the vertex, or commence at the coronal suture. If the fracture line branches, is stellate, crosses suture lines, is bilateral, is multiple with several fractures, is wider than 5 mm at presentation, or expands as a growing fracture, then non-accidental fracture is more likely. A depressed fracture, especially of the occipital bone in a child under 3 years of age, suggests abuse. Any of these features merit a full skeletal survey but none is pathognomonic in itself of abuse.

The minimal radiological survey that should be requested in these situations would be an anteroposterior (AP) and lateral chest, skull, spine and pelvis scan on one large film plus an AP of the arms and legs looking for associated fractures of long bones (Carty 1989).

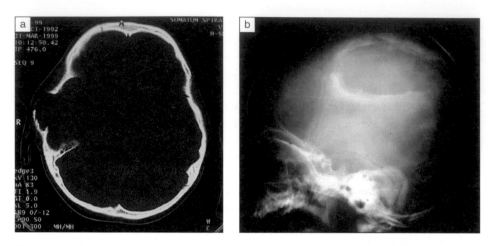

Fig. 1.13. (a) CT with bone windows showing extension of the brain between the fracture ends. (b) Plain skull X-ray showing widening of the cranial defect with growth, requiring bone grafting.

Growing skull fractures

Growing skull fractures (Fig. 1.13) are typical of fractures of the skull occurring in children under 1 year but are not restricted to non-accidental skull fractures. They are often wide at presentation and occur in the first year of life. They occur because of the rapid phase of skull growth; 50% are seen in children aged under 1 year and virtually all are seen before 3 years of age. It is thought that they occur by several possible mechanisms:
- a tear of the dura with trapping of the dura between the fracture ends
- pulsation of the dura, i.e. a meningeal hernia that may contain meninges, CSF (lepto-meningeal cyst or cephalohydrocele) or brain
- the formation of pseudo-arthrosis, i.e. a neo-suture (Scarfo et al. 1989).

The edges gradually become smooth and eroded as the centre expands over several centimetres. The defect may be so large that a bone graft of ribs may be necessary to fill the defect (Fig. 1.13b). The ventricle on the affected side expands and shifts towards the defect (Arseni and Clurea 1981).

Importance of skull fractures

The skull fracture by itself is only medically important if it is depressed into the brain, goes through the anterior fossa and cribriform plate allowing CSF rhinorrhoea and a risk of meningitis, goes through the petrous temporal bone into the ear with a risk of meningitis, or enters the sinuses or is across the base of the skull with a brainstem injury.

Skull fractures are legally important in that they confirm impact and thus indicate forceful impact rather than a simple shake. The excuses offered, e.g. that the infant fell off a couch, can then assume great importance.

Death can occur with no skull fracture, and there may be no symptoms at all with an extensive fracture. Eighty per cent of people of all ages who die from a head injury have a fractured skull (Jennett and Teasdale 1981). It is the associated brain damage that kills, the fracture only indicates the amount of force. Hobbs (1984) studied skull fractures in 89 children under 2 years of age; 29 were due to child abuse, and 19 of these children died.

NON-SKULL FRACTURES

The incidence of fractures in non-accidental injury varies widely between 11% and 55% (Carty 1989). They are commonest in children under 2 years of age. Fractures in the first 4 months are nearly all due to abuse, and if ignored further injury may occur (Skellern et al. 2000). Callus makes them more easily visible, so that acute injuries missed on the initial film may be detected on repeat examination after 2 weeks. Certain lesions such as the radio-lucent metaphyseal lines are difficult to interpret since they may represent definite fractures but also occur in diseases such as leukaemia. A radionucleide bone scan with technetium may show hot healing bone with an increased blood supply, especially in rib, vertebral and flat bone fractures. Some authors feel this is more useful in the acute stage than plain X-rays (Sty and Starshak 1983). Positive scans will also occur with bone tumours or osteo-myelitis. Skull fractures may not show on an isotope scan. There may be a periosteal reaction from gripping the limb tightly over a long bone such as the tibia or humerus. This is due to subperiosteal bleeding, but again by itself it should be interpreted with caution as a similar X-ray appearance occurs from so-called physiological periosteitis between 2 and 8 months of age. Periosteal bleeding can also occur due to traction on the legs in breech extraction. Intraosseous vascular access may also cause an abnormality on subsequent bone scans mimicking abuse (Harty and Kao 2002). Metaphyseal injuries were caused by five different orthopaedic surgeons to eight children when casting for talipes equinovarus (Grayev et al. 2001).

One method of shaking is to grab the child by the shoulders and upper arms; this may cause a spiral humeral fracture or periosteal avulsion (Fig. 1.14a). Spiral fractures of the long bones such as the humerus can occur from twisting the limb. These are rare in a non-mobile child from accidental causes. A transverse fracture (Fig. 1.14b) suggests a direct blow or bending of the limb. However, a spiral fracture of the femur does not mean that abuse is more likely than with a transverse fracture, and a transverse fracture does not lessen suspicion (Scherl et al. 2000). More so than femoral fractures, fractures of the humerus should raise the suspicion of non-accidental injury. Thomas et al. (1991) reviewed the X-rays of 215 children who had sustained fractures under the age of 3 years; of the 14 humeral fractures seen, 11 were found to be due to child abuse. The three accidental ones were all supracondylar elbow fractures after known falls. In other words, humeral fractures other than supracondylar were all found to be due to abuse. Nine out of 25 femoral fractures were due to abuse, and there was nothing specific about the pattern to separate abuse from accident except that 60% of those due to abuse were under the age of 1 year (Rex and Kay 2000). A baby exerciser called the Exersaucer was responsible for distal metaphyseal fractures of the femur in two non-ambulatory infants reported by Grant (2001).

Metaphyseal injuries

The typical fracture of child abuse is the metaphyseal fracture. Metaphyseal fractures are

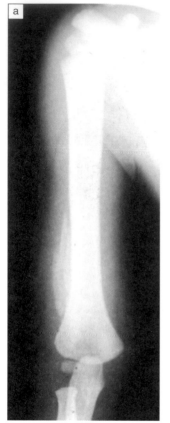

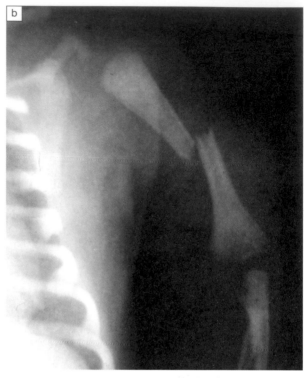

Fig. 1.14. (a) Subperiosteal reaction around lower half of humerus from forcefully grasping the limb. (b) Transverse fracture of left humerus.

caused by twisting the limb and can also occur from birth injury when pulling the arms down in a breech extraction or orthopaedic manoeuvres as described above (Snedecor and Wilson 1949, Shulman and Terhune 1951). They can occur as a disciplinary injury. The tendency to slap, shake the child or grab a limb and twist it appears to be part of the same compulsive act by an exasperated adult (slap, shake and twist injuries). Less easily acceptable as an explanation is the idea that the shaken child who flails his or her limbs can cause metaphyseal injuries from the flailing.

The 'bucket handle' (Fig. 1.15a) and 'corner' type metaphyseal fractures (Fig. 1.15b) are often regarded as very typical of child abuse. The metaphysis is an immature part of the long bone with loose periosteal attachment, which shears and bleeds. They are true microfractures of spongiosa of the metaphysis rather than simple soft tissue avulsion or shearing of the growth plate (Kleinman 1990). Histologic study may show more extensive damage than is appreciated radiologically. Metaphyseal fractures do not appear to cause great pain, and the child often moves the limb quite normally. Oedema, bruising and swelling may be completely absent in the presence of unequivocal recent fractures. Metaphyseal fractures are very difficult to date on X-ray.

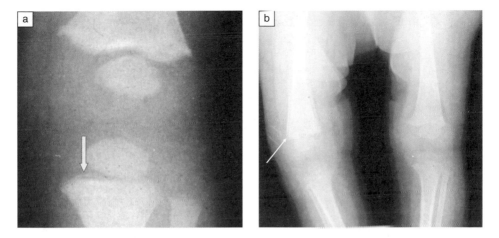

Fig. 1.15. (a) 'Bucket-handle' and (b) 'corner' type metaphyseal fractures (with additional healing periosteal reaction in the femur and distal left tibia) resulting from twisting the limb, which have been regarded as typical of child abuse.

It is thought that twisting shears the epiphysis, fractures the metaphysis and causes sub-periosteal bleeding either as part of, or separate from, the act of shaking the head. They may be more severe on the left than the right (i.e. from right-handed aggressors) but are often bilateral. Holding the child by the feet and swinging is a similar mechanism, and can also tear ligaments and their attachment to periosteum and bone as well as causing a torsion injury to the limb. The fact that shaking injuries are often not a simple disciplinary injury, but rather an impact injury with the child being hit against a floor or wall or other hard surface, means that these are more violent malicious injuries than are often suggested (Aoki and Masuzawa 1986, Duhaime et al. 1987). The metaphyseal fracture was described by Caffey (1972) as part of the typical child abuse picture, along with retinopathy, fractured ribs and subdural haematomas. Kleinman et al. (1989) found 13 metaphyseal injuries and only one shaft fracture in eight fatally abused children.

Rib fractures
Rib fractures are again typical of child abuse, but other causes such as accidents, resuscitation, coughing, birth trauma and bone fragility need to be considered. Of 39 rib fractures in infants studied by Bulloch et al. (2000), 32 were due to child abuse, 3 to accidental injuries, 1 to birth injury, and 3 to bone fragility (1 osteogenesis imperfecta, 1 rickets, 1 osteopenia of prematurity). A controversial mechanism is severe compression by a physiotherapist. Five boys aged 3 months (4 with bronchiolitis and 1 with pneumonia) suffered between 1 and 5 fractures (median 4) between the third and eighth ribs by chest physiotherapy (Chalumeau et al. 2002). Rib fractures were thought to be due to abuse in 15 of 18 children described from Australia by Cadzow and Armstrong (2000).

Rib fractures from abuse may be unilateral or bilateral (Fig. 1.16), and again (with a right-handed abuser) may be more severe on the left side. It is thought that the chest is grabbed

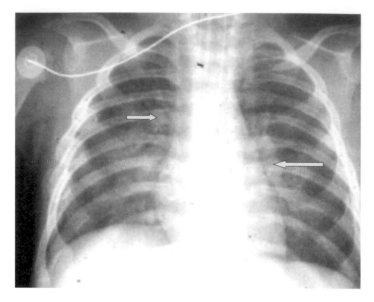

Fig. 1.16. Multiple rib fractures.

and squeezed or the upper arms and shoulder are squeezed in order to shake the infant. The fractures are more commonly posterior near the costo-vertebral junction, especially the fourth to the seventh ribs. Ribs are anchored posteriorly and may lever against the transverse process, and so when pressed anteriorly they are most likely to snap at the posterior convexity. Anterior or other sites of rib fracture can occur and do not suggest an alternative diagnosis. Rib fractures appear as callus on X-ray like a string of beads and to the unwary may be misdiagnosed as rickets (these, however, are not at the costochondral junction). They may not show on X-ray when recent, and may be hidden by cardiac and other soft tissue shadows. Rib ultrasound and bone scans may be required in difficult cases. Rib fractures are very rare in young infants due to falls, cough or birth injury, and even very vigorous cardiac massage and resuscitation does not normally fracture ribs (Feldman and Brewer 1984).

Other bone injuries
The costochondral junctions can be sheared or the sternum fractured and a flail chest produced, if an adult stands on the child. Such unusual fractures, e.g. of the sternum or scapula, and particularly bilaterally fractured clavicles, should always arouse strong suspicion of a non-accidental injury. Multiple metacarpal fractures of the hand are seen if an adult stands on the child's hand (Cameron and Rae 1975).

DIFFERENTIAL DIAGNOSIS OF MULTIPLE FRACTURES
Accidental fractures may occur in young children in situations not immediately thought to be potentially traumatic, for example during vigorous physiotherapy to the chest (but rarely with CPR), after surgical application of casts for talipes, or holding a child for a lumbar

40

TABLE 1.5
Diseases with skeletal lesions simulating abuse

- Rickets of prematurity associated with a low calcium and phosphorus intake is more likely than vitamin D resistant or deficient rickets, which has a later onset
- Congenital indifference to pain and insensitivity to pain
- Myelodysplasia (or spasticity)
- Osteomyelitis (and meningococcaemia)
- Congenital syphilis
- Vitamin C deficiency
- Vitamin A toxicity
- Caffey's disease (infantile cortical hyperostosis)
- Leukaemia (due to invasive disease or nutritional lack)
- Drug induced bone changes (anticonvulsants, methotrexate, desferrioxamine, other cytostatics)
- Copper deficiency (associated with low birthweight, malnutrition and peritoneal dialysis)
- Menkes' kinky hair disease (an X-linked recessive condition with reduced copper absorption associated with seizures, learning disability, failure to thrive, metaphyseal spurs, subperiosteal new bone formation, osteopenia, and SDH)
- Inherited bone dysplasias (e.g. spondylo-metaphyseal dysplasia, metaphyseal chondrodysplasia)
- Sickle cell anaemia
- Prolonged immobilization
- Achondroplasia
- Osteopetrosis
- Hunter syndrome
- Congenital cytomegalovirus (CMV) infection
- Hypertrophic osteoarthropathy
- Osteogenesis imperfecta types 1 and 4

puncture with resultant vertebral collapse fracture. Estimation of calcium, phosphorus, alkaline phosphatase and vitamin D is indicated in all cases of multiple fractures under 1 year of age.

Several diseases have associated skeletal lesions that can simulate abuse (e.g. fractures, irregular metaphysis, osteopenia, subperiosteal new bone formation, and these are listed in Table 1.5.

Osteogenesis imperfecta
One must always remember the pitfalls of multiple fractures of skull and long bones, which may be present from birth in osteogenesis imperfecta . Occasionally parents of these unfortunate children (<2%) have been accused of child abuse prior to the correct diagnosis being made (Paterson and McAllion 1989). It is also used as a routine defence in cases of child abuse with multiple fractures (which can include ribs, long bones, metaphysis and skull), especially as bruising and nosebleeds, and RHs and SDHs can also be seen (Ganesh et al. 2004). Fractures, however, need not be associated with obvious bruising.

Most cases of osteogenesis imperfecta are autosomal dominant with the exception of type 7, which is autosomal recessive. It is due to a disorder of collagen metabolism and occurs with an overall prevalence of 1:20,000 live births.

Type 1 collagen forms the main structural protein of bone, skin and ligaments. Therefore abnormalities of type 1 collagen result in fragile bones, deafness, blue sclera, hypermobility of joints from lax ligaments, and dentinogenesis imperfecta.

Osteogenesis imperfecta results from a more than 200 possible mutations in type 1 collagen genes, although COL1 A1 and COL1 A2 account for more than 90% of cases. The most common defects are point mutations. Milder forms are characterized by a decrease of type 1 collagen, while severe forms result from abnormal synthesis and secretion of type 1 pro-collagen.

Sillence (1979) has classified cases of osteogenesis imperfecta into seven types, as:

Type 1 – milder form, no bone deformity, may not affect stature

Type 2 – lethal type, usually perinatal death

Type 3 – severe, with crippling deformities

Type 4 – mild to moderate bone deformities, variable short stature

Type 5 – similar to 4 but no blue sclera, limited pronation/supination with dislocation of radial head; genetics not elucidated

Type 6 – fractures between 4 and 18 months of age more frequent than in type 4, vertebral fractures occur due to osteoid accumulation; genetics undetermined

Type 7 – moderate to severe, fractures at birth, bluish sclera, deformity and osteopenia; rhizomelia is a prominent feature; autosomal recessive, localized to chromosome 3p22–24.1 (i.e. outside the locus for type 1 collagen).

Type 4 and milder cases of type 1 are the ones that usually result in disagreement in court. Lund et al. (1996) state that mild osteogenesis imperfecta type 4 without other signs than fractures, is very rare. The diagnosis of 'temporary brittle bone disease' is unsustained. Retinopathy, SDH and cerebral oedema cannot be blamed on metabolic bone disease, although a subdural haematoma from birth or minor trauma may occur in the severe form of osteogenesis imperfecta. Taitz (1991a,b) in a series of multiple fractures brought to court as alleged non-accidental injuries, found no single case due to osteogenesis imperfecta (by radiological examination), copper deficiency or other rare metabolic bone disease.

Fractures in young infants are stated to be 24 times more likely to be due to abuse than to osteogenesis imperfecta (Marlowe et al. 2002). However, osteogenesis imperfecta needs to be seriously considered in all infants who present with multiple fractures including skull fractures.

Investigations should include imaging for osteopenia using radiography and bone densitometry, although a negative finding does not necessarily exclude the diagnosis. The skull should be examined radiologically for a mosaic of wormian bones. Joint laxity is a common clinical finding, and in some cases there may be no blue sclera (normal infants often have blue looking sclera). The family history should be investigated for fractures, deafness from otosclerosis, abnormal teeth (dentinogenesis imperfecta), hyperextensile joints, aortic valve disease, and vasculopathy with calcification.

The biochemical analysis of type 1 collagen can be very helpful in confirming the diagnosis of osteogenesis imperfecta. Ninety per cent of cases have demonstrable abnormality of pro-collagen (Wenstrup et al. 1990). In cases with recurrent fractures, or with fractures of long bones after proven minor trauma, biochemical studies of skin fibroblasts and biochemical analysis of collagen are indicated.

Other metabolic bone disease

Vascular markings on the infant's skull are not always easily differentiated from fracture lines. Scurvy, rickets and syphilitic osteitis have all been either blamed or confused. Copper deficiency in preterm infants, infants on parenteral nutrition and those with malabsorption syndromes can result in an osteopenic osteitis with rickets, which is associated with pathological and often very symmetrical fractures. Anaemia and delayed bone age may also accompany the fractures (Shaw 1988) and this is a source of possible confusion with non-accidental injury. Estimation of serum copper and ceruloplasmin make the diagnosis easier than in osteogenesis imperfecta.

Preterm infants pose particular problems: (i) they are often irritable and difficult to manage, and therefore are more prone to abuse; (ii) the immature kidney cannot handle phosphate until about 36 weeks and vitamin D hydroxylation depends on kidney and liver maturity and the milk content, predisposing to rickets of prematurity; and (iii) copper deficiency also effects bone mineralization, so osteopenia of prematurity may predispose to fracture.

The immobile disabled child on anticonvulsants and with feeding problems may show severe osteopenia and may have multiple fractures, such as the case reported by Torwalt et al. (2002) who had fractures of various ages of the left humerus, both femurs, tibia and fibula.

Vascular lesions of the metaphysis following septicaemia with DIC as in meningococcal septicaemia or with sickle cell disease can also resemble bone lesions of abuse.

Mechanisms of injuring and mechanisms of intracranial damage

There are several mechanisms by which a head injury may be sustained: (i) a penetrating injury, (ii) a compression injury, (iii) an impact acceleration injury, (iv) an impact deceleration injury, (v) a shaking injury (rotational shearing injury), (vi) a whiplash injury (Fig. 1.17).

PENETRATING INJURY

Penetrating injuries are high velocity, high energy injuries acting over a small area and can penetrate bone. The most obvious is a gunshot wound, which in the UK is thankfully rare in children. Knife and scissor blades or screwdrivers can penetrate the vault of the skull in a malicious assault.

Accidental penetrating injuries of the orbits with sticks, knitting needles, pencils and toy railway lines are seen. The stick may be broken off leaving a piece still in the frontal lobes as a source of infection. A mechanism of the intracranial damage in this type of injury is a brain laceration with haemorrhage, and since these are open wounds they carry a high risk of secondary CNS infection with cavernous sinus thrombosis.

Objects in the mouth may penetrate the tonsillar fossa and cause carotid artery injury. There may be a delay of a day or more before the onset of neurological signs as a dissecting aneurysm forms. Cavernous sinus thrombosis or carotico-cavernous fistula can result from intracranial injuries to the carotid. Penetrating injuries are non-rotational and so non-concussional, and consciousness may not be lost unless raised ICP supervenes.

COMPRESSION INJURY

If the head is compressed between two surfaces, sat upon or stood on, a bursting fracture

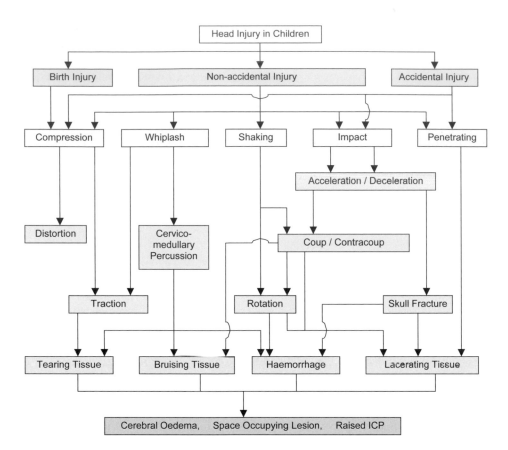

Fig. 1.17. Mechanisms and pathophysiology of head injury in children.

with suture diastases and a fractured base of the skull results. Compression is very rarely seen as the primary mechanism in NAHIs but occasionally the head is stood on or as in one case in our series compressed between the knees of an adult. The classical model for compression head injury in childhood is birth injury. Even today about 3.2% of all deliveries have some degree of birth trauma, most commonly fractures of the clavicle, humerus or femur, depressed skull fracture and facial palsy.

Theoretically, pressure on the head in a normal second stage of labour could result in pressures being transmitted to the brain causing raised ICP, cerebral oedema and low CPP with risk of ischaemia (Mann et al. 1972, Myers and Adamsons 1981). This is not supported by more objective data from Svenningsen et al. (1988), who measured the actual pressures between the fetal head and the birth canal during normal labour (46 spontaneous births, mean birthweight 3500 g) using a pressure transducer. Although the pressures sound alarming – mean 158 mmHg, range 38–390 mmHg) – the neurological outcome was uniformly good. RHs were present in some infants and they also did not correlate with the measured pres-

44

sures. This could be because the pressures are not transmitted to the fetal brain (mean blood pressure 50mmHg), and the fetal skull is offering more protection than its structure suggests, or because the applanation principle does not apply.

The head will be most compressed if there is (i) malpresentation (occipito-posterior, deep transverse arrest or an extended neck), or (ii) disproportion from too big a head, e.g. big baby, infant of diabetic mother, Sotos syndrome or too small an outlet (pelvic contraction). The full picture of a compressive head injury after birth is: (i) a difficult presentation with a prolonged labour; (ii) failed normal delivery with the need for obstetric intervention; (iii) external evidence of head compression.

The external evidence of a traumatic compressive head injury in the newborn infant takes the form of: (i) marked moulding; (ii) caput succedaneum (oedema of the scalp over the presenting part due to an accumulation of fluid in soft tissues above the periosteum, i.e. subcutaneous, secondary to pressure associated with delivery) disappears within 24-48 hours; (iii) cephalohaematomas that appear 24-48 hours after birth due to blood below the periosteum, and are therefore confined to a single bone; (iv) Erb's palsy; (v) radial palsy; and/or (vi) fractures (skull, spine, humerus).

In the vertex presentation the head moulds in the anteroposterior diameter to give a 'Magoo' head where there is no forehead but a large amount of skull behind the ears. This stretches the falx and tentorium beyond their elastic limits so they tear. The vein of Galen and major sinuses in these dural reflections then also tear, causing severe tentorial, middle fossa subdural and posterior fossa bleeding. Thrombosis of the vein of Galen may also result from the traction injury and causes bilateral thalamic infarction with high density on MRI.

Tentorial haemorrhages may be missed even using ultrasonography – in one study, trans-fontanelle ultrasound failed to reveal 50% (Faillot et al. 1990) – but they show readily on CT. In a recent study from Sheffield (Whitby et al. 2003), MRI was performed in 111 normal newborn infants in the first 24 hours of life. Small SDHs, which were clinically silent, were found in nine babies. Five followed ventouse and forceps deliveries and one followed ventouse alone. Three occurred following normal vaginal delivery. All fully resolved by 4 weeks, with subsequent normal development. Posterior fossa subdural bleeding can also result from ventouse extraction, as in 7/15 cases reported by Perrin et al. (1997).

The head is also compressed laterally so that the parietal bones override and pull the sagittal sinus between them (sagittal sinus entrapment syndrome). This puts traction on the veins entering the sinuses and tears them so that a convexity subdural and subarachnoid haemorrhage results. The head ossifies very rapidly after 40 weeks gestation and will not mould, so obstructed labour with the infant failing to descend is more likely, and skull fractures and cephalohaematomas are more common in the post-term infant.

Compression injuries are non-rotational, non-shearing and non-concussional, so the child may be conscious after severe injury. Cerebral oedema with secondary bleeding into the subarachnoid and subdural spaces occurs. The pathology in 82 cases of birth trauma (neonatal compression head injury) seen by the present authors showed 9 had Erb's palsy, 5 radial palsies, 1 fractured cervical spines, 2 fractured skulls, 12 cephalhaaematomas, 48 marked moulding and external trauma to the head, 29 traumatic subarachnoid haemorrhage (29 out of 82), 8 subdural haematoma, 8 traumatic asphyxia (retinal, subconjunctival and facial

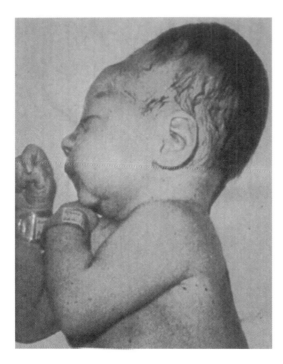

Fig. 1.18. Severe anteroposterior moulding of the head.

petechiae), 8 vertebral artery thrombosis, and 1 intraventricular haemorrhage (Brown 1974). These data demonstrate that before attributing a subdural bleed to birth trauma there must have been a difficult delivery with external signs of injury. Compressive birth injury is now very rare, but modern imaging can pick up lesser degrees, usually asymptomatic (Whitby et al. 2004).

The mechanisms of intra- and extracranial nervous system damage in compression injury are thus:

1. *Compression* (impaired cerebral blood flow, oedema, traumatic asphyxia, coning)
2. *Moulding* – lateral moulding (sagittal sinus entrapment, tearing of bridging veins)
          – anteroposterior moulding (tearing of the vein of Galen and the tentorium and venous sinuses) (Fig. 1.18).
3. *Traction* (cervical spine, brachial plexus, vertebral arteries).

The mechanisms of damage are therefore distortion of the brain, compression and ischaemia with cerebral oedema, moulding of the head with traction and tearing of the veins, and dural reflections. Ingraham and Matson (1954) in their classic series of subdural haematomas were already suspicious that the social problems in some of their infants suggested there was an overemphasis on birth trauma. Retinal haemorrhages may also occur in the neonate from chest compression during delivery, hence the combination of sub-dural haematoma, retinal haemorrhage, subperiosteal bleeding in long bones, cerebral oedema, secondary hypoxic–ischaemic encephalopathy and cervical spine damage may truly mimic SBS.

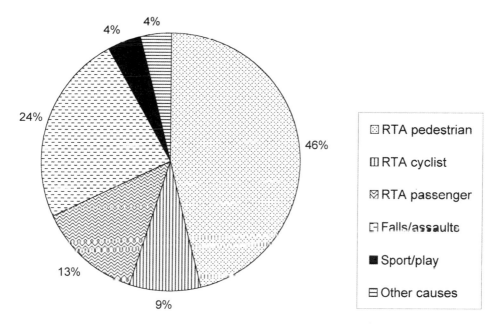

Fig. 1.19. Causes of head injury in children under the age of 16 years admitted with a GCS <12 (N=359) (Brown 1994). Note that falls and assaults are combined into a single category as the history of a 'fall' or a 'push' (i.e. assault) could not be distinguished in the A&E department.

A recent study of uncommon *accidental* compression injuries from Spain also emphasizes a characteristic basal syndrome without concussion (Gonzalez Tortosa et al. 2004). The authors reviewed clinical and radiological features in a series of 11 patients who had sustained a special type of cranial crush injury produced by the bilateral application of compression forces to the temporal region. Patients presented with a characteristic clinical picture consisting of no loss of consciousness (6 patients), epistaxis (9 patients), otorrhagia (11 patients), peripheral paralysis of the VIth and/or VIIth cranial nerves (10 patients), hearing loss (5 patients), skull base fractures (11 patients), pneumocephalus (11 patients, and diabetes insipidus (7 patients). Ten patients survived the injury, and most recovered neurological function. Stretching of the cranial nerves at the skull base explains the nearly universal finding of cranial nerve paralysis, whereas an increase in the vertical diameter of the skull accounts for the occurrence of diabetes insipidus.

IMPACT ACCELERATION AND DECELERATION INJURIES
Impact injuries
The vast majority of accidental injuries in children are impact injuries. From our local children's hospital records of head injury in children under the age of 16 with a GCS of 12 or less (N=359), the child pedestrian accounted for by far the largest number of cases (46%). Falls and assaults combined (it was not possible to distinguish the two based on the recorded history) were the second most common cause (24%) (Fig. 1.19).

Causes may differ in other populations, and in other cultures (e.g. the culture of walking or being driven). Kraus et al. (1990) reviewed US publications on the external causes of brain injury by gender and age from California in 1981. Of a total of 1234 injuries, motor vehicle accidents accounted for 37% (occupant 19%, motor cycle 8%, pedestrian 6%, bicycle 4%). Falls accounted for 24% (from a height 15%, level 9%). Sports/recreation accounted for 21% (bicycle 11%, sports 7%, playground 3%). Assault was responsible for 10% and firearms 2%. Other causes accounted for 12%.

Reporting on the US National Pediatric Trauma Registry 1994–2000, Morrison et al. (2004) found, among a total of 16,437 cases of impact injury in the 0–19 years age-group, an equal number where the child was a vehicle passenger (27%) as where trauma was due to a fall. Other causes (17%) were the next most common category in this series, which excluded penetrating injuries.

Impact injuries may be accidental or non-accidental, and one cannot state which purely from a study of the injury. The explanation may sound unusual, e.g. Bernard et al. (1998) reported 73 injuries and 28 deaths from television sets falling on children, and Di Scala et al. (2001) described similar injuries in 183 children, 68% of which were head injuries.

Acceleration injuries
These occur when a moving object hits the child and so imparts acceleration to the child. The object could be a moving vehicle, fist, foot, hammer, golf club or milk bottle. If the child flies through the air, some of the force is dissipated as the imparted motion.

BOXING AS A MODEL FOR IMPACT ACCELERATION/ROTATIONAL INJURY
A type of impact injury that is interesting in that it is, in essence, a human experimental model for impact/rotational injury, is that caused in boxing. Boxing shares with a few other sports the potential for acute and chronic brain injury. A postal survey of 162 British neurologists in 1976, enquiring about their encounters with chronic traumatic encephalopathy (CTE) and its association with sport, yielded: 12 jockeys, 5 soccer players, 2 rugby players, 2 professional wrestlers, 1 parachutist, and 290 boxers (Corsellis 1989).

The aim in boxing is to produce a rotation swirling injury to cause midbrain dysfunction with concussion, i.e. a knockout. An acute SDH, retinal bleeding (and tears), axonal injury (which may take time to appear as dementia and parkinsonism) and cervical spinal injury are seen. Although the acute shearing/rotation may cause death, it takes at least 25 fights, and usually 50, to be more certain of developing the more long-term neurological syndrome, i.e. it is as though the shaking with impact was done one at a time over years (NHMRC 1994).

When the head is struck by a fist, force is transmitted to the skull and the brain suffers violent acceleration. As the brain is a jelly-like organ surrounded by displaceable fluid it has some capacity for linear and tangential movement within the skull, and also swirling movement within the brain itself, with consequent sudden deformation. The acceleration may be linear or rotational as the head is able to pivot on the joints of the neck.

The sudden rotational acceleration of the brain within the skull may tear the bridging veins that run from the brain to the venous sinuses, resulting in bleeding into the subdural space (Gennarelli and Thibault 1982), a well-known cause of death in boxing contests. Impact/acceleration causes brain deformation, which will damage nerve cells and fibres in the white matter, and this could be the mechanism underlying boxers' chronic encephalopathy when traumatic diffuse axonal injury may resemble histologically the changes seen in Alzheimer's disease. The repeated concussional injuries also cause midbrain damage with severe parkinsonism. MRI abnormalities and minimal memory deficits occur in many boxers who appear otherwise normal.

Gloves significantly reduce the force of impact. Peak linear accelerations up to 160 G, and peak angular accelerations up to 16,000 rad/s^2, were recorded by Pincemaille et al. (1989) in gloved boxers trading punches that did not result in loss of consciousness or disturbed evoked potentials. Schwartz et al. (1986) studied the accelerations induced in a dummy head when kicked or punched by karate experts. Maximum peak accelerations were in the range 90–120 G. The duration of the impact acceleration is important, as very brief pulses of acceleration are better tolerated than pulses in excess of 3 ms.

Ocular injuries are frequent in boxing. In a study by Giovinazzo et al. (1987), vision-threatening injuries, defined as significant damage to the lens, macula or peripheral retina, occurred in 58% of the boxers. A total of 24% had retinal tears, and 66% had at least one ocular injury. Significant correlations were found between the total number of bouts, the total number of losses, and the presence of retinal tears.

Three main mechanisms have been described to explain the ocular complications:
(1) 'coup' injuries caused by a direct blow to the eye that produces local damage
(2) ocular 'contra coup' injuries that occur remote from the area of impact: a direct blow produces a line of force traversing the globe, producing damage at interfaces or to those structures that are borders between tissues of different density
(3) equatorial expansion: as the globe is compressed along the anterior–posterior axis, the circumference of the equator increases, this causes the circumference of the equatorial sclera to increase, and the underlying retina and pars plana detach from the vitreous base resulting in avulsion of this base, with tears in the retinal and ciliary epithelium.

Deceleration injuries

Conversely, a deceleration injury is brought about when the child is moving and comes to a sudden halt, as in a car crash for example. They occur in children who fall from or are pushed from windows, bunk beds, slides and ladders, or when the child is held by the chest or arms, shaken, and the head repeatedly bashed against the floor or wall. The worst impact of all is when the infant is held by the legs, swung around, and the head smashed against the wall. Impact injuries can be dissipated only by bounce or a very forgiving surface. If the impact force cannot be dissipated then these deceleration impact injuries form the most devastating type of head injury. The biomechanics are discussed above under skull fractures.

Biomechanics of accidental falls

Since falls are the commonest cause of accidental impact injuries, and short falls are often given as the cause of injury, we will consider the biomechanics of a fall in more detail.

49

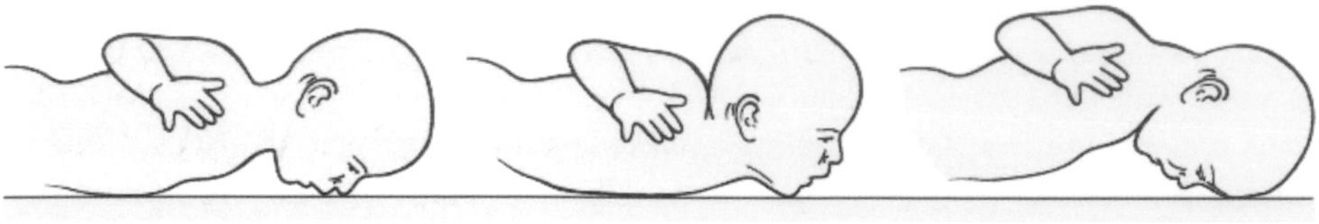

Fig. 1.20. Rotational effect is governed by where the impact to the head occurs in relation to the centre of mass of the head.

If a moving object such as a car travels at a certain speed and hits a wall, a high force will result with a low impact time. If a vehicle with protection, such as a bumper bar, travels at the same speed and hits the wall, the force will be less and the impact time longer, so the peak force and deceleration are less but the overall impulse (mass x velocity) will be the same. Similarly, a skull dropped onto concrete will have a high force and a short impact time. By contrast, plasticine dropped onto concrete will have a low force and a high impact time, such that the peak force is reduced and deceleration is reduced.

A child may hit the fender with his nose (the centre of mass or the centre of gravity is behind the nose and there is not much rotational effect) and this results in the nose crumbling and protecting the brain. If on the other hand the child hits the fender with his forehead, the result is worse because the centre of gravity is lower than the point of impact resulting in a rotational effect. There are therefore two factors: (i) where the head hits in relation to the centre of gravity (Fig. 1.20), and (ii) if there is the possibility of 'crumbling' where the child's head is hit. The torque about the centre of mass will determine the angular acceleration, and the torque or moment of inertia (mass $\times$ radius^2) is the angular equivalent of force.*

Typical falls can be considered firstly *from a standing position*. Let us consider the body as a uniform pole, of length L and mass M, standing on a flat surface, and the child falls over the base of the pole (i.e. the child's feet), which doesn't move, as if the base is hinged at the surface. The final angular velocity just before the head hits the surface varies as $(L/2)^{-1}$. For a 60 cm tall child the angular velocity at impact would be approximately 7 rad/s.

If the child is initially *vertical and moving horizontally*, and the child falls over the base of the pole (the child's feet) as a 'perfect trip', the final angular velocity just before the head hits the surface is rather more complicated. For a 60 cm tall child, running at 1 m/s and tripping, the angular velocity at impact is approximately 7.6 rad/s. Running at 2 m/s it is 9.1 rad/s, and running at 3 m/s it is 11.1 rad/s, i.e. the angular velocity will increase with the speed of the child. These angular velocities are calculated just before impact. The ensuing angular acceleration will depend on how quickly the relevant impulses occur, i.e. soft surface (e.g. the nose) gives a longer time, whereas a harder strike on the forehead could mean higher forces for a shorter time with larger linear and angular accelerations.

Angular impulse or *rotational impulse* is the integral of torque ÷ time (it represents a change in angular momentum).
The angular momentum of a rotating body is the product of the angular velocity times the moment of inertia of the body about the axis of rotation.

Where the impact is near the top of the forehead, such that the head is doubled back on the neck, this will result in a much larger change in angular momentum and hence larger angular accelerations. The body now consists of two parts – a head and a body, hinged at the neck. Assuming a uniform rod body hinged at the neck and with the length of the head assumed to be a quarter the length of the body, and also assuming the impact on the top of the head does not result in any bounce (i.e. the coefficient of restitution equals zero), the angular velocity of the head immediately after the impact is approximately 8 times its angular velocity just prior to impact, but in the opposite direction. This means a change in angular velocity of 8 times the initial angular velocity. This is clearly a much worse situation because the head is rotating in one direction just prior to impact, and rotating 8 times as fast in the opposite direction just after impact.

A typical situation might be an angular velocity before impact of 7 rad/s, and after impact, by calculation, 56 rad/s in the opposite direction. The change is 63 rad/s. The question remains, how long does this take? In this example the impact point is travelling at 4.2 m/s prior to impact, supposing the head distorts 20 mm and then returns to normal, the distance travelled is 40 mm at an average speed of 2.1 m/s, and the time taken would be approximately $40/2100 \approx 20$ ms. For a 20 ms impact the average rotational acceleration would be more than 3000 rad/s^2, and at a 100 ms impact it would be 600 rad/s^2, comparing interestingly with the results from our shaking experiments. Therefore, impacts that 'throw' the head backwards result in angular accelerations which could exceed those measured during shaking.

Case 1. A father had been standing in the kitchen holding his 5-week-old child one-handed over his shoulder while using the other hand on another task, when the child fell to the floor, sustaining skull fractures, brain contusion and soft tissue injury. The father was well over 6 ft (185 cm) tall, so the child's head height was approximately 180 cm above the floor, i.e. not a short fall. The floor was a tiled surface and there was no bounce (coefficient of restitution = 0). The impact time will have been short. The infant had arched backwards, effectively throwing himself in a diving fashion from his father's arm, providing an additional kinetic energy to the fall. Therefore the height, the surface and the initial velocity resulted in an increased deceleration force, causing his injuries (Fig. 1.21). There was no evidence of rotational injury or concussion.

Case 2. This child, at 7 months of age, had fallen down a flight of 15 stairs in a baby walker. There was no loss of consciousness and the child cried immediately; he remained alert with normally reactive pupils, moving his limbs, although a boggy swelling was noted at the side of his head. CT showed a large right extradural haematoma (maximum width 18 mm) with a mixed attenuation pattern consistent with active bleeding (Fig. 1.22). There was some effacement of the right lateral ventricle. The scan demonstrated a linear fracture in the left frontal region extending to the supraorbital area, and a second fracture in the right parietal region that was associated with a subperiosteal haematoma overlying the extradural haemorrhage. The extradural haemorrhage was evacuated surgically, and apart from some immediate postoperative bruising about the eye and swelling of the scalp, he made a subsequent good recovery.

51

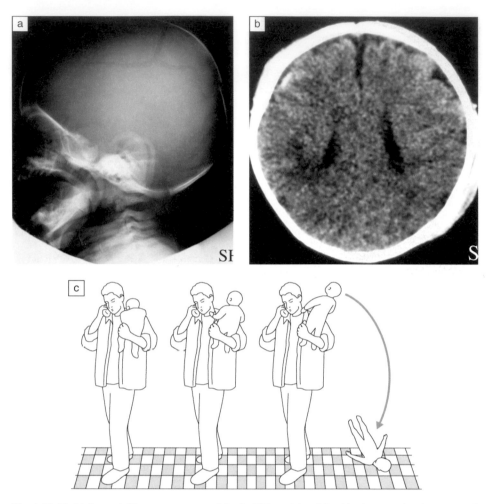

Fig. 1.21. Multiple cranial fractures seen on plain skull X-ray (a) and focal brain contusion (contracoup) on CT (b) of infant who fell a distance of 180 cm onto a tiled floor. The schematic (c) shows how the father had an inadequate grasp on the infant, who arched and fell, landing on his head.

Case 3. A 3-month-old boy was being nursed by his mother when she tripped over a stair-gate and fell with the child 150–180 cm down carpeted stairs. The child sustained an immediate left parietal skull fracture but CT showed no parenchymal injury. He remained irritable for weeks later, and the head circumference crossed the centiles from below the 50th to above the 97th. MRI at 5 months of age shows extensive subdural haematoma (Fig. 1.23).

Pathophysiology of impact injuries
The pathophysiology of impact injuries includes injuries sustained by (1) contusion and laceration, (2) brain compression, and (3) shearing or rotational injury.

52

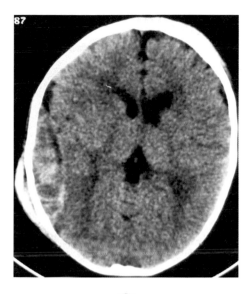

Fig. 1.22. (Left) CT of 7-month-old child who fell down a flight of stairs in a 'baby walker', sustaining a large right extradural haematoma with mixed attenuation pattern indicative of continued bleeding. There were additional frontal and parietal skull fractures.

(Below) Up to 30% of baby walker injuries result in serious injury including fatalities.

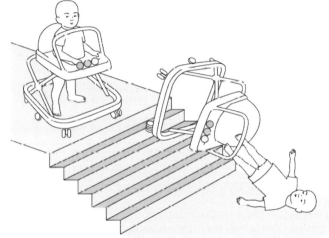

• *Contusional and laceration injuries.* These include: (i) skin bruising, (ii) scalp/subgaleal contusion, (iii) skull fracture, (iv) epidural haematoma, (v) focal subdural haematoma, (vi) cortical contusion, and (vii) contracoup injuries.

Contusion or bruising of the brain occurs at the site of impact (coup injury) and then at the opposite side as the brain forcibly hits the other side of the skull (contra coup). The frontal and temporal lobes swirl and hit the bony buttress such as the sphenoid wing and ethmoidal plate, so contusions are particularly likely on the under surface of the frontal and temporal lobes and the anterior temporal pole (Fig. 1.24). It is said that occipital impact is more likely to cause these contusions than frontal or lateral impact (Jennett and Teasdale 1981). These swirling and contra coup movements against sharp bony buttresses, if severe,

53

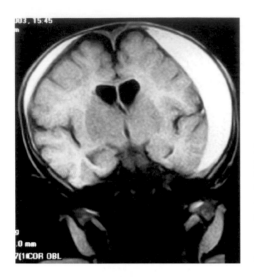

Fig. 1.23. While carrying her 3-month-old child a mother fell over a stair gate and down the stairs. The child sustained only a parietal skull fracture. Two months later he appeared irritable, with an increasing head circumference. (Left) MRI shows extensive bilateral subdural haematoma. (Below) Schematic illustrates the eight-fold increase in angular velocity following a change in the direction of head rotation.

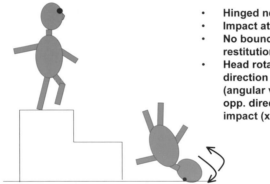

- Hinged neck
- Impact at top of head
- No bounce (coefficient of restitution = 0)
- Head rotates one direction prior to impact (angular v) – head rotates opp. direction after impact (x8 angular v)

will also cause brain laceration. In a simple contusion, blood vessels rupture, allowing red cells into the tissue spaces. However, the brain architecture is preserved so that although there is temporary interference with function, good recovery is possible. Suggestions that liberated iron and haemosiderin can cause severe local metabolic upset and brain damage do not appear to be borne out by clinical observation. Localized haematomas, however, will act as space-occupying lesions and materially alter local blood flow, causing focal ischaemia and so greater subsequent focal atrophy than expected for the size of the haematoma (Jenkins et al. 1990).

If the brain is actually lacerated due to sphenoid impaction or tearing from impounded bone fragments, then local atrophy and gliosis with less complete recovery is to be expected. Severe contusions can occur without any loss of consciousness. It is surprising how little disturbance of function may seem to occur on superficial examination with unilateral focal frontal atrophy. However, with proper neuropsychological examination the effects are often found to be devastating.

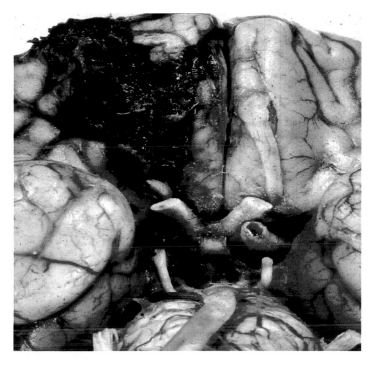

Fig. 1.24. Extensive contusion on the inferior surface of the frontal lobe from swirling engagement with the ethmoid plate.

• *Brain compression.* Compression head injury as a mechanism of injury has already been described and is due to a compressive force external to the skull, whilst the compression of the brain in impact injuries is due to a compressive force generated inside the skull. The brain is mainly water and so is highly incompressible (it takes 10,000 tons of pressure to reduce brain volume by 50% – Shapiro 1975). Boyle's Law (i.e. pressure varies inversely with volume at a constant temperature) means that if the volume of brain cannot reduce and the volume of skull cannot increase, then for any added intracranial volume the pressure must rise. The subsequent rise in ICP seriously impairs cerebral perfusion pressure and so cerebral blood flow, and again the end result is cerebral ischaemia. Even though the infant skull has sutures and fontanelles and so the head can increase in volume (increasing head circumference), the brain is encased in a relatively non-elastic dura that can stretch only gradually and so the pressure will rise to serious ischaemic levels with acute increases in intradural volume.

The usual cause of brain compression is space occupation by too much blood, brain or cerebrospinal fluid (CSF). Blood clot, either extradural or subdural, cerebral oedema (increase in brain water), cerebral congestion (an increase in cerebral blood volume, i.e. an increase in the amount of blood in the vessels within the brain) and excess CSF (hydrocephalus or hygroma) will all cause a rise in ICP and so brain compression.

TABLE 1.6
Confirmed rotational/inertial injuries

Interhemispheric subdural haemorrhage
Tearing surface veins – subdural, subarachnoid haemorrhage
Concussion – midbrain shear
Fronto/temporal rotational sphenoid impact
Gliding contusions, lacerations at grey–white interface
Traumatic axonal injury
Corpus callosum and cerebellar peduncle white matter shearing
Cranio-cervical junction injuries
Diffuse retinal haemorrhage/retinoschisis

Cerebrovascular autoregulation implies an alteration in the cerebral vascular volume in order to maintain the cerebral perfusion. In cerebral congestion there may be pooling of blood within the brain vasculature due to vasoparalysis and therefore an increase in the total volume of blood within the brain, which acts as a space occupation. Carbon dioxide is the most potent overrider of autoregulation, and a rise in pCO_2 causes cerebral congestion.

A rise in ICP impairs cerebral perfusion by reducing CPP as described later. A second effect is to cause shifts and cones. In a tentorial herniation the rise in supratentorial pressure forces the medial temporal lobe structures (uncus) through the tentorial hiatus. This impaction of tissue or cone impairs the blood supply to the midbrain and brainstem, causing secondary midbrain infarction and haemorrhages, the so-called Duret haemorrhages. These are to be differentiated at autopsy from primary brainstem haemorrhage, which may accompany high falls or other head trauma.

If pressure is not relieved, or particularly if a lumbar puncture is performed, a cone occurs at the foramen magnum. This can cause secondary ischaemia of the medulla and upper cervical cord as well as cerebellar tonsillar necrosis, and needs to be differentiated from a primary whiplash injury.

Immediate death after injury is more likely from primary brainstem injury, massive basal fractures, chest injury or systemic haemorrhage. The secondary injury will cause later death from cerebral infarction secondary to perfusion failure and coning.

• *Shearing or rotational injury*. Rotation of the brain within the skull, and shearing of vessels and dural attachments at points of fixation, cause subarachnoid and subdural bleeding. The right and left cerebral hemispheres also rotate at a different rate and amount, so tearing of the veins between them causes an interhemispheric SDH. Because of the differential densities – and hence the inertias – of grey and white matter, the axons tear, causing shearing at the grey–white interface. The tracts within the white matter may show tearing, bleeding and axonal shearing, characteristic of a rotational injury: the pathognomonic sites are the middle cerebellar peduncle and the corpus callosum. The eye also shows retinoschisis from shearing between vitreous and retina. The cerebral hemispheres rotate on the midbrain causing primary midbrain injury and so concussion and coma. Injuries due to rotational/inertial forces are summarized in Table 1.6, and are discussed in more detail in the following section.

Shaking as a mechanism of non-accidental head injury in infants

In this section we will consider shaking as one mechanism of inducing brain injury rather than as a generic term covering all inflicted head injuries.

There are five major mechanisms by which brain damage may occur:

1. Shaking, causing rotation of the brain inside the skull resulting in rotational shearing injuries as well as repeated percussion/cavitation.
2. Impact against a 'soft surface', resulting in acute deceleration of the brain and vastly increasing the rotational torque forces inside the skull.
3. Hyperflexion and hyperextension injury from the whiplash, causing repetitive subluxation of the cervical vertebrae resulting in injury to the cervical cord and medulla.
4. Shaking with hard impact, causing skull fractures and contusional injuries in addition to the rotational injuries.
5. Primary hypoxic–ischaemic brain injury resulting from stem apnoea from stem injury.

Sufficient numbers of parents and carers have admitted and described the manner of shaking to establish it as an unequivocal cause of NAHI. Duhaime et al. (1987) and Kleinman et al. (1989) were doubtful that shaking alone was the mechanism because of the high incidence of associated findings indicating impact seen in the shaken infant. If there is associated impact – for example by the head being banged against a hard surface repeatedly during the shaking, or the infant being thrown or dropped on the floor after the shaking (shake and throw away) – then the clinical features will confirm the impact injury. However, soft impact may be more devastating and yet leave no mark.

PREDISPOSING FACTORS

A number of factors predispose the infant to injury from shaking.

1. The young infant has *a relatively large and heavy head* in relation to body size (the brain represents 10% of the infant weight but only 2% of adult weight).

2. *The neck muscles are weak and with little head control* so that even picking the infant up requires a hand behind the occiput to prevent the head flopping back. The force required need only be sufficient to overcome the neck muscles and allow the head to whiplash with each shake. Strong neck muscles prevent a boxer being easily knocked out or a footballer being concussed every time he heads the ball (Shapiro 1975). In experiments on monkeys, wearing a collar prevented 'knockouts' (Denny Brown and Russell 1941) and also physical trauma from shaking (Ommaya et al. 1968). As the child gets older, body weight increases in relation to the head, the neck muscles become stronger so that the head moves with the body, and the greater body weight means it takes more force to accelerate the child so that shaking whiplash injuries are rare after the second year of life and are characteristic of the child in the first year of life.

3. The skull grows secondary to brain growth, and the brain weighs 350 g at birth and 1350 g at 4 years; the skull therefore has to increase in volume over this period by 1000 cm^3. The brain grows and stretches the suture lines encouraging skull growth. The brain does not exert pressure on the skull bones directly, but the wider CSF filled subarachnoid space of the young infant has the effect of distributing pressure evenly through a hydrostatic bag of water. *The extracerebral space is relatively large* in the normal infant, as shown by CT,

and in the first year of life it can be up to 1cm deep (Nickel and Gallenstein 1987). This is more marked in males and maximal at about 5 months of age. This acts as a hydrostatic cushion to allow skull growth to keep pace with the brain growth, i.e. physiological cranio-cerebral disproportion, by which we mean that either the brain is too big for the skull, or more importantly, in a shaking context, the skull is too big for the brain. CSF acts as a buffer, and the brain as it were floats in the CSF (removal makes the brain heavier), adding inertia against starting any movement but allowing the brain to carry on moving once the external force is removed. If CSF is removed or shunted, or decreased by giving mannitol, this predisposes to a subdural fluid collection.

There is disagreement about whether the larger extracerebral space in the young infant will by itself increase the risk of subdural bleeding with lesser degrees of rotational force (Reece 2002). A large extracerebral space would allow the brain to rattle in the head and so rotate more easily, and there would be more space for extracerebral blood to accumulate. Old age, steroids, mannitol, uraemia and diuretics may all cause an increase in the extracerebral space at other ages.

4. There is a *physiological laxity of the meninges* (falx and tentorium) in infancy compared to older children. This, taken in conjunction with the greater extracerebral space, means that there is relatively more space and less tethering of the brain, thus allowing more movement within the infant's skull.

5. There is a *higher water content in the infant brain* in the absence of myelination in white matter, while at the same time the grey matter has a full complement of neuronal cell bodies, causing an increased difference in the specific gravity between the grey and the white matter of the infant compared to the adult brain. That is, for a given force there will be a greater difference between the getting moving (inertia) and the subsequent speed of movement (tangential accelerations at different radial positions) of grey vs white matter, which will be more likely to produce major shearing.

Biomechanical Determinants of Shaking Injury

A number of physical parameters determine the risk of injury from an episode of shaking. These are: (i) force, (ii) speed, (iii) duration, (iv) fulcrum, (v) deceleration (at hit stop), (vi) degree of rotation, (vii) differing viscosity and inertias (see above), and (viii) craniocerebral disproportion (see above).

Force

In order to set up the forces within the skull that result in the brain injury, the external force has first of all to overcome the neck muscles and induce whiplashing with rotation. Shaking the child causes the head to whiplash 'to and fro', causing the brain to swirl first in one direction and then the reverse, setting up shearing forces within the skull and within the brain itself (rotational shearing forces). This would be the equivalent to repeated knockouts by a boxer. As discussed above, the head must be free both to whiplash backwards and forwards, and to show rotation. A boxer will get a knockout by hitting his opponent to the side of the chin and not by simply causing an anteroposterior linear force. Linear movement not causing rotation is less damaging to the brain but may still cause a hyperextension injury to the cervical cord and brainstem. There is also alternately deformation of the brain as it percusses the inside of the skull, then cavitation with a relative negative (suction) pressure as it moves in the opposite direction, deforming the jelly-like brain as it tries to flow.

An interesting traditional therapy, in certain Hispanic communities, is used for 'fallen fontanelle syndrome' ('caida de mollera'), where a supposed flat or depressed fontanelle in an infant is treated by holding the child upside down and vertically shaking them, without rotation, and this is not known to cause any harm (Hansen 1998).

The CSF, blood, grey matter and white matter of the brain are all fluids (or at least have a high water content), meaning that they will tend to flow compared to the rigid non-fluid non-viscous skull. They vary in viscosity and inertia, so that various compartments will accelerate and decelerate at different speeds and with different amounts of shift (flow). These differential rates of movement between the skull and the brain, between the grey and white matter, and between the skull and the CSF, set up shearing forces, i.e. sliding strain at interfaces. This can be illustrated by placing water and oil in a flask and gently tilting or tapping. The less viscous water moves more quickly than the oil, so that there is a differential movement at the interface. With more vigorous movements, marked incoordinate waveforms occur at the interface.

The maximum tangential accelerations will be at the outer edge of the arc from the pivot point, decreasing in intensity as one approaches the pivot along the axis of rotation. There will therefore be a tendency, because of the different densities of skull, CSF, grey matter, white matter, etc., for shearing to occur to the blood vessels, axons and midbrain. The outer hemispheres move through an arc with four times the displacement of that at the pivot point. The injury to the brainstem at the axis of pivot (where the tangential accelerations are theoretically nil) is a hyperflexion–hyperextension injury, which results from repetitive subluxation and a water hammer effect of the cord against the spinal canal.

As with impact injuries, the amount of damage will depend upon the rate of acceleration/deceleration before the direction is reversed. Soft impact brings the skull to a sudden halt but the brain may continue to rotate with maximum stretching of the bridging veins, and deformation from viscous flow stretching and rupturing axons. Torque (angular) forces are set up that cause the brain to rotate within the skull as if round a central midbrain pivot, while the head itself pivots on the cervical spine. It is the sudden angular acceleration then deceleration experienced by the brain and cerebral vessels, not the specific contact forces applied to the surface of the head, that results in intracranial injury, i.e. shaking impact syndrome (Duhaime et al. 1998). With soft impact, therefore, because the damage is caused by the deceleration and not the force of impact against the surface, there need be no surface injury to scalp or skull.

It is impossible to simulate the actual forces sustained by an infant's brain by shaking, and biomechanical studies using mannequins must be relied upon to approximate these forces. Studies by Duhaime et al. (1987) and Minns et al. (2004) found the angular acceleration to be of the order of 1139 rad/s^2 (mean) and 87–892 rad/s^2 (range of peak values) respectively. The forces exerted by the shaker are dependent on the age, height, gender and strength of the individual shaking, so that young children (3 years) are unable to lift, let alone shake a weight equivalent to a 2-month-old child, and sustained acceleration patterns gradually increase to adult values by the age of 10. By 10–15 years the children can shake weights equivalent to human infants of 2 months, 5 months and 1 year equally as well as adults.

Speed (frequency of shaking)

If one moves a part of the body that can only move in one plane (a hinged joint) with increasing frequency, the amount of movement (excursion) for a given force gradually increases to a maximum at the resonant frequency, and then gets less so that at a very fast frequency very little excursion occurs at all. Each joint has a different resonant frequency, but that for the movement of the infant's cranium on the cervical spine is not yet determined. Theoretically for a given force, a rate of shaking that is at resonance produces maximum excursion, which is likely to result in the greatest rotational accelerations and hence potential brain injury.

In a study by one of the present authors (RAM, unpublished), the mean frequency of shaking for adult volunteers shaking different weight dolls (3.5–10 kg) was between 3.5 and 3.1 per second, and for children 2.1 to 1.8 per second, with males shaking significantly faster than females (p<0.0001). Interestingly, the frequency is independent of the load.

Duration of shaking

There is obviously a necessary minimum duration of shaking to produce brain damage; there is also a maximum duration of shaking that is possible by the shaker before fatigue prevents further shaking. The experimentally determined maximum possible duration for adults shaking dolls was a median of 21.5 s for a doll of equivalent mass to that of a 2-month-old baby, 19.8 s for a doll equivalent to a 5-month-old, and only 16.0 s for a doll with the physical dimensions of a 12-month-old. Males were able to shake significantly longer than females (p<0.0001), and the duration of shaking was related to the strength of the weakest arm and to the height of the individual. For a rate of 3.5 shakes per second and a duration of 21.5 s, this represents a possible maximum of 75 whiplashes. It would be highly unlikely that anyone would shake to exhaustion, and likewise a brief shake to the older child is unlikely to produce injury; however, we suspect that shaking for as little as a few seconds (9–10 whiplashes) would be sufficient to induce the forces necessary to cause injury. One important result from these experiments is that it is not generally possible for an adult to shake an infant of 2, 5 or 12 months for the prolonged periods of 30–60 s sometimes suggested in court cases, although for someone in a rage situation, all the biomechanical parameters may be increased compared to the experimental situation.

Fulcrum

In the infant, we consider the fulcrum for head movement in the anteroposterior direction to be in the upper cervical spine, i.e. C2, rather than the C5/6 site where adult whiplash injuries are usually sustained. The fulcrum around which the brain pivots (i.e. the midbrain) is discussed later, in the section on whiplash shaken medullary syndrome.

Deceleration (at hit stop)

If the head is whiplashed on the cervical spine it is not a pendulum type motion as the head

TABLE 1.7
Pathological mechanisms of rotational injury

- Surface shearing – cortical emissary veins – subdural haematoma
- Differential hemisphere rotation – interhemispheric SDH
  (The origin of interhemispheric SDH could have been from (i) an original convexity
  SDH, (ii) rupture of bridging veins between the occipital poles, or (iii) asymmetrical
  movement of the hemispheres because of angular acceleration–deceleration forces)
- Parenchymatous shearing
     Shearing of grey–white interface, axonal shearing
     Shearing of long white matter tracts (percussion/cavitation)
     Midbrain shearing injury
- Cervico-medullary whiplash injury
- Hypoxia–ischaemia – secondary shock, and cerebral oedema with raised ICP
     Vascular injury – carotid compression and vertebral artery trauma in whiplash
- Contusion from impact injury
- Optic nerve concussion, retinoschisis

is brought to a stop by the anatomy of the spine and elasticity of the ligaments which bring
the head to a slower halt than if impacted. The to and fro motion causes a repeated 'coup–
contracoup' type situation. If the skull is brought to a sudden halt by impact, even soft impact
as already described, the forces generated within the skull are greatly amplified, up to 50
fold (Duhaime et al. 1987).

Degree of rotation
The excursion or degree of rotation through which the infant's cranium moves is a function
dependent on the speed of shaking, i.e. with fast shakes a small excursion is possible and
vice versa. It is not known if a slower shake with a wider excursion is more injurious than
a faster shake over a shorter excursion. From the above two determinants it is clear that
shaking with 'soft impact' will reduce the excursion of head on neck movement, offering
some protection against hyperextension cervico-medullary syndrome, but increases the
supratentorial rotational forces.

PATHOPHYSIOLOGY OF SHAKING INJURIES
The pathological features will vary from case to case as there are many intermediary pathophysiological mechanisms, the choice of which will determine the final pattern of brain
damage (Tables 1.7–1.9).

Vascular (surface) shearing injuries
An extradural haematoma is usually due to arterial bleeding, and a subdural one from
venous bleeding. The extradural is commonest in true accidental injuries complicated by
skull fractures from falls with direct impact, which tears the middle meningeal artery, in
its canal, where it is anchored to the inner table of the skull. Although the child is shocked
with acute brain compression, if diagnosed early and treated effectively the outlook is
excellent with no residual brain damage.

61

TABLE 1.8	TABLE 1.9
Mechanisms of shearing injuries	**Pathology of rotation–shearing injuries**
• At interfaces the density of tissues may vary (brain/CSF, grey/white matter, vitreous/retina) so that they accelerate at different rates (inertia) and so move against each other at different speeds. Friction and traction at these interfaces causes shearing of tissue	• Right on left hemisphere – interhemispheric shear – SDH
	• Surface rotation and shearing – bridging and emissary veins – surface SDH
	• Corpus callosum tear
• At other sites one part of the brain may be anchored and so not able to rotate as freely as the adjacent part	• Hemispheres on midbrain and anchored cerebellum – midbrain injury
	• Cerebellar peduncle tear
	• Grey–white interface, gliding contusions, axonal tears
• Because of the easily deformable but incompressible nature of brain it can change shape and flow, setting up traction strains in fibres running in the direction of the flow	• Percussion/cavitation – 'jelly flow' – longitudinal association fibre tears
	• Retina – retinoschisis

• *Subdural haematoma.* A subdural haematoma is not a common accompaniment of accidental head injury in children, and among 6700 children with head trauma described by Choux et al. (1986) it was present in only 4.3% of cases. This was very similar to the figure of 2.5–5% in all head injuries in Guthkelch's (1971) earlier series. Kravitz et al. (1969) found only one case of subdural haematoma in 536 children who had accidently fallen a distance of 20–60 inches (50–150 cm).

If one considers all types of child abuse, a subdural haematoma is equally rare, present in only 8% of cases reported by Lauer et al. (1974). Selection of cases with head injuries will increase this percentage: Smith and Hanson (1974) found 30 cases among 47 children with NAHI from a total of 134 cases of child abuse. Of our 124 cases, 89% had a subdural haematoma, and in the big Canadian series of 364 cases, 96% of which underwent CT, 86% had an identified SDH. Hoskote et al. (2002) were referred 36 subdural haematomas, of which 9 were considered accidental and 4 iatrogenic. Twenty-three were suspected to be due to abuse, but after further investigations, 14 of these were confirmed with a diagnosis of NAHI, 1 was diagnosed with lateral sinus thrombosis, 2 were accepted as accidental, and 6 remained unexplained. In their radiographic (CT/MRI) study of the inflicted trauma group, 6 had interhemispheric bleeds along with loss of grey–white differentiation.

Subdural haematomas in the first 2 years of life are more commonly acute and due to child abuse than to birth injury or accidental injury. Following normal delivery, around 4% of infants demonstrate small asymptomatic SDHs on MRI, and this figure increases after ventouse extraction or forceps delivery (Whitby et al. 2004).

• *Intradural bleeding.* Duhaime et al. (1992) reported that the presence of an intradural (subdural) haemorrhage was highly significantly related to inflicted injury (p<0.0002). Intradural haemorrhages are, however, not specific for NAHI. They are usually microscopic and venous in origin, and equivalent to intradural petechiae. They are seen in a wide variety of conditions such as spontaneous abortions, intrauterine death, perinatal death, neonatal deaths and deaths in infancy. Geddes et al. (2003) suggest that these intradural haemorrhages

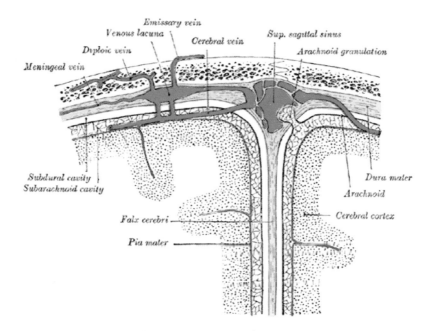

Fig. 1.25. Graphical illustration of venous channels in and around the dura mater (bridging veins are seen crossing the subarachnoid and subdural space). (Reproduced by permission from Warwick and Williams 1973.)

are secondary to hypoxia in the presence of a raised central venous pressure and question the hypothesis that infant SDHs are a result of the traumatic tearing of bridging veins in all cases, although they accept that they are compatible with trauma but not diagnostic of it. We contend that hypoxia is the commonest agonal event explaining these intradural petechiae. The conversion of a microscopic intradural haemorrhage into a macroscopic SDH occurred in only one of 36 cases, which was a known case of septicaemia (Smith et al. 2003). In our experience of hundreds of cases of perinatal asphyxia, a macroscopic SDH is an exceptional rarity in the absence of birth trauma. Similarly they are not seen with cot deaths.

An acute SDH in adults with accidental head injury invariably is associated with severe contusional brain injury. Intradural haematomas resulting from head injury in adults affect the temporal pole in 80% of cases and the frontal pole in the remainder. They are confined to subdural or intracerebal haematoma/contusion sites (Jennett and Teasdale 1981).

• *Pathophysiology of SDH.* The venous drainage of the brain (Fig. 1.25) is collected by surface veins, which then directly enter one of the venous sinuses. From the base, venous blood is collected into the great vein of Galen and then into the lateral sinuses. The cortical veins have to cross the subarachnoid and subdural spaces as bridging veins in order to enter the superior and inferior saggital sinuses (Fig. 1.26). There are also emissary veins that cross these spaces and then penetrate the bone to enter the scalp circulation. It is at this point of crossing between brain and sinus or skull that they are most liable to tearing and injury.

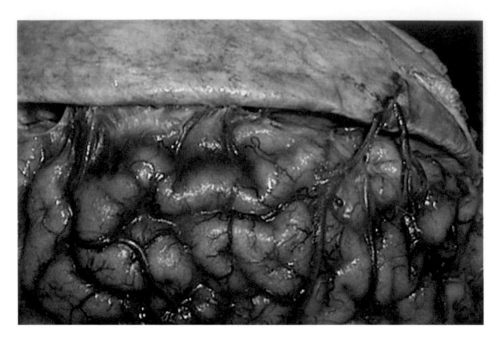

Fig. 1.26. Necropsy specimen showing bridging veins from the cortical surface, traversing the subdural space and penetrating the dura. (Reproduced courtesy of WebPath Internet Pathology Laboratory for Medical Education © Edward C Klatt, University of Utah, Salt Lake City.)

Elongation of the head in the anteroposterior diameter as in birth trauma stretches and ruptures the galenic veins, while rotation of the brain within the skull tears the bridging cortical surface and interhemispheric veins. The shearing force described above causes tearing of the 18–20 posteriorally directed bridging veins running from the surface of the brain to the saggital sinus, which in turn causes a surface and interhemispheric subdural and subarachnoid bleeding without any fracture being present (Fig. 1.27).

Posterior fossa subdural haematomas seen on CT were reported in 7 of 26 term or near-term non-asphyxiated infants with SDH, born vaginally (13/26 required forceps assistance). The haematomas were all less than 3 mm in transverse dimension. Ten of the 26 had other evidence of traumatic delivery (including cephalohaematoma, subgaleal haemorrhage, Erb's palsy, diaphragmatic paralysis, clavicular fracture, facial palsy, and depressed skull fracture) (Chamnanvanakij et al. 2002).

A further study of 15 posterior fossa subdural haematomas in neonates (Perrin et al. 1997) found that 7 followed instrument-assisted delivery (forceps and/or vacuum extraction). Symptoms developed within 24 hours in most, and included irritability, seizures, apnoea and bradycardia. Six were anaemic, and five had low platelets. Causes other than trauma (coagulation disturbances and posterior fossa medulloblastoma) were aetiologic in 4 cases.

Posterior fossa haematomas may follow mild or severe accidental traumatic brain injury, where there is often a fracture of the occipital bone and often scalp marks, stiff

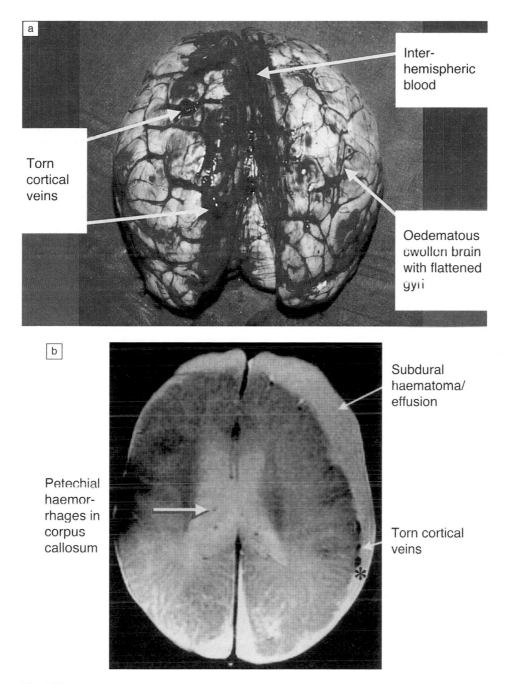

Fig. 1.27. (a) Oedematous swollen brain with subdural and interhemispheric blood resulting from torn cortical (bridging) veins.

(b) T$_2$ axial MRI showing torn cortical veins with large SDHs and petechial haemorrhages in the corpus callosum.

neck, etc. Deterioration may be rapid, with respiratory depression without motor or pupil changes, and later signs of a posterior fossa lesion. Such haematomas are associated on occasions with contrecoup lesions in the frontal and temporal lobes.

Following non-accidental injury the posterior fossa haematoma could theoretically result from (i) subtemporal, supratentorial haemorrhage tracking through the tentorial hiatus into the posterior fossa, where it will be seen on imaging below the tent; (ii) numerous infra-tentorial bridging veins may be ruptured following occipital impact, but given the confined nature of the posterior fossa structures, are probably not sheared in the same way as supra-tentorial rotational injury; (iii) a less likely postulate would be increased venous pressure from elevated thoracic pressure or impaired venous return.

• *Pressure effects on the overlying calvarium.* Apart from the secondary effects of the subdural haematoma on the underlying brain parenchyma, as outlined above, a further potential secondary effect is for the elevated surface pressure to be exerted on the overlying cranial bones with resultant erosion.

Exceptionally this erosion may penetrate the inner table with leakage of marrow cells, such as red cell precursors, into the extradural space. Subsequent tapping of the subdural haematoma, via the fontanelle, may create a tract that allows primitive marrow cells to leak into the subdural fluid (Minns et al. 2004). This may prolong the SDH, necessitating shunting, and may also cause confusion diagnostically, as to whether there is a possible malignancy. Peripheral haematological malignancies will need to be excluded.

If the brain under pressure is in contact with the inner table it may cause a pattern of cranial lacunae with a 'ping pong skull', i.e. craniotabes, if severe. This may appear on X-ray as a copper beaten skull. The brain itself pulsates more than a surface haematoma or effusion, and the erosion is more likely to be due to direct pressure than to pulsatile erosion.

• *Differentiation of acute, subacute and chronic subdural haematomas.* Subdural haematomas are usually classified as acute (subdural haemorrhage), subacute (subdural haematoma) and chronic (subdural effusion), although there is no universally agreed definition as to the exact timing that differentiates one from the other. Choux et al. (1986) define them as: acute, occurring within 3 days of the injury; subacute, from 3 days to 3 weeks; and chronic, more than 3 weeks post-injury. The reason for dividing the condition in this way is that an acute subdural haematoma is usually associated with shock and a severe contusional brain injury progressing to severe necrotic cerebral oedema. The brain is covered with a layer of 'redcurrant jelly' (undiluted blood clot with a high haematocrit), which may not itself be of great space-occupying volume yet is fatal due to the associated brain injury in 50% of cases. Over the next 10 days haemodilution occurs and haematocrit falls to less than 10%, and denaturation of haemoglobin changes the colour from bright red to brown (subacute or subdural haematoma). The increase in volume now causes symptoms of space occupation to dominate. In contrast, a chronic subdural haematoma is liquid (even lower haematocrit; more water than blood, i.e. effusion) and insidious in onset with few signs of pressure as an enlarging head accom-modates the increased intracranial volume. It is usually 3–4 weeks before a diagnosis is made when the preceding trauma is known. Despite a large space-occupying volume there is an excellent prognosis, 80% making a complete recovery, with 17% morbidity and a low mortality of 3% in 131 cases described by Kotwica and Brzezinski (1991).

• *Causes of subdural haematomas.* If an acute subdural haematoma occurs in the family and social setting described, with the full medical clinical syndrome and an infant in the first 6 months of life, the diagnosis may not be difficult. On the other hand the infant who presents with an enlarging head, vomiting or failing to thrive, and who is found to have an isolated chronic subdural effusion or haematoma, poses much more diagnostic difficulty. One does not know when it occurred, or how. In general, a subdural haematoma in infancy is far more likely to be an inflicted traumatic lesion – of 16 cases of acute subdural haematoma reported by Duhaime et al. (1992) in children under 2 years, 13 were due to non-accidental injury and 3 to high speed road traffic impact injuries. *Depressed skull fractures* that penetrate vessels, a primary *penetrating injury hitting a sinus*, or *contusion causing oozing of surface veins* are rare. A depressed fracture is a surprisingly rare cause of subdural haematoma (Choux et al. 1986).

Arteriovenous malformations* can bleed into the subdural space, and theoretically *haemorrhagic diatheses* can cause spontaneous subdural bleeding, but this is very rare without trauma. Vitamin C deficiency, the use of aspirin, hypoprothrombinaemia from vitamin K deficiency common in adult alcoholics or during warfarin therapy, congenital platelet abnormalities, genetic coagulation disorders and virus induced thrombocytopenia are all possible causes but occur only as occasional sporadic 'interesting cases' in children. We have seen spontaneous subdural haematomas arise in defibrinated infants with cortical thrombophlebitis. There was no subdural haematoma in the study of non traumatic spontaneous intracranial haemorrhages in children reported by Livingstone and Brown (1986). Many causes of an isolated subdural haematoma without the other features of SBS need to be considered and relevant investigations performed to exclude them. These are listed in Table 1.10.

• *Imaging and subdural haematomas.* Seventy-five per cent of subdural haematomas are bilateral, 90% are supratentorial and 10% infratentorial (Ingraham and Matson 1954, Harwood Nash and Fitz 1976). In non-accidental injury they are most likely to be posterior, i.e. parieto-occipital or interhemispheric (Zimmerman et al. 1979). Eighty per cent of interhemispheric subdural haematomas also have a retinopathy. An extradural haematoma can be recognized as a biconvex disc on CT; the crescentic subdural haematoma is more easily missed.

In the early acute stage when the blood clot is solid over the hemispheres it may not appear impressive, and may be just a thin crescentic density on CT. As it breaks down by fibrinolysis and water is drawn into the haematoma to form an effusion there is marked expansion, so that by 7 days one is disturbed by the apparently enormous expansion of a lesion that may not have impressed initially. This may be accompanied not by slit ventricles from compression but by marked ventriculomegaly. The dynamic nature of the pathology means that sequential brain imaging is essential in order to capture the evolution of the different lesions (Fig. 1.30).

TABLE 1.10
Conditions associated with or predisposing to subdural haemorrhage
or effusion

Birth trauma
Accidental trauma
Non-accidental head injury
Defibrination with infection, necrotizing encephalitis, e.g. herpes simplex
Aspergillosis
Kawasaki disease
Osteogenesis imperfecta
Idiopathic
Glutaric aciduria type 1 (Woelfe et al. 1996) (Fig. 1.28)
Menkes' disease
Meningitis (pneumoccoccal or group B streptococcus)
Septicaemia (including meningococcal)
Haemophilia/factor 5 deficiency/anticoagulant treatment
Vitamin K deficiency in newborn infants (50% have intracranial bleeding)
    (von Kries and Gobel 1992)
Idiopathic thrombocytopenia purpura (Fig. 1.29)
Malignancy, including leukaemia and brain tumours
Arteriovenous malformation or aneurysm
Post-cardiopulmonary bypass
Post-ventriculoperitoneal shunting
Alagille syndrome (arteriohepatic dysplasia)
Disseminated intravascular coagulation
Slit ventricle syndrome
Hyperosmolar dehydration from mannitol
Pericerebral enlargement
Renal dialysis
Severe dehydration ± sino-venous thrombosis
Congenital subarachnoid cyst

Biousse et al. (2002) showed the value of diffusion-weighted MRI (DWMRI) in detecting cerebral ischaemia in 26 infants with subdural haematoma aged 6 weeks to 24 months. All 18 patients with "confirmed SBS" had an abnormal DWMRI that suggested diffuse or posterior cerebral ischaemia in addition to the subdural haematoma. In 13 patients the scan showed lesions that were larger than on conventional MRI.

Barlow et al. (1999) described the MRI findings in acute NAHI in 14 children with and without clinical and radiological evidence of impact (Table 1.11). Datta et al. (2005) report the imaging features from both MRI and CT in a larger group of 49 children with confirmed NAHI, and found a convexity subdural collection in 44, interhemispheric fissure bleeds in 38, posterior cranial fossa bleeds in 14, and middle cranial fossa bleeds in 9. SDHs were found in multiple sites in 32 of the 49 cases. They additionally found oedema (focal in 9 and generalized in 3), parenchymal changes in 12, and subarachnoid haemorhage in 7. Both of these studies have shown relatively little diffuse axonal injury.

Shearing axonal injuries and skull fractures are more common in accidental injuries. Torn bridging veins are sometimes visible on the original MRI.

An acute SDH is denser than brain, but after 2 weeks it becomes isodense and so is

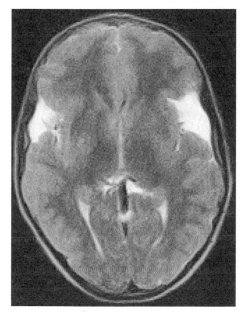

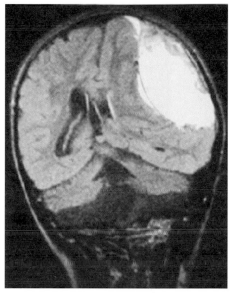

Fig. 1.28. T₂ axial MRI in a case of glutaric aciduria type 1 with bilateral sylvian subdural effusions.

Fig. 1.29. Coronal MRI of persistent large volume acute on chronic subdural haemorrhage resulting from thrombocytopenia.

easily missed on CT or ultrasound (Faerber 1986). After 3 weeks the colour turns from red to brown due to formation of methaemoglobin, and the fluid is very xanthochromic on centrifugation. Ageing of haematomas depends upon the protein content gradually increasing for the first 21 days and then gradually decreasing. The acute subdural haematoma, if a thin layer, will liquify from fibrinolysis and be absorbed unless death occurs from the associated cerebral injury. There are very high concentrations of fibrin degradation products, plasminogen activators and plasminogens in the fluid (Ito et al. 1978).

• *Chronic subdural haematoma.* A chronic subdural haematoma is in most cases due to failure to resolve an acute haematoma. It has two components: (1) a liquid low haematocrit 'haematoma', and (2) evidence of continued fresh bleeding, and a membrane. The membrane, which is vascular and easily bleeds, encapsulates the haematoma and binds it to the dura where it undergoes degradation and invasion by fibroblasts. Calcification may be detected by 3 months. Incorporation of the haematoma into the dura as a membrane is the basis of the healing process. A chronic subdural haematoma is not a true haematoma but a subdural effusion in that it is mainly water not blood, the haematocrit rarely exceeding 10%. Heavy water and labelled albumin can move freely in and out of the haematoma and blood stream (Rabe 1967). There is also free movement between CSF in the subarachnoid spaces, and across the arachnoid into the subdural effusion (Zouros et al. 2004), i.e. there is no compartmentalization.

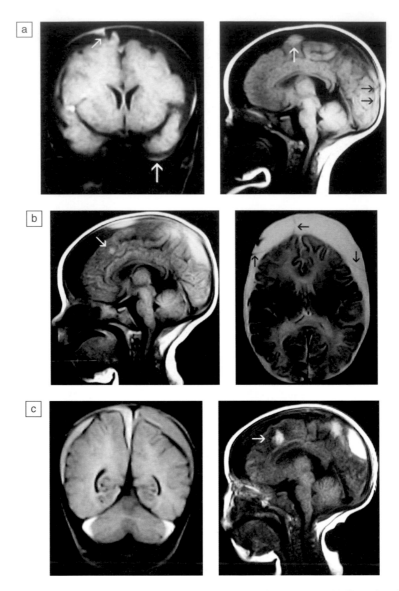

Fig. 1.30. Sequential MR cranial images of a 6-week-old infant who presented with fits and a spiral fracture of the tibia.

(a) At presentation, a coronal FLAIR scan (left) shows widening of the subdural spaces with high intensity seen in the subtemporal region bilaterally (large arrow). In the right parafalcine region there is a linear high intensity, suggestive of a clot around a bridging vein (small arrow). The T_1 sagittal view (right) shows layering of the high intensity posteriorly (black arrows). A suggestive focal clot formation is seen over the frontoparietal convexity.

(b) On day 6 after presentation a T_1 sagittal view (left) shows persistence of high signal over the convexity and posterior layering. There is an ill-defined high intensity at the grey–white matter junction representing a white matter tear (arrow). On the T_2 transverse view (right), stranding is now visible bilaterally in the subdural space anteriorly. ↗

70

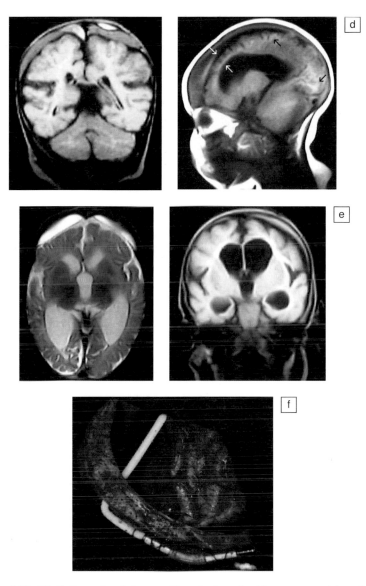

(c) Coronal FLAIR (left) on day 6 shows widened subarachnoid spaces containing clear CSF, indicating early atrophy. T_1 sagittal view (right) at 2 weeks after presentation shows the white matter tear is more prominent (arrow).

(d) At 2 weeks the coronal FLAIR (left) shows foci of high intensity within the subdural collections. T_1 sagittal view (right) 2 months after presentation shows marked atrophy particularly in the frontoparietal white matter in the region of the previous tear (white arrows). High intensity in the cortex of the occipital lobe may represent changes following haemorrhagic cortical contusion (black arrows).

(e) 2 months after presentation a T_2 transverse view (left) shows widespread atrophy with dilated ventricles and prominent sulci. Coronal FLAIR (right) shows low intensity CSF signal in the subarachnoid space, contrasting with the high intensity subdural collections.

(f) Pathology specimen showing subdural space despite subduro-peritoneal shunting.

TABLE 1.11
Frequency of observations on MR brain scan in acute NAHI*

	All cases	Without clinical/radiological evidence of impact
Subdural haemorrhage	14/14	7/7
Subtemporal	10/14	5/7
Interhemispheric	7/14	4/7
Subdurals with varying signal intensity	6/14	2/7
Tearing the surface veins	4/14	2/7
Compartmentalized	3/14	1/7
Suboccipital	2/14	1/7
Contusion	4/14	1/7
Haemorrhagic contusion	3/14	1/7
Cerebral laceration	3/14	1/7
Petechial haemorrhages at the grey–white matter junction	4/14	2/7
Petechial haemorrhages in the corpus callosum	1/14	—
Local asphyxial insult	2/14	1/7
Cerebral oedema	1/14	1/7
Intraventricular haemorrhage	3/14	—
Subarachnoid haemorrhage	3/14	—
Gliotic changes in parenchyma	1/14	1/7

*Data from Barlow et al. (1999).

The way in which an acute haemorrhage becomes chronic may depend upon the volume of blood in the haemorhage. There may be a critical mass that defeats the repair process. The size of the subarachnoid space would then be critical. The older theory was that there was an increase in osmolality due to breakdown of blood products drawing water into the haematoma. This is not now generally accepted, as the osmolality of haematoma fluid is usually isotonic with blood and CSF (Weir 1980). Osmotic equilibration as described above, however, may be more or less instantaneous. The liberation of idiogenic osmols by protein degradation, as well as the high protein content and osmotic forces, may still apply in converting the initial thin haemorrhage into a much larger effusion.

There are always fresh uncrenated red blood cells in the fluid of even very chronic haematomas with persistent xanthochromia, suggesting that there is continued fresh bleeding. There may be repeated bleeding from distraction of the brain from the inner table of the skull and so continued traction of the bridging veins, in addition to bleeding from the vascular membrane. There is a true pachymeningitis with a chronic inflammatory response in the meninges initiated by the continued breakdown of erythrocytes. This inflammatory process is thought to cause the vascular proliferation with formation of sinusoids, fibrin deposition and fibrosis, and so the formation of a membrane. Continued bleeding will maintain the inflammatory process and so gradually thicken the membrane. If this is repeated it shows on MRI as an 'onion skin' membrane like the annual rings of a tree from each bleed. The high fibrinolytic activity in the fluid may in turn prevent the vessels sealing properly with a good clot. The proponents of this theory feel that dexamethasone would suppress lymphokines and prostaglandins and so the inflammatory response and should form part

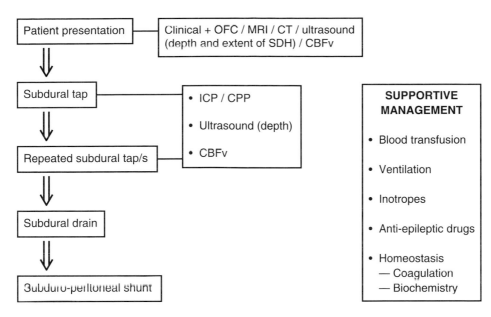

Fig. 1.31. Flow diagram showing the specific management of subdural haemorrhage (left), and additional supportive management (right).

OFC = occipitofrontal circumference; CBFv = cerebral blood flow velocity; ICP = intracranial pressure; CPP = cerebral perfusion pressure.

of routine treatment. The presence of a membrane confirms a 'chronic' subdural collection (usually traumatic). Absence of a membrane, however, does not exclude a chronic SDH.

• *Treatment of subdural haematoma.* Treatment is considered in detail in Chapter 7. The algorithm in Fig. 1.31 illustrates the main principles.

• *Subarachnoid haemorrhage.* Nineteen per cent of infants with NAHI have a significant subarachnoid bleed as well as SDH. This causes further expansion of the subarachnoid space due to blockage of the arachnoid granulations – really an external hydrocephalus. This can often be seen on MRI as a 'double shadow' of differing density, with the outer subdural effusion and the inner external hydrocephalus. Fluid in the subarachnoid space is mobile and communicates with the spinal subarachnoid space. Occasionally the obstruction to CSF absorption (by parasaggital subdural collection of blood compressing the subarachnoid space and arachnoid granulations at the vertex) also causes ventricular dilatation, and a pressure hydrocephalus requiring shunting. The blood in the CSF may also cause ischaemia to the brain itself by inducing arterial vasospasm, and the ventricular dilatation may also be due to the rapid destruction of white matter with passive ventricular enlargement.

Parenchymal shearing injuries
• *Midbrain shearing injury.* Consciousness depends upon intact reticular nuclei at the

midbrain/pontine junction. Coma is more likely to result from pathology of the tegmentum of the midbrain than from a focal cortical lesion. The tentorium and cerebellum anchor the brainstem and so the midbrain acts as pivot upon which the cerebral hemispheres can rotate. The sudden acceleration of the head must again cause rotation in order to be concussional, i.e. a primary stem injury (Ommaya and Gennarelli 1974). Concussion will then come on immediately after the accident without any lucid interval. A lucid interval occurs while a clot or cerebral oedema develops. Concussion can be short-lived or merge into a vegetative state with prolonged coma (Symonds 1962). The midbrain may be damaged from the primary injury or as part of a tentorial herniation from raised ICP. A tentorial pressure cone will also cause midbrain and brainstem haemorrhage, Duret type secondary haemorrhages, which develop some time after the primary injury. Pupil dilatation or loss of visual awareness, extensor–decorticate postures, akinetic mutism, and autonomic dysfunction of blood pressure, pulse and respiration occur in both primary and secondary midbrain injury.

The reticular formation is very energy dependent, and consciousness is also rapidly lost with lowered oxygen tensions, i.e. hypoxia or hypoglycaemia.

• *White matter shearing injuries.* The infant head is larger than the adult's in proportion to the body surface area, and stability of the head on the cervical spine is dependent on the ligaments and muscles rather than bony structure. The infant's brain has a higher water content, 88% vs 77% in adults, which makes the brain softer and more prone to acceleration–deceleration injury and cerebral oedema. The water content is inversely related to the myelinization process. The increase in weight of the brain is mainly in white matter myelin. The cells in the grey matter are all present at birth but more densely packed, and become spread out only as the area of the cerebral cortex increases. There is thus a change in the density of cells in grey matter and in the amount of lipid in white matter during development, so the infant brain is different from the adult's. Grey matter is firm and cellular, while poorly myelinated white matter is more gelatinous and of slightly different density and inertia, and so they swirl at different velocities.

The brain, because of this water content, is incompressible but very easily deformable (by a finger at operation), in a non-deformable skull. It has jelly-like characteristics, i.e. when wobbled on a plate the top wobbles more than the base, or has been likened to pushing a pack of playing cards where the top and bottom shift at different rates. This allows shearing forces to be set up within the white matter when the brain rotates within the skull as well as at interfaces with different inertial properties.

Holbourn (1943), using 2-dimensional gelatine moulds, was first in the field whose work led to the understanding that shear injury is caused by rotational forces. The injury to tissue is greatest in areas where the density difference is greatest. For this reason, approximately two thirds of traumatic 'axonal injury' lesions occur at the grey–white matter junction.

Strich (1961) drew attention to primary shearing of white matter. In child abuse, tears in the white matter of the orbital, first and second frontal convolutions and temporal lobe are seen (Calder et al. 1984).

Long axons, as in the commissural fibres (running transversely from right to left hemisphere) and long association tracts (running longitudinally from occipital to frontal

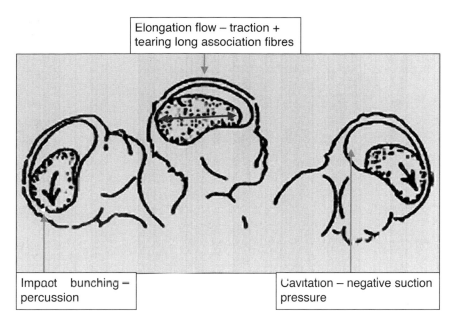

Elongation flow – traction +
tearing long association fibres

Impaot bunching –
percussion

Uavitation – negative suction
pressure

Fig. 1.32. The deforming brain 'bunches' at percussion and elongates at cavitation.

lobes) can be avulsed by traction as the deforming brain tries to flow (i.e. bunches at percussion and elongates at cavitation – Fig. 1.32), as well as by shearing. This results in a traumatic diffuse axonal injury. Axonal damage may also occur following hypoxia–ischaemia, when it is seen at the margins of the ischaemic zones. Differentiating traumatic from hypoxic origin is not possible except inasmuch as the traumatic axonal injury is seen in the cerebral peduncle and internal capsule.

Projection fibres from the cortex running vertically may be sheared at the grey–white interface and show as petechiae on imaging (Barlow et al. 2000,). There may be slit-like cavities in white matter called gliding contusions, and the ependyma may be torn so that necrotic brain extrudes into the ventricles (Rorke 1990). There need not be any skull fracture.

Particularly characteristic shearing injuries of the white matter are those in the corpus callosum (Fig. 1.33), and cerebellar peduncle (Fig. 1.34). Midbrain injury may be unilateral or bilateral but is always larger on one side (Fig. 1.35), and the lesions are always multi locular and not just confined to the midbrain (Adams et al. 1977). By comparison, secondary pontine haemorrhages (Duret haemorrhages) are delayed, secondary brainstem haemorrhages that are typically located in the ventral and paramedian aspects of the upper brainstem (mesencephalon and pons) (Fig. 1.36). Typically, in the cerebral hemispheres, the process is diffuse and bilateral, involving the lobar white matter at the grey–white matter interface. The most commonly involved area is the frontotemporal white matter, followed by the posterior body and splenium of the corpus callosum. Internal capsule lesions are associated more frequently with haemorrhage, which is due to the proximity of the lenticulostriate vessels.

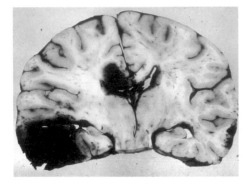

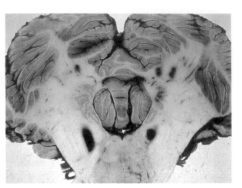

Fig. 1.33. Haemorrhage seen in the temporal lobe and corpus callosum resulting from shear forces.

Fig. 1.34. Bilateral cerebellar peduncle haemorrhages resulting from shear forces.

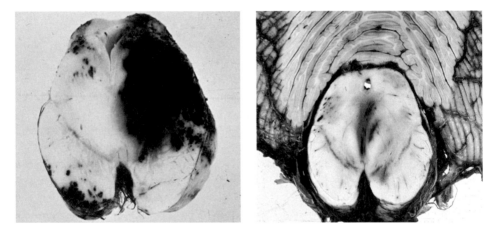

Fig. 1.35. Extensive primary midbrain haemorrhages.

The following stages of axonal injury have been described (according to the anatomic location of the lesions) by Adams et al. (1989):

Stage I involves the parasagittal regions of the frontal lobes, periventricular temporal lobes, and, less likely, the parietal and occipital lobes, internal and external capsules, and cerebellum.

Stage II involves the corpus callosum, in addition to the white matter areas in stage I. This is observed in approximately 20% of patients. Most commonly, the posterior body and splenium are involved; however, the process is believed to advance anteriorly with increasing severity. Both sides of the corpus callosum may be involved; however, involvement more frequently is unilateral and may be haemorrhagic. The involvement of the corpus callosum carries a poorer prognosis.

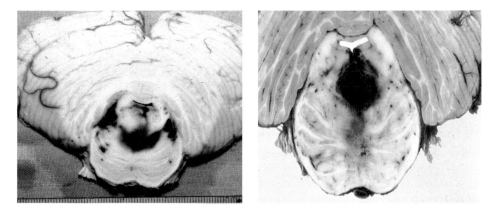

Fig. 1.36. Pontine haemorrhages secondary to intracranial pressure cones.

Stage III involves the areas associated with stage II, with the addition of the brainstem, and with a predilection for the superior cerebellar peduncle.

Axons can withstand enormous compressive forces but are easily sheared by traction. It is suggested that the poorly myelinated axons of the young child may stretch more than fully myelinated adult fibres (Crompton 1985). The shearing forces on the axons result in tearing with local oedema and axoplasmic leakage that is most severe during the first 2 weeks after injury. Swelling ensues, and the axon then splits in two. A retraction ball forms, which is the pathologic hallmark of shearing injury. After several weeks the axon then undergoes wallerian degeneration. Dendritic restructuring may occur, with some regeneration possible in mild-to-moderate injury. The sheared axons ooze axoplasm which can be stained by silver stains. There then appears a whole series of black blobs along the white matter. These retraction balls last for 2 weeks and then microglia migrate around the tear to form microglial stars (Vowles et al. 1987). This is now more clearly demonstrated immunohistochemically by amyloid precursor protein (APP). Blood vessels may also stretch, and if they do not rupture can act like a wire cheese-cutter and cause local cutting of white matter tracts so that blobs then appear along the line of blood vessels.

DAI classically was believed to represent a primary injury (occurring at the instant of the trauma). Currently, however, it is apparent that the axoplasmic membrane alteration, transport impairment and retraction ball formation may represent secondary (or delayed) components to the disease process. It may therefore not be seen in infants dying within 24 hours of the insult. At autopsy pure cases are rare, as necrotic oedema, secondary hypoxic–ischaemic damage and secondary infarction from cones overshadow these more subtle primary injuries. Shearing injuries of white matter occur independently of contusion, oedema, hypoxia, ischaemia or evidence of raised ICP (Adams et al. 1977). It is now thought that hypoxic–ischaemic damage rather than axonal shearing is the dominant pathology in some cases. In a study by Geddes et al. (2001a) of the brains of 37 infants less than 9 months dying from NAHI, 75% of whom presented with apnoea and so had an unequivocal additional hypoxic insult, only two cases had the typical axonal traumatic shearing as opposed to vascular axonal damage (13 cases). They were most likely due to the hyperacute cervico-medullary syndrome due to whiplash (see above), as they died rapidly, rather than the mainly supratentorial repetitive rotational shearing syndrome of NAHI.

In surviving patients, axonal damage may account for a large percentage of residual morbidity with a vegetative state including gross cerebral atrophy with shrinkage of white matter and ex vacuo ventricular dilatation. The frightful long-term prognosis (Barlow et al. 2004) does appear to correlate with damage to white matter with shrinkage and atrophy. This is due to a combination of trauma and hypoxic–ischaemic damage. White matter atrophy and secondary ventriculomegaly are now known to be more rapid in onset, as shown by sequential MRI, and can appear in less than 10 days from the insult. DAI has been demonstrated on ultrasound imaging of suspected shaken infants as tears in the parenchyma between grey and white matter (Jaspan et al. 1992). It is now easier to see these shearing injuries on MRI (Barlow et al. 1999). The initial scan may show haemorrhage, which on follow-up imaging is found to be due to crescentic tears.

Cerebral oedema

In the Canadian SBS study (King et al. 2003), 42% were identified as having cerebral oedema on imaging, and in post-mortem studies this was doubled (80%). In impact and shaking injuries cerebral oedema is often very severe. In the Geddes et al. (2001a) study of 37 infants less than 9 months and 16 children over 9 months, cerebral oedema was confirmed as a major cause of death in 82%.

Cerebral oedema is thought to take about 6 hours to appear after the injury in infants (Crompton 1985), compared to 4-6 days post-injury in older children and adolescents. It has many different mechanisms of production, including vasogenic, osmotic, hydrostatic, cytotoxic and necrotic (Brown 1991). The cause of the oedema in the shaken infant is probably multifactorial (Fig. 1.37) with vascular damage (as in the eye) causing vasogenic oedema, white matter damage, disrupted venous drainage, damage to the blood–brain barrier, high central venous pressure from chest compression, brain necrosis from shock and impaired perfusion and secondary hydrocephalus causing hydrostatic oedema from obstruction of the arachnoid granulations by blood.

We shall consider cerebral oedema in some detail as it is present in most cases of acute traumatic encephalopathy and often contributes to death. Cerebral oedema is defined as an increase in volume in the whole (generalized) or part (focal oedema) of the brain due to an increase in the water content (Pappius and Feindel 1976). The increase in water may be in one or several compartments:

(1) *intracellular* (cytotoxic), affecting grey matter (particularly astrocytes), and often associated with energy failure or hypo-osmolar states and fluid shifts into cells (Bruce 1983)

(2) *extracellular/extravascular* (vasogenic), affecting the extracellular fluid compartment of the brain, particularly white matter, and resulting from increased permeability due to direct vascular endothelial damage and albumin leakage, as in hypoxic–ischaemic states

(3) *intramyelinic* (myelinoclastic), as a direct effect of toxicity, e.g. in galactosaemia, hexachlorophane toxicity and due to some drugs and metabolic disorders.

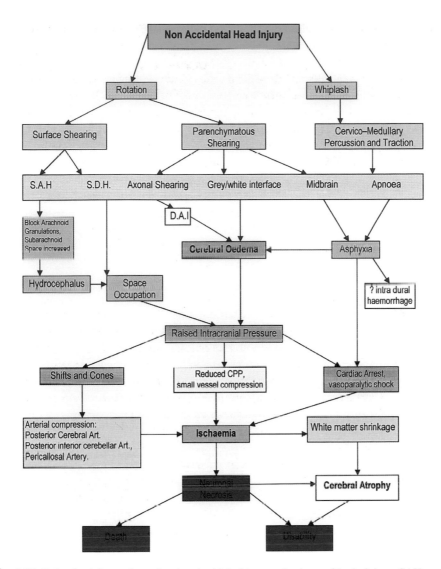

Fig. 1.37. Pathophysiology of rotational and whiplashing mechanisms of brain injury. SAH = sub-arachnoid haemorrhage; SDH = subdural haemorrhage; DAI = diffuse axonal injury; CPP = cerebral perfusion pressure.

- *Intracellular oedema.* Accumulation of water within the cells of the brain usually denotes astrocytic rather than neuronal oedema. The oligodendroglia may also swell. Hypoxia leads to swelling of the mitochondria and accumulation of glycogen within the cell, which is seen as an early sign on electron microscopy. Glucose is broken down to produce energy in the form of adenosine triphosphate (ATP), which is necessary to energize the membrane pumps in order to pump sodium out of the cell. The end result of complete aerobic glycolysis is

79

carbon dioxide and water. The cell has to excrete this water so as not to develop severe hydrops. Interference with energy supply will therefore cause water retention in two main ways, i.e. failure to exclude sodium and failure to excrete water. If the cell is damaged, intracellular proteolysis releases idiogenic osmols, which will then also encourage water to be drawn into the cells by osmosis.

• *Extracellular oedema*. This can be further subdivided into (a) vasogenic oedema, (b) hydrostatic oedema, (c) hydrocephalic oedema, (d) osmotic oedema, and (e) necrotic oedema.

(a) Vasogenic oedema.

The endothelial cells in the brain do not have the gaps between adjacent cells seen in other organs, i.e. they have tight junctions. The footplate of the astrocyte is applied to the neuronal side, helping form the blood–brain barrier. The endothelial cell is also very metabolically active, with as many mitochondria as muscle cells. Damage to the endothelial cells or their junctions can result in breakdown of the blood brain–barrier, which then allows substances normally present in the blood stream such as glycine, glutamate and noradrenaline to penetrate into the brain. Capillary damage can result from many causes such as asphyxia and head injury (especially in non-accidental shaking injuries when vascular damage is severe).

Albumin leaks out of the intravascular space into the extracellular space, and this may also selectively bind water molecules in addition to the osmotic effect. If the albumin is broken down by proteases into peptides this can increase the osmotic effect more than a hundredfold. In the presence of a severe vasogenic leak, the proteins in the CSF should resemble a plasma protein profile rather than the very selective protein pattern from choroid plexus CSF. Occasionally there is continued vascular leak of protein and fluid, which flows through the brain and into the CSF without any impedance so that there is 'bulk extracellular flow'.

(b) Hydrostatic oedema.

If the blood pressure is steadily increased in a normal child, there is increasing cerebral vasoconstriction, i.e. protective vasoconstriction or autoregulation. If the blood pressure is progressively lowered, then vasodilatation occurs in order to decrease cerebral vascular resistance and maintain perfusion. There is therefore a range of blood pressure over which cerebral blood flow is maintained – the autoregulation range. There comes a point of maximum protective vasoconstriction after which autoregulation is overcome and a vastly increased perfusion pressure is transmitted to the microcirculation (Van Vught et al. 1976).

Hydrostatic oedema means that the fluid content of the brain is increased as a result of fluid being forced under pressure from one compartment to another. A very high perfusion pressure blows sodium and water through the endothelial junctions like a filter causing hydrostatic oedema.

Hypoxic–ischaemic damage paralyses this local protective autoregulation, allowing a normal systemic blood pressure to be transmitted to the microcirculation and this can also be seen by the effect on ICP when drugs such as nitroprusside or halothane are given: ICP can become pressure passive, i.e. it follows blood pressure.

If the normal protective autoregulation is lost (due to paralysis from hypoxia–ischaemia, prolonged seizures, trauma, severe hypercarbia or the use of drugs such as nitroprusside or papaverine) then even a normal blood pressure will be transmitted in full to the microcirculation and can result in oedema (Johansson 1974).

(c) Hydrocephalic oedema.

CSF is partly formed from the choroid plexus, but 40% is really brain lymph that is brain ECF and enters the ventricle via pores in the ependymal lining. Obstruction to the ventricular outflow will cause a rise in intraventricular pressure and reverse this transependymal flow of CSF back through the pores in the ependyma. This causes an increase in extracellular fluid easily visible on MRI or CT as hypodensities around the lateral ventricles.

(d) Osmotic oedema.

There are several compartments within the brain across which an osmotic gradient can develop, encouraging fluid shifts from one to the other. It can take several hours for osmotic gradients to equilibrate as between blood and CSF: (i) across the endothelium between blood and extracellular fluid; (ii) across the arachnoid between blood and CSF; (iii) across the ependyma between brain CSF and extracellular fluid (ECF); (iv) across the cell membrane between ECF and intracellular fluid.

A sudden increase in plasma water can occur in true inappropriate ADH secretion, which often complicates meningitis, asphyxia, encephalitis, head injury, status epilepticus or acute encephalopathies. The ADH secretion is appropriate for brain but inappropriate for the kidney, especially if there is a further increase in plasma water from intravenous infusions that the kidney cannot then excrete. This failure to excrete water by the kidneys results in 'strong' hyperosmolar urine and diluted hypo-osmolar plasma. There is oedema (of eyelids, dorsum of hands, pretibia and ankles), dilutional hyponatraemia, weight gain from water intoxication, and severe brain swelling from cerebral oedema. A fall in serum sodium below 120 mmol/l results in fits, whether the sodium is low due to salt loss or dilution. An osmolality below 255 milliosmoles is nearly always associated with severe cerebral oedema. Seizures, coma and decerebration may therefore be due to the electrolyte upset.

Water intoxication will also result if the osmolality of the plasma is suddenly reduced, as in the over-use of electrolyte-free intravenous fluids (dextrose is rapidly mopped up by the liver into glycogen, leaving osmotically free water). The water intoxication resulting from careless fluid balance regimens is often wrongly attributed to inappropriate ADH secretion. Infusion of normal saline and glucose does not change ICP, and infusion of 5% glucose raises ICP (Fishman 1953, Bakay et al. 1954). Excessive haste in reducing plasma concentration of osmotically active substances such as sodium, glucose or urea causes a dysequilibrium syndrome. This is because the lag in equilibration leaves the brain relatively hyperosmolar and causes severe brain oedema by drawing water into it. Excess administration of hypo-osmolar fluids after prior treatment with hyperosmolar agents such as mannitol, the use of dialysis to reduce high blood urea, and the sudden reduction of hyperglycaemia in diabetes can all result in fatal cerebral oedema (Duck and Wyatt 1988).

(e) Necrotic oedema.

Apoptosis is cell suicide, and cells die but are removed without exciting an inflammatory reaction. In cell necrosis (cell murder) there is a marked inflammatory response that excites the classical signs of Celsus: rubor from increased local blood flow, calor (local heat,

81

tumour), local swelling, and dolor (pain). In children, when there is widespread infarction of the brain caused by serious impairment of the CPP, either secondary to raised ICP, a drop in systemic arterial pressure or vessel occlusion (Bruce et al. 1981), cells die and lysosomes burst, releasing enzymes and vasoactive peptides that are also osmotically active and cause local oedema. The endothelium is damaged, and autoregulation to the area is lost. Thromboplastin is rich in the brain, and liberation from the damaged tissue causes thrombosis in the microcirculation and veins draining the tissue, thus further impairing blood supply and increasing the swelling due to an increase in blood volume in the infarct.

The loss of autoregulation means that the ICP will follow systemic blood pressure. There may be a rise in ICP, which is totally resistant to hyperventilation and to mannitol. This situation represents a stage of brain death, and the oedema is in essence brain liquefaction. A fatal outcome is usually to be expected; survival is inevitably with severe intellectual and physical disability (Bannister 1983).

• *Diagnosis of cerebral oedema.* These various pathophysiological types of cerebral oedema are rarely discriminated on clinical grounds and several types may be seen in the same patient. The commonest clinical scenario is of deteriorating consciousness with signs of brainstem dysfunction in pulse, respiration, blood pressure and pupils. The signs and symptoms of coning are looked for as the clinical evidence of raised ICP in the Glasgow Coma Scale or nursing 'neuro obs'. It must be remembered, however, that coma after head injury may be due to a primary midbrain injury or cervico medullary injury as well as raised ICP. Monitoring ICP is the only sure way of diagnosing its presence.

Furthermore, the diagnosis of cerebral oedema can be made with varying degrees of certainity, dependent on the urgency of the situation and the ready availability of imaging and neurophysiological tests. For example, if a child develops symptoms and signs such as those of tentorial herniation, suggesting raised ICP, it is reasonable to assume that cerebral oedema is the cause and to institute treatment without any further investigation (Batzdorf 1976, Bruce 1983). Extensor hypertonus following asphyxia may be due to oedema, but is more often a dystonia due to basal ganglia involvement, so-called post-asphyxial rigidity. This is not influenced by treatment to reduce ICP, which is often normal (Minns 1991). In cases of head injury, raised ICP may be due to a mass lesion (space occupation) or cerebral compression rather than oedema. Treatment of presumed oedema without imaging could then result in a dangerous delay in removing a mass lesion.

• *Imaging and cerebral oedema.* CT scans initially demonstrate a reduction in lateral ventricular size, then the third ventricle and finally the ambiens cistern are obliterated. This last sign of the loss of the 'smiling face' means that a lumbar puncture must never be performed as there is already some tentorial herniation. CT shows hydrocephalic oedema as a hypodense 'bat wing' around the lateral horns of the ventricles. The MR scan is now the mainstay of diagnosis. MRI ,and especially diffusion weighted images, show the cerebral oedema to be more extensive than that recognized on CT scanning. It is possible to measure brain water using MR technology, but this is rarely available in the acute clinical situation.

TABLE 1.12
Primary, secondary, tertiary and quaternary injury in non-accidental head trauma

PRIMARY INJURY	SECONDARY INJURY
• Subdural haemorrhage	• Hypoxaemia
• Extradural haemorrhage	• Hyper/hypotension
• Shearing injuries	• Anaemia
• Cerebral oedema	• Tachy/bradycardia
• Cortical tears	• Hypo/hypercarbia
• Contusion	• Pyrexia
• Subarachnoid haemorrhage	• Hyponatraemia
• Intraparenchymal/petechial haemorrhage	• Hypo/hyperglycaemia
• Cervical cord	• Raised intracranial pressure
• Skull fractures	• Low cerebral perfusion pressure
	• Hypoperfusion/ischaemia
	• Vasospasm
	• Seizures
	• Infection
	• Loss of cerebrovascular autoregulation
	• Loss of metabolic autoregulation
	• Excitotoxic stress

TERTIARY INJURY	QUATERNARY INJURY
• Chronic subdural haemorrhage	• Secondary positional deformity
• Post-haemorrhagic hydrocephalus	• Scoliosis and windsweeping
• Growing skull fracture	• Contractures
• Cerebral atrophy	• Persistent vegetative state
• Microcephaly	• Family dynamics
• Chronic cytokine encephalopathy	• Wasting (diencephalic and parietal wasting)
	• Subnutrition
	• Bed sores
	• Soft tissue calcification

The head injury cascade

Up to now we have been discussing the mechanics and pathological mechanisms of the primary injury but once this has occurred it sets off a cascade of secondary, tertiary or quaternary events so the end result is a combination of all these factors (Table 1.12).

HYPOXIC–ISCHAEMIC DAMAGE

In accidental head injuries the vast majority (90%) of children who die are found to have severe hypoxic–ischaemic brain damage (Adams et al. 1977). It is responsible for neuronal death and determines the pattern of long-term impairment. In NAHI a figure of 77% is reported (Geddes et al. 2001a). Hypoxic–ischaemic damage may occur immediately at the time of the primary injury due to apnoea or medullary damage. The secondary injury is more common and consists of hypotensive shock, raised ICP, decreased CPP, and increased consumption from fits. The basis of management of head injury is to prevent this secondary damage. The infant with NAHI may present with shallow breathing, hypoventilation, apnoea, anaemia, and sometimes medullary or spinal injury affecting respiration. Shock with hypotension in the presence of raised ICP reduces CPP. Subdural haematomas and cerebral oedema get worse, and at the same time the infant has intractable seizures, consuming energy. The presence of severe hypoxic–ischaemic damage on sequential imaging or at autopsy is not surprising.

The presence of diffuse hypodensities on imaging, the 'big black brain' (reversal sign), on MRI, carries a very poor prognosis, usually indicating hypoxic–ischaemic damage rather than purely white matter shearing and traumatic axonal injury. This may be unilateral or bilateral but with relative sparing of the cerebellum. It may be due to hypoxia–ischaemia, raised ICP or excitotoxic stress, and may be an indication of the need for decompression. The rapid development of cerebral atrophy (progressive development of extracerebral and ventricular fluid spaces) within a week to 10 days (Lo et al. 2003), together with the loss of brain parenchyma secondary to ischaemia as shown on diffusion-weighted MRI, demonstrate the importance of hypoxia–ischaemia as causing the severe long-term brain damage. Fifty per cent of infants will suffer arrest of brain development as shown by a falling head circumference with microcephaly, and arrest of cognitive development with learning disability.

It is also often suspected that the child may have been suffocated to stop them crying, and one may see bruising under the chin from a thumbprint as the hand is put forcibly over the child's mouth. Care must be taken when evaluating post-mortem studies as nowadays it is unusual for resuscitation not to have taken place and the child reanimated, then kept alive for hours or days in an intensive care unit. Death from any cause is usually in the final stages a hypoxic–ischaemic event.

Impairment of cerebral circulation
Adequate perfusion of the brain is essential to its structural and functional integrity, and cerebral ischaemia is the commonest and most devastating cause of neuronal necrosis and so death or persisting disability (Fig. 1.38).

The cerebral blood flow depends upon (a) the CPP (which is not the same as aortic blood pressure), (b) inversely, cerebral vascular resistance (radius of vessel, length of vessel), (c) viscosity of the blood, (d) venous back pressure, and (e) the ICP.

The CPP will be opposed by any rise in ICP, and there comes a point when the ICP is of such a magnitude that it can totally prevent cerebral perfusion. Cerebral blood flow (CBF) can be expressed as mean arterial pressure minus intracranial pressure, divided by cerebrovascular resistance:

The normal CBF is around 50 ml per 100 g of brain tissue per minute (Lassen and Christensen 1976). In the adult with a brain weight of 1500 g this means that 750 ml of a total cardiac output of 3500 ml goes to the brain each minute. The percentage of cardiac output that goes to the brain is very much higher in the small infant.

Blood flow varies from region to region and is normally five times higher in grey (100 ml per 100 g) than white matter (20 ml per 100 g). The order of flow, from highest to lowest, can be placed in a league table: (1) inferior colliculus, (2) sensory cerebral cortex, (3) motor cerebral cortex, (4) geniculate bodies, (5) superior colliculus, (6) caudate nucleus, (7) thalamus, (8) cerebellum, and (9) cerebral white matter.

Clinically, impairment of the cerebral circulation may show as distension of scalp and retinal veins, exaggerated and then decreased pulsation of the fontanelle, or the appearance

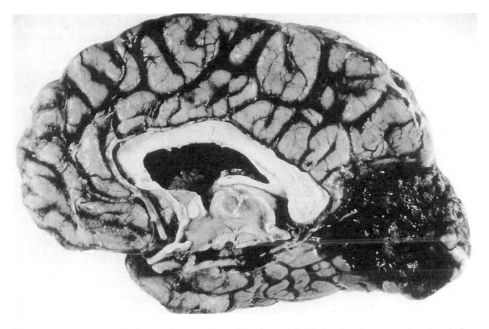

Fig. 1.38. Posterior cerebral artery ischaemia resulting in occipital infarction from tentorium herniation.

of a loud systolic bruit over the fontanelle. The bruit arises when ICP exceeds diastolic blood pressure. The pitch of the bruit rises as cerebral circulation slows; when circulation is finally arrested, the bruit disappears. The impairment of diastolic flow is now best seen, at the bedside, using cranial Doppler ultrasound. The resistance index is the most commonly used clinical measure of CBF velocity and this correlates with ICP. Newer methods of transcranial colour Doppler imaging that allow the diameter of the vessel to be determined will enable measurement of true flow and not just velocity. Perfusion MRI is again a very sensitive method of looking at flow in a non-acute situation but is not available at the bedside and consecutive rather than one-off measurements are desirable.

The interrelationship between ICP, CPP, mean arterial pressure (MAP), CBF and cerebral metabolic rate (CMR) in the normal brain can be represented as an algorithm as shown in Figure 1.39.

Cerebral perfusion pressure
Cerebral perfusion pressure is the difference between the mean arterial pressure and intracranial pressure, i.e. CPP = MAP – ICP. Systolic blood pressure at birth may be only 40mmHg, rising to systolic/diastolic averages of 80/55mmHg in the first year, 85/60 in the preschool years, 90/60 during the school years, and 120/80 in the adult, meaning that CPP is more easily encroached upon in children than in adults.

CPP is, in true physiological terms, the difference between the arterial pressure in the vessels entering the subarachnoid space and the pressure in the veins leaving it. The

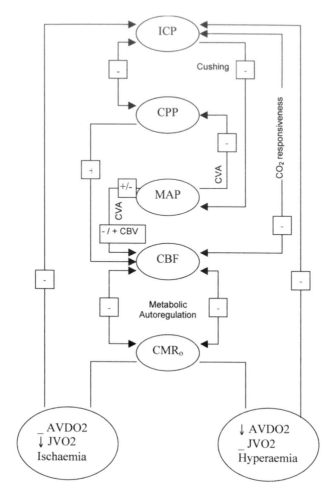

Fig. 1.39. The interrelationship of pressure, flow and metabolism in normal intracranial homeostasis.

ICP = intracranial pressure; CPP = cerebral perfusion pressure; MAP = mean arterial pressure; CBF = cerebral blood flow; CMR0 = cerebral metabolic rate; AVDO2 = arteriovenous oxygen difference; JVO2 = jugular venous oxygen saturation; CVA = cerebrovascular autoregulation; CBV = cerebral blood volume.

+ = positive or direct effect; − = negative or inverse effect.

relationship between ICP and CPP is complex. The normal ICP is usually given in the adult as 12–15 mmHg (~2 kpa). In children, the upper limit of normal ICP is lower, at 5 mmHg below 2 years of age and 7 mmHg below 5 years.

The brain is a slave to the heart, and failure of oxygen supply to the myocardium causes bradycardia and a fall in cardiac output and blood pressure. Many hypoxic episodes may have a central origin but if there is insufficient oxygen for myocardial demands a devastating ischaemic cascade is set up; this is equally true with perinatal asphyxia and status epilepticus.

TABLE 1.13
**Critical cerebral perfusion pressure levels
in children**

Age	Desirable CPP values
2–6 years	≤53mmHg
7–10 years	≤63mmHg
11–16 years	≤66mmHg

In the adult, CBF is maintained between blood pressure fluctuations of 60–160 mmHg. At blood pressures below 60 mmHg no further compensation is possible, i.e. cerebral vasodilation, and the CBF falls in parallel with any further drop in systemic perfusion pressure. If auto-regulation is lost, as after an ischaemic event, then one has a pressure-passive circulation and CBF follows changes in blood pressure at all blood pressure levels. In practical terms the mean blood pressure level equates to the critical CPP level (i.e. diastolic flow will be impaired below this critical level). The levels of CPP we strive for in practice (which are likely to be higher than the absolute critical CPP thresholds) are seen in Table 1.13 (Chambers et al. 2005).

When CPP falls below 40 mmHg there is absolute reduction in cerebral perfusion, and at flows below 18–20 ml per 100 g of brain per minute, infarction will result. The CPP is possibly the single most important measurement in the acute neurologically ill child, and certainly in traumatic head injury, NAHI and acute encephalopathies it most relates to outcome.

Autoregulation
In the intact brain a CBF adequate to meet local metabolic demand is maintained by auto-regulatory mechanisms that induce changes in cerebrovascular resistance in response to changes in local metabolic (e.g. lactate) changes (metabolic autoregulation) – metabolism match. Flow can change as metabolic demands increase either focally within the brain or generally. These physiological changes in flow are thought to be regulated by the small arteries and arterioles and not by the major vessels. However, the major vessels are capable of intense vasospasm, such as to cause infarction as seen in the intense vasospasm following subarachnoid bleeding, migraine or trauma.

The vessels have a sympathetic innervation, possibly from the locus coeruleus, which allows changes in flow not only with use of a particular part of the brain but also with vari-ations in state of alertness, e.g. 40% increase in CBF with REM sleep. Blood flow to an epileptic part of the brain may need to rise several hundred per cent in order to meet meta-bolic demands. Nitric oxide is now known to have a powerful effect on control of local blood flow. In response to raised ICP, the pump pressure (systemic) is increased by the Cushing response. Cushing's phenomenon comprises a progressive rise in blood pressure once the ICP approaches the resting arterial diastolic pressure, and it is thought that this is mediated via brainstem reflexes, depending upon adequacy of blood flow to the locus coeruleus.

When both compensatory mechanisms, i.e. autoregulation by cerebral arteriolar dilatation and Cushing's hypertensive response, operate during rises in ICP, a three step pattern of blood pressure change has been observed:

1. As the ICP rises above the normal range, cerebral arteriolar vasodilatation occurs, with no change in MAP and a steady fall in CPP;
2. When the Cushing range is attained, the MAP rises steadily and CPP is maintained;
3. When this compensatory rise in blood pressure is eventually exhausted, MAP and CPP both fall, the latter often into the negative range (Kaiser and Whitelaw 1988).

Cerebral infarction from impaired perfusion

The cerebral metabolic rate for oxygen is 3.2–3.8 ml/min/100g, with glucose (60 mg/min/100g) the predominant energy source. Each molecule of glucose yields 38 molecules of ATP by complete aerobic metabolism, but only two under anaerobic circumstances. This latter amount of ATP production is enough to prevent any severe damage but is totally dependent on the continued supply of glucose substrate and removal of the lactic acid so produced. ATP is used in neurotransmitter synthesis, transport mechanisms, and maintenance of membrane pumps and polarization potentials. The oxygen availability to the brain is the product of CBF and the oxygen content of arterial blood. The amount of oxygen carried depends upon not only the pO_2 but also the haemoglobin, so children with congenital heart disease and intense cyanosis, because of the compensatory polycythaemia, still carry more oxygen than anaemic patients and, although cyanosed, do not suffer from cerebral hypoxia. Polycythaemia increases plasma viscosity, and so with an haematocrit over 55% there may be a significant effect upon CBF. If the blood flow falls below metabolic demand then this is far more devastating than hypoxia, as there is now no substrate, glucose or ketones, and no way of removing lactic acid, so a severe intracellular acidosis results. *The brain can withstand periods of hypoxia but cannot withstand ischaemia, which rapidly causes neuronal necrosis.*

Neuropathology of ischaemic brain damage

Brain infarction can be caused by (i) interference with CBF (hypotension), (ii) raised ICP, (iii) vessel compression (shifts, coning), (iv) vessel occlusion, (v) vessel spasm, or (vi) venous obstruction.

Ischaemia is divided into phases by neuropathologists:

In *phase 1*, the mitochondria in neurons swell, and the brain swells as astrocytes and neurons swell from water retention (cytotoxic oedema). The anoxic neurons rapidly release potassium, which is mopped up by the astrocytes. Glycogen accumulates in the astrocytes. This may also alter the osmolality of cytoplasm, causing swelling (Fujimoto et al. 1976).

In *phase 2*, the endothelial cells, rich in mitochondria, lose their tight junctions and leak, allowing protein to escape into the extracellular space, and in severe cases allowing blood into the tissues (i.e. a haemorrhagic infarct). In these cases, the plasma escapes as extra-cellular brain lymph, and red cells become packed, crenated, and break down causing iron and bilirubin to be formed in the tissues. This ferruginization is used to date the infarct. The leakage of protein into the infarct can last up to 10 days so that radioactive technetium is taken up by a relatively old infarct.

Phase 3 is characterized by death of cells in the infarcted area with lysosomal rupture, resulting in breakdown of tissue proteins with swelling of the infarct, breakdown of the blood–brain barrier, loss of autoregulation, sludging of the microcirculation and liquefaction of the tissues. The swelling of astrocytes and endothelial cells compresses the capillaries, and electron microscopy shows the erythrocytes to be stuck. A further cause of sludging is the release of thromboplastic substances (which can be measured in the CSF). The resulting necrotic tissue may then be absorbed by macrophages to leave a cyst or cysts, as in multicystic encephalomalacia or infarctive periventricular leukomalacia, or one large porencephalic cyst. In other cases, an astrocyte reaction gradually replaces the dead tissue forming a glial scar. Capillaries proliferate and new ones grow into the damaged area.

The therapeutic window of cerebral ischaemia

Children who die following a cardiac arrest or head trauma often appear to be recovering, and may even speak after the event, and yet appear to suddenly deteriorate 6–12 hours later. At autopsy they show extensive cerebral ischaemia. This gap between event and deterioration offers a possibility of therapeutic intervention, i.e. the 'therapeutic window', in order to try to arrest whatever pathophysiological mechanism is responsible. Cerebral oedema may be responsible in some cases, but a biochemical cascade mechanism with triggering of apoptosis is thought more likely in most cases. There are mechanisms (e.g. adenosine and ACTH) whereby the brain can 'switch off' and reduce its metabolic demands, i.e. cellular hibernation occurs.

Mechanisms of hypoxic–ischaemic brain damage

A cascade of biochemical abnormalities follows hypoxia–ischaemia; all probably play some part in causing permanent brain damage, but it is not possible in the clinical situation to say which ones, and at present the therapeutic possibilities are limited:

- consumptive asphyxia, i.e. local metabolic demand outstrips supply
- excitotoxicity – glutamate stimulation of cells beyond energy supply
- glutamate causes toxic calcium entry into the cell
- substrate failure (hypoglycaemia, failure of ketone production)
- intracellular acidosis (aggravated by excess substrate supply, e.g. glucose)
- ATP depletion
- rupture of lysosomes
- calcium invasion of the cell with cytotoxicity
- release of S-S/S-H groups
- free radical toxicity (e.g. epoxides)
- failure of microcirculation from thromboplastin release
- osmotic disruption – release of idiogenic osmols and failure to excrete metabolic water.

Mechanisms of cellular injury

The final common pathway of head injury is energy failure and ATP depletion, which leads to further cell necrosis or apoptosis. Free radicals play an important role in the brain injury following hypoxic–ischaemic encephalopathy. They cause damage to endothelial cells,

89

receptors, synaptosome structure and astrocyte function. Asphyxia, reperfusion following ischaemia, arachidonic acid cascade, and activation of phagocyte and catecholamine metabolism result in mitochondrial dysfunction. This results in induction of peroxidation by Fenton/Haber Weiss reaction or via iron–oxygen complexes. Non-protein-bound iron is essential for the induction of lipid peroxidation. There is a build-up of iron in the white matter (due to disrupted axonal iron transport). Significant positive correlation has been found between plasma-free iron and the number of nucleated red cells in cord blood, which is currently considered a reliable index of lasting intrauterine asphyxia and a predictor of poor neurodevelopmental outcome (Bracci et al. 2001). Elevated levels of protein-S100ß and brain-specific creatine-kinase reliably indicate moderate and severe hypoxic–ischaemic encephalopathy as early as 2 hours after birth (Nagdyman et al. 2001).

Factors determining site of infarction
1. *Vascular anatomy.* A fall in systemic blood pressure does not result in uniform infarction of the whole brain (Bruce et al. 1973). The basal ganglia may catch the brunt on one side, and cortical grey matter on the other; the leg area may be more affected than the arm.

The circle of Willis is supplied from four feeding arteries; this means that there must be areas where the pressures even out, or there would be retrograde flow. These areas of no flow focus the ischaemia, so one may see a pattern of predominant middle cerebral artery infarction from a general drop in perfusion pressure. Loss of autoregulation can also be localized. This accounts for the fact that on follow up of infants with NAHI, 19% have a hemiplegia, although total infarction with a quadriplegia is more common (35%).

2. *Watershed zones.* Severely impaired CBF causes 'cerebral peripheral circulatory failure', so the watershed zones between adjacent vascular territories are more susceptible. This may shift with age from between centrifugal and centripetal arteries in the newborn, causing periventricular leukomalacia, to the territory between middle and posterior cerebral arteries in older infants, causing infarcts in the pericentral white matter of the optic radiation and posterior temporal lobe or between anterior and middle cerebral arteries, causing a wedge-shaped infarct in the leg area or the motor cortex. This susceptibility is due to the cerebral arterioles being 'end arteries' that do not anastomose.

3. *Selective vulnerability* to cerebral hypoxia exists not only between different cellular elements in the brain (neurones being most sensitive, and microglia and blood vessel cells least sensitive), but also between different types of neurone. Ischaemic damage occurs predominantly in the most recently evolved areas of the brain – neocortex, basal ganglia, hippocampus and cerebellar Purkinje cells (Dearden 1985). Jennett and Teasdale (1981) showed that in head injuries there was hypoxic–ischaemic damage to these selective areas as well as watershed zone infarction (hippocampus 81%, basal ganglia 79%, cerebral cortex 46%, cerebellum 44%).

4. The selective *compression of intracranial vessels by shifts and cones*, e.g. pericallosal (subfalcine shifts), posterior cerebral (tentorial herniation) and posterior inferior cerebellar

artery (foramen magnum cone), will cause focal ischaemia secondary to generalized raised ICP.

5. *Other reasons* why there may be focal damage in what at first appears a global insult include: (i) asymmetrical bridging vein rupture due to asymmetrical rotation of the hemispheres and tearing of the weakest bridging vein and ipsilateral RH; (ii) asymmetrical extracerebral vascular injury (direct carotid compression or whiplash injury to the vertebral arteries); (iii) focal impact including 'tin ear syndrome' (Hanigan 1987), which occurs after kicks or bangs unilaterally to the side of the head and result in ear bruising, unilateral cerebral oedema, and ipsilateral subdural and retinal haemorrhages.

INJURIES TO CERVICAL SPINE AND MEDULLA

Accidental injuries to the cervical spine occur rarely in childhood, with a mean age of about 10 years from motor vehicle accidents (50%) and sports injuries (25%) (Brown et al. 2001). Hanging injuries and hangman's fractures of the cervical spine may be caused by car seat harnesses and (now more widely recognized) by window cords

Birth trauma to the cervical spine is well documented in breech delivery and was not a rare clinical diagnosis at the time when birth trauma was common, estimated to be present in 10–33% of neonatal deaths (Towbin 1970). Lifting the baby's body over the mother's abdomen with the head still engaged may cause fractures of the occipital bone and cerebellar haemorrhage. A true spinal injury from such hyperextension causes sudden death in labour or tetraparesis, bilateral Erb's palsy, or diaphragmatic and respiratory paralysis. Root pocket haemorrhage, spinal root avulsion, spinal epidural haemorrhage and intraparenchymatous cord haemorrhages were seen at autopsy (Towbin 1970). Yates (1959) was one of the first neuropathologists to describe vertebral insufficiency in the elderly but he also looked at the cervical spines of 60 infants dying in the neonatal period from various types of delivery (only 9 breech) and confirmed that spinal injury was more common than expected: 27/60 showed spinal subdural and extradural bleeding, torn ligaments, torn dura and joint capsules; and 9/60 showed bruised or torn spinal nerve roots (Fig. 1.40).

The vertebral arteries are anchored in the transverse processes of the cervical vertebrae as they pass through foramina in the bone. Yates showed bruising of the adventitia with intramural clots or occlusion in 24 of the 60 infants. This study was important as all too often the cervical spine and certainly the vertebral arteries were not examined at autopsy. It also explains the frequent association with brainstem dysfunction known to be common in these infants. Until recently the cervical spine was also not studied on routine cranial MRI.

Caffey (1972) originally described NAHI as whiplash shaking injury. The whiplash has since been forgotten and the shaking dominates. One would have expected that a so-called whiplash shaking injury might cause cervical spinal injury to the very young infant, especially as they are so vulnerable during delivery. It is surprising that it is only relatively recently that the root pocket haemorrhages and trauma to the cervical cord and medulla have been recognized as an integral part of the syndrome and probably a major cause of sudden death. The subdural spinal haemorrhages, spinal infarction and root avulsions from

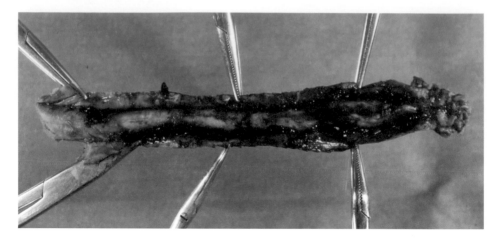

Fig. 1.40. Necropsy specimen showing spinal subdural haemorrhage.

non-accidental trauma, shown by Leestma (1995) in Duckett's excellent text on paediatric neuropathology, are very reminiscent of the spinal pathology shown by Yates. Both types, i.e. birth trauma and whiplash, are hyperextension injuries. Concurrent injuries to the cervical spine with epidural spinal haemorrhage and bruising of the cervicomedullary junction are probably underestimated; they were found in 5 of 6 fatal cases of whiplash shaking injury by Hadley et al. (1989). Cases with apnoea and those who die without SDH or cerebral oedema should be particularly suspect (Towbin 1967, Swischuk 1969). Geddes et al. (2001b) have revisited and increased the profile of the spine and medulla; their cases showed epidural spinal bleeding, localized axonal damage to the cranio-cervical junction and damage to the spinal nerve roots and brainstem in 11 of 37 infants dying of NAHI.

As previously mentioned, the infant head pivots at the cranio-cervical junction, but in the older child in the mid-cervical region. This may be why cervicomedullary damage tends to occur in infants and a C5 level lesion in older children. The posterior ligaments and joint capsule are more elastic in the infant than in the adult. The cervical spine, i.e. vertebral column, is extensile and traction will allow elongation, while the spinal cord itself cannot stretch and would avulse. The spinal nerves move within the sheaths. Equally, the cervical vertebral column can move in the anteroposterior direction allowing a degree of slippage (spondylolisthesis), the facet joints slope in a different direction from the adult spine, and there is a wide atlanto–dens space. Whiplashing can therefore result in cord concussion from repeated partial subluxations causing 'waterhammering' and traction with bruising, as well as possible vertebral artery and anterior spinal artery lesions, resulting in a 'cervico-medullary syndrome'.

The presentation in the very young infant, i.e. up to 3 months, is with apnoea. This, together with the high incidence of hypoxic damage reported in acutely fatal cases by Geddes et al. (2001a), suggests another syndrome different from the supratentorial rotation injury from shaking. Death from suddenly stopping breathing or a period of hypoventilation, especially if accompanied by vasoparalytic shock from loss of vasomotor tone, also due to the medullary injury, will cause severe hypoxic–ischaemic damage with oedema. These infants can be expected to be over-represented in pathology series; many die immediately or within 24 hours. Subdural haematomas are small and not greatly space occupying at this time, as seen on initial CT scans, and only expand if the child survives. Ten to 20 per cent of infants with NAHI die. The 80% who survive and are seen by paediatricians with severe damage show a different picture of acute atrophy of the cerebral hemispheres and expanding large subdural spaces. Sudden death before large subdural haematomas appear could be mistaken as cot death. The recent increased awareness of the vulnerability of the cervical spine in the infant causing spinal cord damage without fracture highlights the need for MRI to include the cervical spine in all suspected cases, including post-mortem study in cases of sudden death.

Timing of injury

In court the paediatrician is often asked to give an estimate of the timing or age of the injury and it must be appreciated as with all biological variables that this is not exact. Table 1.14 gives an approximation of the timing of the primary and secondary injuries. Bruising, fractures, brain imaging, tissue pathology and spectrophotometry of the subdural aspirate provide the best estimates of timing.

TABLE 1.14
Timing of injury

Feature	Observation	Time
Body temperature	Hypothermia in normal ambient temperature	2.5°C/hour (for 5 hours)
Skin bruising (Langlois and Gresham 1991, Stephenson and Bialas 1996)	Yellow colour	>18 hours
	Most disappear	1–4 days
Retinal haemorrhages	Colour changes as skin bruising	Variable depending on retinal tissue layer and extent
Fractures (Carty 1993)	Soft tissue resolution	2–10 days
	Early periosteal reaction (to haemorrhage):	
	Long bones and ribs	4–21 days
	Loss of fracture line definition:	4–21 days
	Soft callus	4–21 days
	Hard callus	14–90 days
	Remodelling	3 months – 2 years
Brain repair process (autopsy) (Anderson and Opeskin 1998)	Neuronal ischaemic death:	
	Microvacuolation	Minutes/hours
	Red neurons (eosinophilic)	<1 hour
	Axonal swelling	1 hour
	Neuronal incrustation	3 hours

continued ↗

TABLE 1.14
(continued)

Feature	Observation	Time
Brain repair process (autopsy) (Anderson and Opeskin 1998)	Glial, microglial, vascular reaction to ischaemic injuries:	
	Astrocytic swelling	12– 36 hours
	Gliosis	48 hours – months
	Macrophages:	
	Appear	48 hours
	Peak	14 days
	Present	Months – years
	Granulocytes – present	<1 hour
Spectrophotometry (Tallur et al. 2005)	Subdural aspirate: crenated red cells	Several hours
	Brown and no intact red cells	Days to weeks
	Oxyhaemoglobin	2–12 hours
	Bilirubin	1–3 days

Timing by imaging

Imaging	Findings	Timing
Primary injury		
CT (Lee et al. 1997)	Subdural haemorrhage (SDH)	
	Hyperdense	<7 days (acute)
	Hypo/isodense	8–22 days (subacute)
	Iso/hypodense	>22 days (chronic)
	Increasing hyperdensity	30–90 days (enlarging chronic)
	Hypodensity (resolution)	>90 days (neomembrane)
MRI (FLAIR, T_1, T_2) (McPhillips 2002)	Acute: SDH low intensity	1–3 days
	Late: SDH high intensity	1–2 weeks
Secondary injury		
MRI/CT (Dias et al. 1998)	Parenchymal hypodensities / oedema / contusion	<3 hours following report of injury
MRI (McPhiilips 2002)	Diffuse brain swelling (hyperaemic, unilateral or bilateral) ↓	Immediate or delayed
	Oedema – grey matter low intensity on T_1 and high intensity on T_2 and FLAIR (i.e. increased water) ↓	3 days
	Atrophy	>1 week
	Hypoxic–ischaemic injury (loss of grey–white differentiation – reversal sign)	Immediate or delayed
	Subcortical hyperintensity on T_1, hypointensity on T_2	>1 week, may persist for months
MRI (Rutherford 2002)	Asphyxial brain oedema (T_1 spin echo)	24–48 hours; not evident by 2nd week
	Hydrocephalus	Days – weeks

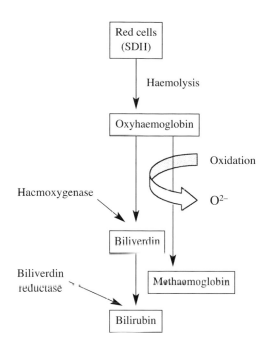

Fig. 1.41. Genesis of oxyhaemoglobin, methaemoglobin and bilirubin from red blood cell breakdown.

Sequential brain imaging (both MRI and CT) is essential as it shows the evolution of the pathology. An infant with a fresh small surface and interhemispheric SDH on admission but large subdural effusions, ventriculomegaly and parenchymatous infarcts with atrophy by 10 days must have an acute lesion, and birth injuries, old falls or injury at the time of old fractures can be discounted. CT best shows blood and fractures, whereas MRI is better for infarction, tears and parenchymatous damage. The changes are so dramatic over such a short time as to be almost unbelievable and very few other pathologies show this rapid and dramatic change. Sequential scanning gives a more dynamic picture of the pathology than a single view from autopsy hours or days after the event and after periods of resuscitation and reanimation.

SPECTROPHOTOMETRY

When red cells enter the subarachnoid space, they are visible by microscopy for a few days to several weeks (Tourtelotte et al. 1964). They then become crenated. Lysis of red cells results in release of oxyhaemoglobin, usually between 2 and 12 hours but continuing up to 48 hours. A microsomal enzyme haemoxygenase released from macrophages (and the arachnoid membrane) converts oxyhaemoglobin to bilirubin. Bilirubin usually appears after 3–4 days but may exceptionally occur as early as 9–10 hours. The 'bilirubin transforming capacity' is a limiting reaction, and when the concentration of oxyhaemoglobin rises rapidly additional amounts are oxidized non-enzymatically to methaemoglogin (Wahlgren and Lindquist 1987) (Fig. 1.41).

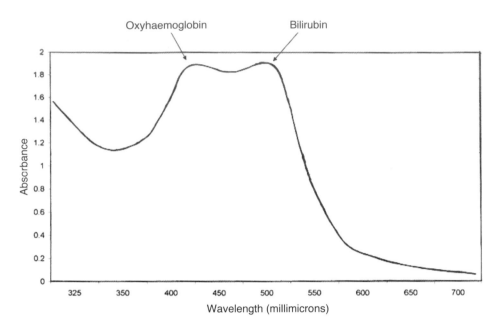

Fig. 1.42. Spectrogram showing absorbance of oxyhaemoglobin at 413–415 nm, and bilirubin at 450–460 nm, undertaken on the subdural aspirate from a 2-month-old infant who presented with scalp bruising, full fontanelle, 'sun-setting' and retinal haemorrhages. Her twin sister had died 3 days earlier and was found at autopsy to have bilateral subdural haematomas.

The spectrophotometry is carried out on centrifuged CSF, and the supernatent is scanned using a double beam Unicam spectrophotometer at wavelengths between 350 nm and 650 nm. Oxyhaemoglobin has an absorption at 413–415 nm. Oxyhaemoglobin and bilirubin together have a shoulder at 450–460 nm at the down slope of the oxyhaemoglobin curve. Bilirubin alone has a broad peak at 450–460 nm, and methaemoglobin has an absorption peak at 405 nm (methaemoglobin absorbance moves towards 413 nm when oxyhaemoglobin is concurrently present) (Fig. 1.42).

Physiological jaundice of the newborn may be present clinically until 7 days (longer in the preterm infant); however, xanthochromia may persist in the CSF and the serum bilirubin may still be elevated for 5–6 weeks. Care should therefore be exercised if there is xanthochromia without red cells.

A recent study of the haemoglobin index and the haemoglobin coefficient has shown that it is not possible to time the original haemorrhage by using data from existing models for subarachnoid haemorrhage (Tallur et al. 2005). This is because the haemorrhage within the subarachnoid is dispersed within the CSF and may well dilute and disappear faster than haemorrhage from an encapsulated subdural space without a natural circulation. So while spectrophotometry can identify fresh blood, oxyhaemoglobin, bilirubin or methaemoglobin in the aspirate, the presence of bilirubin merely indicates bleeding has occurred between 24 hours and 3 days prior to the aspiration.

TABLE 1.15
Investigations in head trauma due to suspected child abuse

- Brain imaging:
  MRI within 48 hours and repeat at 1 week
  CT immediately on admission including bony windows
  Ultrasound
  Doppler imaging daily to monitor cerebral blood flow velocity (resistance index)
- Skeletal survey.
  The Royal College of Radiologists (2003) recommends:
  Age 0–2 years, skeletal survey together with mandatory CT of head.
  Age 3–5 years, X-ray clinically suspicious area.
  Age over 3 years, skeletal survey not generally indicated.
  Bone scintigraphy indicated in children over 2 years if the skeletal survey is equivocal
- Photography: needs good technique to show bruising in true colours
- EEG – needed 24–48 hours if in ITU
- Exclude other causes of acute encephalopathy – blood culture, CSF examination, virology, lactate, ammonia, organic acids, amino acids, as indicated
- Examination of biochemical predisposition to fractures, calcium, phosphorus, copper, alkaline phosphatase, vitamin D, parathormone, as indicated
- Spectrophotometry
- Intracranial pressure measurement
- Coagulation screen
- Other inborn errors of metabolism (IBEM) investigations
- Child protection team (paediatrician, social work, police, forensic)

Investigations

For any case presenting with suspected NAHI, a series of investigations needs to be carried out. These are summarized in Table 1.15.

Role of the paediatrician

A difficulty with multidisciplinary teams is defining expertise and boundaries in order to prevent friction, confusion or domination. The media report cases where different agencies acted alone without communicating with each other while the child slipped through the net. At the same time, long drawn out case conferences with people giving personal opinions without fact and with no intention of repeating them in court can be regarded as time wasting.

The child with 'suspected NAHI' usually presents initially to the hospital, and in such cases the paediatrician has a duty to notify the child protection team when s/he reaches a diagnosis of 'possible NAHI' (although it may be many days before all investigations to confirm or refute the diagnosis are available), but at the same time will reap condemnation from all sides if parents are wrongly accused of abuse when there is another explanation.

We would list the duties of the paediatrician as follows.

- Prime advocacy is for the child and his/her protection and not, in these cases, the parents – the paediatician must be willing to put the child's point of view and his/her safety first.
- Document the nature and extent of the injuries.

- Organize imaging to delineate injuries and their subsequent development.
- Treat the child's acute encephalopathy.
- Treat any subdural bleeding.
- Make a diagnosis of 'suspected NAHI' / accidental head injury, or other diagnosis.
- Consider the possible mechanisms of the injury.
- Try to make an assessment of the timing of the injury.
- Investigate possible differential diagnoses.
- Maintain working relationship with parents (may need to work with them for years caring for a disabled child).
- Be non-judgmental, without prejudice, and do not assume that the abuser is necessarily the male in the family (although if there is also sexual abuse, the male is the more likely).
- Never attempt to make accusations of guilt unless there is a confession.
- Share information with police and social work department through case conferences.
- Give clear opinion in court relating to known facts – it is not the paediatrician's job to get a conviction, and if the case does not succeed it should not be regarded as failure.
- Advise 'frustration counselling' for carers if appropriate.
- Safety of the child is paramount.

Conclusions

Non-accidental head injury is not a single entity, and the classical 'shaken baby syndrome' of Caffey is but one aspect. There is a cascade of possible mechanisms, biomechanics and pathophysiology, and hence the type of brain damage varies widely. Modern MR imaging has allowed a more dynamic approach to antemortem pathology. The primary injury is far more devastating than the majority of accidental head injuries, with only 11% completely normal on follow-up. At the same time only 20% of infants are protected by a subsequent successful prosecution.

REFERENCES

Adams JH, Mitchell DE, Graham DI, Doyle D (1977) Diffuse brain damage of immediate impact type. *Brain* **100**: 489–502.

Adams JH, Doyle D, Ford I, Gennarelli TA, Graham DI, McLellan DR (1989) Diffuse axonal injury in head injury: definition, diagnosis and grading. *Histopathology* **15**: 49–59.

Aldershlade R, Bellman MH, Rawson NSB, Ross EM, Miller DL (1981) The National Childhood Encephalopathy Study. In: *Whooping Cough: Reports from the Committee on Safety of Medicine and The Joint Committee on Vaccination and Immunisation*. London: HMSO, pp. 79–169.

American Academy of Pediatrics: Committee on Child Abuse and Neglect (2001) Shaken baby syndrome: Rotational cranial injuries – technical report. *Pediatrics* **108**: 206–210.

Anderson RMcD, Opeskin K (1998) Timing of early changes in brain trauma. *Am J Forensic Med Pathol* **19**: 1–19.

Aoki N, Masuzawa H (1986) Subdural haematomas in abused children: report of six cases from Japan. *Neurosurgery* **18**: 475–477.

Arseni C, Clurea AV (1981) Clinicotherapeutic aspects in the growing skull fracture. *Child's Brain* **8**: 161–172.

Bakay L, Crawford JD, White JC (1954) The effects of intravenous fluids on cerebrospinal fluid pressure. *Surg Gynecol Obstet* **99**: 48–52.

Bannister R (1983) Clinical studies of autonomic function and dysfunction. *J Auton Nerv Syst* **7**: 233–237.

Barlow KM, Minns RA (1999) The relation between intracranial pressure and outcome in non-accidental head injury. *Dev Med Child Neurol* **41**: 220–225.

Barlow KM, Minns RA (2000) Annual incidence of shaken impact syndrome in young children. *Lancet* **356**: 1571–1572.

Barlow KM, Gibson RJ, McPhillips M, Minns RA (1999) Magnetic resonance imaging in acute non-accidental head injury. *Acta Paediatr* **88**: 734–740.

Barlow KM, Spowart JJ, Minns RA (2000) Early posttraumatic seizures in non-accidental head injury: relation to outcome. *Dev Med Child Neurol* **42**: 591–594.

Barlow K. Thompson E. Johnson D. Minns RA (2004) The neurological outcome of non-accidental head injury. *Pediatr Rehabil* **7**: 195–203.

Bax M (1983) Child abuse and cerebral palsy. *Dev Med Child Neurol* **25**: 141–142 (editorial).

Batzdorf U (1976) The management of cerebral edema in pediatic practice. *Pediatrics* **58**: 78–87.

Berger, D (1979) Child abuse simulating "near miss" sudden infant death syndrome. *J Pediatr* **95**: 554–556.

Bernard PA, Johnston C, Curtis SE, King WD (1998) Toppled television sets cause significant pediatric morbidity and mortality. *Pediatrics* **102**: e32.

Biousse V, Suh DY, Newman NJ, Davis PC, Mapstone T, Lambert SR (2002) Diffusion-weighted magnetic resonance imaging in shaken baby syndrome. *Am J Ophthalmol* **133**: 249–255.

Bracci R, Perrone S, Buonocore G (2001) Red blood cell involvement in fetal/neonatal hypoxia. *Biol Neonate* **79**: 210–212.

Brown JK (1974) Systemic neurology. In: Cockburn F, Drillien CM, eds. *Neonatal Medicine*. Oxford. Blackwell Scientific, pp. 556 626.

Brown JK (1991) Mechanisms of production of raised intracranial pressure. In: Minns RA, ed. *Problems of Intracranial Pressure in Childhood. Clinics in Developmental Medicine No. 113/114*. London. Mac Keith Press, pp. 13–37.

Brown JK (1994) CNS trauma. In: Millichap JG, ed. *Progress in Pediatric Neurology, 2nd edn*. Chicago: PNB, pp. 387–391.

Brown RL, Brunn MA, Garcia VF (2001) Cervical spine injuries in children: a review of 103 patients treated consecutively at a level 1 pediatric trauma center. *J Pediatr Surg* **36**: 1107–1114.

Bruce DA (1983) Management of cerebral edema. *Pediatr Rev* **4**: 217–224.

Bruce DA, Langfitt TW, Miller JD, Schutz H, Vapalahti MP, Stanek A, Goldberg HI (1973) Regional cerebral blood flow, intracranial pressure, and brain metabolism in comatose patients. *J Neurosurg* **38**: 131–144.

Bruce DA, Alavi A, Bilaniuk L, Dolinskas C, Obrist W, Uzzell B (1981) Diffuse cerebral swelling following head injuries in children: the syndrome of "malignant brain edema". *J Neurosurg* **54**: 170–178.

Bulloch B, Schubert CJ, Brophy PD, Johnson N, Reed MH, Shapiro RA (2000) Cause and clinical characteristics of rib fractures in infants. *Pediatrics* **105**: e48.

Cadzow SP, Armstrong KL (2000) Rib fractures in infants: red alert! The clinical features, investigations and child protection outcomes. *J Paediatr Child Health* **36**: 322–326.

Caffey J (1946) Multiple fractures in the long bones of infants suffering from subdural haematoma. *AJR* **56**: 163–173.

Caffey J (1972) On the theory and practice of shaking infants: its potential residual effects of permanent brain damage and mental retardation. *Am J Dis Child* **124**: 161–169.

Caffey J (1974) The whiplash shaken infant syndrome: manual shaking by the extremities with whiplash-induced intracranial and intraocular bleedings, linked with residual permanent brain damage and mental retardation. *Pediatrics* **54**: 396–403.

Calder IM, Hill I, Scholtz CL (1984) Primary brain trauma in non-accidental injury. *J Clin Pathol* **37**: 1095–1100.

Cameron JM, Rae IJ (1975) *Atlas of the Battered Child Syndrome*. London: Churchill Livingstone.

Carrigan TD, Walker E, Barnes S (2000) Domestic violence: the shaken adult syndrome. *J Accid Emerg Med* **17**: 138 139.

Carty H (1989) Skeletal manifestations of child abuse. *Bone* **6**: 3–7.

Carty HM (1993) Fractures caused by child abuse. *J Bone Joint Surg Br* **75**: 849–857.

Chalumeau M, Foix-L'Helias L, Scheinmann P, Zuani P, Gendrel D, Ducou-le-Pointe H (2002) Rib fractures after chest physiotherapy for bronchiolitis or pneumonia in infants. *Pediatr Radiol* **32**: 644–647.

Chambers IR, Stobbart L, Jones PA, Kirkham FJ, Marsh M, Mendelow AD, Minns RA, Struthers S, Tasker RC (2005) Age-related differences in intracranial pressure and cerebral perfusion pressure in the first 6 hours after children's head injury: association with outcome. *Child's Nerv Syst*, **29**: 195–199.

Chamnanvanakij S, Rollins N, Perlman J (2002) Subdural haematoma in term infants. *Pediatr Neurol* **26**: 301–304.

Choux M, Lena G, Genitori L (1986) Intracranial haematomas. In: Raimondi A, Choux M, di Rocco C, eds. *Head Injuries in the Newborn and Infant*. Heidelberg: Springer Verlag, pp. 203–216.

99

Claydon SM (1996) Fatal extradural hemorrhage following a fall from a baby bouncer. *Pediatr Emerg Care* **12**: 432–434.

Cohen S, Warren RD (1987) Preliminary survey of family abuse of children served by United Cerebral Palsy centers. *Dev Med Child Neurol* **29**: 12–18.

Copeland AR (1985) Homicide in childhood. The Metro-Dade County experience from 1956 to 1982. *Am J Forensic Med Pathol* **6**: 21–24.

Corsellis JA (1989) Boxing and the brain. *BMJ* **298**: 105–109. Erratum in: *BMJ* **298**: 247.

Crompton R (1985) *Closed Head Injury in Children*. London: Edward Arnold.

Dashti SR, Decker DD, Razzaq A, Cohen AR (1999) Current patterns of inflicted head injury in children. *Pediatr Neurosurg* **31**: 302–306.

Datta S, Stoodley N, Jayawant S, Renowden S, Kemp A (2005) Neuroradiological aspects of subdural haemorrhages. *Arch Dis Child*, in press.

Dearden NM (1985) Ischaemic brain. *Lancet* **2**: 255–259.

Denny-Brown D, Russell WR (1941) Experimental cerebral concussion. *Brain* **64**: 93–164.

de San Lazaro C, Harvey R, Ogden A (2003) Shaken infant trauma induced by misuse of a baby chair. *Arch Dis Child* **88**: 632–634.

Dias MS, Backstrom J, Falk M, Li V (1998) Serial radiography in the infant shaken impact syndrome. *Pediatr Neurosurg* **29**: 77–85.

Di Scala C, Sege R, Li G, Reece RM (2000) Child abuse and unintentional injuries: a 10 year retrospective. *Arch Pediatr Adolesc Med* **154**: 16–22.

Di Scala C, Bartel M, Sege R (2001) Outcome from television sets toppling onto toddlers. *Arch Pediatr Adolesc Med* **155**: 145–148.

Duane TD (1973) Valsalva hemorrhagic retinopathy. *Am J Ophthalmol* **75**: 637–642.

Duck SC, Wyatt DT (1988) Factors associated with brain herniation in the treatment of diabetic ketoacidosis. *J Pediatr* **113**: 10–14.

Duhaime AC, Gennarelli TG, Thibault LE, Bruce DA, Margulies SS, Wiser R (1987) The shaken baby syndrome. A clinical, pathological, and biomechanical study. *J Neurosurg* **66**: 409–415.

Duhaime AC, Alario AJ, Lewander WJ, Schut L, Sutton LN, Seidl TS, Nudelman S, Budenz D, Hertle R, Tsiara W, Loporchio S (1992) Head injury in very young children: mechanisms, injury types, and ophthalmologic findings in 100 hospitalized patients younger than 2 years of age. *Pediatrics* **90**: 179–185.

Duhaime AC, Christian CW, Moss E, Seidl T (1996) Long-term outcome in infants with the shaking-impact syndrome. *Pediatr Neurosurg* **24**: 292–298.

Durham SR, Clancy RR, Leuthardt E, Sun P, Kamerling S, Dominguez T, Duhaime AC (2000) CHOP Infant Coma Scale ("Infant Face Scale"): a novel coma scale for children less than two years of age. *J Neurotrauma* **17**: 729–737.

Eden OB, Brown JK (1977) Hypertension of acute neurological diseases of childhood. *Dev Med Child Neurol* **19**: 437–445.

Elder JE, Taylor RG, Klug GL (1991) Retinal haemorrhage in accidental head trauma in childhood. *J Paediatr Child Health* **27**: 286–289.

Ellaway BA, Payne EH, Rolke K, Dunstan FD, Kemp AM, Butler I, Sibert JR (2004) Are abused babies protected from further abuse? *Arch Dis Child* **89**: 845–846.

Emery JL (1983) The necropsy and cot death. *BMJ* **287**: 77–78.

Ewing-Cobbs L, Brookshire B, Scott MA, Fletcher JM (1998a) Children's narrative following traumatic brain injury: linguistic structure, cohesion and thematic recall. *Brain Lang* **61**: 395–419.

Ewing-Cobbs L, Kramer L, Prasad M, Canales DN, Loius PT, Fletcher JM, Vollero H, Landry SH, Cheung K (1998b) Neuroimaging, physical, and developmental findings after inflicted and non-inflicted traumatic brain injury in young children. *Pediatrics* **102**: 300–307.

Ewing-Cobbs L, Prasad M, Kramer L, Louis PT, Baumgartner J, Fletcher JM, Alpert B (2000) Acute neuro-radiologic findings in young children with inflicted or non-inflicted traumatic brain injury. *Child's Nerv Syst* **16**: 25–33; discussion 34.

Fackler JC, Berkowitz ID, Green WR (1992) Retinal hemorrhages in newborn piglets following cardiopulmonary resuscitation. *Am J Dis Child* **146**: 1294–1296.

Faerber EN (1986) Trauma. In: *Cranial Computed Tomography in Infants and Children. Clinics in Developmental Medicine No. 93*. London: Spastics International Medical Publications, pp. 99–120.

Faillot T, Sichez JP, Brault JL, Kapell L, Kujas M, Bordi L, Boukobza M (1990) Lhermitte–Duclos disease (dysplastic gangliocytoma of the cerebellum). Report of a case and review of the literature. *Acta Neurochir* **105**: 44–49.

Fazen LE, Felizberto PI (1982) Baby walker injuries. *Pediatrics* **70**: 106–109.

Feldman KW, Brewer DK (1984) Child abuse, cardiopulmonary resuscitation and rib fractures. *Pediatrics* **73**: 339–342.

Fishman RA (1953) Effects of isotonic intravenous solutions on normal and increased intracranial pressure. *AMA Arch Neurol Psychiatry* **70**: 356–360.

Frank Y, Zimmerman R, Leeds NMD (1985) Neurological manifestations in abused children who have been shaken. *Dev Med Child Neurol* **27**: 312–316.

Fujimoto T, Walker JT, Spatz M, Klatzo I (1976) Pathophysiologic aspects of ischaemic edema. In: Pappius HM, Feindel W, eds. *Dynamics of Brain Edema*. Heidelberg: Springer, pp. 171–180.

Ganesh A, Jenny C, Geyer J, Shouldice M, Levin AV (2004) Retinal haemorrhage in type I osteogenesis imperfecta after minor trauma. *Ophthalmology* **111**: 1428–1431.

Garrettson LK, Gallagher SS (1985) Falls in children and youth. *Pediatr Clin North Am* **32**: 153–162.

Geddes JF, Hackshaw AK, Vowles GH, Nickols CD, Whitwell HL (2001a) Neuropathology of inflicted head injury in children. I. Patterns of brain damage. *Brain* **124**: 1290–1298.

Geddes JF, Vowles GH, Hackshaw AK, Nickols CD, Scott IS, Whitwell HL (2001b) Neuropathology of inflicted head injury in children. II. Microscopic brain injury in infants. *Brain* **124**: 1299–1306.

Geddes JF, Tasker RC, Hackshaw AK, Nickols CD, Adams GGW, Whitwell HL, Scheimberg I (2003) Dural haemorrhage in non-traumatic infant deaths: does it explain the bleeding in 'shaken baby syndrome'. *Neuropathol Appl Neurobiol* **29**: 14–22.

Gennarelli TA, Thibault LE (1982) Biomechanics of acute subdural hematoma. *J Trauma* **22**: 680–686.

Gilles EE, Nelson MD (1998) Cerebral complications of nonaccidental head injury in childhood. *Pediatr Neurol* **19**: 119–128.

Gilliland MG, Luckenbach MW (1993) Are retinal hemorrhages found after resuscitation attempts? A study of the eyes of 169 children. *Am J Forensic Med Pathol* **14**: 187–192.

Giovinazzo VJ, Lannuzzi J, Sorenson JA, Delrowe DJ, Campbell EA (1987) The ocular complications of boxing. *Ophthalmolgy* **94**: 587–596.

Goldstein B, Kelly MM, Bruton D, Cox C (1993) Inflicted versus accidental head injury in critically injured children. *Crit Care Med* **21**: 1328–1332.

Gonzalez Tortosa J, Martinez-Lage JF, Poza M (2004) Bitemporal head crush injuries: clinical and radiological features of a distinctive type of head injury. *J Neurosurg* **100**: 645–651.

Grant P (2001) Femur fractures in infants: A possible accidental aetiology. *Pediatrics* **108**: 1009–1012.

Grayev AM, Boal DK, Wallach DM, Segal LS (2001) Metaphyseal fractures mimicking abuse during treatment for clubfoot. *Pediatr Radiol* **31**: 559–563.

Griffin MR, Ray WA, Mortimer EA, Fenichel GM, Schaffner W (1990) Risk of seizures and encephalopathy after immunization with diphtheria–tetanus–pertussis vaccine. *JAMA* **263**: 1641–1645.

Gurdjian ES, Webster JE, Lissner HR (1949) Studies on skull fracture with particular reference to engineering factors. *Am J Surg* **78**: 736–742.

Guthkelch AN (1971) Infantile subdural haematoma and its relationship to whiplash injuries. *BMJ* **2**: 430–431.

Hadley MN, Sonntag VKH, Rekate HL, Murphy A (1989) The infant whiplash–shake injury syndrome: a clinical and pathological study. *Neurosurgery* **24**: 536–540.

Hall JR, Reyes HM, Horvat M, Meller JL, Stein R (1989) The mortality of childhood falls. *J Trauma* **29**: 1273–1275.

Hanigan WC, Peterson RA, Njus G (1987) Tin ear syndrome: rotational acceleration in pediatric head injuries. *Pediatrics* **80**: 618–622.

Hansen KK (1998) Folk remedies and child abuse: a review with emphasis on caida de mollera and its relationship to shaken baby syndrome. *Child Abuse Negl* **22**: 117–127.

Harty MP, Kao SC (2002) Intraosseous vascular access defect: fracture mimic in the skeletal survey for child abuse. *Pediatr Radiol* **32**: 188–190.

Harwood Nash DC, Fitz CR (1976) *Neuroradiology in Infants and Children*. St Louis: CV Mosby.

Helfer SA, Slovis TL, Black M (1977) Injuries resulting when small children fall out of bed. *Pediatrics* **60**: 533–535.

Hobbs CJ (1984) Skull fracture and the diagnosis of abuse. *Arch Dis Child* **59**: 246–252.

Holbourn AHS (1943) Mechanics of head injuries. *Lancet* **2**: 438–441.

Holbourn AHS (1945) The mechanics of brain injuries. *Br Med Bull* **3**: 147–149.

Hooper R (1969) Injuries of the skull. In: Hooper R, ed. *Patterns of Acute Head Injury*. Edward Arnold, pp. 21–30.

Hoskote A, Richards P, Anslow P, McShane T (2002) Subdural haematoma and non-accidental head injury in children. *Child's Nerv Syst* **18**: 311–317.

Ingraham FD, Matson DD (1954) *Neurosurgery of Infancy and Childhood*. Springfield, IL: Charles C Thomas, pp. 328–347.

Ito H, Komai T, Yamamoto S (1978) Fibrinolytic enzyme in the lining walls of chronic subdural haematomas. *J Neurosurg* **48**: 197–200.

Jaspan T, Narborough G, Punt JA, Lowe J (1992) Cerebral contusional tears as a marker of child abuse – detection by cranial sonography. *Pediatr Radiol* **22**: 237–245.

Jenkins A, Mendelow AD, Graham DI, Nath FP, Teasdale GM (1990) Experimental intracerebral haematoma, the role of blood constituents in early ischaemia. *Br J Neurosurg* **4**: 45–52.

Jennett B, Teasdale GM (1981) Intracranial hematoma. In: *Management of Head Injuries*. Philadelphia: FA Davis, pp. 153–191.

Jenny C, Hymel KP, Pitzen A, Reinert SE, Hay TC (1999) Analysis of missed cases of abusive head trauma. *JAMA* **281**: 621–626. Erratum in: *JAMA* 1999 **282**: 29.

Joffe M, Diamond P (1990) Letter to the Editor (V). *J Trauma* **30**: 1421–1422.

Johansson B (1974) Blood–brain barrier dysfunction in acute hypertension after papaverine-induced vasodilatation. *Acta Neurol Scand* **50**: 573–580.

Kaiser AM, Whitelaw AG (1988) Hypertensive response to raised intracranial pressure in infancy. *Arch Dis Child* **63**: 1461–1465.

Kanter RK (1986) Retinal hemorrhage after cardiopulmonary resuscitation or child abuse. *J Pediatr* **108**: 430–432.

Kaur B, Taylor D (1992) Fundus hemorrhages in infancy. *Surv Ophthalmol* **37**: 1–17.

Keenan H (2003) Nomenclature, definitions, incidence and demographics of inflicted childhood neurotrauma. In: Reece RM, Nicholson CE, eds. *Inflicted Childhood Neurotrauma*. Elk Grove City, IL: American Academy of Pediatrics, pp. 3–11.

King WJ, MacKay M, Sirnick A (2003) Shaken baby syndrome in Canada: clinical characteristics and outcomes of hospital cases. *CMAJ* **168**: 155–159.

Kivlin JD (2001) Ophthalmic manifestations of SBS. In: Lavoritz S, Palusci VJ, eds. *The Shaken Baby Syndrome*. New York: Haworth Press, pp. 137–154.

Kivlin J, Simons KB, Lazoritz S, Ruttum MS (2000) Shaken baby syndrome. *Ophthalmology* **107**: 1246–1254.

Kleinman PK (1990) Diagnostic imaging in infant abuse. *AJR* **155**: 703–712.

Kleinman PK, Blackbourne BD, Marks SC, Karellas A, Belanger PL (1989) Radiological contributions to the investigatin and prosecution of cases of fatal infant abuse. *N Engl J Med* **320**: 507–511.

Kotwica Z, Brzezinski J (1991) Chronic subdural haematoma treated by burr holes and closed system drainage: personal experience in 131 patients. *Br J Neurosurg* **5**: 461–465.

Kraus JF, Rock A, Hemyari P (1990) Brain injuries amoung infants, children, adolescents and young adults. *Am J Dis Child* **144**: 684–691.

Kravitz H, Driessen G, Gomberg R, Korach A (1969) Accidental falls from elevated surfaces in infants from birth to one year of age. *Pediatrics* **44**: 869–876.

Lane WG, Rubin DM, Monteith R, Christian CW (2002) Racial differences in the evaluation of pediatric fractures for physical abuse. *JAMA* **288**: 1603–1609.

Langlois NE, Gresham GA (1991) The ageing of bruises: a review and study of colour changes with time. *Forensic Sci Int* **50**: 227–238.

Lantz PE, Sinal SH, Stanton CA, Weaver RG (2004) Perimacular retinal folds from childhood head trauma. *BMJ* **328**: 754–756.

Lassen NA, Christensen MS (1976) Physiology of cerebral blood flow. *Brit J Anaesth* **48**: 719–734.

Lauer B, Broeck ET, Grossman M (1974) Battered child syndrome: review of 130 patients with controls. *Pediatrics* **54**: 67–70.

Lee KS, Bae WK, Bae HG, Doh JW, Yun IG (1997) The computed tomographic attenuation and the age of subdural hematomas. *J Korean Med Sci* **12**: 353–359.

Leestma JE (1995) Forensic neuropathology. In: Duckett S, ed. *Pediatric Neuropathology*. Baltimore: Williams & Wilkins, pp. 243–283.

Levin A (2000) Retinal haemorrhage and child abuse. In: David T, ed. *Recent Advances in Paediatrics*. London: Churchill Livingstone, pp. 151–219.

Levin A (2002) Ophthalmic manifestations of inflicted childhood neurotrauma. In: Reece RM, ed. *Inflicted Childhood Neurotrauma*. Elk Grove City, IL: American Academy of Pediatrics, pp. 127–159.

Livingstone JH, Brown JK (1986) Intracerebral haemorrhage after the neonatal period. *Arch Dis Child* **61**: 538–544.

Lo TYM, McPhillips M, Minns RA, Gibson RJ (2003) Cerebral atrophy following shaken impact syndrome and other non-accidental head injury (NAHI). *Pediatr Rehabil* **6**: 47–55.

Ludwig S, Warman M (1984) Shaken baby syndrome: a review of 20 cases. *Ann Emerg Med* **13**: 104–107.

Lund AM, Schwartz M, Skovby F (1996) Variable clinical expression in a family with OI type IV due to deletion of three base pairs in COL1A1. *Clin Genet* **50**: 304–309.

Lyons TJ, Oates RK (1993) Falling out of bed: a relatively benign occurrence. *Pediatrics* **92**: 125–127.

Mann LI, Carmichael A, Duchin S (1972) Effect of head compression on FHR, brain metabolism and function. *Obstet Gynecol* **39**: 721–726.

Margulies SS, Thibault KL (2000) Infant skull and suture properties: measurements and implications for mechancs of pediatric brain injury. *J Biomech Eng* **122**: 364–371.

Marlowe A, Pepin MG, Byers PH (2002) Testing for osteogenesis imperfecta in cases of suspected non-accidental injury. *J Med Genet* **39**: 382–386.

Maxeiner H (2001) [Evaluation of subdural hemorrhage in infants after alleged minor trauma.] *Unfallchirurg* **104**: 569–576. (German.)

McPhillips M (2002) Non-accidental head injury in the young infant. In: Rutherford M, ed. *MRI of the Neonatal Brain*. London: WB Saunders, pp. 261–269.

Meadow R (1984) Fictitious epilepsy. *Lancet* **2**: 25–28.

Meadow R (1987) Video recording and child abuse. *BMJ* **294**: 1629–1630.

Milhorat TH (1978) Pediatric neurosurgery. *Contemp Neurol Ser* **16**: 1–389.

Minns RA (1991) Infectious and parainfectious encephalopathies. In: Minns RA, ed. *Problems of Intracranial Pressure in Childhood. Clinics in Developmental Medicine Nos 113/114*. London: Mac Keith Press, pp. 170–282.

Minns RA (2005) Shaken baby syndrome: theoretical and evidential controversies. *J R Coll Phys Edinb* **35**: 5–15.

Minns RA, Thomas A, Lo TYM, Gilkes CE, Tallur KK (2004) Inner calvarial erosion from traumatic subdural haematoma in infancy. *Child's Nerv Syst*, e-pub ahead of print.

Morison CN (2002) The dynamics of shaken baby syndrome. PhD thesis, University of Birmingham, UK.

Morrison WE, Arbelaez JJ, Fackler JC, De Maio A, Paidas CN (2004) Gender and age effects on outcome after pediatric traumatic brain injury. *Pediatr Crit Care Med* **5**: 145–151.

Mushin AS (1971) Ocular damage in the battered baby syndrome. *BMJ* **14**: 402–404.

Myers RE, Adamsons K (1981) Obstetric considerations of perinatal brain injury. In: Scarpelli EM, Cosmi EV, eds. *Reviews in Perinatal Medicine, vol. 4*. New York. Raven Press, pp. 221–245.

Nagdyman N, Komen W, Ko HK, Muller C, Obladen M (2001) Early biochemical indicators of hypoxic–ischemic encephalopathy after birth asphyxia. *Pediatr Res* **49**: 502–506.

National Clearinghouse on Child Abuse and Neglect Information (2004) Child Maltreatment 2002: Reports from the States to the National Child Abuse and Neglect Data Systems – National statistics on child abuse and neglect. Online publication: http://www.acf.hhs.gov/programs/cb/publications/cmreports.htm.

NHMRC (1994) *Boxing Injuries*. Canberra: National Health and Medical Research Council, Australian Government Publishing Service.

Nickel RE, Gallenstein JS (1987) Developmental prognosis for infants with benign enlargement of the subarachnoid spaces. *Dev Med Child Neurol* **29**: 181–186.

Nimitjongskul P, Anderson LD (1987) The likelihood of injuries when children fall out of bed. *J Pediatr Orthoped* **7**: 184–186.

Odom A, Christ E, Kerr N, Byrd K, Cochran J, Barr F, Bugnitz M, Ring JC, Storgion S, Walling R, Stidham G, Quasney MW (1997) Prevalence of retinal hemorrhages in pediatric patients after in-hospital cardiopulmonary resuscitation: a prospective study. *Pediatrics* **99**: e3.

Ommaya AK, Gennarelli TA (1974) Cerebral concussion and traumatic unconsciousness, correlations of experimental and clinical observations on blunt head injuries. *Brain* **97**: 633–654.

Ommaya AK, Hirsche AE (1971) Tolerances for cerebral concussion from head impact and whiplash in primates. *J Biomech* **4**: 13–21.

Ommaya AK, Faas F, Yarnell P (1968) Whiplash injury and brain damage: an experimental study. *JAMA* **204**: 285–289.

Pape KE, Wigglesworth JS (1979) *Haemorrhage, Ischaemia and the Perinatal Brain. Clinics in Developmental Medicine No. 69/70*. London: Spastics International Medical Publications, pp. 61–84.

Pappius HM, Feindel W (1976) *Dynamics of Brain Edema*. Springer: Heidelberg.

Paterson CR, McAllion SJ (1989) Osteogenesis imperfecta in the differential diagnosis of child abuse. *BMJ* **299**: 1451–1454.

Perrin RG, Rutka JT, Drake JM, Meltzer H, Hellman J, Jay V, Hoffman HJ, Humphreys RP (1997) Management and outcomes of posterior fossa subdural hematomas in neonates. *Neurosurgery* **40**: 1190–1199; discussion 1199–1200.

103

Pincemaille Y, Trosseille P, Mack L, Tarriere C, Breton F, Renault P (1989) Some new data related to human tolerance obtained from volunteer boxers. In: *Proceedings of the 33rd STAPP Car Crash Conference, Washington DC*, pp. 177–190.

Plunkett J (2001) Fatal pediatric head injuries caused by short-distance falls. *Am J Forensic Med Pathol* **22**: 1–12.

Pounder DJ (1997) Shaken adult syndrome. *Am J Forensic Med Pathol* **18**: 321–324.

Rabe EF (1967) Subdural effusions in infants. *Pediatr Clin North Am* **14**: 831–850.

Rao P, Carty H, Pierce A (1999) The acute reversal sign: comparison of medical and non-accidental injury patients. *Clin Radiol* **54**: 495–501.

Reece RM (2002) Differential diagnosis of inflicted childhood neurotrauma. In: Reece RM, ed. *Inflicted Childhood Neurotrauma*. Elk Grove City, IL: American Academy of Pediatrics, pp. 17–31.

Reiber JD (1993) Fatal falls in childhood. How far must children fall to sustain fatal head injury? Report of cases and review of the literature. *Am J Forensic Med Pathol* **14**: 201–207.

Rivara FP, Alexander B, Johnston B, Soderberg R (1993) Population based study of fall injuries in children and adolescents resulting in hospitalization or death. *Pediatrics* **92**: 61–63.

Rex C, Kay PR (2000) Features of femoral fractures in nonaccidental injury. *J Pediatr Orthop* **20**: 411–413.

Roberts J, Gildong J, Keeling J, Sutton B, Lynch MA (1984) Is there a link between cot death and child abuse? *BMJ* **289**: 789–791.

Rogers D, Tripp J, Bentovim A, Robinson A, Berry D, Goulding R (1976) Non-accidental poisoning: an extended syndrome of child abuse. *BMJ* **1**: 793–796.

Rorke LB (1990) Neuropathology of homicidal head injury in infants. *Child's Nerv Syst* **6**: 295.

Rosen CL, Frost Jr JD, Bricker T, Tarnow JD, Gillette PC, Dunlavy S (1983) Two siblings with recurrent cardio-respiratory arrest: Munchausen syndrome by proxy or child abuse? *Pediatrics* **71**: 715–720.

Royal College of Radiologists (2003) *Making the Best Use of a Department of Clinical Radiology. Guidelines for Doctors. 5th edn.* London: Royal College of Radiologists.

Rutherford MA (2002) The asphyxiated term infant. In: Rutherford M, ed. *MRI of the Neonatal Brain.* London: WB Saunders, pp. 99–128.

Sandramouli S, Robinson R, Tsaloumas M, Willshaw HE (1997) Retinal haemorrhages and convulsions. *Arch Dis Child* **76**: 449–451.

Sasaki N, Enyo A (1995) Viscoelastic properties of bone as a function of water content. *J Biomech* **28**: 809–815.

Scarfo GB, Mariottini A, Tomaccini D, Palma L (1989) Growing skull fractures: progressive evolution of brain damage and effectiveness of surgical treatment. *Child's Nerv Syst* **5**: 163–167.

Schenker JG, Gombos GM (1966) Retinal hemorrhage in the newborn. *Obstet Gynecol* **27**: 521–524.

Scherl SA, Miller L, Lively N, Russinoff S, Sullivan CM, Tornetta P (2000) Accidental and nonaccidental femur fractures in children. *Clin Orthop* **376**: 96–105.

Schwartz ML, Hudson AR, Fernie GR, Hayashi K, Coleclough AA (1986) Biomechanical study of full-contact karate contrasted with boxing. *J Neurosurg* **64**: 248–252.

Sezen F (1970) Retinal haemorrhages in newborn infants. *Brit J Ophthalmol* **55**: 248–253.

Sankaran K, Wiebe H, Seshia MM, Boychuk RB, Cates D, Rigatto H (1979) Immediate and late ventilatory response to high and low O2 in preterm infants and adult subjects. *Pediatr Res* **13**: 875–878.

Shapiro HA (1975) Adult skull fracture – the magnitude of forces and the mechanism involved. In: Gordon I, ed. *Medico-Legal Mythology.* Johannesburg: High Keartland, pp. 267–277.

Shaw JC (1988) Copper deficiency and non-accidental injury. *Arch Dis Child* **63**: 448–455.

Shulman BH, Terhune CB (1951) Epiphyseal injuries in breech deliveries. *Pediatrics* **8**: 693–700.

Sillence D, Senn A, Danks D (1979) Genetic heterogeneity in osteogenesis imperfecta. *J Med Genet* **16**: 101–116.

Skellern CY, Wood DO, Murphy A, Crawford M (2000) Non-accidental fractures in infants: risk of further abuse. *J Paediatr Child Health* **36**: 590–592.

Smith C, Bell JE, Keeling JW, Risden RA (2003) Dural haemorrhage in nontraumatic infant deaths: does it explain the bleeding in 'shaken baby syndrome'? Geddes JE et al. A response. *Neuropathol Appl Neurobiol* **29**: 411–412; author reply 412–413.

Smith SM, Hanson R (1974) 134 battered children: a medical and psychological study. *BMJ* **3**: 666–670.

Snedecor ST, Wilson HB (1949) Some obstetrical injuries to the long bones. *J Bone Joint Surg Am* **31**: 378–384.

Southall DP, Stebbens V, Shinebourne EA (1987) Sudden and unexpected death between 1 and 5 years. Arch Dis Child 62: 700–705.

Stephenson T, Bialas Y (1996) Estimation of the age of bruising. *Arch Dis Child* **74**: 53–55.

Strich SJ (1961) Shearing of nerve fibres as a cause of brain damage due to head injury – a pathological study of 20 cases. *Lancet* **2**: 443–448.

Sty J, Starshak R (1983) The role of bone scintigraphy in the evaluation of the suspected abused child. *Radiology* **146**: 369–375.

Svenningsen L, Lindemann R, Eidal K (1988) Measurements of fetal head compression during bearing down and their relationship to the condition of the newborn. *Acta Obstet Gynecol Scand* **67**: 129–133.

Swischuk LE (1969) Spine and spinal cord trauma in the battered child syndrome. *Radiology* **92**: 733–738.

Symonds CP (1962) Concussion and its sequelae. *Lancet* **1**: 1–5.

Tallur KK, Belton N, Stephen R, Minns RA (2005) Is timing of haemorrhage by spectrophotometry similar for haemorrhages in the subdural and subarachnoid space? *Arch Dis Child* (in press).

Thomas AS, Rosenfield NS, Leventhal JM, Markowitz RI (1991) Long bone fractures in children: distinguishing accidental injuries from child abuse. *Pediatrics* **88**: 471–476.

Tomasi LG, Rosman NP (1975) Purtscher retinopathy in the battered child syndrome. *Am J Dis Child* **129**: 1335–1337.

Tourtelotte W, Metz LN, Bryan ER, DeJong RN (1964) Spontaneous fluid after intracranial haemorrhage. *Neurology* **14**: 302–306.

Towbin A (1967) Sudden infant death (cot and crib death) related to spinal injury. *Lancet* **2**: 940 (letter).

Towbin A (1970) Central nervous system damage in the human fetus and newborn infant. Mechanical and hypoxic injury incurred in the fetal–neonatal period. *Am J Dis Child* **119**: 529–542.

Torwalt CR, Balachandra AT, Youngson C, de Nanassy J (2002) Spontaneous fractures in the differential diagnosis of fractures in children. *J Forensic Sci* **47**: 1340–1344.

US Department of Health & Human Services, Administration for Children & Families (2001) Child Maltreatment 2001. (Online publication: www.acf.hhs.gov/programs/cb/publications/cm01/outcover.htm.)

van Vught AJ, Troost J, Willemse J (1976) Hypertensive encephalopathy in childhood. Diagnostic problems. *Neuropadiatrie* **7**: 92–100.

von Kries R, Gobel U (1992) Vitamin K prophylaxis and vitamin K deficiency bleeding (VKDB) in early infancy. *Acta Paediatr* **81**: 655–657.

Vowles GH, Scholtz CL, Cameron JM (1987) Diffuse axonal injury in early infancy. *J Clin Pathol* **40**: 185–189.

Wahlgren NG, Lindquist C (1987) Haematological derivatives in the cerebrospinal fluid after intracranial haemorrhage. *Eur Neurol* **26**: 216–221.

Warwick R, Williams PL (1973) *Gray's Anatomy. 35th British edn.* Philadelphia: WB Saunders.

Weber W (1984) Experimentelle Untersuchungen zu Schadelbruchverletzungen des Säuglings. *Z Rechtsmedizin* **92**: 87–94.

Weber W (1985) Zur biomechanischen Fragilität des Sauglingsschädels. *Z Rechtsmedizin* **94**: 93–101.

Weir B (1980) Oncotic pressure of subdural fluids. *J Neurosurg* **53**: 512–515.

Wenstrup RJ, Willing MC, Starman BJ, Byers PH (1990) Distinct biochemical phenotypes predict clinical severity in nonlethal variants of osteogenesis imperfecta. *Am J Hum Genet* **46**: 975–982.

Whitby EH, Paley MN, Smith MF, Sprigg A, Woodhouse N, Griffiths PD (2003) Low field strength magnetic resonance imaging of the neonatal brain. *Arch Dis Child Fetal Neonatal Ed* **88**: F203–F208.

Whitby EH, Griffiths PD, Rutter S, Smith MF, Sprigg A, Ohadike P, Davies NP, Rigby AS, Paley MN (2004) Frequency and natural history of subdural haemorrhages in babies and relation to obstetric factors. *Lancet* **363**: 846–851.

Williams RA (1991) Injuries in inants and small children resulting from witnessed and corroborated free falls. *J Trauma* **31**: 1350–1352.

Woelfe J, Kreft B, Emons D, Haverkamp K (1996) Subdural hemorrhage as an initial sign of glutaric aciduria type 1: a diagnostic pitfall. *Pediatr Radiol* **26**: 779–781.

Yates PO (1959) Birth trauma to the vertebral arteries. *Arch Dis Child* **34**: 436–441.

Zangwill SD, Strasburger JF (2004) Commotio cordis. *Pediatr Clin North Am* **51**: 1347–1354.

Zhou C, Khalil TB, King AL (1996) Viscoelastic response of the human brain to sagittal and lateral rotational acceleration by finite element analysis. Paper presented at the International IRCOBI Conference on the Biomechanics of Impacts.

Zimmerman RA, Bilaniuk LT, Bruce D, Schut L, Uzzell B, Goldberg HI (1978) Interhemispheric acute subdural haematoma: a computed tomographic manifestation of child abuse by shaking. *Neuroradiology* **16**: 39–40.

Zimmerman RA, Bilaniuk LT, Bruce D, Schut L, Uzzell B, Goldberg HI (1979) Computed tomography of craniocerebral injury in the abused child. *Radiology* **130**: 687–690.

Zouros A, Bhargava R, Hoskinson M, Aronyk KE (2004) Further characterization of traumatic subdural collections in infancy. Report of five cases. *J Neurosurg Spine* **100**: 512–518.

2
THE BIOMECHANICS OF SHAKING

Chris N Morison and Robert A Minns

If all component parts of the intracranial cavity were the same density, when the head was accelerated every molecule would be subjected to the same acceleration and there would be no reason for one molecule to move in relation to its neighbour. However, although the brain is similar in terms of density throughout, the grey and white matter are of very slightly different densities which results in movement of one molecule towards the next, depending on the type of acceleration, particularly at the grey–white interface. This may be exemplified by a set 'jelly' which, when moved, is seen to vibrate more at the top than at the base where it is more dense.

For a model with two densities subjected to linear acceleration there is little change at the interface, e.g. an oil-on-water combination moving in one plane does not disrupt the interface. Rotation, however, produces rotational accelerations with much disruption at the interface between the two densities. Tangential acceleration is evident when a mass is submerged in a liquid which is rotated. The greatest differential movement is seen near the outer boundary and the minimal differential movement near the centre of the mass (Fig. 2.1). There is therefore a gradient of accelerations and forces that are not the same in adjacent planes and this gradient results in a 'shear strain' which in the cranium results in vascular shearing (subdural haematoma), white matter shearing (tears and axonal injury), and shearing of dural attachments at places of fixation of the brain to the skull.

Subdural haematoma in shaken baby syndrome

Although shaken baby syndrome (SBS) is a collection of various injuries including retinal haemorrhages, subdural haematoma, hypoxia, and fractures/bruising, the subdural haematoma, acute or otherwise, is usually the main presenting injury and therefore is commonly the primary diagnostic evidence of shaking.

Subdural haemorrhages (SDHs) are caused when the motion of the brain within the skull stretches and tears the bridging veins (Fig. 2.2a). There are between 15 and 20 of these veins which drain backwards from the surface of the cerebral cortex, through the pia mater, across the subarachnoid space, through the arachnoid, across the subdural space and finally through the dura mater and into the venous sinus. The arachnoid is closely apposed to the dura mater and hence the subdural space is only a 'potential' space, compared to the 1–10 mm wide subarachnoid space. However, it has been shown (Yamashima and Friede 1984) that bridging veins are weaker in the subdural space, which perhaps explains why SDH is more common than subarachnoid haemorrhage in SBS (Fig. 2.2b).

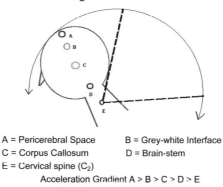

Tangential Acceleration

A = Pericerebral Space   B = Grey-white Interface
C = Corpus Callosum   D = Brain-stem
E = Cervical spine (C_2)
Acceleration Gradient A > B > C > D > E

Fig. 2.1. Schematic diagram of acceleration gradients in an infant head during anteroposterior rotation.

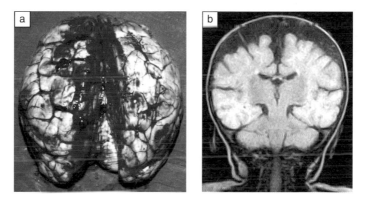

Fig 2.2. (a) Torn bridging vein in the parasaggital region with associated interhemispheric and convexity subdural haemorrhage. (b) Flair coronal MRI of a 12-month-old child who was born at 28 weeks gestation. In the second half of infancy the head circumference had increased from the 25th to the 98th centile. The ventricles are at the upper limit of normal size and there is a mild delay in myelination. A marked increase in the subarachnoid space is visible, particularly superiorly, with a taut bridging vein traversing the subarachnoid space, seen over the right hemisphere in this image. The widened subarachnoid space may reflect the extreme end of benign macrocrania or external communicating hydrocephalus.

When one or more bridging veins bleed into the subdural space the resulting subdural haematoma can either be acute or subacute. An acute subdural haematoma causes severe interruption of blood flow through the cerebrum as well as pressure on the cerebral cortex. Symptoms are immediate, and require swift treatment if the chances of brain damage and death are to be minimized. A subacute subdural haematoma may not cause immediate symptoms since the volume of blood loss is smaller and symptoms may develop over a longer period of time. However, absorption of water as the haematoma breaks down causes a gradual increase of pressure on the cerebral cortex and a deterioration in health which, if left undiagnosed, and treated can again result in serious brain damage or death.

107

THE STRENGTH OF BRIDGING VEINS

The severity of injury caused by bridging vein failure has led to several studies into their mechanical failure properties (Löwenhielm 1974, Lee and Haut 1989, Meaney 1991, Morison 2002). As well as determining the stretch ratio (λ, defined as the ratio of extended length to initial length) at failure, one question these studies tried to answer was whether or not the failure properties are dependent upon strain rate (ε, defined as the ratio of speed to initial length). That is to say, do they change as the speed of the applied stretch is varied? To answer this question the bridging vein testing equipment used in the studies must have the ability to stretch the veins at a wide range of speeds, and importantly they must ensure that the required speed is attained within a negligible stretch of the vein samples, and that the steady speed is maintained throughout each test.

The first three published studies of bridging vein failure criteria all used different methods of mounting and stretching the vein samples, and also extracted their bridging vein samples from cadavers of different age ranges using different methods. A brief summary of the studies follows.

Löwenhielm (1974)

The first mechanical tests of human parasagittal bridging veins were performed by Löwenhielm (1974). He successfully tested 22 samples taken from 11 persons aged between 13 and 87 years and who had no previous brain injury. The veins were held at each end by clips, with one end connected to a rigidly held force transducer and the other end attached to a massive steel cylinder which was free to move axially, with the axis of the cylinder parallel to the axis of the vein. This cylinder was impacted by a second cylinder which was mounted in a tube and accelerated to a steady velocity by compressed air. It was shown that the loss of velocity during one trial was less than 4% and the speed was therefore considered constant. In the 22 successful tests, the rupture of the bridging veins occurred at random positions, but in about one-quarter of the conducted trials the bridging veins were torn at their insertion at the clip and these were considered void and discarded.

The vein samples were tested at strain rates between 2/s (i.e. the vein would be stretched by twice its original length every second) and 1000/s which resulted in ultimate stretch ratios between 1.14 and 1.83 respectively, with a negative logarithmic relation in between. This suggests that the bridging vein properties exhibit strong strain-rate dependence.

Lee and Haut (1989)

Lee and Haut (1989) were the next to perform mechanical tests to investigate the strain-rate dependence of human bridging vein properties, and their results challenge those of Löwenhielm (1974). They tested a total of 139 parasagittal bridging veins from eight unembalmed human cadavers aged between 62 and 85 years without noticeable head trauma or cerebrovascular disease. The veins were tested in a servo-controlled hydraulic testing machine at low strain rates of 0.1–2.5/s or high strain rates of 100 to 250/s while bathed in saline at 37°C.

The authors reported that "no gross damage of the vessel was observed up to the ultimate stretch [ratio of approximately 1.5], thereafter necking of the specimen appeared." From their plot of ultimate stretch ratio versus strain rate, the ultimate stretch appears to vary between 1.15 and 1.88 at strain rates of 0.2/s, between 1.24 and 2.00 at strain rates of 2/s, and between 1.32 and 2.00 at strain rates of 200/s. In the text the ultimate stretch is quoted as 1.5 ± 0.24 at low strain rates and 1.55 ± 0.15 at high strain rates. This led to the conclusion that strain rate had no significant effect on the measured failure properties.

Meaney (1991)

In his PhD thesis, Meaney (1991) also performed dynamic tests of human bridging veins, mainly due to the disagreement between the previous two studies. Meaney's testing system consisted of a solenoid connected to the specimen though a linkage which produced strain rates up to 250/s. The samples were mounted on stainless steel tubing, which allowed them to be perfused with saline during testing. Parasagittal bridging veins were obtained within 24 hours post-mortem from 59 unembalmed cadavers ranging in age from 9 to 62 years and which showed no sign of head injury. The results indicate a lack of dependency of the ultimate stretch ratio upon strain rate, with average stretch ratio of 1.55 for all strain rates used.

Morison (2002)

Although the previous three studies resulted in consistent failure stretch ratios of around 1.5, the question remains as to whether the failure properties are dependent upon strain rate. A possible reason for the difference in strain rate dependence found by each study is their respective methods of applying the strain to the vein samples. Calculations show that it would be very difficult for a direct current (DC) motor to apply enough acceleration to one end of the veins to ensure that the required strain rate is achieved within a negligible strain. The reports by Lee and Haut and Meaney do not confirm the ability of their equipment to reach the required strain rates before the veins break. Perhaps the only method of achieving the high accelerations necessary is to use a form of impact, as did the original experiments by Löwenhielm which demonstrated clear strain-rate dependence. Furthermore, none of the previous experiments investigated the failure properties of human infant bridging veins.

Therefore, as part of his PhD research into the biomechanics of SBS, this author along with others at the University of Birmingham in the UK built a bridging vein testing rig designed to stretch human infant bridging veins using a DC motor at the lower speeds, but using an impact with a pendulum to achieve the higher speeds and accelerations. The testing rig is shown in Figure 2.3, set up for use with the DC motor (shown in the left of the figure). When released from horizontal, the pendulum would impact against the rig causing it to accelerate to 3 m/s within only 10% strain of average length human infant bridging veins.

The timing of these experiments happened to coincide with the enquiry into organ retention at Alder Hey Children's Hospital in Liverpool, UK. Therefore, the local ethics committee determined that an additional consent form should be presented to the parents giving details of the experiments, why they were necessary, exactly what would be taken from their child during the post-mortem examination (a maximum of four bridging veins) and how they would be disposed of afterwards. Parents proved to be very unwilling to give their consent, perhaps because of the negative publicity circulating at the time, resulting in

TABLE 2.1
Results of all four attempts to measure the failure properties of human bridging veins

Study	Samples	Age range	Result	Range
Lee and Haut (1989)	139	62–85 y	$\lambda_{ult} = 1.513$	±0.35
Löwenhielm (1974)	22	13–87 y	$\lambda_{ult} = 1.767 - 0.88 \ln \varepsilon$	±0.15
Meaney (1991)	59	9–62 y	$\lambda_{ult} = 1.550$	±0.25
Morison (2002)	3	0–12 wk	$\lambda_{ult} = 1.433$	±0.31

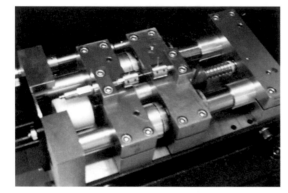

Fig. 2.3. Bridging vein testing rig used for the University of Birmingham research into bridging vein failure properties.

access to only three cadavers from which seven samples were excised. This made it impossible to examine the effect of strain rate. Instead all the samples were tested at a constant, relatively low speed to determine whether or not the equipment was capable of producing consistent results at equal strain rates. Furthermore, difficulties in mounting the extremely small and viscous veins to the testing rig meant that only three of the vein samples were successfully tested.

Although the very limited number of samples meant that these experiments could not produce statistically relevant results, Table 2.1 shows that the results fell within the ranges reported by the previous research. One point these experiments did clearly demonstrate is that bridging veins are very small and extremely delicate and their properties can vary significantly between individuals. This makes it very difficult to rely on tolerance criteria quoted in previous research which are themselves just the averages of a wide range of values. Table 2.1 indicates that for some veins stretches of as little as 1.15 may be enough to cause failure, therefore SBS tolerance criteria based on the commonly quoted average ultimate stretch of 1.5 may be significantly overestimated. It must also be remembered that SBS is usually caused when bridging veins fail, but is most likely to occur when the weakest veins fail.

ROLE OF THE CEREBROSPINAL FLUID

Until Holbourn (1943) demonstrated the importance of rotation in head injury, it was assumed that most internal head injuries were caused by impacts and translational accelerations of the head. Holbourn explained that linear acceleration forces tend to produce

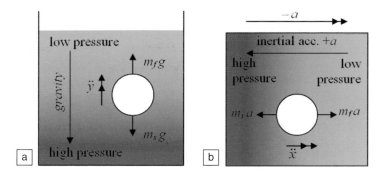

Fig. 2.4. Inertial and buoyancy forces acting on submerged bodies.

compressional strains in the brain tissue, while rotational accelerations produce shear strains. Brain tissue is much stronger in compression than it is in shear, therefore Holbourn concluded that rotational accelerations are much more likely to cause injury than linear accelerations. This was demonstrated by filling a narrow-necked flask with water and adding shredded cotton wool in order to highlight any movement of the water. This approximately represents the cranial contents if one assumes that nerve tissue, blood and cerebrospinal fluid (CSF) all have approximately the same density as water. When this flask was accelerated purely linearly there was no discernible movement of the water; however, when the flask was suddenly rotated the water tended to stay behind and only the flask rotated.

Despite this hypothesis, the effect that the CSF might have on the motion of the brain has been largely ignored or perceived to be merely acting as a 'shock absorber'. In nearly all previous computer models of the head, the CSF has either been totally omitted or modelled as a solid with low shear modulus.

Further to Holbourn's explanation for the increased risk of injury from rotational accelerations, Hodgson et al. (2001) describe a consequence of Archimedes' principle that explains the different role played by the CSF during rotational and translational accelerations. Archimedes' principle states that a body immersed in a fluid is buoyed up by a force equal to the weight of the displaced fluid. This can be inserted into Newton's Second Law of Motion for the body (neglecting fluid resistance) shown in Figure 2.4a as the final term in the equation:

$$m_s \ddot{y} = -m_s g + m_f g \qquad \textbf{equation 1}$$

or

$$\ddot{y} = -g \left(1 - \frac{\rho_f}{\rho_s}\right) \qquad \textbf{equation 2}$$

where m_s and m_f are the masses of the submerged body and displaced fluid, ρ_s and ρ_f are the densities of the body and fluid, g is the gravitational acceleration (downwards) and $\ddot{y}$ is the vertical acceleration of the submerged body (upwards). This buoyancy force is present because

111

the gravitational field produces a pressure gradient in the fluid with a high pressure below the submerged body and a lower pressure above it resulting in a net vertical force on the body. If the solid is denser than the fluid ($\rho_s > \rho_f$) then its acceleration will be negative and it will sink. Conversely if the solid is less dense than the fluid then it will rise, and if the solid and fluid have equal densities then the solid will remain stationary within the fluid.

'Buoyancy' forces will exist in any fluid which contains a pressure gradient, whether or not it is caused by gravity. Figure 2.4b shows a container completely filled with a fluid in which a sphere is submerged. If the container is accelerated to the right then a high pressure will be produced in the fluid to the left of the body graduating to a low pressure to the right of the body. Viewing the contents of the container from a frame of reference moving with it, every particle of matter within the container will experience an inertial acceleration to the left. This inertial acceleration is equivalent to the gravitational acceleration in Figure 2.4a, and hence equation 2 can be modified to give:

$$\ddot{x} = - a \left(1 - \frac{\rho_f}{\rho_s} \right) \qquad \textbf{equation 3}$$

where a is the inertial acceleration experienced within the moving container, and x is the horizontal acceleration of the body relative to the moving container. Therefore, if the solid is denser than the fluid ($\rho_s > \rho_f$) then its acceleration (relative to the moving container) will be negative and it will move to the left within the container. Viewing from a fixed (inertial) frame of reference, the container will be moving to the right with acceleration a and the solid will also be moving to the right but with the reduced acceleration $a + \ddot{x}$ (where $\ddot{x}$ is negative). Again, if the solid and fluid have equal densities then the solid will remain stationary relative to the container.

This perfectly explains the 'cushioning effect' of the CSF on the brain during translational accelerations, since an accelerated head can be simplified to the system in Figure 2.4b, with the skull, brain and CSF represented by the rigid container, the submerged solid and the fluid respectively. As the skull is accelerated backwards as a rigid body in pure translation (e.g. after an impact to the forehead with a padded surface), the brain will accelerate forwards within the skull by an amount given in equation 3. If the brain and CSF were to have equal densities, then the acceleration of the brain within the skull would be zero and bridging veins would not be stretched. Unfortunately the brain is slightly denser than the CSF, with a mean brain density of $1040\,kg/m^3$ (Ruan and Prasad 1996) vs a CSF density of $1005\,kg/m^3$ (Saladin 1998). Equation 3 then gives a relative brain acceleration of $\ddot{x} = -0.337a$, meaning that the buoyancy force produced by the CSF would have the effect of reducing the acceleration of the brain within the skull to only 3.4% of the acceleration of an unsupported brain with no CSF. Furthermore, this acceleration reduction is achieved without applying any high localized forces to any part of the brain. Unfortunately, this buoyancy force offers no protection against rotational accelerations, and as the container is rotated, the solid would remain stationary (neglecting viscous drag forces). Perhaps this more adequately explains the findings of those researchers whose experiments have shown a vulnerability of various species to brain injury caused by rotation compared to an ability to withstand large translational acceleration without injury. For example, the primate experiments of Ommaya and Gennarelli (1974) involved applying pure rotation to the heads of 12 squirrel monkeys, and pure translation to a further 12 monkeys. Peak positive accelerations ranged between 665G and 1230G over an angle of 45° or a displacement of 1 inch (2.5cm). All the animals in the rotated group exhibited evidence of cerebral concussion or traumatic unconsciousness, while none of the translated group showed this effect. Also, the rotated groups all suffered subdural and subarachnoid haematomas, compared to only five focal subdural and one focal subarachnoid haematomas in the translated group.

Similarly, May et al. (1979) observed that woodpeckers can withstand prolonged repetitive decelerations of the order of 1000G without experiencing any concussion, yet can be knocked unconscious by inadvertently flying head first into a window. Analysis of high-speed footage of woodpecker drilling showed that the strike trajectory of the tip of the beak was straight, and that the trajectories of the vertex and the centre of the head were also essentially translational.

Can shaking alone really cause SBS?

The medico-legal community is still painfully aware of a lack of conclusive evidence either for or against the capacity for SBS to be caused by shaking alone. In fact, specialists in the diagnosis and treatment of SBS find contradiction between the currently accepted publications which seem to prove the necessity of impact to cause such severe injuries, and their own clinical observations and investigations which seem to produce many occurrences of SBS symptoms in which they themselves are convinced that there was no impact.

Therefore the question remains as to whether or not shaking alone can kill a baby, and if it can, what degree of shaking is necessary? Furthermore, can the contradiction between the cumulative clinical observations which support SBS and the biomechanical investigations which support the notion of shaken impact syndrome be explained?

This chapter has already explained the history and prominent symptoms of SBS and has demonstrated the importance of rotation, the bridging veins, and CSF. It will now critically review the published literature on the subject of shaking versus impact and will then report the results of new investigations into the biomechanics of the shaker (i.e. the extent to which humans of various ages could shake a baby), and also the results of the first three-dimensional computer model of SBS which was specifically designed to include the real effects of the CSF.

Literature review

IN SUPPORT OF SBS

The literature in support of SBS consists largely of clinical observations, starting with Guthkelch (1971) who was perhaps the first to explain the unusually high incidence of subdural haematoma occurring in battered children compared to head injuries of other origin. Guthkelch also remarked on the similarity between injuries caused by severe whiplash in an automobile accident (with no head impact) and those which are known to exist in the many cases of so-called 'battered child syndrome'. He studied 23 cases of proven or suspected parental assault on children, and found no evidence of direct violence to the head in five of the 13 cases involving SDH. In addition he described two cases in which there was a very strong reason to suppose that the mechanism of production of the SDH had been shaking rather than battering. He also remarked that "'a good shaking' is felt to be socially more acceptable and physically less dangerous than a blow on the head or elsewhere."

The term 'whiplash shaken infant syndrome' was probably first coined by Caffey in 1974 to differentiate injuries sustained from the habitual shaking of infants – where there is no evidence of external trauma to the head – from the 'battered child syndrome' which had previously been used to categorize most cases of suspicious infant death or injury. Caffey's research (1972, 1974) collated many previous reported cases of bilateral subdural haematomas, intraocular haemorrhages and multiple traction changes in the long bones where there was no evidence of external head trauma and/or strong testimony suggesting that the injuries could only have been the product of shaking.

A study of 134 battered children was published by Smith and Hanson (1974) from the University of Birmingham, UK only a few months before Caffey (1974) defined 'whiplash shaken infant syndrome'. Intracranial haemorrhages were found in 47 children, consisting of 30 subdural, nine subarachnoid, and eight cerebral haemorrhages. Of these, 15 had no skull fractures, and seven had no head bruises but instead showed finger and thumb shaped bruises on the trunk and arms. The authors believe that these children were violently shaken and are in support of Guthkelch's (1971) suggestion that whiplash injury rather than direct blows accounts for intracranial bleeding.

McClelland et al. (1980) examined 21 patients with cerebral injury as a result of child abuse. SBS was suspected in six of these cases (median age 5.5 months) due to the presence of subdural haematoma, retinal haemorrhage, severe central nervous system dysfunction, bulging fontanelle, hemiplegia (paralysis affecting only one side of the body), or extensor posturing (stiffly extended and internally rotated arms and/or legs). X-rays showed normal skulls in five of these six patients and an occipital skull fracture in the remaining case. Unfortunately bruising is not mentioned in this study, so it is difficult to isolate pure shaking from shaking with soft impact.

A biomechanical study by Gennarelli and Thibault (1982) proved that impact is not necessary to cause acute subdural haematoma in primates. In this study, the heads of rhesus monkeys were securely fitted into a helmet that was attached to a pneumatic actuator and linkage system. The system was programmed to deliver a single acceleration–deceleration pulse to the head by rotating it though a 60° arc in times varying from 5 to 25 milliseconds with magnitudes between 100 and 3000 G. Angular acceleration produced acute subdural haematoma of sufficient size to cause the animal's death in 37 of 128 cases. The haematomas were usually bilateral overlying the ruptured parasagittal bridging veins, although most often much larger on one side. It should be noted, however, that the acceleration magnitudes and especially the frequencies used in this study were much higher than could probably be produced by an adult manually shaking an infant. The definition of acute subdural haematoma used in this study is also noteworthy, since acute subdural haematoma was considered present only if there was sufficient blood in the subdural space to cause death. There was no separate classification for non-fatal subdural haematomas which could eventually have led to brain damage. The choice of the magnitude of the deceleration phase of the loading as the criterion has also been criticised by various authors (Lee et al. 1987, Lee and Haut 1989), who correctly highlight the fact that the majority of bridging veins have been shown to drain forwards from the brain into the venous sinus and hence they would be stretched more during forward acceleration, whereas forward deceleration would cause compression before tension. Therefore, even though the deceleration used by Gennarelli and Thibault was several times the magnitude of the prior acceleration, use of the deceleration magnitude as the failure criterion may have significantly overestimated the tolerances for subdural haematoma.

Hadley et al. (1989) found 13 individuals suspected of having a clinical history of shaking injury without direct cranial trauma in 36 infants identified as having non-accidental head injury. This was a prospective study over a period of 6 years. The criteria met by these 13 patients were (1) a documented history of infant shaking as admitted by the perpetrator, and (2) no historical, clinical or radiographic evidence of direct impact trauma to the cranio-facial region. Eight of these 13 patients died. Computed tomography (CT) findings reported the presence of subdural haematoma in all 13 patients judged as 'present' in three, 'moderate' in seven and 'severe' in three patients. The authors conclude that direct cranial impact is 'not always' required, especially in the very young.

A study by Alexander et al. (1990) was specifically designed to determine the presence of external signs of head trauma in suspected cases of SBS. Over a 4 year period, 24 infants between the ages of 3 and 59 weeks were diagnosed as having injuries consistent with the intracranial injuries attributed to shaking. All participants in the study underwent physical examination, or autopsy examination if the child died, which looked specifically for signs of direct head trauma. It was found that 12 of these children had no signs of external head trauma; and from a total of nine fatal cases, five had no signs of external head trauma. This supports the hypothesis that shaking alone is sufficient to cause serious intracranial injury. Furthermore, the lack of a correlation between mortality and evidence of impact suggests that severe injury can occur with shaking alone.

A review of the non-accidental head injury literature by Brown and Minns (1993) mentions 30 children with non-accidental head injury seen by the authors. Shaking was thought to be the cause of 17 of these cases, with impact attributed to the other 13. A subdural haematoma was diagnosed in 16 of the 30 cases, and was the only finding in three cases.

Gilliland and Folberg (1996) performed a prospective study of 169 child deaths, and found 80 deaths due to head trauma. Evidence of shaking was considered present if two or more of the following criteria were met: (1) finger marks and/or rib fractures; (2) subdural and/or subarachnoid haemorrhage; (3) a history of vigorous shaking. Direct head trauma was defined as either scalp or skull injuries. They found that nine (11.3%) of the deaths had evidence only of shaking, 30 (37.5%) had evidence of shaking and impact, and the remaining 41 (51.3%) had evidence only of impact. Their evidence supports the theory that "shaking alone is a lethal mechanism of injury"; however, they do point out that in their study most infants believed to have been shaken had some evidence of impact injury.

Lazoritz et al. (1997) noticed that Caffey's original definition of 'whiplash shaken infant syndrome', and today's 'shaken baby syndrome' or 'shaken impact syndrome' is now commonly used in cases which clearly involve impacts and even in some cases of impact without shaking, and so he undertook a study for comparison with Caffey's original study (1974). Seventy-one individuals identified as having a subdural haematoma caused by non-accidental means were included in the study. The incidence of subdural haematoma with no evidence of impact trauma is not explicitly stated, although shaking was admitted initially in nine (12.7%) cases and after the conclusion of an investigation in two additional cases. No explanation was given for the injuries in 24 (33.8%) cases, with falls or head impacts being reported in the remaining cases. Skull fractures were found in 13 (18.3%) cases, and rib or long-bone fractures in 23 (32.4%) cases. Scalp bruising without underlying fractures is not reported. The report concludes that "the term shaken impact syndrome should be avoided, and . . . it should be acknowledged that shaken infant syndrome is a syndrome of severe head injury to infants caused by either shaking alone or by shaking plus impact."

Tzioumi and Oates (1998) found a very high incidence of shaking-only cases in their 10-year retrospective study of subdural haematomas in children under 2 years. They found subdural haematomas in 38 children, 21 of which were ascribed to non-accidental causes, with a mean age of 5.3 months. Shaking – diagnosed when there were no associated injuries to the head or where there was an admission by the caregiver – accounted for 16 of these 21 cases. Surprisingly, 6 of the 'shaken' children were found to have only unilateral SDHs, whereas shaking is usually thought to produce bilateral haemorrhages as reported by Caffey (1974) and Gennarelli and Thibault (1982). However, the authors refute the possibility that child abuse was over-diagnosed in children with unilateral subdurals since in one of these cases the mother admitted to shaking the infant.

In a report on four pairs of twins, five children of whom experienced SBS, Becker et al. (1998) reported that shaking was admitted to in three of the cases. Also, confirming one of Guthkelch's (1971) observations, they reported that "Two parents believed that the shaking was a less violent approach than striking."

Research by Barlow and Minns (1999) relating intracranial pressure to outcome in non-accidental head injury focused on 17 individuals with an average age of 5.1 months. Seven of these individuals had subdural haematomas, retinal haemorrhages and rib fractures but no evidence of impact and so were thought to be victims of pure whiplash-shaking. Evidence of impact was defined as bruising to the head, subgaleal haematoma (found either clinically or with imaging), or skull fracture.

Research by DiScala et al. (2000) examined the cases of 1997 abused and 16831 un-intentionally injured children under the age of 5 years, extracted from a database covering the 10 years between 1988 and 1997. The sex, age, history, nature and severity of injury, diagnostic procedures used, and outcomes were compared between both groups. The median age for child abuse was 8 months, compared with 28 months for accidental injury, also 53% of abused infants had a previous medical history compared with 14.1% of accident victims. Battering was reported in 53% of the abuse cases and shaking in 10.3%. Children in the abuse group were significantly more likely to sustain injury to the thorax (12.5% versus 4.5%) and abdomen (11.4% versus 6.8%). Both groups sustained similar numbers of injuries to the head (62% for abused, 59.9% for accidental), and of those subgroups, the abused children experienced more intracranial injury (42.2% versus 14.1%) but less skull fracture without intracranial injury (13.7% versus 19.2%) and less concussion or other unspecified closed

116

head injury (6.2% versus 26.6%). Unfortunately those are the only head injuries distinguished in this report — there are no data for scalp bruising which makes it difficult to isolate pure shaking cases from cases with shaking and soft impact.

A review of all intracranial haemorrhages seen by a child protection team during 1997 was performed by Morris et al. (2000), extracted from more than 400 cases of alleged physical abuse. A total of 32 cases of intracranial haemorrhage (subarachnoid, epidural and subdural) were found, 19 of which were possible child abuse. Eight of these 19 cases were excluded from further study because they had inflicted bruises and/or fractures of abuse and/or retinal haemorrhages, leaving nine infants with pure subdural haematoma who lacked external bruises, fractures, and retinal haemorrhages. This gives an incidence of 9/19 subdural haematomas with no evidence of head impact, a figure which excludes cases which may have had retinal haemorrhages and bruising of the thorax, both of which are common in classical SBS.

A report by Maxeiner (2001) mentions 10 cases of subdural haematoma in which four children had no external or internal injuries on the face or head. In one of these cases a detailed confession of violent shaking was made which was consistent with the findings.

Recent studies by Geddes et al. (2001a,b) confirm the presence of acute subdural haematoma in infants who have been shaken. Their neuropathological study of 53 cases of non-accidental head injury in infants (37, age <1 year) and children (16, age ≥1 year) revealed only eight cases, all infants, where no bruising or fracture was found at autopsy. These infants were assumed to have been shaken, and in one case the carer confessed to having shaken the infant. Eighty-one percent (43 of 53) of the total cases (including 31 of the infants) were found to have subdural haematomas, including seven of the eight shaken infants.

In Support of Shaken Impact Syndrome

The main proponents of 'shaken impact syndrome' are a team in Philadelphia (Duhaime et al. 1987) whose study concluded that it was unlikely that shaking alone could generate enough force to cause acute subdural haematoma. Their initial hypothesis was based on the review of 48 individuals identified with suspected SBS, ranging in age from 1 month to 2 years. Only 12 of these cases had intracranial damage without any evidence of impact trauma, and all of the 13 fatal cases had some evidence of blunt head trauma (although in seven of these cases the impact findings were noted only at autopsy and had not been apparent prior to death).

They tested their hypothesis by fixing accelerometers inside the head of lifelike dolls of 1 month-old infants and subjecting these dolls to repetitive violent shaking followed by an impact against either a metal bar or a padded surface. The mean peak tangential acceleration of the shaking and impacts were 9.29G and 428.18G respectively, with mean time intervals of 106.6ms and 20.9ms respectively. When these values were compared with scaled tolerance criteria for brain injury in primates (Thibault and Gennarelli 1985, see below), the angular acceleration and velocity associated with shaking were below the injury range, while the values for impacts spanned concussion, subdural haematoma, and diffuse axonal injury (DAI) ranges. This led to the conclusion that "shaken baby syndrome, at least in its most severe acute form, is not usually caused by shaking alone" (Duhaime et al. 1987).

Evidence of impact was found in all 10 cases reported by Elner et al. (1990). This paper primarily reports the incidence of ocular injuries (which were present in seven of 10 sequential cases of suspected child abuse) but also highlights the difficulty of spotting evidence of direct head impact, which, although present in all 10 cases, was sometimes subtle or hidden beneath the hair. In two of the seven detailed cases with ocular injuries, evidence of blunt head trauma was apparent only at autopsy, during which one of these cases was found to have a skull fracture.

A retrospective study by Howard et al. (1993) considered 28 cases of infantile subdural haematoma over 20 years and also found little or no evidence to suggest that shaking alone is enough to cause subdural haematoma. This evidence is presented in a variety of formats:

- Ten of the cases resulted in legal action, five of which had history of assault or evidence of impact injury, with carers of the five remaining infants claiming that their child had fallen but with no unbiased witnesses to verify their history. On physical examination of the five claimed fall cases, all were found to have retinal haemorrhages, with minimal scalp injury seen in one case and no evidence of scalp injury in four cases. However, CT appeared to show skull fracture in two of these final four cases. In other words, only two of the 28 subdural haematomas could possibly have been caused by shaking alone, because they could not be satisfactorily explained by witnessed injury or evidence of head impact.
- Three of the 28 infants were reported to have been shaken; however, in all three cases the history and clinical findings revealed that the infant had also sustained a direct impact injury.
- In total, 14 of the 28 subdural haematoma cases showed no external signs of head injury, a figure in line with those reported by Guthkelch (1971) and Alexander et al. (1990) among others. However, 13 of these 14 infants with normal scalp examination sustained a fall observed by multiple unbiased witnesses (6), had an underlying skull fracture (2) or scalp contusion on post-mortem examination (1), or were likely to have suffered an impact injury more than 1 week prior to evaluation (4).

Issues raised by the Duhaime study

The 1987 publication by Duhaime et al. summarized above appears to provide strong evidence to support their conclusion that severe SBS symptoms are unlikely to be caused by shaking alone, and is often quoted in the prosecution of those alleged to have battered children as proof that the level of violence must be higher than that perhaps admitted to. However, deeper research into the primate experiments used as a basis for the tolerance criteria, and the scaling function used to scale the tolerance criteria to the brain mass of a human infant, reveals several factors which bring into doubt the validity of this conclusion.

The primate experiments (Thibault and Gennarelli 1985) involved subjecting monkeys' heads to known accelerations and velocities, thereby inducing varying degrees of cerebral damage ranging from concussion through to acute subdural haematoma and diffuse axonal injury. This produced tolerance criteria in the form of minimum accelerations and velocities required to cause different levels of damage in the monkey. The frequencies used in the primate experiments are not known; however, the same Philadelphian team

118

consistently used frequencies between 50 and 100 Hz in their experiments (Ommaya and Gennarelli 1974, Gennarelli et al. 1982, Margulies et al. 1985, *inter alia*), and if such high frequencies were used to develop these tolerance levels then they may not be directly applicable to manual shaking which was found to produce frequencies of only around 4 Hz (Duhaime et al. 1987).

The scaling function used by Duhaime et al. (1987) to scale the rhesus monkey tolerance criteria found by Thibault and Gennarelli (1985) to tolerance criteria for human infants was presented by Ommaya et al. (1967) after it was proposed in a private communication from Holbourn in 1956. The function was originally developed to scale tolerance criteria for diffuse axonal injury and cerebral concussion, both of which are injuries to the brain matter caused by high shear strains. The function was based on seven assumptions, two of which are: (1) both brains are geometrically similar, through one scale factor; and (2) injury is the result of shear strains exceeding a certain value.

Both of these assumptions would individually invalidate the use of the scaling function for converting rhesus monkey tolerance criteria to human infant tolerance criteria, the latter more so than the former. Although rhesus monkeys' brains are a similar shape to those of human babies, they are not geometrically similar through one scale factor. More significantly, moreover, subdural haematoma is not the result of high shear strains within the brain tissue itself; rather, it is caused by relative motion between the surface of the brain and the skull resulting in bridging vein rupture. Therefore it does not seem realistic to apply this scaling function to tolerance levels for subdural haematoma. Indeed, applying this scaling function without taking into account the much lower shear modulus (viscosity) of the CSF compared to brain tissue, and the much wider layer of CSF in infants than adults and monkeys would result in grossly overestimated tolerance criteria.

Cory and Jones (2003), in an attempt to test the validity of the Duhaime biomechanical 1-month-old baby model, constructed a replica, tested it, and found that in 80% of cases, the angular head acceleration results exceeded the original results from Duhaime et al. (1987) and spanned two scaled tolerance limits for concussion. Results from the Cory and Jones study were closer to the internal head injury, subdural haematoma, tolerance limits. A series of end-point impacts were identified in the shake cycles, therefore an impact-based head injury measure (head injury criterion: HIC) was used to assess the severity. Seven of 10 tests conducted resulted in HIC values exceeding the tolerance limits (critical load value, Stürtz 1980) suggested for children.

Problems they identified with the biomechanical study by Duhaime et al. were first that evidence suggests the tolerance limits used to assess the shaking simulation in that study may not have been reliable. Second, the results of all shake tests conducted during the Cory and Jones study identified clear impact of the chin-to-chest and occiput-to-back sections of the shake cycle, therefore the tolerance limits used by Duhaime et al. may not be applicable in the assessment of shaking simulations due to impacts identified in this study. Third, although the Cory and Jones model was not biofidelic, the impact tolerance limits should be assessed with impact-based tolerance limits. Fourth, the cumulative effect of multiple impacts cannot be assessed as the tolerance limits are based on single impacts, and the effects of repeated, consecutive sub-lethal loading are unknown.

119

TABLE 2.2
Summary of SBS research in which clear distinction is made between shaking and impact

Authors	Year	Non-accidental head injury cases	Shaking only cases n	Shaking only cases %	Median age (mo)
Guthkelch	1971	15	7		
Smith and Hanson	1974	47	7		
McClelland et al.	1980	21	5		5.5
Duhaime et al.	1987	48	24		7.85
Hadley et al.	1989	36	13		3
Alexander et al.	1990	24	12		
Elner et al.	1990	10	0		
Howard et al.	1993	28	2		
Brown and Minns	1993	30	17		5
Gilliland and Folberg	1996	80	9	11.3	
Lazoritz et al.	1997	71	11	15.5	
Tzioumi and Oates	1998	21	16		5.3
Barlow and Minns	1999	17	7		5.1
Barlow et al.	1999	12	7		5.7
Gleckman et al.	1999	17	7		4.5
DiScala et al.	2000	1997	206	10.3	8
Morris et al.	2000	19	9		5
Geddes et al.	2001	37	8		
Maxeiner et al.	2001	10	4		
Averages:				32.7	5.5

SUMMARY

The above literature review presents the results of many clinical studies in which incidences of subdural haematoma with and without evidence of shaking are reported. These studies are summarized in Table 2.2. When combined, the data show that almost one-third of non-accidental subdural haematomas have no evidence of impact, which is in itself strong evidence in favour of the existence of the syndrome.

Biomechanics of the 'shaker'

One is often asked in court how much shaking is required to damage a baby. While that is a pertinent question, we have attempted to answer a more basic question about how long and how fast it is possible to shake, i.e. what are the upper limits of duration, frequency and acceleration in a 'shaker'. Also, because children are occasionally the target of accusations, we have included 3- to 15-year-olds in our study (Minns 2005). We do not know for a fact that children can shake or even lift the necessary weights. Obviously the amount of shaking required to cause damage will be less than that which is maximally possible. The discussion below describes the characteristics of the 'shaker'.

The aim of this first simulation study was to determine the maximum duration a person is able to shake dolls of 3, 5.1, 7.1 and 10.7 kg, representing average baby weights at 1, 2, 5 and 12 months respectively, by young adult volunteers, and to measure the frequency (of shakes per second), angular displacement, peak velocity and linear acceleration, and to calculate the theoretical force exerted on the heads of the models, and the peak-to-peak velocity for each shake. Children were not asked to shake dolls but only to shake 'dead weights' of the equivalent size.

Construction of doll models and 'dead weights' were to reflect infant proportions, and it was the 'shaker' who was instrumented. The doll bodies were made from a linen material filled with nylon beads and the heads were of plastic construction. The head was not continuous with the body in order to allow 'whiplashing'. In order to reduce the overall volume, but to maintain the requisite infant weight some nylon beads were replaced with lead-shot. The heads were weighted to approximate those of infants. Although correct proportions were maintained, the construction required a durability to withstand vigorous shaking. The dimensions for the dolls' construction were obtained from 50th centiles on standard growth charts for infants. For the 2-month equivalent doll the mean weight was 5.1 kg, head circumference 37 cm, and length 56 cm. For the 5-month equivalent doll, the weight was 7.1 kg, head circumference 42 cm, and length 64 cm. The 12-month equivalent doll weighed 10.7 kg, head circumference was 51 cm, and length 76.5 cm.

In the construction of the doll models several principles were followed – the limbs were required to flail, the neck was unhinged so that there was no head control, the head-to-body ratio which is relatively increased compared to older children and adults was maintained, and the centre of gravity for the model was kept at a point in a plane above the 'umbilicus'. No reference information was available for such anthropometric data, although it is clear that the centre of mass (gravity) is considerably proximal for an infant compared to that for an adult: that is to say, prone positioning required the examiner's hand in the low chest–upper abdominal region to balance. These principles were followed in the construction of the doll models because it was uncertain what influence they might have on the ability of the shaker to shake.

A total of 94 adult volunteers was recruited (62% of whom were male) at a median age of 23 years. Ninety per cent were students. There were 40 children at a median age of 9 years (range 3–15 years), 19 of whom were boys. The age, sex, height, weight, and left- and right-hand strength were recorded for each of the volunteers. Hand strength was measured by a Martin Vigorometer (analogue sphygmomanometer), and a video recording made of all shakers to allow their preferred method of shaking and their grasp of the doll to be assessed without attention being drawn to it at the time.

Each shaker had a linear accelerometer strapped to the dorsal aspect of the right wrist and a single-axis goniometer fixed over the right elbow joint. Both the goniometer and the accelerometer were calibrated for each volunteer by means of a 90° pronating movement at the wrist indicating 1 G (9.81 m/s) and 90° flexion at the elbow representing an angle of 90°. The measurements were displayed on a chart recorder via an angle display unit and separate G force measuring system.

The method of grasping infants may be by (1) grasping the rib cage/abdomen, (2) grasping the shoulder/upper arms, (3) grasping around the neck, and (4) grasping the ankles. Most volunteers used the first of these by preference.

Using their self-selected grasp each volunteer was requested to shake the doll maximally for the longest duration possible, i.e. to their physical limit, in two different planes (horizontal and vertical) for all doll weights and 'dead weights' for comparison. The volunteers were not asked to shake with impact as pilot data showed the linear accelerations were outside the range of this accelerometer. While this scenario does not equate with a domestic scene and real shaking of infants because it lacks the anger or frustration, it probably does represent a close approximation of what is physically possible. A short sharp burst of intense shaking is likely to be more representative of an *in vivo* episode rather than the subjective physical limits in the experimental situation. Volunteers had timed rest breaks between successive shakes.

Measurements were made from the recording of the duration of shaking of each doll (or weight), peak-to-peak acceleration changes over time, frequency changes over time, and angular displacement changes over time.* The frequency (numbers of shakes per second), acceleration, and angle for each 5-second period was calculated and the average frequency, acceleration, and angle were calculated over the whole period. Analyses were conducted on these averages. Typical examples are shown from the recordings from adults, teenagers and children shaking (Fig. 2.5).

The recordings of the shaking movements have much similarity to a sine wave when maximum effort was applied. This could allow one to calculate the peak velocity:

Velocity$_{peak}$ $= 2\pi f a$ (where f = frequency and a = acceleration)

Descriptive statistics are provided for each variable to give an idea of the distribution of the variable, the majority of which were not normally distributed, and the median and quartiles are thus reported.

$$\text{Average force} = \frac{\text{mass} \times \text{average acceleration}}{100}$$

Average peak velocity over the duration = $2\pi f a$, where f = average frequency, and a = average acceleration, for the duration.

$$\text{Average peak-to-peak velocity} = \frac{\text{average acceleration} \times \text{average frequency}}{2\pi}$$

Multiple linear regression was used to examine which volunteer factors influenced the duration, frequency and acceleration averaged over the whole duration. Regression was considered only for adult shakers and was conducted on the most commonly shaken baby equivalent (2 months/5.1 kg).

Definitions used:

Linear velocity is the distance covered per unit of time: v = distance/time (m/s).

Linear acceleration is the rate of change of velocity: $a = dv/dt$ (m/s^2; also expresssed in relation to gravitational pull, G).

Angular velocity is the rate of rotation: $\omega = d\theta/dt$ (rad/s).

Angular acceleration is the rate of change of angular velocity with respect to time: $\alpha = d\omega/dt$ (rad/s^2).

Tangential acceleration – if the instantaneous angular velocity of a disc is ω, a point at displacement r from the centre will have tangential acceleration: $a_{tang} = \alpha \times r$ (m/s^2)

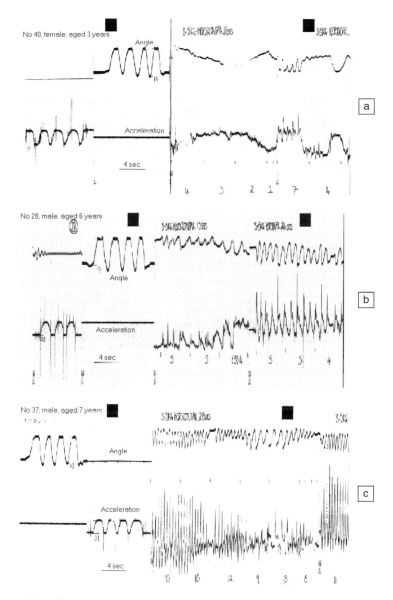

Fig. 2.5. (a–i) Recordings of joint angle at the elbow (upper trace) and acceleration measured at the wrist (lower trace) with preceding signal calibrations are seen in these examples from volunteers, maximally shaking doll models and dead weights, horizontally and vertically to the point of fatigue for only the 3.5 kg weights.

(a) Recording from a 3-year-old girl showing an inability to produce any shaking accelerations horizontally but an interrupted 7 s low-amplitude vertical shake.

(b) A 6-year-boy again found vertical shaking of dead weights considerably easier and produced larger accelerations (over 24 s) than the slow, low-amplitude horizontal shaking over 15 s.

(c) A 7-year-boy shaking horizontally for a lengthy 28 s, but with decreasing acceleration amplitude and slowing after 9 s.

123

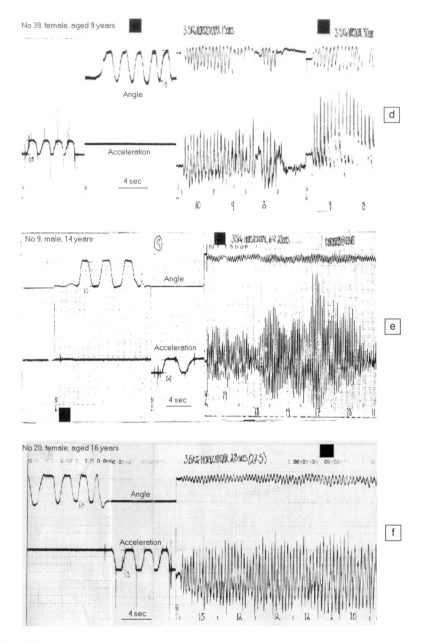

Fig. 2.5 (cont'd)

(d) A 9-year-old girl, with larger accelerations over a longer period vertically (30 s) compared to a 15 s horizontal shake.

(e) A 14-year-old boy, shaking a dead weight for a total of 28 s but with fluctuating intensity of acceleration.

(f) A 16-year-old female shook a 3.5 kg doll horizontally for a total of 27.5 s. Minor fluctuation in intensity occurred throughout, although the rate remained virtually constant.

124

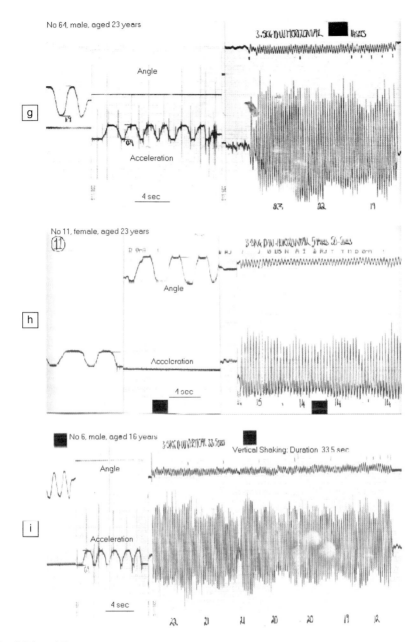

Fig. 2.5 (cont'd)

(g) A 23-year-old male shows a constant high acceleration and fast rate (5/s) of shaking of a dead weight horizontally, over 14 s.

(h) A 23-year-old female managed a long duration horizontal shake of a dead weight for 56.5 s at constant rate of 3/s.

(i) A 16-year-old male with an interrupted shake, minor fluctuations in accelerations vertically (at 4/s) and lasting 33.5 s in total.

TABLE 2.3
Summary table of duration, frequency, mean acceleration and mean angle for adults and children, horizontally shaking dolls and dead weights respectively

	Duration (s)	Frequency (Hz)	Mean acceleration (cm/s^2)	Mean angle (°)
Adults shaking dolls horizontally				
5 kg (2-mo-old equivalent)	23.0	3.5	4360	34.6
7 kg (5-mo-old equivalent)	18.5	3.4	3954	28.0
10 kg (12-mo-old equivalent)	15.0	3.1	4076	26.0
Significance	$p<0.001$	$p<0.001$	ns	$p<0.001$
Children shaking 'weights' horizontally				
3.5 kg (newborn equivalent)	20.0	2.1	2975	38.8
5 kg (2-mo-old equivalent)	16.3	1.9	2087	31.8
7 kg (5-mo-old equivalent)	14.0	1.8	2125	24.0
10 kg(12-mo-old equivalent)	9.5	1.8	1358	28.1
Significance	$p<0.001$	ns	$p<0.002$	$p<0.028$

ADULT SHAKERS

When the 5.1 kg doll was shaken horizontally, the left-hand strength predicted both duration and mean acceleration, i.e. both these measures are predicted by the strength of the weakest arm. This also predicted acceleration when the doll was shaken vertically. Sex also predicted the mean frequency when the doll was shaken vertically, with females shaking at a lower average frequency. We might have anticipated that taller, heavier and stronger people, and males in particular, would be able to shake for a longer duration and with a higher horizontal frequency, but this proved not to be the case in this data set.

Table 2.3 illustrates the differences in duration, mean frequency, acceleration and angle over the whole period by the weight shaken, and it can be seen that for adults shaking dolls of different sizes, the duration of shaking decreased with the increasing load. The load, however, had little influence of the frequency. This is an interesting observation and suggests that the limitation on frequency is likely to be related to muscle and musculoskeletal properties, rather than inertia. It can be seen that the linear accelerations are fairly similar across the different weights. Not unexpectedly, the angular excursion is decreased when shaking a large doll weight. With large weights there is a tendency to 'splint' and 'lock' the wrist and flex the elbow, which results in a smaller angle and therefore tends to underestimate the acceleration.

For adults shaking different 'dead weights' of the same size, results showed a similar effect on duration, i.e. there was a slight decrease with increasing weight, and there was a definite reducing frequency of the shake with larger 'dead weights'. Linear accelerations were similar to those seen during shaking of dolls. The angles were considerably less when shaking 'dead weights' than dolls.

In summary, for adults there was a significant difference in duration, mean frequency and mean angle among the different weights shaken for both dolls and weights ($p < 0.001$) but no differences for mean acceleration for either weights or dolls. No significant differences

Age bands of children who shook weights

Weight	3.2–3.8 yr	4.0–5.8 yr	5.9–9.1 yr	9.2–12.8 yr	12.9–15.7 yr
10.7 kg					
7.1 kg				*	
5.1 kg					
3.0 kg					

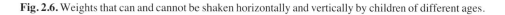

☐ Ages of children, 100% of whom were able to shake specific dead weights
☐ Ages of children, 100% of whom were unable to shake weight

*One child aged 13.1 years was unable to shake a weight of 7.1 kg in the vertical direction

Fig. 2.6. Weights that can and cannot be shaken horizontally and vertically by children of different ages.

were found for adults shaking weights in different directions but there were some differences for dolls shaken in different directions (duration, $p-0.04$; mean angle $p=0.002$; mean acceleration, $p=0.05$) (Minns 2005).

CHILDREN SHAKERS

The 40 children ranged in age from 3 to 15 years. Some of the younger children could not lift or shake the heavier dead weights. The ability to lift the various weights and shake them horizontally and/or vertically by age bands is shown in Figure 2.6.

For children there is a significant difference in duration ($p<0.001$), mean acceleration ($p=0.002$) and mean angle ($p=0.028$) among the four weights, and a significant difference in duration, mean acceleration and mean angle (all $p<0.0001$) between the shaking directions. There was no significant difference in the mean frequency among the weights or between the directions. Table 2.3 shows the reduced duration with shaking heavier weights, and children, like adults, shake with a frequency which seems independent of the weight. Their linear accelerations declined with an increasing load, as did the angles but to a lesser degree (RA Minns, unpublished observations)

ACCELERATION IN THE BABY COMPARED WITH MEASURED ACCELERATION ALONG THE SHAKER'S ARM

When shaking a doll in space, both the doll and the shaker are moving. For shaking to occur horizontally the shaker has either to move the shoulder (otherwise the direction of the shake would be a downward arc) or the wrist angle has to change. Videos show that most of the movements that keep the doll horizontal are at the shoulder, and the wrist is maintained in a 'locked' position at approximately 45° to the doll (this is especially the case if the doll or weight is heavy). This wrist position results in flexion of the elbow and causes a sharper, smaller angle and wave (of acceleration), i.e. as previously mentioned this tends to under-

127

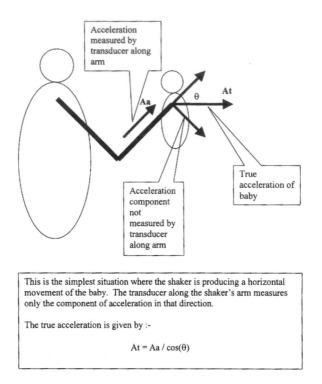

Acceleration measured by transducer along arm

Aa

θ

At

Acceleration component not measured by transducer along arm

True acceleration of baby

This is the simplest situation where the shaker is producing a horizontal movement of the baby. The transducer along the shaker's arm measures only the component of acceleration in that direction.

The true acceleration is given by :-

$$At = Aa / \cos(\theta)$$

Fig. 2.7. Acceleration produced in a baby compared with measured acceleration along shaker's arm.

estimate acceleration when shaking a heavier weight, which causes the body to tip forward. In practical terms, a large baby would need to be held closer to the body and slightly tilted.

The translational acceleration measured in the shaker's arm is in the direction of the arm and the linear acceleration that would be experienced in the doll's head could be calculated by taking into account the angle θ as shown in Figure 2.7. Calculation of the force (in Newtons) that would be experienced in the doll's (baby's) head could be assessed by application of the simple formula:

force = mass × acceleration

With knowledge of the 'time' and the 'length of the arm' and 'angle' one could theoretically project a maximum amplitude acceleration:

Acceleration$_{(peak)}$ = $(2\pi f)^2$ × peak excursion of angle

that is, acceleration is proportional of the square of the frequency. The acceleration experienced by the head of the doll is more accurately measured by means of direct application of accelerometers than by this indirect calculation.

Shaking an object is always a trade-off between frequency and angle, i.e. one can shake fast with a smaller very acute angle or slower with a larger angle. In practical terms we do

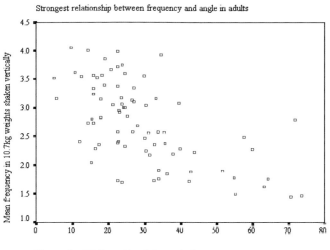

Strongest relationship between frequency and angle in adults

Fig. 2.8. Relation between cubital angle and frequency of shake.

not know what is worse for the infant brain (either a larger acceleration over a shorter time, or a smaller acceleration for a longer time. A more accurate measure would be:

Impulse = force × time

Impulse, however, was not determined in our study as the volunteers were asked to shake as fast and as hard as they possibly could. Figure 2.8 shows the strong relation between frequency and elbow angle in adults who shook a 10.7 kg weight vertically, showing the clear relation between the fast frequency of shake with a narrow angle and a slower frequency over a larger angle.

In the above studies weights were shaken longer than corresponding doll sizes ($p < 0.001$), and dolls were shaken with a higher frequency ($p < 0.001$). These results confirm our suspicion that the infant's anthromorphometry does have an effect on the shaking characteristics over and above the weight similarity and justifies our construction of dolls where the head moves on the trunk, and the arms are allowed to flail.

To construct an identical infant replica would require a substantial research programme as it would need to take into account: the intricate characteristics of the infant neck; the presence of varying degrees of head lag; the precise relation between head and body size; the presence of primitive reflexes involving the neck, e.g. asymmetrical tonic neck reflex, symmetrical tonic neck reflex; the centre of mass of the infant; the pivot point (at approximately C2); and the relative length and weight of the limbs compared to the trunk; all for different stages of infant growth and development.

Biomechanics of the 'shaken'
Early research performed on a gelatine brain model by Holbourn (1943) concluded that

129

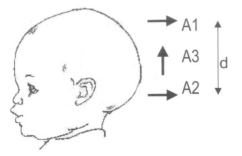

Fig. 2.9. Alignment of accelerometers on doll's head. As shown, accelerometer A3 was mounted with its sensitive axis parallel to the doll's 'vertical' axis which was taken to be the axis of the neck. Accelerometers A1 and A2 were mounted orthogonally to A3 and separated by a distance d metres as shown. All significant movements were assumed to be in the plane of the paper and no measurements were made along the third axis. The calibrated outputs of the accelerometers A1, A2, and A3 were a1 m/s^2, a2 m/s^2, and a3 m/s^2, respectively.

rotational injury was an important determinant in producing concussion and brain injury. Further studies 25 years later by Ommaya et al. (1968) accepted Holbourn's findings; these authors also documented that brain injury could be caused by whiplash without impact.

In the early 1970s, Guthkelch (1971) and Caffey (1972) proposed that rotational acceleration injury was the underlying physical cause of diffuse brain trauma in abused infants. However, Duhaime et al. (1987), as discussed above, concluded that "shaking alone in an otherwise normal baby is unlikely to cause the shaken baby syndrome."

We investigated the maximum angular acceleration and linear acceleration produced on the head of a doll model during repetitive shaking by healthy adult volunteers. A new doll model was constructed by the Medical Physics Department, Edinburgh, with dimensions similar to an average 2-month-old infant. The doll's total weight was 5 kg, with the head and neck weighing a total of 1.75 kg. For the purpose of this study the doll had a solid neck and head, filled with filler material used for car body work, and there was no movement of the top of neck relative to the head. The neck was able to support the head when the doll was placed in an upright position. The neck joint allowed for the head to move in the antero-posterior plane, stopping when the head hit either the model's chest or back.

CALIBRATED SYSTEM FOR THE MEASUREMENT OF LINEAR AND ANGULAR
ACCELERATIONS IN A SHAKEN DOLL

Results from previous measurements on lifelike dolls shaken without impact indicated that measured linear accelerations were unlikely to exceed about 14 G (~140 m/s^2) (Duhaime et al. 1987). The measuring system developed for our tests employed three Analog Devices type ADXL150 accelerometers (Analog Devices, Norwood, MA, USA), which were configured for a maximum range of ±2.5 G (~±25 m/s^2). These accelerometers were originally designed for use in the automotive industry and provide accurate measurements of acceleration along their sensitive axis.

The accelerometers A1, A2 and A3 were mounted within a protective aluminium case on the back of the doll's head. This unit was readily dismounted for calibration. The arrangement of the accelerometers and the directions of their sensitive axes relative to the doll's head and neck are shown in Figure 2.9.

The 'vertical' (v) acceleration of the centre of the transducer assembly was given by a3, while the corresponding 'horizontal' (h) acceleration was given by (a1 + a2)/2. The

130

angular acceleration of the doll's head was given by $(A1-A2)/d$ rad/s^2.

For a given movement of a solid head, the measured linear accelerations will vary according to the point of measurement but the angular acceleration will be the same wherever it is measured.

To obtain accurate values for linear and angular accelerations it was essential that the accelerometers were calibrated regularly using a specifically designed calibration turntable which rotated steadily about a horizontal axis subjecting each accelerometer to a sinusoidal gravitational equivalent acceleration of amplitude of 1 G ($g = 9.81$ m/s^2, the acceleration due to gravity in Edinburgh).

Labview software (National Instruments 'Labview' Austin, TX, USA) was used for data capture and recording and later analysis, resulting in a file that contained all the data for all the volunteers, enabling full statistical analysis.

'FEASIBLE' VALUES FOR ANGULAR ACCELERATION WITH A SHAKEN BABY

If an object is moved back and forth sinusoidally, simple mathematics gives us corresponding values for the angular velocity and acceleration. For example, consider a sinusoidal movement where the angle of the object is given by:

$$\theta = \theta_0 \sin(2\pi ft)$$

where θ is the angle in radians, θ_0 is the angular amplitude in radians, f is the frequency of movement in Hz, and t is the elapsed time in seconds. After differentiating twice with respect to t, the angular acceleration ξ is given by

$$\xi = -\theta_0 4\pi^2 f^2 \sin(2\pi ft) \text{ rad/s}^2$$

When shaking a doll, the amplitude of angular movement of the head, θ_0, is unlikely to exceed 1 radian.

A very vigorous and muscular volunteer might achieve a shaking frequency of 4 Hz, giving a peak value for the angular acceleration, ξ, of 632 rad/s^2 (assuming an amplitude of 1 rad). This value is similar to the peak values that were achieved during our tests.

For the above calculation, we have assumed that the movement and the acceleration are sinusoidal. In practice, the observed waveforms are not quite sinusoidal as most shakers have more muscle available for 'pulling' than 'pushing'. Fourier analysis of typical acceleration waveforms shows that the waveforms are very close to sinusoidal. This is not surprising as most maximal effort physiological repetitive movements turn out to be close to sinusoidal, provided that no impacts are involved.

Some experimenters have reported angular accelerations in excess of 10,000 rad/s^2 (without impact) during whiplash experiments. If we assume a shaking amplitude of 1 rad, such an angular acceleration would require a sinusoidal shaking frequency in excess of 15 Hz, which is physiologically impossible for an adult human.

Volunteers

Fifty healthy adult volunteers between the ages of 16 and 46 years with a mean age of 25 years were selected.

Results

Results for males show the maximum and average values for angular acceleration were 326–892 rad/s^2 and 300 rad/s^2 respectively. The maximum and average values for resultant acceleration were 4–15 G and 3.5 G respectively.

For females, the maximum and average for angular acceleration were 475 rad/s^{-2} and 196 rad/s^{-2}. The maximum and average values for resultant acceleration were 3–10 G and 2.4 G respectively.

The majority (76%) of maximum accelerations reached were between 4 and 7 G, and the majority (86%) of maximum angular accelerations reached were between 200 and 500 rad/s^2.

The average frequency of the shake was seen to be around 4 Hz (mean of average frequency of shake was 3.9 Hz for males, and 3.5 Hz for females)

Comparison of our acceleration values with those of Duhaime et al. (1987) shows that the peak value of our angular acceleration was 87–892 rad/s^2 when using a 'plastic neck' for the doll, compared to a mean angular acceleration of 1139 rad/s^2 for models employing different neck designs.

The linear accelerations were comparable, a peak value of 3–15 G from our studies compared with mean peak values of 13.85 G for the 'hinged neck', 5.7 G for the 'flexible rubber neck', and 9.86 G for the 'stiff rubber neck' obtained by Duhaime et al. (1987). A recent further doll model (De San Lazaro et al. 2003) records peak acceleration values approximately 3 G for 'normal' shaking and approximately 7 G for 'violent' shaking.

Modelling SBS

Recent research undertaken by the University of Birmingham in the UK (Morison 2002) resulted in the first three-dimensional computer model that was specifically designed to accurately represent the CSF. It was used to simulate the movement of a child's brain within the skull for various amplitudes and speeds of shaking and thus provided a valuable insight into the likelihood of causing subdural haematoma from shaking.

Computer, or 'finite element', modelling involves representing the solid model as a mesh of a finite number of discrete elements, for which the governing equations of mass, momentum, and energy can be built into a matrix and solved analytically. Since finite element modelling techniques entered the research field of head biomechanics in the early 1970s there have been many attempts to model head injury. The first decade of research is reviewed by Khalil and Viano (1982) and comprises two- and three-dimensional models. These models consisted mainly of an elastic shell skull completely filled with brain material modelled as an inviscid fluid using a bulk modulus $K = 2.1$ MPa or elastic modulus $E = 66.7$ kPa, Poisson ratio $\upsilon = 0.49$, and density of $\rho = 104$ kg/m^3. These early models were all used to simulate impact response.

The second decade of finite element modelling of head impact is reviewed by Sauren and Claessens (1993). This also includes both two- and three-dimensional models, generally using a more complex geometry with a greater number of elements than the earlier models, some including dura, falx, tentorium, and even CSF, albeit modelled as a soft solid. Unfortunately, most finite element models of head injury to date concentrate on impact loading during road traffic accidents, and therefore very few give results applicable to the development of subdural haematoma.

Perhaps the closest model to date is that of Zhou et al. (1996) whose three-dimensional model of a 50th centile male human head consisted of scalp, skull, dura, falx, tentorium, pia, CSF, venous sinuses, ventricles cerebrum (grey and white matter), cerebellum, brainstem and bridging veins. They converted the complex shear moduli from the shear experiments of Shuck and Advani (1972) to achieve their brain material parameters, and modelled the CSF as a solid material with low shear modulus. They loaded the model with an impulsive angular acceleration in both the sagittal and lateral planes, scaled from the monkey experiments of Abel et al. (1978), resulting in peak angular acceleration of $7030 \, \text{rad/s}^2$ occurring at 4 ms and peak angular deceleration of $9192 \, \text{rad/s}^2$ occurring at 32 ms. The stress and strain in the brain and the stretch of bridging veins were compared during rotation in the sagittal and lateral planes. Their bridging vein elements experienced stretch ratios of 1.383 during sagittal rotation.

Previous models either ignored the CSF or modelled it as a soft solid for the simple reason that the modelling software available at the time was unable to combine the different physics of fluid and solid behaviour. However, some modern software does have the ability to model both fluids and solids as well as their interactions, hence the recent work of the present author (CM) to build the first three-dimensional model of SBS to include accurate representation of the CSF.

CAN FLUID/SOLID INTERACTIONS BE MODELLED ACCURATELY?
The modelling software chosen was MSC.Dytran (MSC.Software Corp., Santa Ana, CA, USA) which is one of the few modern packages claiming to be able to model fluid/solid interactions. However, before the results of a model of SBS can be relied on, the ability of the modelling software to accurately model the interactions between fluids and solids must be demonstrated. Therefore a model of a simple fluid/solid interaction problem was built and its results compared with the known theoretical result for that system.

The simplest such model is a rigid sphere submerged in an infinite fluid reservoir, similar to the system in Figure 2.1. The effect of buoyancy upon the motion of the sphere is contained within equation 3. However, there is another important fluid/solid interaction force which must be taken into account before the theoretical and modelling results can be compared, and that is the 'acceleration reaction force'.

Acceleration reaction forces
As a submerged body accelerates it also has to accelerate the surrounding fluid, by pushing the fluid in front of it and 'sucking' the fluid in behind it. This requires the body to apply a force on the fluid which, by Newton's Third Law of Motion, will apply an equal and opposite reaction force on the body. Hence this force is known as the 'acceleration reaction force'. It has been shown (Milne-Thompson 1968) that this force is proportional to the acceleration of the body, and hence has the effect of increasing the inertia of the solid. Therefore, it is convenient to quote this force in terms of an added mass coefficient (α), whereby the effective inertial mass (m'_s) is given by:

$$m'_s = m_s + \alpha m_f \qquad \textbf{equation 4}$$

Replacing the inertial mass (i.e. the mass that is multiplied by the body's own acceleration to give the net force acting upon the body, not the mass that is multiplied by the acceleration due to gravity to give the body's weight) of equation 1 with equation 4 gives:

$$\left(m_s + \alpha m_f\right) \ddot{y} = -m_s g + m_f g \qquad \textbf{equation 5}$$

And since the sphere and displaced fluid are of equal volume,

$$\ddot{y} = -g \left(\frac{\rho_s - \rho_f}{\rho_s + \alpha \rho_f}\right) \qquad \textbf{equation 6}$$

The added mass coefficient is dependent on the shape of the submerged body, the shape of the fluid reservoir and the direction of motion. Milne-Thompson (1968) gives the added mass of a sphere in an infinite fluid reservoir as $\alpha = \frac{1}{2}$. The sphere submerged in a semi-infinite fluid was modelled for various combinations of densities and gravitational accelerations, and MSC.Dytran reliably produced accurate results.

However, for further verification of MSC.Dytran's abilities and to produce a model more akin to a head within a skull filled with CSF, the infinite fluid reservoir of the previous example can be replaced with a concentric fluid-filled sphere. For a sphere of radius a inside a spherical fluid reservoir of radius b the added mass coefficient is given by:

$$\alpha = \frac{2a^3 + b^3}{2b^3 + 2a^3} \qquad \textbf{equation 7}$$

This gives a sphere acceleration of:

$$\ddot{y} = -g \left(\frac{\rho_s - \rho_f}{\rho_s + \frac{2a^3 + b^3}{2b^3 + 2a^3} \rho_f}\right) \qquad \textbf{equation 8}$$

Again, MSC.Dytran produced accurate results for various combinations of densities, gravitational accelerations, and sphere and reservoir radii. Therefore the model of SBS could be build with confidence in the software's ability to include the fluid/solid interaction forces.

An interesting result can be found if the fluid region in these previous models is replaced with a soft solid as was done in previous models of head injury. The result given by equation 6 and achieved by MSC.Dytran with a fluid boundary is that of a constant acceleration and therefore a smooth parabolic displacement (assuming $\rho_s > \rho_f$). However, if the fluid is replaced with a soft solid, the solid sphere oscillates with simple harmonic motion within the fluid. This clearly demonstrates that these substitute fluid models are extremely unrepresentative of the original fluid–solid system, which is to be expected because unlike the fluid, the solid material cannot flow to relieve stress and absorb energy. Hence, as the rigid sphere accelerates, the elastic material in front of and behind it is compressed and extended

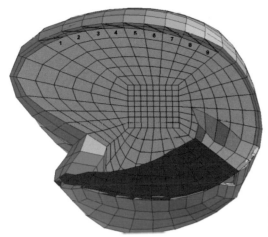

Fig. 2.10. The finite element model showing the brain, CSF, tentorium cerebelli and bridging veins.

respectively until the spring energy it acquires is enough to bounce the sphere back to its initial position, at which point the cycle repeats.

DEVELOPMENT OF FINITE ELEMENT MODEL

The geometry of the brain and inner skull surfaces was derived from a series of 11 magnetic resonance imaging (MRI) scans of sagittal sections of the right-hand half of the head of an 11-week-old male infant. In reality the inner cavity of the skull is subdivided into three cavities by the falx cerebri which runs forwards and backwards, and the tentorium cerebelli which runs side to side across the back of the head. The anterior cavities are occupied by the left and right cerebral hemispheres, and the posterior cavity by the cerebellum, all joined by the brainstem. For the purposes of this model, however, the two cerebral hemispheres and the cerebellum were considered to be one continuous body, which greatly simplified the geometry digitization and mesh generation processes and should not have a great impact on the results of the model since it will mainly be used to investigate relative forwards/backwards (sagittal) brain movement at the vertex.

The final model is shown in Figure 2.10, with the brain and CSF elements of the left-hand side hidden to reveal the tentorium. The model consists of 3 592 viscoelastic brain elements (including eight brainstem elements which connect the base of the brain to the skull surface), 993 CSF elements, 128 elastic membrane elements to represent the tentorium, 512 rigid shell elements to represent the skull, and nine elastic non-linear spring elements to represent the bridging veins (programmed with a typical force-displacement curve found from the bridging vein testing).

The falx cerebri was not included in the model because it was assumed that it would have little effect on the translation or rotation of the brain in the sagittal plane. This assumption was based on the fact that the falx is not in direct contact with the sides of the brain hemispheres; instead it is separated by a thin layer of fluid which, in the absence of viscosity, would provide little resistance to the motion of the brain parallel to it. Conversely, the tentorium cerebelli is effectively perpendicular to the sagittal plane and hence will apply direct forces to the surrounding brain tissue as it moves. If lateral motion were to be included then the effect of the falx cerebri would be more significant, and thus it should be included in such models.

Boundary conditions

Interface conditions between the CSF and the brain and skull surfaces are calculated automatically by MSC.Dytran, hence the only external boundary condition that needs to be applied to the model is the rigid body motion of the skull. This motion was based on purely sinusoidal sagittal (forwards–backwards) translation and rotation of the skull about a pivot at the base of the neck. The motion of the skull was programmed into the model such that the amplitude and frequency of the oscillations could be varied at will with frequencies between 2 and 10 Hz and amplitudes of 20°, 40°, and 60°. The choice of 4 Hz as the input frequency was taken from Duhaime et al. (1987) in which the angular acceleration histories of the baby doll shaking experiments are plotted. The input amplitude of ±60° was determined to be representative of the maximum range of passive motion of 20 infants' heads, as measured using a goniometer by Dr Sunderland, Consultant Paediatrician at Birmingham Children's Hospital (2001, personal communication).

Sliding contact was enabled between the brain and skull in case they came into contact with each other during the analyses.

Material properties

The skull surface was defined as a rigid body and hence needed no material properties. The CSF was given a density of $\rho_{csf} = 1005$ kg/m^3 (Saladin 1998) and the bulk modulus of water $K_{csf} = 2.25$ GPa. The tentorium cerebelli was given a density of $\rho_{tent} = 1130$ kg/m^3, Young's modulus $E_{tent} = 31.5$ MPa, and Poisson's ratio $\rho_{tent} = 0.45$ (McElhaney et al. 1973). The brain and brainstem were given the density of $\rho_{brain} = 1040$ kg/m^3 (Ruan and Prasad 1996), and eventually the viscoelastic properties of short-term shear modulus $G_0 = 38$ kPa, long-term shear modulus of $G_\alpha = 7$ kPa and decay constant $\beta = 700$/s (Zhou et al. 1996).

The choice of brain material properties was non-trivial since previous finite element models of brain injury have used proprieties that differ by several orders of magnitude, and experiments on brain tissue which yield viscoelastic material properties compatible with finite element software are few. Indeed, of the most significant previous finite element models of brain injury:

- Ruan et al. (1993) use shear moduli scaled from the experiments performed by Galford and McElhaney (1970), which were in fact performed in compression, not shear
- Galbraith and Tong (1988) used the properties of a silicone gel which was used in an associated series of physical models, hence their properties are not of brain tissue
- DiMasi et al. (1991) do not quote the original source of their material properties
- Kuijpers et al. (1995) use the properties (incorrectly) calculated as the average of those quoted in Sauren and Claessens (1993), which include those mentioned above.

This leaves the models of Zhou et al. (1996) and Kang et al. (1997), who both converted their model from the torsional shear experiments of Shuck and Advani (1972), in which

136

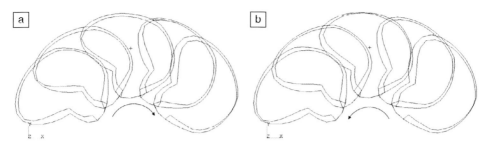

Fig. 2.11. (a) Backwards and (b) forwards motion of the head for one cycle.

the variation of the complex shear moduli with frequency is clearly tabulated to facilitate the conversion of these properties into other representations of viscoelastic properties. Zhou et al. used the interconversion equations of Christensen (1982), while Kang et al. do not explain how they arrived at their converted values, which are slightly different from those of Zhou et al. The present author (CM) reapplied the Christensen equations and found that the properties derived by Zhou et al. are correct and those used by Kang et al. are not (at least using this method). Therefore it was decided to adopt the material properties of Zhou et al. (1996) in this new model since these are the only properties for which the sources of both the physical experiments and the method of conversion are known to be reliable.

RESULTS

Figure 2.11 shows the movement of the mid-sagittal section of the skull and brain for an input frequency of 4 Hz and amplitude of 60°. Figure 2.11a shows the head moving backwards during the first half of the cycle, and Figure 2.11b shows the head moving forwards during the rest of the cycle. The crossed line in Figure 2.12 shows the stretch of the bridging vein which experiences the most stretch during the complete oscillation. The motion of the brain and the extension of the bridging veins goes through several stages:

1. As the skull starts translating and rotating backwards the brain lags forward since it is denser than the CSF. Since the bridging veins drain forwards from the brain into the mid-sagittal sinus they are relaxed as the brain moves forwards within the skull producing a stretch ratio less than 1.

2. Then as the skull decelerates towards the rear extremity of its motion, the brain continues accelerating backwards until the back of the brain approximates with the skull and the brain is compressed against it. Figure 2.12 (see discussion below) shows the peak stretch ratio at this point in the motion.

3. As the skull rotates forwards the brain begins to move forwards reducing the strain on the bridging veins.

4. The skull starts to decelerate as it rotates forwards while the brain continues moving forwards, further relaxing the bridging veins.

Added mass coefficients of the brain/skull

The added mass coefficients of the brain and skull geometry were determined by replacing

137

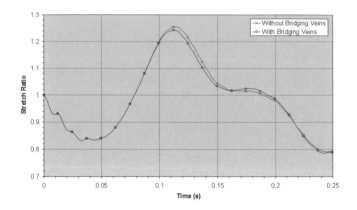

Fig. 2.12. Effect of bridging vein elasticity on bridging vein stretch ratio.

the soft brain material with a rigid body and applying constant accelerations in the sagittal, vertical and lateral directions. The resulting relative acceleration of the brain allowed the three added mass coefficients to be calculated from equation 6. This gave coefficients of 13.62, 12.55 and 17.43 in the sagittal, vertical and lateral directions respectively, with a mean added mass coefficient of 14.54. This means that, on average, the combined effect of the buoyancy and acceleration reaction forces is to reduce the translational acceleration of the brain with the skull to only 0.22% of the translational acceleration applied to the skull, as shown in equation 9.

$$a = 100 \left(\frac{1040 - 1005}{1040 + 14.54 \times 1005} \right) \qquad \textbf{equation 9}$$

$$= 0.22 \ m/s^2$$

Effect of bridging vein elasticity
Figure 2.12 compares the results of the standard model during one oscillation at a frequency of 4 Hz and amplitude 60° with those achieved when the nine bridging vein spring elements are removed from the model. This shows that the bridging vein elasticity causes only a small reduction in bridging vein stretch ratio from 1.256 to 1.243, a 5% reduction in strain.

Effect of the tentorium cerebelli
Figure 2.13 shows the effect of running the model with and without the tentorium cerebelli during one oscillation. The tentorium has the dramatic effect of reducing the maximum stretch ratio from 1.608 to 1.243, a 60% reduction in strain. Therefore it is of great importance that the tentorium cerebelli is included in finite element models of heads, especially when there is movement in the sagittal plane. Similarly, if lateral or oblique motions are to be modelled then the falx cerebri will have a significant effect and should also be included in such models.

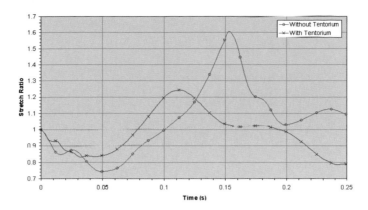

Fig. 2.13. Effect of the tentorium cerebelli on the bridging vein stretch ratio.

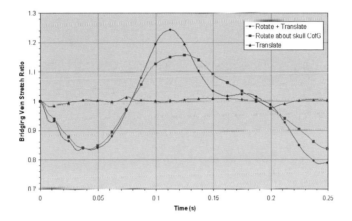

Fig. 2.14. Effect of isolated rotation and translation on the bridging vein stretch ratio.

Translation versus rotation

Figure 2.14 shows the stretch ratio caused by isolated translation, isolated rotation about the skull centre of mass, and the full combined rotation and translation (i.e. rotation about the neck pivot). This clearly demonstrates the influence of the fluid forces acting to protect the brain from translational accelerations, since the isolated translational component of the motion causes stretch ratios of only 1.016 compared to 1.243 for the full motion at a frequency of 4 Hz and amplitude 60°. Thus the rotation is responsible for over 93% of the bridging vein strain.

Effect of input frequency and amplitude

Figure 2.15 shows the stretch ratio of vein 4 (which was stretched the most in all models) during the first cycle for an amplitude of 60° at frequencies of 2–10 Hz. Figure 2.16 shows

139

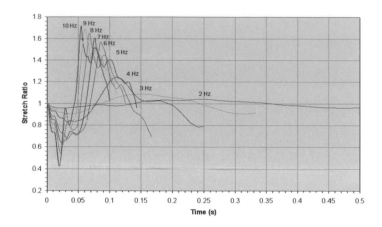

Fig. 2.15. Effect of input frequency on the bridging vein stretch ratio for an input amplitude of 60°.

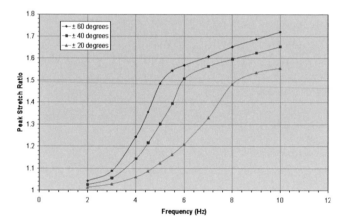

Fig. 2.16. Effect of input frequency and amplitude on the peak bridging vein stretch ratio.

the maximum of all these stretch ratios plotted against frequency, along with those for oscillations of 20° and 40°. As expected, oscillations of higher amplitude or frequency produce higher stretch ratios, with a high degree of sensitivity between frequencies of 2–6 Hz and with lower sensitivity at higher frequencies. The curves seem to flatten out consistently at stretch ratios of around 1.5. This is because the initial vein strain is caused by movement of the brain as a whole, but at higher frequencies or amplitudes the brain comes into contact with the skull and further vein strain can only be caused by brain compression against the back of the skull.

These curves can be plotted against peak angular acceleration (i.e. the angular velocity of the skull at either extremity of the shaking motion) instead of frequency by using the relationship:

140

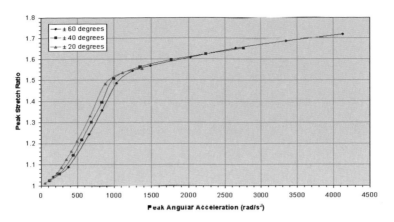

Fig. 2.17 Effect of input frequency and amplitude on the peak bridging vein stretch ratio

$$\ddot{\theta}_p = \omega^2 \theta_0 \qquad \text{equation 10}$$

where $\ddot{\theta}_p$ is the peak angular acceleration (rad/s²), ω is the angular frequency (rad/s) and θ_0 is the amplitude of the oscillations (rad). Figure 2.17 shows that plotting the peak stretch ratio against peak angular acceleration gives almost superimposed curves for various amplitudes, with two distinct near-linear regions within the results. This allows the input oscillation to be categorized by a single, lumped parameter instead of two independent parameters, and for the following relations to be stated:

$$\lambda = \begin{cases} 1 + 4.5 \times 10^{-4} \, \ddot{\theta}_p & \text{for} \quad 0 \le \ddot{\theta}_p \le 1234 \text{ rad/s}^2 \\ 1.476 = 6.3 \times 10^{-5} \, \ddot{\theta}_p & \text{for} \quad 1234 \le \ddot{\theta}_p \le 4000 \text{ rad/s}^2 \end{cases} \qquad \text{equation 11}$$

Modelling impacts
Impacts of the head against both hard and soft surfaces were also modelled. Since the skull is a rigid body in this model, any impact has to be applied either through the modelling of the resulting inertial forces or as enforced motion of the skull. The acceleration histories presented by DiMasi et al. (1991) were used as the inputs, and consisted of effectively half-sine wave accelerations with amplitude 300 G and duration 8 ms for the hard impact and amplitude 160 G, duration 10 ms for the soft impact. These translational accelerations were converted to angular accelerations about the neck pivot, with the head rotating in the more dangerous forwards direction representing an occipital impact. Figure 2.18 shows peak stretch ratios of 1.226 and 1.137 for the hard and soft impacts respectively, and 1.243 for the shaking. This suggests that shaking can be just as dangerous as hard impacts, and considerably more dangerous than soft impacts.

Internal brain stresses
Figure 2.19 shows the Von Mises stress distribution in the brain at the instant of maximum

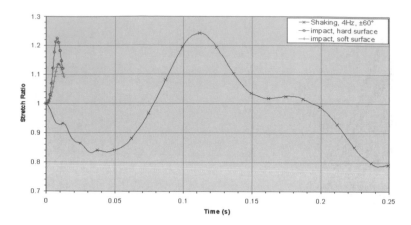

Fig. 2.18. Bridging vein strain as caused by hard and soft impacts, compared to shaking.

stress for shaking at 4 Hz and all three amplitudes. As expected they show the stress increasing from the brainstem to the vertex, up to almost 800 Pa.

Figure 2.20 shows the stress distributions for the hard and soft impacts, with peak coup stress occurring shortly after impact under the impact site and peak contrecoup stress occurring shortly after the angular acceleration input is removed. In these models the peak stresses are approximately 2 kPa and 1.6 kPa respectively for the coup and contrecoup stresses during the hard impact, and 1.2 kPa and 0.8 kPa respectively for the coup and contrecoup stresses during the soft impact.

Previous finite element models of head injury (as mentioned previously) report brain stresses in the order of 80 kPa, considerably higher than those found in this research; however, this is to be expected since the inclusion of the CSF will allow increased whole brain movement instead of transferring the impact force directly into the brain tissue.

CONCLUSIONS OF THE FINITE ELEMENT MODELLING

This new model of SBS has resulted in several important conclusions. First, it has shown that the combined effect of the buoyancy and acceleration reaction forces is to reduce the relative translational acceleration of the brain within the skull to only 0.22% of the translational acceleration applied to the skull. This explains why impacts and inertial accelerations which produce mainly translational head accelerations are unlikely to cause severe brain injury. For example, the literature is peppered with clinical observations (and animal experiments, including Ommaya and Gennarelli 1974) of straight-line head impacts with fast-moving rigid bodies causing severe skull fractures in which the patients do not even experience concussion.

This first conclusion leads to the next, which is that the rotational component of the shaking motion is responsible for approximately 93% of the bridging vein strain. The tentorium cerebelli which probably provides the brain with most of its protection against sagittal rotation – and was shown by this model to reduce the bridging vein strain by 61% – is still

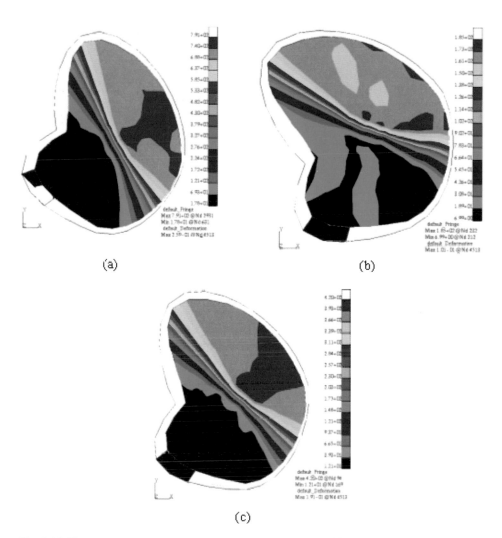

Fig. 2.19. Von Mises stress distributions for shaking the head at 4 Hz and amplitudes of (a) ± 60°, (b) ± 40°, and (c) ± 20°.

not as effective as the CSF is at providing protection against translation, and therefore rotational accelerations are extremely dangerous to humans and animals. The relative danger of rotation compared to translation has been well acknowledged since Holbourn (1943) and has been demonstrated in primate experiments by Ommaya and Gennarelli (1974) and observations of woodpeckers by May et al. (1979). However, all these previous researchers have attributed this difference to brain tissue's very high ratio of bulk modulus to shear modulus as highlighted by Holbourn (1943), but this research gives support to the hypothesis of Hodgson et al. (2001) which is that the CSF almost perfectly protects the brain against translational accelerations but effectively acts as a lubricant to brain rotation.

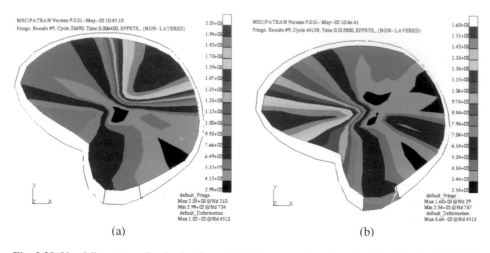

| (a) | (b) |

Fig. 2.20. Von Mises stress distribution for occipital impact against a hard surface showing (a) initial coup stress and (b) consequent contrecoup stress.

The stretch ratio histories presented show that maximum bridging vein strain is experienced as the skull is at the rear extremity of its motion and accelerating forwards. At this point in the motion the higher density brain rotates backwards relative to the skull (which is starting to rotate forwards), stretching the bridging veins which drain forwards from the brain surface to the midsagittal sinus. This is in agreement with the general understanding that the brain is more susceptible to injury from occipital impacts than frontal impacts, and hence when characterizing head motion for comparison with or development of head injury tolerance criteria care should be taken since lower magnitude forwards rotational acceleration may cause more damage than higher magnitude backwards rotational acceleration.

Most importantly this model has shown that the maximum bridging vein stretch ratio is very sensitive to shaking frequency, especially at frequencies between 2 and 5 Hz. This means that a relatively small increase in shaking frequency will cause a disproportionate increase in bridging vein stretch ratio and hence dramatically increase the likelihood of bridging vein rupture and subdural haematoma. The review of the previous bridging vein testing and the new tests described above showed that while the average ultimate stretch ratio of bridging veins was found to be approximately 1.5, some veins may fail at ratios of as little as 1.15. These results show that shaking at a frequency of 4 Hz and amplitude of ± 60° can produce a stretch ratio of approximately 1.26, therefore this model shows that subdural haematoma may well be a possible result of manually shaking a baby. Furthermore, the amplitude of ± 60° was measured without applying any excessive force to the heads of healthy babies, therefore it is likely that forced shaking may cause oscillations of a higher amplitude and hence proportionately higher bridging vein strain.

REFERENCES

Abel JM, Gennarelli TA, Segawa H (1978) Incidence and severity of cerebral concussion in the Rhesus monkey following sagittal plane angular acceleration. In: *Proceedings of 22nd Stapp Car Crash Conference*. Warrendale, PA: Society of Automotive Engineers, pp. 35–53.

Alexander R, Sato Y, Smith W, Bennett T (1990) Incidence of impact trauma with cranial injuries ascribed to shaking. *Am J Dis Child* **144**: 724–726.

Barlow KM, Minns RA (1999) The relation between intracranial pressure and outcome in non-accidntal head injury. *Dev Med Child Neurol* **41**: 220–225.

Becker JC, Liersch R, Tautz C, Schlueter B, Andler W (1998) Shaken baby syndrome: report on four pairs of twins. *Child Abuse Negl* **22**: 931–937.

Brown JK, Minns RA (1993) Non-accidental head injury, with particular reference to whiplash shaking injury and medico-legal aspects. *Dev Med Child Neurol* **35**: 849–869.

Caffey J (1972) On the theory and practice of shaking infants. *Am J Dis Child* **124**: 161–169.

Caffey J (1974) The whiplash shaken infant syndrome: manual shaking by the extremities with whiplash-induced intracranial and intraocular bleedings, lined with residual permanent brain damage and mental retardation. *Pediatrics* **54**: 396–403.

Christensen RM (1982) *Theory of Viscoelasticity, 2nd edn*. New York: Academic Press.

Cory CZ, Jones MD (2003) Can shaking alone cause fatal brain injury? A biomechanical assessment of the Duhaime shaken baby syndrome model. *Med Sci Law* **43**: 317–333.

De San Lazaro C, Harvey R, Ogden A (2003) Shaking infant trauma induced by misuse of a baby chair. *Arch Dis Child* **88**: 632–634.

DiMasi F, Marcus J, Eppinger HC (1991) 3-D anatomic brain model for relating cortical strains to automobile crash loading. In: *Proceedings of the 13th International Technical Conference on Experimental Safety Vehicles, vol. 2*. Washington, DC: US Dept of Transportation, National Highway Traffic Safety Administration, pp. 915–923.

DiScala C, Sege R, Li G, Reece RM (2000) Child abuse and unintentional injuries: a 10-year retrospsective. *Arch Pediatr Adolesc Med* **154**: 16–22.

Duhaime A-C, Gennarelli TA, Thibault LE, Bruce DA, Margulies SS, Wiser R (1987) The shaken baby syndrome: a clinical, pathological and biomechanical study. *J Neurosurg* **66**: 409–415.

Elner SG, Elner VM, Arnall M, Albert DM (1990). Ocular and associated systemic findings in suspected child abuse: a necropsy study. *Arch Ophthalmol* **108**. 1094–1101.

Galbraith CG, Tong P (1988) Boundary conditions in head injury finite element modeling. In: *16th Annual International Workshop on Human Subjects for Biomechanical Research*. Washington, DC: US Dept of Transportation, National Highway Traffic Safety Administration, pp. 179–193.

Galford JE, McElhaney JH (1970) A viscoelastic study of scalp brain and dura. *J Biomech* **3**: 211–221.

Geddes JF, Hackshaw AK, Vowles GH, Nickols CD, Whitwell HL (2001a) Neuropathology of inflicted head injur in children. I. Patterns of brain damage. *Brain* **124**: 1290–1298.

Geddes JF, Vowles GH, hackshaw AK, Nickols CD, Scott IS, Whitwell HL (2001b) Neuropathology of inflicted head injury in children. II. Microscopic brain injury in infants. *Brain* **124**: 1299–1306.

Gennarelli TA, Thibault LE (1982) Biomechanics of acute subdural hematoma. *J Trauma* **22**: 680–686.

Gennarelli TA, Thibault LE, Adams MB, Graham DI, Thompson CJ, Marcincin RP (1982) Diffuse axonal injury and traumatic coma in the primate. *Ann Neurol* **12**: 564–574.

Gilliland GF, Folberg R (1996) Shaken babies – some have no impact injuries. *J Forensic Sci* **14**: 114–116.

Gleckman AM, Bell MD, Evans EJ, Smith TW (1999) Diffuse axonal injury in infants with nonaccidental craniofacial trauma. *Arch Pathol Lab Med* **123**: 146–151.

Guthkelch AN (1971) Infantile subdural hematoma and its relationship to whiplash injury. *BMJ* **2**: 430–431.

Hadley MN, Sonntag KH, Rekate HL, Murphy A (1989) The infant whiplash-shake injury syndrome: a clinical and pathological study. *Neurosurgery* **24**: 536–540.

Hodgson DC, Shippen JM, Sunderland R (2001) Protective role of cerebrospinal fluid in brain injuries. *Arch Dis Child* **84**: 187. (Letter).

Holbourn AHS (1943) Mechanics of head injuries. *Lancet* **2**: 438–441.

Howard MA, Bell BA, Uttley D (1993) The pathophysiology of infant subdurals. *Br J Neurosurg* **7**: 355–365.

Kang H-S, Willinger R, Diaw BM, Chinn B (1997) Validation of a 3D anatomic human head model and replication of head impact in motorcycle accident by finite element modeling. In: *Proceedings of the 41st Stapp Car Crash Conference*. Warrendale, PA: Society of Automotive Engineers, pp. 329–338.

Khalil TB, Viano DC (1982) Critical issues in finite element modeling of head impact. In: *Proceedings of the 26th Stapp Car Crash Conference*. Warrendale, PA: Society of Automotive Engineers, pp. 87–102.

Kuijpers AHWM, Claessens MHA, Sauren AAHJ (1995) The influence of different boundary conditions on

145

the response of the head to impact: A two-dimensional finite element study. *J Neurotrauma* **12**: 715–724.

Lazoritz S, Baldwin S, Kini N (1997) The whiplash shaken infant syndrome: has Caffey's syndrome changed or have we changed his syndrome? *Child Abuse Negl* **21**: 1009–1014.

Lee M-C, Haut RC (1989) Insensitivity of tensile failure properties of human bridging veins to strain rate: implications in biomechanics of subdural hematoma. *J Biomech* **22**: 537–542.

Lee M-C, Melvin JW, Ueno K (1987) Finite element analysis of traumatic subdural hematoma. In: *Proceedings of the 31st Stapp Car Crash Conference*. Warrendale, PA: Society of Automotive Engineers, pp. 67–77.

Löwenhielm P (1974) Dynamic properties of the parasagittal bridging veins. *Z Rechtsmedizin* **74**: 55–62.

Margulies SS, Thibault LE, Gennarelli TA (1985) A study of scaling and head injury criteria using physical model experiments. In: *International IRCOBI Conference on the Biomechanics of Impacts*. Lyon: International Research Council on the Biomechanics of Impacts (IRCOBI), pp. 223–234.

Maxeiner H (2001) Demonstration and interpretation of bridging vein ruptures in cases of infantile subdural bleedings. *J Forensic Sci* **46**: 85–93.

May PR, Fuster JM, Haber J, Hirschman A (1979) Woodpecker drilling behaviour: an endorsement of the rotational theory of impact brain injury. *Arch Neurol* **36**: 370–373.

McClelland CQ, Rekate H, Kaufman B, Persse L (1980) Cerebral injury in child abuse: a changing profile. *Child's Brain* **7**: 225–235.

McElhaney JH, Melvin JW, Roberts VL, Portnoy HD (1973) Dynamic characteristics of the tissues of the head. In: Kenedi RM, ed. *Perspectives in Biomedical Engineering*. London: Macmillan, pp. 215–222.

Meaney DF (1991) Biomechanics of acute subdural hematoma in the subhuman primate and Man. PhD thesis, University of Pennsylvania.

Milne-Thompson LM (1968) *Theoretical Hydrodynamics, 5th edn*. London: MacMillan.

Minns RA (2005) Shaken baby syndrome: theoretical and evidential controversies. *J R Coll Physicians Edinb* **35**: 5–15.

Morison CN (2002) The dynamics of shaken baby syndrome. PhD thesis, University of Birmingham, England.

Morris MW, Smith S, Cressmen J, Ancheta J (2000) Evaluation of infants with subdural hematoma who lack external evidence of abuse. *Pediatrics* **105**: 549–553.

Ommaya AK, Gennarelli TA (1974) Cerebral concussion and traumatic unconsciousness. *Brain* **97**: 633–654.

Ommaya AK, Yarnell P, Hirsch AE, Harris EH (1967) Scaling of experimental data on cerebral concussion in sub-human primates to concussion threshold for Man. In: *Procedings of the 11th Stapp Car Crash Conference*. New York: Society of Automotive Engineers, pp. 47–52.

Ommaya AK, Faas F, Yarnell P (1968) Whiplash injury and brain damage. *JAMA* **204**: 75–79.

Ruan JS, Prasad P (1996) Study of the biodynamic characteristics of the human head. In: *International IRCOBI Conference on the Biomechanics of Impacts*. Lyon: IRCOBI, pp. 63–74.

Ruan JS, Khalil TB, King AI (1993) Finite element modeling of direct head impact. In: *Proceedings of the 37th Stapp Car Crash Conference*. Warrendale, PA: Society of Automotive Engineers, pp. 69–81.

Saladin KS (1998) *Anatomy and Physiology*. New York: McGraw-Hill.

Sauren AAHJ, Claessens MHA (1993) Finite element modelling of head impact: The second decade. In: *International IRCOBI Conference of Biomechanics of Impacts*. Lyon: IRCOBI, pp. 241–253.

Shuck LZ, Advani SH (1972) Rheological response of human brain tissue in shear. *ASME Journal of Basic Engineering* Dec: 905–911.

Smith S, Hanson R (1974) 134 battered children: a medical and psychological study. *BMJ* **3**: 666–670.

Stürtz G (1980) Biomechanical data of children. In: *Proceedings of the 24th Stapp Car Crash Conference*. Warrendale, PA: Society of Automotive Engineers, pp. 513–559.

Thibault LE, Gennarelli TA (1985) Biomechanics of diffuse brain injuries. In: *Proceedings of the Fourth Experimental Safety Vehicle Conference*. New York: American Association of Automotive Engineers. *Reprinted in:* Backaitis S, ed. (1993) *Biomechanics of Impact Injury and Injury Tolerances of the Head Neck Complex*. Warrendale, PA: Socity of Automotive Engineers, pp. 555–561.

Tzioumi D, Oates RK (1998) Subdural haematomas in children under 2 years. Accidental or inflicted? A 10-year experience. *Child Abuse Negl* **22**: 1105–1112.

Yamashima T, Friede RL (1984) Why do bridging veins rupture into the virtual subdural space?. *J Neurol Neurosurg Psychiatry* **47**: 121–127.

Zhou C, Khalil TB, King AI (1996) Viscoelastic response of the human brain to sagittal and lateral rotational acceleration by finite element analysis. In: *International IRCOBI Conference on the Biomechanics of Impacts*. Lyon: IRCOBI, pp. 35–48.

3
THE EPIDEMIOLOGY OF NON-ACCIDENTAL HEAD INJURY

John H Livingston and Anne-Marie Childs

Non-accidental head injury (NAHI) encompasses a spectrum of inflicted injuries ranging from trivial superficial injuries through to severe brain injuries that are often fatal. NAHI must be seen in the overall context of child abuse.

Child abuse is common In the USA the reported incidence is 16.3 per 1000 children (Monteleone 1998). In England and Wales in 1987 there were 8000 registered cases of abuse, 720 (9%) of which were classified as 'serious' (Creighton and Noyes 1989) These figures are undoubtedly an underestimate of the true scale of the problem.

Fatal child abuse occurs in 8 per 100,000 children under the age of 1 year in the USA (Monteleone 1998). In the UK, the National Society for the Prevention of Cruelty to Children (NSPCC) has stated that three children per week die from child abuse. Creighton and Noyes (1989) reported a higher figure of 200–230 non-accidental deaths per year in the UK. At least 50% of deaths due to abuse are NAHI cases.

NAHI is the commonest cause of acquired brain injury in infancy after the neonatal period (Table 3.1).

Identification of NAHI
There are several difficulties with ascertainment for studies of NAHI. Identification of patients may come from several different sources and may be clinical, radiological or pathological (Table 3.2).

Particular problems with ascertainment arise because: (1) the brain is not always examined in children with extracranial NAHI; (2) NAHI is not always considered in infants presenting clinically with acute encephalopathy; and (3) imaging and in particular brain scans may be misinterpreted Any reported figures are therefore likely to be underestimates.

Skull fractures
Skull fractures are relatively common in NAHI, particularly in infants. The prevalence of skull fractures in all cases of abuse is 10–13%. In children under 2 years of age around 30% of skull fractures are due to abuse (Hobbs 1984, Merten and Osborne 1984, Meservy et al. 1987, Leventhal et al. 1990, Kleinman 1998).

Simple linear fractures commonly occur in accidental and non-accidental trauma. No pattern of skull injury is diagnostic of abuse. However, multiple, complex, bilateral or diastatic fractures are strongly associated with abuse, as are occipital fractures (Hobbs 1984, Meservy et al. 1987).

147

TABLE 3.1	TABLE 3.2
Causes of acquired brain injury in infancy	Sources of identification of NAHI in infants

Causes of acquired brain injury in infancy	Sources of identification of NAHI in infants
Trauma	
Meningitis/encephalitis	**Clinical**
Hypoxic–ischaemic encephalopathy	NAI
Septicaemia	Head trauma
Cardiac arrest	Acute encephalopathy
Drowning/electrocution	**Radiological**
Other asphyxial causes including	Head trauma
smothering	Intracranial haemorrhage
Cerebrovascular	Cerebral oedema
Tumour	Extracerebral collections
Metabolic (including hypoglycaemia)	**Pathological**

Skull fractures are present in many children with intracranial injury due to abuse but the correlation is relatively poor. Skull fractures are seen in only 25–56% of children with intracranial injury due to abuse (O'Neil et al. 1973, Zimmerman et al. 1979, Merten and Osborne 1984).

Severe non-accidental head injury
Although there are many ways in which inflicted brain injury can occur, the commonest manifestation of severe NAHI is the so-called shaken baby syndrome. This syndrome could be described as a syndrome looking for a name. It would be preferable if the name to describe this entity did not presuppose the underlying mechanism of injury. However, given that the syndrome comprises many different clinical and radiological features (see below) none of which is absolutely pathognomonic of NAHI, it is unavoidable that such terms have evolved to describe the whole syndrome. Other similar terms have been employed, including battered child syndrome (Kempe et al. 1962), whiplash shaken infant syndrome (Caffey 1974), and the shaking–impact syndrome (Duhaime et al. 1987).

With the above reservations we will use the term shaken baby syndrome (SBS) to describe this clinico-radiological syndrome.

The shaken baby syndrome: definition
There are three components of the SBS: a clinical syndrome, a radiological syndrome, and usually a lack of a compatible history to explain the clinical and radiological features.

The clinical syndrome of SBS comprises:
• a severe acute encephalopathy with a characteristic clinical course that is considered elsewhere in this volume
• extracranial features of NAHI are present in up to 70% of cases; these include the whole spectrum of physical abuse such as bruises, bites and fractures
• retinal haemorrhages occur in 65–90% of cases (Taylor 2000) and, while not pathognomonic, are highly suggestive.

Different forms of abuse often coexist and there may be a combination of physical, sexual and emotional abuse.

148

The radiological syndrome of SBS comprises:
- characteristic extra-axial haemorrhage with or without an extra-axial fluid collection; this haemorrhage is usually subdural but may in addition be subarachnoid
- diffuse parenchymal changes, in particular cerebral oedema or haemorrhagic contusions
- subcortical tears if present are probably pathognomonic (Jaspan et al. 1992)
- there may be skull fractures and soft tissue swelling.

There is usually no compatible history to account for these injuries, indeed there is often no history of injury having occurred at all. Sometimes there is a history of minor injury, such as a fall from a sofa or a bump into furniture. This history may be developmentally incompatible. As with non-accidental injury in general, the history often changes over time and between historians. There is virtually never a history of shaking at the time of presentation.

SBS is the commonest form of severe NAHI in infancy, but other injuries may occur, such as single blows without haemorrhage. Extradural haemorrhage due to non-accidental injury is rare. Smothering and/or strangulation may coexist with a shaking injury or may occur in isolation.

Radiological definitions

Ascertainment of cases often depends on radiological findings. Unfortunately, there are many different terms used to describe abnormal extra-axial fluid collections. These terms are often used imprecisely and sometime interchangeably. Thus, subdural collections may be called: haemorrhage, haematoma, effusion, hygroma or simply collections. Chronic subdural haemorrhages (SDHs) may be erroneously called hygromas. A hygroma, strictly speaking, is an extra-axial collection composed of CSF usually thought to have been caused by a laceration in the arachnoid (Gean 1994). A subdural effusion is a collection of fluid in the subdural space with a higher protein content than the CSF.

Severe brain injury due to shaking may occur without a radiologically apparent SDH. The SDH is usually much less important as a mass lesion than as a marker for a shearing injury. This is important because SDH is sometimes erroneously seen as synonymous with NAHI, and in its absence NAHI may not be considered.

A further difficult and controversial area arises over unexplained SDHs occurring without other features of shaking injury or NAHI. Some consider all such cases as NAHI, whereas others allow the possibility of some as yet undetermined risk factor or precipitating event, for example minor trauma in a child with a previously large extra-axial space.

Pericerebral collections may have other explanations, for example the syndrome of benign external hydrocephalus (synonyms: benign subdural effusions, benign pericerebral collections, benign communicating external hydrocephalus). These children present with rapidly enlarging heads and sometimes are erroneously thought to have been victims of NAHI. This is usually because the radiological appearance of the pericerebral fluid collection is misinterpreted. A similar syndrome may occur in infants with superior vena cava or jugular obstruction.

The inconsistent definitions of these radiological and clinical terms need to be taken into consideration in interpreting the currently available data on the epidemiology of NAHI.

149

TABLE 3.3		TABLE 3.4	
Head injury cases in which inflicted injury was confirmed*		Subdural haemorrhage in infants under 2 years*	
N = 24		N = 33	
15 male, 9 female		23 male, 10 female	
Mean age = 8.7 months		Age range 3w–17 mo (median 3 mo)	
Reported history:		Incidence: 12.8/100,000 under 2 years	
fall less than 4 feet	8	21.0/100,000 under 1 year	
admitted assault	2	Outcome:	
no history	14	Death	9
Subdural haemorrhage	13	Severe disability	15
Retinal haemorrhage	9	Normal after 1 year	9
Death (4 in whole series)	3		

*Jayawant et al. (1998).

*Duhaime et al. (1992)

Published population studies of NAHI

Duhaime et al. (1992) carried out a hospital based, prospective study of 100 consecutive admissions to three teaching hospitals of children under 2 years of age with a primary diagnosis of head injury. All children had a standardized evaluation that included a biomechanical profile where the nature of the injuries and the history were evaluated in a standardized way; skull X-ray, CT/MRI and skeletal survey; ophthalmologic assessment; and a social interview by a child abuse specialist. If no history was available, multiple interviews were performed. An algorithm was devised to determine whether the injuries were felt to be inflicted or accidental. This was independent of the ophthalmological or social findings.

Twenty-four of the 100 cases were classified as inflicted injuries (Table 3.3) and an additional 32 were suspicious of abuse, neglect or social problems.

SDH was much more likely to occur from inflicted brain injury and motor vehicle accidents than any other mechanism. Inflicted injury was the commonest cause of death. In this series subdural haematomas occurred in only three children following accidental injury, all as a result of a motor vehicle accident.

The authors concluded that accidental blunt head injuries in children younger than 2 years of age were very common, but except for falls from extreme height and head injury due to motor vehicle accidents, these were almost always benign. Inflicted head injury accounted for nearly one quarter of patients in this series.

Two studies have considered specifically SDHs (Jayawant et al. 1998) or subdural haematoma and effusion (Hobbs et al. 2005).

Jayawant et al. (1998) conducted a population based study of SDH in infants under 2 years of age. This was a three year retrospective study based in the South Wales and South Western regions of the UK. Diagnosis was by CT, MRI or autopsy, and multiple routes of case identification were utilized. Neonatal and post-surgical cases were excluded. The results of their study are shown in Table 3.4.

Of the 33 cases identified, only one was the victim of a major road traffic accident. Surprisingly, a clear history of shaking was obtained in 14 children, although this was never the first history given.

150

TABLE 3.5
**Suggested mandatory investigations for an infant
with a subdural haemorrhage***

Full multidisciplinary social assessment
Ophthalmoscopy by an ophthalmologist
Skeletal survey with a bone scan or a repeat skeletal
   survey at around 10 days
Coagulation screen
Radiological assessment by CT or MRI

*Jayawant et al. (1998).

TABLE 3.6
BPSU study of subdural haematoma and effusions (SDH/E) in infancy*

N = 186
Male 123, female 63
Age: 0–82 weeks (mean 17 weeks, median 13 weeks)
Annual incidence (all aetiologies): 12.7/100,000 under 2 years
                                     24.3/100,000 under 1 year
Incidence of non-accidental SDH/E: 7.28/100,000 under 2 years
                                   14.8/100,000 under 1 year

Aetiology:
NAHI	106
Accidental trauma	7
Meningitis	23
Perinatal	26
Other disease	7
Unknown	17

Outcome in NAHI group:
Died	18 (17%)
Significant neurodevelopmental problems (evident at 6 months follow-up)	29 (28%)
Normal at 6 months follow-up	46 (43%)
Unknown outcome	13 (12%)

*Hobbs et al. (2004).

In 18 children no history of injury was given. Coexisting trauma, mostly fractures, was documented in 19 cases. After full evaluation it was concluded that abuse had definitely occurred in 21 children and was highly probable in six. The authors extrapolated an incidence of non-accidental SDH in infants of 10.13 per 100,000 children per year. There was a high mortality and morbidity associated with non-accidental SDH. This study documented the high probability of abuse in infants with SDH. It was emphasized, however, that this was not always recognized, and a mandatory screen of investigations for infants with SDHs was suggested (Table 3.5).

All of the children in the Duhaime et al. (1992) study (see above) were evaluated in this way, and the authors emphasized that future prospective studies need to employ such a systematic evaluation.

151

The most recent epidemiological study is that of the British Paediatric Surveillance Unit (BPSU) into subdural haematomas and/or effusion (SDH/E) in infancy (Hobbs et al. 2005).

Cases of SDH/E were notified through the BPSU. Paediatricians, neurosurgeons and forensic pathologists identified, via a card reporting system, cases they had seen in the previous month. A questionnaire was then sent to the reporting doctor for completion. A follow-up questionnaire was sent out at 6 months. In addition, the Office of National Statistics reporting scheme identified fatal cases and the coroner was approached for information.

Data were collected from April 1998 for 12 months. Entry criteria were: (i) age under 2 years, (ii) fatal or non-fatal SDII/E, and (iii) diagnosis by imaging or post-mortem examination. Only three children were diagnosed by ultrasound alone; most children had CT, MRI or both. Twelve cases were diagnosed at autopsy. The results of the study are shown in Table 3.6.

This study comprised a heterogeneous group including children with effusions as well as haemorrhages. The diagnosis of NAI was based on the reporting clinician's opinion. Some of the unknown cases may have been non-accidental. The study suggests an incidence of non-accidental SDH/E of 7.28 per 100,000 children under the age of 2, or 14.8 per 100,000 children per year under the age of 1.

A further recent study (Barlow and Minns 2000) suggests an incidence of NAHI of 24.6 per 100,000 children under 1. The confidence intervals, however, overlap those of the above studies. This study treats NAHI and shaken–impact injury as synonymous. There is little detail as to how NAHI was defined, investigated or confirmed.

In all of the above studies the male to female ratio was 2:1.

Conclusion

NAHI is a major cause of mortality in infancy and of acquired brain injury and disability. The 'shaken baby syndrome' refers to an easily recognized or suspected constellation of clinical and radiological features. Recent epidemiological studies suggest an incidence of non-accidental SDH in infants of around 10 per 100,000 per year with a higher incidence in the first year of life. In view of the different forms that NAHI may take and the difficulties with ascertainment and definition, future prospective studies need to employ a systematic approach to the evaluation of head injury in infants that would include a full social assessment by a child abuse specialist as well as appropriate radiological and ophthalmological assessment.

REFERENCES

Barlow K, Minns RA (2000) Annual incidence of shaken impact syndrome in young children. *Lancet* **356**: 1571–1572.
Caffey J (1974) The whiplash shaken infant syndrome: manual shaking by the extremities with whiplash induced intracranial and intraocular bleedings, linked with residual permanent brain damage and mental retardation. *Pediatrics* **54**: 396–403.
Creighton SJ, Noyes P (1989) *Child Abuse Trends in England and Wales 1983–1987.* London: NSPCC.
Duhaime AC, Gennarelli TA, Thibault LE, Bruce DA, Marguiles SS, Wiser R (1987) The shaken baby syndrome. A clinical, pathological, and biomechanical study. *J Neurosurg* **66**: 409–415.

Duhaime AC, Alario AJ, Lewander WJ, Schut L, Sutton LN, Seidl TS, Nudelman S, Budenz D, Hertle R, Tsiaras W, Loporchio S (1992) Head injury in very young children: mechanisms, injury types, and ophthalmologic findings in 100 hospitalized patients younger than 2 years of age. *Pediatrics* **90**: 179–185.

Gean AD (1994) *Imaging of Head Trauma*. New York: Raven Press.

Hobbs CJ (1984) Skull fracture and the diagnosis of abuse. *Arch Dis Child* **59**: 246–252.

Hobbs C, Childs AM, Wynne J, Livingston J, Seal A (2005) Subdural haematoma and effusion in infancy. An epidemiological study. *Arch Dis Child* **90**: 952–955.

Jaspan T, Narborough G, Punt JAG, Lowe J (1992) Cerebral contusional tears as a marker of child abuse – detection by cranial sonography. *Pediatr Radiol* **22**: 237–245.

Jayawant S, Rawlinson A, Gibbon F, Price J, Schulte J, Sharples P, Sibert JR, Kemp AM (1998) Subdural haemorrhages in infants: population based study. *BMJ* **317**: 1558–1561.

Kempe CH, Silverman FN, Steele BF, Droegemueller W, Silver HK (1962) The battered-child syndrome. *JAMA* **181**: 105–112.

Kleinman PK, Barnes PD (1998) Head trauma. In: Kleinman PK, ed. *Diagnostic Imaging of Child Abuse*. St Louis: Mosby, pp 290–291.

Leventhal JM, Thomas SA, Rosenfield NS, Markowitz RI (1990) Skull fractures in young children: do characteristics of the fractures clearly distinguish child abuse from accidental injuries? *Am J Dis Child* **144**: 429.

Merten DF, Osborne DRS (1984) Craniocerebral trauma in the child abuse syndrome: Radiological observations. *Pediatr Radiol* **14**: 272–277.

Meservy CJ, Towbin R, McLaurin RL, Myers PA, Ball W (1987) Radiographic characteristics of skull fractures resulting from child abuse. *AJNR* **149**: 173–175.

Monteleone J (1998) *Child Maltreatment: A Clinical Guide and Reference*. St Louis: GW Medical.

O'Neil JAJ, Meacham WF, Griffin PP, Sawyers JL (1973) Patterns of injury in the battered child syndrome. *J Trauma* **13**: 332–339.

Taylor D (2000) Unnatural injuries. *Eye* **14**: 123–150.

Zimmerman RA, Bilaniuk LT, Bruce D, Schut L, Uzzell B, Goldberg HI (1979) Computed tomography of craniocerebral injury in the abused child. *Radiology* **130**: 687–690.

4
NON-ACCIDENTAL HEAD INJURY IN SCOTLAND: THE SCOTTISH DATABASE

Robert A Minns, Caroline Millar, Fiona C Minns, TY Milly Lo, Patricia A Jones and Karen M Barlow

A prospective study was initiated in 1998 to assess the incidence and demography of non-accidental head injury (NAHI) in Scotland. All previously known, as well as new cases of suspected NAHI throughout Scotland were registered on a database. The number currently totals 129 cases.

Participating centres

All hospital paediatric wards/units in Scotland, paediatric intensive care units and neuro-surgical units admitting children (Table 4.1) are contacted fortnightly by a clerk liaising with the unit secretary. When notification of a new case of 'suspected NAHI' is made, demographic, clinical, and social details are requested (Table 4.2).

Validation

Validation of the data is done by biannual questionnaires to the participating centres, and a separate search of the 'Information and Statistics Division of the Scottish Health Service' ICD10 coding system is undertaken. To ensure that as many children as possible who die prior to admission with NAHI are registered, we further search the registrar general database for childhood deaths in Scotland. Further verification of the information obtained is attempted by liaising with the Region's lead child protection paediatrician and at other times by visits to these units and their medical records by the data collector.

This database contains only anonymous details and has both local and multicentre research ethics committee approval.

Limitations of database

Although attempts are made to ensure that no case of suspected NAHI is missed and none doubly recorded, there are undoubted limitations to complete accuracy of the database as follows.

• As all reported cases are suspected NAHI, it is essential that information pertaining to the suspected cases is not accepted as proven unless non-accidental origin has been acknowledged or has resulted in a criminal conviction.
• Information is obtained from multiple paediatric units and other sources thus increasing the chance of errors or omissions.

TABLE 4.1
List of participating Scottish hospitals with paediatric wards

Aberdeen Royal Infirmary, Aberdeen
Ayrshire General Hospital, Ayr
Borders General Hospital, Melrose, Roxburghshire
Dumfries and Galloway Royal Infirmary, Dumfries
Inverclyde Royal Hospital, Greenock
Ninewells Hospital, Dundee
Perth Royal Infirmary, Perthshire
Raigmore Hospital, Inverness
Royal Alexandra Hospital, Paisley, Renfrewshire
Royal Hospital for Sick Children, Edinburgh
Royal Hospital for Sick Children, Glasgow
Southern General Hospital, Glasgow
St John's Hospital, Livingston, West Lothian
Stirling Royal Infirmary, Stirlingshire
Victoria Hospital, Kirkcaldy, Fife
Wishaw General Hospital, Lanarkshire

TABLE 4.2
Demographic, clinical and social details collected for each case

Sex	Date of birth	
Address, town/city, postcode	Social class	
Date of admission	Admitted via GP?	
Hospital(s)	Consultant	Speciality
Diagnosis	Presenting symptoms	Inappropriate history/change in history
Preterm birth?	Twin birth?	Single parent?
Age of parents	Biological parents?	
Past history of child abuse	Past history of drug/alcohol abuse	
Past history of domestic abuse	Past history of social worker involvement	
Mental health history	Recurrent consultations/admissions	
Subdural/subarachnoid/intraparenchymal/intracranial haemorrhage		Unilateral
Raised intracranial pressure	Initial pressure	Brain swelling	EPTS (fits)
MRI (number)	CT (number)	Head ultrasound (number)
Haemorrhagic retinopathy	Skeletal injury	
Malicious injury	Impact – skull/haematoma/bruising	
Inpatient duration	Intensive care duration	Intermittent positive pressure ventilation
Outcome – dead/alive (GOS)	Discharged/transferred	
Court case – child protection/criminal proceedings	Admitted injury?	Conviction?
Perpetrator – male or female	Relation of perpetrator to child	Age of perpetrator

- Information is relayed by non-medical personnel, although potential errors are minimized by requesting specific answers to database questions.
- Information may be missing or unavailable. The most significant cause of missing data is the frequently protracted nature of both treatment procedures and child protection/criminal proceedings, which means that information may not be available at the time of contact.
- In some cases children die from NAHI prior to admission or in the accident and emergency department, when staff may liase directly with forensic pathologists.

155

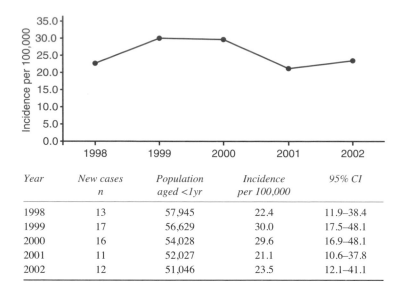

Year	New cases n	Population aged <1yr	Incidence per 100,000	95% CI
1998	13	57,945	22.4	11.9–38.4
1999	17	56,629	30.0	17.5–48.1
2000	16	54,028	29.6	16.9–48.1
2001	11	52,027	21.1	10.6–37.8
2002	12	51,046	23.5	12.1–41.1

Fig. 4.1. Incidence of 'suspected non-accidental head injury' in Scotland in children aged 0–12 months, per 100,000 population.

- Cases in which a non-accidental origin originally enters the differential diagnosis but is subsequently excluded may not always be notified.
- Details of the legal processes and their outcome are frequently recorded in social work records and not medical case files.

Incidence

From July 1998 to December 1999, 19 new cases of suspected NAHI in children less than 1 year old were identified (12 boys and 7 girls), giving an annual incidence of 24.6 per 100,000 (95% confidence interval 14.9–38.5). The median age at acute admission was 2.2 months (range 4 weeks to 8.8 months). No child was older than 12 months. Three quarters of admissions during that period were in the autumn and winter months, and a higher incidence was found in the urban areas of Greater Glasgow and Edinburgh (45.7 and 43.8 per 100,000 children under 1 year respectively). Three children died as a result of child abuse during that 18 month period, one from brain injury (Barlow and Minns 2000).

The annual incidence of suspected NAHI in Scotland from 1998 to 2002 is shown in Figure 4.1.

Acknowledged (confessed) and convicted cases

There are a number of cases where the perpetrator has acknowledged injuring the child. Assuming uncoerced confessions, these cases represent an invaluable cohort providing a 'gold standard' for clinico-pathological data. A further cohort (but not mutually exclusive) of cases where the perpetrator has been criminally convicted of injuring the child has been

156

TABLE 4.3
Presenting features of abuse victims where the perpetrator is known to have, or not to have, confessed

	Known to have confessed (Total N=29)	Known not to have confessed (Total N=33)	Confidence intervals	Significance
SDH (bilateral or unilateral)	25/28	29/33	–0.144 to 0.172	ns
Bilateral RH	19/28	14/31	–0.013 to 0.467	ns
Any skeletal injury	10/28	14/32	–0.323 to 0.163	ns
Bruising	6/28	8/29	–0.275 to 0.152	ns
Malicious injuries	13/28	12/30	–0.183 to 0.311	ns
Inappropriate history	22/24	27/32	–0.087 to 0.233	ns
Recurrent admissions	7/24	17/31	–0.494 to 0.020	ns
Early post-traumatic fits	18/27	19/33	–0.150 to 0.331	ns
Skull fracture	4/28	14/32	–0.507 to 0.083	ns
Risk factors	8/22	5/28	–0.033 to 0.404	ns
Encephalopathy	16/28	19/33	–0.251 to 0.242	ns
Past history of child abuse	9/26	8/27	–0.183 to 0.283	ns

SDH = subdural haemorrhage; RH = retinal haemorrhage.

TABLE 4.4
Presenting features of abuse victims where the perpetrator is known to have, or not to have, been convicted

	Known to have been convicted (Total N=25)	Known not to have been convicted (Total N=30)	Confidence intervals	p
SDH (bilateral or unilateral)	24/25	25/30	–0.019 to 0.272	ns
Bilateral RH	16/25	15/27	–0.159 to 0.328	ns
Any skeletal injury	13/25	11/28	–0.120 to 0.374	ns
Bruising	9/25	6/27	–0.087 to 0.363	ns
Malicious injuries	18/25	10/28	0.132 to 0.574	ns
Inappropriate history	21/24	22/28	–0.095 to 0.274	ns
Recurrent admissions	5/23	16/27	–0.600 to 0.150	ns
Early post-traumatic fits	20/25	19/30	–0.053 to 0.386	ns
Skull fracture	6/25	9/29	–0.292 to 0.151	ns
Risk factors	14/22	2/26	0.362 to 0.757	$\chi^2 = 9.64$, $p<0.01$
Encephalopathy	18/25	17/29	–0.101 to 0.368	ns
Past history of child abuse	12/25	8/28	0.044 to 0.433	ns

SDH = subdural haemorrhage; RH = retinal haemorrhage.

identified. The database therefore contains groups who have confessed, a group known not to have confessed, a group who have been convicted, and a group known not to have been convicted.

Table 4.3 shows the percentages of subdural haemorrhage (SDH; bilateral or unilateral), bilateral retinal haemorrhage, skeletal injuries, bruising, malicious injuries, inappropriate history, recurrent hospital admissions, epileptic seizures, skull fractures, risk factors, encephalopathy (seizures, coma, decerebration, loss of homeostatis, central apnoea), and past history of child abuse in the acknowledged (confessed) group compared with the group known not to have confessed. The only significant difference (at the 5% level) was in the percentage of skull fractures between the two groups (14% in the confessed and 44% in the non-confessed). This database contains cases of different types of inflicted brain injury to infants and children, and while shaking alone or shaking against a soft surface would not have associated skull fracture, shaking against a hard surface or other forms of deceleration impact injuries would be associated with a high frequency of skull fracture. The confessed group appears to include more instances of pure shaking without impact (or onto a soft surface) than the non-confessed groups.

In all other respects the confessed and non-confessed groups are not statistically significantly different as reflected by the chi-square levels. However, this does not mean that the groups are significantly the same. The nonsignificant chi-square means there is no statistically significant difference in many of these items between the two groups, but to prove they are identical is trying to prove a negative (equivalence). The 95% confidence intervals were therefore used for these categorical data and are superior to percentages in comparing the groups. The confidence intervals and p-values are shown in the accompanying table for the confessed versus non-confessed groups. The confidence intervals are very wide, reflecting the small sample size.

There was a statistically significant difference between two further groups of cases from the database where a perpetrator is known to have been criminally convicted compared with those where no criminal conviction had been obtained, although it is accepted that some of the latter may still have criminal proceedings pending. Significance accrued between various items in the two groups, such as malicious injuries, recurrent hospital admissions and the presence of 'risk factors'. It is likely that these were the features instrumental in obtaining a conviction (Table 4.4).

Given the similarity of the clinical features between the confessed and non-confessed groups, and the clinical features of the convicted and non-convicted groups, it is reasonable to postulate that the whole of the database is likely to be similar in clinical features. However, further statistical rigidity is required to compare the 95% confidence intervals in the group of cases where the perpetrator has confessed and the group of those who did not confess, with the incidence of these features (SDH, retinal haemorrhage, etc.) as they occur from causes other than NAHI in different study populations reported in the medical literature. The medical literature has therefore been searched extensively, and studies that indicate both the population size and the numbers affected have been selected and included in a simple population incidence. From some of the papers, the numbers affected had to be extracted or calculated from the data provided. This has been undertaken for retinal haemorrhages, SDHs, fractures of different types, bruising and skin injuries.

RETINAL HAEMORRHAGES
Confessed cases versus the literature
Table 4.5 lists all the studies found where retinal haemorrhages are reported in conditions other than NAHI. The age of the population is noted and brief relevant details given. A selected number of studies (highlighted), where both the number of cases affected with

TABLE 4.5

Retinal haemorrhages (RH) in conditions excluding non-accidental injury: reports from the literature

Reference	Series	Age of study population	Details	RH %	RH n	Population N
Bergen and Margolis (1976)	Consecutive births	Newborn	Various methods of delivery	35%	35	100
Besio et al. (1979)	Consecutive births	Newborn	Various methods of delivery	30.3%	71	234
Egge et al. (1980)	Consecutive births	Newborn	Quantitative study of RH		74	200
			Vacuum	50%	25	51
			Forceps	16%	8	49
			Natural	41%	41	100
Levin et al. (1980)	Birth	Newborn	Within 24 hours after birth	37.3%	153	410
O'Leary et al. (1986)	Birth		Overall		8	38
	Vacuum extraction		19 vacuum assisted delivery		6	19
			19 spontaneous (controls)		2	19
Elder et al. (1991)	Trauma	1.2–14.5yr	25 children <15yr		0	25
			Documented accidental injury, incl. 5 hit by cars and 3 passengers in RTAs			
			4/25 <2yr		0	4
Buys et al. (1992)	Head trauma	<3yr (mean = 16mo)	79 HI children had ophthalmological exam		0	75
			75 accidental HI		0	75
			3 NAHI		3	3
			1 cause of injury unknown		0	1
Duhaime et al. (1992)	Trauma	<2yr	100 had ophthalmological exam			
			NAHI (admission diagnosis)		9	13
			Accidental TBI (excluding RTA)		0	69
			RTA		1	3
			"After investigations ...24 NAHI; 32? inflicted, therefore 44 accidental"			
			RH found in 10 cases of which 9 'abused'		1	44
			"Can therefore infer RH in trauma"			

TABLE 4.5
(cont'd)

Reference	Series	Age of study population	Details	RH %	RH n	Population N
Gilliland and Luckenbach (1993)	Unsuccessful resuscitation (deaths)	Mean = 17mo (152 <3yr)			70	169
	131 prolonged attempts		CPR of 30 mins in 131		61	131
			Of whom 70 had prolonged resuscitation		0	70
			Head injury or CNS diseases		0	21
			SIDS, asphyxia, respiratory illness		0	
	38 short attempts		38 controls		9	38
Goldstein et al. (1993)	TBI (moderate/severe)	1.9–12.7yr	26 trauma (?ages)		0	26
Johnson et al. (1993)	Trauma		200 children admitted with head injury			
			30 excluded, suspected child abuse			
			Of remaining 170, 140 seen by ophthalmologist	1.4%	2	140
Liu et al. (1993)	Birth Various delivery methods	Within 1wk of delivery	Fundal exam (54 cases had RH, from 78 eyes)		54	527
Gilliland et al. (1994)	Trauma	2wk – 9yr 11mo (54% <1yr)	169 child deaths (natural causes, injuries to head/trunk, asphyxia)			
			RH in 70 (62 HI, 4 CNS causes, 4 n/k)			
			62 HI (9 severe RTA, 53 NAHI)			
			Thus 108 [169–(53+4+4)] were from trauma		9	108
			If CNS and n/k causes included		17	116
Pollack and Tychsen (1996)	ECMO	All	35 neonates, 2 1-yr-olds		5	37
Olumese et al. (1997)	Cerebral malaria	6mo – 6yr		23%	17	73
Odom et al. (1997)	Post-CPR	Mean = 23mo (1mo – 15.8yr) 36/43 <2yr				
Varn et al. (1997)	ECMO	Infants	Small punctate haemorrhages only found	12%	1	36
			171 patients, 342 eyes		40 eyes	342 eyes

160

Study	Population / cause	Age	Findings		
Young et al. (1997)	ECMO	Term or near-term infants	91 infants (182 eyes)	8	91
	Congenital diaphragmatic hernia		Asymmetric retinopathy	6	9
	Meconium aspiration syndrome			1	35
	Respiratory distress syndrome			1	10
Ewing-Cobbs et al. (1998)	Inflicted and non-inflicted	1mo – 6yr	Accidental injuries (moderate/severe)	14	20
			Infants with accidental injuries	0	20
				0	5
Jayawant et al. (1998)	Population based case series of SDH (all causes) RTA (n=1)	3w – 17mo	SDH	33	257,812
Tyagi et al. (1998)	Convulsions	<2yr	SDH but no RH	0	1
Christian et al. (1999)	Household trauma	<15mo	All had detailed ophthalmological exam	0	32
			3 cases of unilateral trauma resulting in a few unilateral RH:		
			(1) 13-mo-old fell down 13 steps to concrete basement in baby walker		
			(2) 9-mo-old being swung by father fell 30–60cm (observed by another adult)		
			(3) 7-mo-old fell through railing onto concrete floor		
			All had unilateral RH, confined to the posterior pole		
			None had peripheral or diffuse RH		
			None had retinoschisis		
Dashti et al. (1999)	Study pop'n 405; 38 inflicted 99/405 were <2yr Accidental trauma Inflicted trauma	Median age = 5.5mo	RH RH	0 17	68 32
Stein et al. (1999)	RTA/air-bag injuries	Adults and children	Airbag injuries - causing RH	24	97
			Retinal tears or detachments	15	97
			25%		
			15%		

161

TABLE 4.5
(cont'd)

Reference	Series	Age of study population	Details	RH %	RH n	Population N
DiScala et al. (2000)	Blunt trauma					
	Unintentional injury (16,831 cases)	<3yr	RH	0.07%	3	4,568
Johanson and Menon (2000)	Child abuse (1997 cases)	Newborn	RH	27.8%	159	571
	Vacuum/forceps delivery		More RH in vacuum extraction group, fewer with forceps delivery			
Reece and Sege (2000)	Trauma	1w – 6.5yr				
		Mean = 2.5yr	RH	2%	5	232
		Those <3yr only	RH	3%	4	144
	NAHI			35%	18	51
Anteby et al. (2001)		Gestational age <32wk	Incidence of RH in low birthweight neonates		2	22
Emerson et al. (2001)	Birth	Newborn	Indirect ophthalmoscopy	34%	51	149
	Various methods of delivery		Single dot haemorrhage to widespread bilateral RH			
			Resolved by 1 month			
Feldman et al. (2001)		≤36mo				
	NAHI	0.6–16.8mo	RH		28	66
	(RTA, or other documented major trauma)	9.1–29.0mo	RH (only 3 examined)		1	39
	Indeterminate cause		RH		?	12

Study	Cause/topic	Age	Details		
Plunket (2001)	Short fall	12mo – 13yr (no infants)	18 deaths from short falls (out of total CPSC* database of 75,000 reports of accidents)		
		Few <3yr	Several noted to have RH, but none had post-mortem exam of eyes		
		5 <2yr	1 23-mo-old fell 60–120cm onto carpeted floor	4	18
			Only 6 had fundoscopic exam, ages n/k Bilateral RH, ages n.k		
White et al. (2001)	Cerebral malaria or coma of other causes or malarial anaemia	Ages not given	Clinical exam and histopathology 35 children who died	10	33
Asproudis et al. (2002)	ROP	Gestational age <32wk	Birthweight <1500g 7.7%	15	194
Dinakaran et al. (2002)	Meningococcal septicaemia	Mean = 4.5yr	All had had a convulsion	5	12
Mei-Zahav et al. (2002)	Convulsions	2mo – 2yr	Retinal exam by ophthalmologist	1	153
Reed et al. (2002)	Soccer Biomechanics of globe movements/forces	13–16yr	21 soccer players, 30 controls	0	21
Schloff et al. (2002)	Intracranial haemorrhage (Terson syndrome n=2)	5mo – 16.1yr	Case 1. 7-yr-old RTA thrown 30m Case 2. 8-yr-old with nephropathy, seizures and sepsis	1 1	57
Vinchon et al. (2002)	Trauma (RTA)	0–2yr	18 cases, 16 examined for RH 9/18 had severe head injury, 12/18 moderate head injury or comatose) All were flame shaped and in posterior pole	3	16

Highlighted data have been used in summaries.
*US Consumer Product Safety Commission.

TABLE 4.6
Occurrence of retinal haemorrhage (RH) from all causes except NAHI –
population data from the literature

Reference	RH n	Population N
Trauma		
Elder et al. (1991)	0	4
Buys et al. (1992)	0	75
Duhaime et al. (1992) – accidental (excluding RTA)	0	69
– RTA	1	3
Johnson et al. (1993)	2	140
Gilliland et al. (1994)	9	116
Ewing-Cobbs et al. (1998)	0	5
Jayawant et al. (1998)	0	1
Dashti et al. (1999)	0	68
DiScala et al. (2000)	3	4,568
Reece and Sege (2000)	4	144
Feldman et al. (2001)	1	3
Vinchon et al. (2002)	3	16
Birth		
Bergen and Margolis (1976)	35	100
Besio et al. (1979)	71	234
Egge et al. (1980)	74	200
Liu et al. (1993)	54	527
Emerson et al. (2001)	51	149
Retinopathy of prematurity		
Asproudis et al. (2002)	15	194
Preterm birth		
Anteby et al. (2001)	2	22
Post-CPR		
Gilliland and Luckenbach (1993) (unsuccessful CPR)	70	169
Odom et al. (1997)	1	36
ECMO		
Pollack and Tychsen (1996)	5	37
Young et al. (1997)	8	91
Convulsions		
Tyagi et al. (1998)	0	32
Mei-Zahav et al. (2002)	1	153
Total	410	7,156

retinal haemorrhages and the population from which they were drawn is known, have been used in our calculations and have been displayed in a second summary table (Table 4.6).

Summated numbers show 410 cases of retinal haemorrhage in a combined population of 7156. There was a significant difference between the frequency of retinal haemorrhage in other conditions reported in the medical literature and that found in our confessed database cohort (p<0.001, χ^2 = 237.31, 95% CI 0.532–0.853).

In summary, there is a very significant difference in the proportion of cases in the confessed group of our database (19/28) compared to other populations and to other

TABLE 4.7

Subdural haemorrhages (SDH) in conditions excluding non-accidental injury: reports from the literature

Reference	Series	Age of study population	Details	SDH (%)	SDH (n)	Population
Aoki and Masuzawa (1984)	"Minor head trauma" No loss of consciousness	3–13mo	SDH Most had seizures, and all had retinal and preretinal haemorrhages		26	(not given)
Aoki and Masuzawa (1984)	"Alleged minor trauma"	3–13mo	All had SDH and RH		26	26
Oi et al. (1986)	Cerebrovascular disorders	Admitted to children's hospital Preterm – older children	All intracranial haemorrhage		79	13,131
Hayashi et al. (1987)	Birth injury survivors	Newborn	SDH RH 12/48		48	(not given)
Nimityongskul and Anderson (1987)	Falls 30–100cm from bed/crib/chair while in hospital	0–5yr	SDH		0	76
Saito et al. (1987)	Middle fossa arachnoid cyst	13/24 were aged 11–20yr	3 cases, 21 others from literature		3	24
Partington et al. (1991)	HI and baby walkers Baby walkers + stairs in 18/19 accidents	<2yr	SDH		0	19
Duhaime et al. (1992)	Trauma	<2yr				100
	NAHI		SDH		13	24
	Probable NAHI		SDH		?	32
	Accidental TBI (excluding RTA)		SDH		0	36
	RTA (passengers)		SDH		3	8

TABLE 4.7
(cont'd)

Reference	Series	Age of study population	Details	SDH (%)	SDH (n)	Population
de Tezanos Pinto et al. (1992)	CNS bleeding		156 episodes of bleeding			156
	Haemophilia	Mean = 14.8yr	Haemophilia A = 131 episodes			
		Mean = 9yr	Haemophilia B = 15 episodes			
			Intracranial bleeds		154	156
			SDH	29.9%	46	154
Goldstein et al. (1993)		Children <5yr	14 NAHI		3	26
		1.9–12.7yr	26 trauma			
Reiber (1993)	Witnessed high falls (>3m)	0 – ≤5yr	All fatal, autopsy found SDH in 2 children <2yr		2	2
	"Unwitnessed short fall"	0 – ≤5yr	Fatal, with SDH		2	19
Berney et al. (1994b)	Head trauma	Children <15yr				
		0–3yr	SDH (all were <14 mo old) (3/4 were attributed to "miscellaneous" cause, which included NAHI)		4	348
Chiaviello et al. (1994)	Baby walkers	3–17mo	SDH		1	65
Shugerman et al. (1996)	Head injury N=759	0–3yr	EDH/SDH		93	759
	NAHI		SDH		28	
	Neglect		SDH		0	⎫
	Cause not identified		SDH		6	⎬ 59
	Trauma		SDH		25	⎭
	NAHI		EDH 2/93			
	Neglect		EDH 1/93			
	Cause not identified		EDH 0/93			
	Trauma		EDH 31/93			
			Total SDH		25	759

166

Study	Category	Age	Finding	n	Total
Ewing-Cobbs et al. (1998)		1mo – 6yr			
	Accidental trauma	Mean = 35.5mo	SDH	9	20
	NAHI	Mean = 10.6mo	SDH	16	20
	Accidental trauma	Mean = 35.5mo	EDH	4	20
	NAHI	Mean = 10.6mo	EDH	0	20
Jayawant et al. (1998)	All known admissions	3wk – 17mo	SDH (all non-inflicted causes, including 1 RTA)	6	257,812
		<2yr	Incidence of 12.8/100,000 per year		
		<1yr	Incidence of 21/100,000 per year		
			Risk of developing SDH by 1yr of age was 1:4761%		
			Association of 80% between RH and SDH		
	NAHI (confirmed or highly suggested)		RH + SDH	19	27
Tzioumi and Oates (1998)	Trauma + non-trauma Disease (haemophilia A)	2–23mo		15	37
				1	1
	NAHI	4wk – 20mo	NAHI	21	38
	Cause n/k (chronic SDH)			1	38
Dashti et al. (1999)	Study pop'n 405; 38 inflicted 99/405 were <2yr				
	Inflicted trauma	Median = 5.5mo	SDH (4/5 RTAs)	5	68
	Accidental trauma		SDH	22	32
Towner et al. (1999)	Birth	Live-born singletons	SDH (incidence = 4.46/10,000)	260	583,340
DiScala et al. (2000)	Blunt trauma	<5yr			
	Unintentional (n=16,831)		24% <1yr (n=4007); 43% <2yr (n=7291) <2yr, any intracrania injury: 4.1% (1078)		
	Child abuse (n=1997)		63% <1yr (n=1253); 81% <2yr (n=1624) <2yr, any intracrania injury: <2.4% (685)		
Ewing-Cobbs et al. (2000)	Non-inflicted injury	<6yr	SDH	9	29
Morris et al. (2000)	"Investigations on children without external evidence of child abuse"	11d – 15mo	19 suspected child abuse cases; all had SDH 8 NAHI (SDH + trauma/bruises/fractures) 2 had tiny SDH adjacent to linear skull # 9 SDH, no other history		

TABLE 4.7
(cont'd)

Reference	Series	Age of study population	Details	SDH (%)	SDH (n)	Population
Reece and Sege (2000)	All head injuries	1w – 6.5yr				287
	Accidental trauma (n=233)	Mean = 2.5yr	SDH	10%	23	232
			SAH	8%	19	232
	NAHI (n=54)	Mean = 0.7yr	SDH	46%	25	54
			SAH	31%	17	54
	Accidental trauma (n=144)	<3yr only	SDH	10%	14	144
	NAHI (n=54)	<2.3yr	SDH	50%	25	51
Feldman et al. (2001)	NAHI	≤36mo	All SDHs		17	66
	RTA, or other documented major trauma	0.6–16.8mo	SDH (chronic, or mixed acute/chronic)		0	39
		9.1–29.0mo	SDH (chronic, or mixed acute/chronic)			15
	Indeterminate cause		SDH (chronic, or mixed acute/chronic)		8	12
	RTA, or other documented major trauma	9.1–29.0mo	Acute SDH	23%	15	66
Maxeiner (2001)	Deaths from trauma with SDH	<1yr	Unclear condition/RTA/high fall		14	24
			NB: No deaths with SDH after short fall			
Vinchon et al. (2001)	Subduroperitoneal drainage for SDH, all causes	<2yr				244
	RTA	<2yr	SDH		21	244
Gradnitzer et al. (2002)	Birth	Term newborn	SDH		13	2019
Hirsch et al. (2002)	Severe head trauma	0.1–14yr	SDH		14	100
			EDH		22	100
Hoskote et al. (2002)	Admission diagnosis		SDH			36
	Accidental/iatrogenic/other		After full clinical/radiological investigation		16	36
	NAHI	Mean <4mo			14	36
	Unexplained				6	36

Study	Population	Age	Finding	n	N
Loh et al. (2002)	Trauma causing SDH	6d – 12mo	SDH		21
	Fall			7	21
	Birth trauma			1	21
	Coagulopathy			1	21
	RTA			1	21
	Shaken baby syndrome			11	21
Vinchon et al. (2002)	Trauma (RTA), all witnessed	36d – 21.4mo	Selected for SDH, radiological/clinical features and time course	18	
Geddes et al. (2003)	Infant deaths, non-trauma (incl. intrauterine deaths, spontaneous abortions)	<5mo (1 age corrected for preterm birth)	SDH	36	50
	Infection n=6				
	Hypoxia n=26				
	Infection + hypoxia n=3				
	SIDS n=4				
	Unexplained n=6 (includes 5 intrauterine)				
Whitby et al. (2003)	Delivery	Newborn	SDH – clinically silent, resolved in 4wk	3	93

Abbreviations: EDH = extradural haemorrhage; NAHI = non-accidental head injury; RH = retinal haemorrhage; RTA = road traffic accident; SAH = subarachnoid haemorrhage; TBI = traumatic brain injury.

Highlighted data have been used in summaries.

169

TABLE 4.8
Occurrence of subdural haemorrhage (SDH) in children <2 years old from all causes except NAHI – population data from the literature

Reference	SDH n	Population N
Trauma		
Nimityongskul and Anderson (1987)	0	76
Duhaime et al. (1992)	3	44
Reiber (1993)	2	2
Berney et al. (1994)	4	348
Chiaviello et al. (1994a)	1	65
Shugerman et al. (1996)	25	759
Ewing-Cobbs et al. (1998)	9	20
Jayawant et al. (1998) (RTAs)	6	257,812
Tzioumi and Oates (1998)	16	37
Dashti et al. (1999)	5	68
Reece and Sege (2000)	14	144
Feldman et al. (2001)	15	66
Hoskote et al. (2002) (witnessed)	16	36
Loh et al. (2002)	10	21
Haemophilia		
de Tezanos Pinto et al. (1992)	46	154
Tzioumi and Oates (1998)	1	1
Birth		
Partington et al. (1991)	0	19
Towner et al. (1999)	260	583,340
Gradnitzer et al. (2002)	13	2,019
Whitby et al. (2003)	3	93
"Alleged minor trauma" deaths		
Reiber (1993)	2	19
Maxeiner (2001)	14	24
Infant deaths		
Geddes et al. (2003)	36	50
Total*	**501**	**845,217**

*Highlighted data have been used in summaries.

conditions causing retinal haemorrhage (410/7156). It is therefore possible to state that there is no statistically significant difference between the confessed and non-confessed groups (14/31), with respect to retinal haemorrhages, and their confidence intervals indicate that they are not dissimilar.

Convicted cases versus the literature
The proportion of cases having a retinal haemorrhage in the convicted group (16/25) was significantly different from that in the cumulated population within the literature of retinal haemorrhage due to other conditions (410/7156) ($p < 0.001$, $\chi^2 = 244.11$, 95% CI 0.577–0.908). Similarly there was no statistically significant difference between the convicted and non-convicted (15/27) groups with respect to retinal haemorrhages, and their confidence intervals indicate that they are not dissimilar.

TABLE 4.9
Injuries from causes other than NAHI – reports from the literature

Reference	Cases n	Population N	Ages	Injuries
Skull fracture				
Kravitz et al. (1969)	2	101	0–12 mo	Accidental falls
Helfer et al. (1977)	2	219	<5 yr	Fall out of bed/crib/table, at home
Helfer et al. (1977)	1	85	<5 yr	Fall in hospital, uncarpeted floor
McClelland and Heiple (1982)	8	15	0–12 mo	Accidental trauma
Stoffman et al. (1984)	3	52	0–2 yr	Baby walkers + stairs
Worlock and Stower (1986)	8	10,989	0–18 mo	Trauma
Nimityongskul and Anderson (1987)	1	76	0–5 yr	Falls from bed in hospital
Joffe and Lugwig (1988)	4	55	0–6 mo	Stairway injuries
Tursz et al. (1990)	13	641	<2 yr	Home accidents
Partington et al. (1991)	9	19	<2 yr	Baby walkers + stairs
Berney et al. (1994)	164	318	0–3 yr	Head trauma
Bhat et al. (1994)	5	34,946	Newborn	Delivery → depressed skull fracture/orbital fracture
Chiaviello et al. (1994b)	10	65	3–17 mo	Baby walkers ± stairs
Chiaviello et al. (1994a)	2	5	<12 mo	Stairway accidents excluding baby walkers
Gruskin and Schutzman (1999)	39	278	<24 mo	Head trauma
Gruskin and Schutzman (1999)	0	31	<24 mo	Head trauma from low falls
Greenes and Schutzman (2001)	45	422	0–24 mo	Asymptomatic head injury
	318	48,347		
Concussion				
Chiaviello et al. (1994a)	8	65	3–17 mo	Baby walkers ± stairs
Chiaviello et al. (1994b)	11	69	<5 yr	Stairs, excluding all baby walker related accidents or possible NAHI
	19	134		
Clavicle fracture				
Sieben et al. (1971)	1	12	<2 yr	Fall from height
Helfer et al. (1977)	3	219	<5 yr	Fall out of bed/crib/table, at home
Worlock and Stower (1986)	1	10,989	0–18 mo	Trauma
Bhat et al. (1994)	16	34,946	Newborn	Delivery
	20	46,166		
Rib fractures				
Sieben et al. (1971)	1	12	<2 yr	Fall from height
Worlock and Stower (1986)	0	10,989	0–18 mo	Trauma
Joffe and Lugwig (1988)	0	363	1 mo – 18.7 yr	Stairway injuries
Bulloch et al. (2000)	3	39	<12 mo	Forceful accidental trauma
Bulloch et al. (2000)	1	39	<12 mo	Birth trauma
Bulloch et al. (2000)	3	39	<12 mo	Bone fragility
Feldman et al. (2001)	1	15	<36 mo	RTA/documented unintentional injuries
	9	11,496		

TABLE 4.9
(cont'd)

Reference	Cases n	Population N	Ages	Injuries
Humerus fracture				
Helfer et al. (1977)	1	219	<5 yr	Fall out of bed/crib/table, at home
Thomas et al. (1991)	3	14	0–35 mo	Falls onto elbow
Bhat et al. (1994)	7	34,946	Newborn	Delivery
Trunk, thorax, abdomen, pelvis fractures				
Worlock and Stower (1986)	0	10,989	0-18 mo	Trauma
Joffe and Lugwig (1988)	7	363	1 mo – 18.7 yr	Stairway injuries
Chiaviello et al. (1994a)	2	65	3–17 mo	Baby walkers ± stairs
Labbe and Caouette (2001)	0	246	0–8 mo	
Lower limb fractures				
Kravitz et al. (1969)	0	101	0–12 mo	Accidental falls
Joffe and Lugwig (1988)	1	212	<4 yr	Stairway injuries
Thomas et al. (1991)	14	25	0–35 mo	All types of femoral fractures from accidental trauma
	15	338		
"Extremities"				
McClelland and Heiple (1982)	7	15	0–12 mo	Accidental trauma
Worlock and Stower (1986)	10	10,989	0–18 mo	Trauma
Chiaviello et al. (1994a)	4	65	3–17 mo	Baby walkers ± stairs
Bhat et al. (1994)	7	34,946	Newborn	Delivery
"Fracture" – not specified				
Lyons and Oates (1993)	2	81	<2 yr	Falls from cribs/beds
Warrington et al. (2001)	21	11,466	<6 mo	Low falls
	23	11,547		
Bruising				
Helfer et al. (1977)	20	85	<5 yr	Fall in hospital, uncarpeted floor
Lyons and Oates (1993)	8	81	<2 yr	Falls from cribs/beds
Carpenter (1999)	22	177	6–12 mo	Bruising on normal babies
Sugar et al. (1999)	2	366	<6 mo	
Warrington et al. (2001)	262	11,466	<6 mo	Low falls
Labbe and Caouette (2001)	3	246	0–8 mo	Bruise
	317	12,421		
Skin lesions (bruises, abrasions, scratches) in normal children				
Labbe and Caouette (2001)	38	246	0–8 mo	Skin lesion/bruise/scrape
Head/face	33			
Wrists	2			
Thighs	2			
Legs	1			
"Lacerations"				
Lyons and Oates (1993)	1	81	<2 yr	Falls from cribs/beds
Labbe and Caouette (2001)	27	246	0–8 mo	Scratch
	3	246	0–8 mo	Abrasions, skin lesions in normal children

SUBDURAL HAEMORRHAGES

Confessed cases versus the literature
Similar literature searches for subdural SDH associated with other causes such as accidental trauma and birth injuries, cerebral vascular disorders, coagulopathy, etc., are shown in Table 4.7. The literature incidences (numbers and study population), again extracted and summated, are given in Table 4.8. In total the literature records 501 cases from a total population of 845,217 (0.059%), compared to 25/28 in our confessed population ($p<0.01$, $\chi^2 = 3584.26$, 95% CI 0.778–1.007).

Convicted cases versus the literature
SDHs were again highly significantly different between the two groups (24/25 vs 501/845217 respectively; $p<0.001$, $\chi^2 = 3707.04$, 95% CI 0.888–1.031).

SKULL AND OTHER SKELETAL FRACTURES (Tables 4.9, 4.10)

Skull fractures
The literature has been tabulated for the frequency of fractures in population based literature studies reporting accidental injuries, birth injuries, etc. A total of 318 cases of fracture occurred in a population of 48,347 (0.66%) compared to 4/28 in the confessed cohort ($p<0.001$, $\chi^2 = 78.60$, 95% CI 0.007–0.266).

Six out of the 25 cases that resulted in a conviction were associated with a skull fracture, compared to 31% when no conviction occurred. The frequency of skull fracture in these convicted cases (and in non-convicted cases) was significantly different from the expected frequency of fractures from other causes ($p<0.001$, 95% CI 0.076–0.391).

Other fractures
Rib fractures have been reported in 0.8%, fractures of the humerus in 0.02%, lower limb fractures in 4.4%, extremity fractures in 0.02%, and unspecified fractures in 0.2% of populations of accidental injury in children, with no cases of fractures of trunk, thorax, abdomen or pelvis, all significantly different from our database population groups of the confessed and convicted cohorts.

BRUISING AND SKIN LESIONS (Tables 4.9, 4.10)
Where the medical literature reports the incidence of bruising in otherwise normal children, it occurs in only 2.55%, compared to 6/28 cases in our confessed cohort and 28% in the non-confessed cohort ($p<0.001$, $\chi^2 = 39.39$, 95% CI 0.036–0.340). Similar differences were seen between the convicted cohort where 9/25 cases had bruising versus 6/27 in the non-convicted group ($p<0.001$, $\chi^2 = 109.43$, 95% CI 0.152–0.517).

These results for SDH, retinal haemorrhage, skull and skeletal injuries, and bruising represents the first element of our evidence base for the diagnosis of NAHI including shaken baby syndrome.

Principle of 'transposed conditional'
If a child dies from or is known to suffer from a specific medical condition with a certain

TABLE 4.10
Other injuries from causes other than NAHI: reports from the literature

Reference	Series	Age of study population	Details	%	n	Population
Home accidents						
Kravitz et al. (1969)	Accidental falls	0–12mo	Falls in 101/436 infants			
			Skull fracture		2	101
			Extremity fractures		0	101
Helfer et al. (1977)	Falls occurring at home from bed or sofa	≤5yr				
			No observable injuries		176	219
			Non-serious (bump, lump, bruise, scratch)		37	219
			Slightly more severe (clavicle # 3, skull # 2, humerus # 1)		6	219
			Life threatening		0	219
	Incidents in hospital (uncarpeted floor)					85
			No injury		57	85
			Small cuts/scratches, bloody nose		17	85
			Bump/bruise		20	85
			Skull fracture		1	85
Pascoe et al. (1979)	Soft tissue accidental injuries	1–18yr	Lacerations more common in accidental injury than in NAI. Fewer injuries over cheek, trunk, genitals, upper legs in accidental injuries			196
	Soft tissue NAIs	1–18yr				154
Stoffman et al. (1984)	Baby walkers + head injuries	0–2yr	All with head injury (HI)			52
			Skull fractures (fall on stairs with baby walker, all <1yr)		3	52
Nimityongskul and Anderson (1987)	Falls of 30–100cm from bed/crib/chair while in hospital	0–5yr	Severe injuries extremely rare; most injuries were minor (scalp hematoma and facial lacerations)		57	76

Study	Age/group	Description	%	n	Total
Joffe and Ludwig (1988)	Stairway injuries				
	In o – 18.7yr	Attended A&E with injuries		55	363
	1-12mo	In baby walkers/fell with carer		10	363
	Infants (?0–6mo)	Skull fracure from fall with carer		4	55
	Infants (?0–6mo)	Baby walkers involved		24	55
	6-12mo	Independent walking		16	40
		Rare for crawling children to fall down stairs; makes no difference how many stairs as energy discharged in one moderate impact and many subsequent minor impacts			40
		For all ages: truncal, thorax abdomen, pelvis injuries rare	2%	7	363
		For all ages: no rib, vertebral or pelvic fractures seen		0	363
		For all ages: head and neck injuries – mostly very minor and most were in <4-yr-olds	73%	263	363
		For all ages: extremities	28%	101	363
		Only 1 lower limb fracture in <4-yr-old group		1	212
Tursz et al. (1990)	Home accidents				
	<2yr 1-2yr ~379 0-1yr ~262	Attending A&E			641?
		Annual rate 6.6 per 100			
		Annual rate 2.7 per 100			
		Skull fracture		15	641
		Deaths		2	641
		Severe sequelae		2	641
		122 (19%) admitted to hospital			
Partington et al. (1991)	H and baby walkers				
	<2yr	Baby walker caused accident in 14.7% of cases		19	129
		SDH		0	19
	Baby walkers + stairs in 18/19 accidents	Skull # (no surgical intervention required)		9	19

175

TABLE 4.10
(cont'd)

Reference	Series	Age of study population	Details	%	n	Population
Lyons and Oates (1993)	Falls out of bed (n=83) or crib (n=124)	<6yr				207
		<12mo	Contusions		3	33
			Lacerations		0	33
			Fracture		1	33
			(All the above were head area)			
		12–23mo	Contusions		5	48
			Lacerations		1	48
			Fracture		1	48
			(6 head area, 1 other region)			
		<24mo	"Fracture"		2	81
			"Laceration"		1	81
			"Contusion/bruise"		8	81
Chiaviello et al. (1994a)	Infant walker related injuries		Extremities	6%	4	65
			Truncal injuries	3%	2	65
			Serious injuries	29%	19	65
			Skull fracture		10	65
			Concussion		8	65
			ICH (including 1 SDH)		5	65
			C-spine fracture		1	65
	Baby walkers down stairs 46/65		Serious injuries (all as above)		17	46
Chiaviello et al. (1994b)	Stairway accidents (not walker-related injuries)	≤5yr				69
		<12mo	2/5 had significant injuries, both with skull fracture, and 1 SDH		5	
		<24mo	5/23 had significant injuries			23
Greenes et al. (2001)	Unintentional HI	0–3mo	More likely to be boy	75%	54	88
			Left alone on furniture and fell		39	88
			Parent dropped child (20/27 boys)		27	88

Long bone fractures

Study	Category	Age	Finding		
Worlock and Stower (1986)	Trauma causing fractures	1–12yr 0–18mo	Incidence of any fracture, 1:1000	19	10,989
			Children with any fracture (RTA = 3, home = 16)	19	826
			Spine/pelvis fracture	0	19
			Linear skull fracture	8	19
			Clavicle fracture	1	19
			Extremities (forearm 2, hand 1, femur 2, tibia 5, ribs, 0)	10	19
			Mostly greenstick; 1/20 # Salter (epiphyseal)		
Thomas et al. (1991)	Long bore fractures from trauma	0–5mo	All fractures (252) found in 215 children		
	NAHI		Diaphyseal/metaphyseal	11	14
	Accidental (falls onto elbow)		Supracondylar humeral	3	14
	NAHI		Femur (all types)	9	25
	Accidental		Femur (all types)	14	25
	Cause not known		Femur	2	25
	Accidental	0–11mo	Humerus	1	8
	Accidental	0–11mo	Femur	3	10
Bhat et al. (1994)	Delivery, live births		Overall incidence of bony injuries, 1:1000	35	34,946
			Clavicle	16	34,946
			Humerus	7	34,946
			Depressed fracture	4	34,946
			Orbital fracture		34,946
			Femur	5	34,945
			Epiphyseal separation lower 3rd femur	1	34,945
			Dislocated elbow	1	34,946

Fractures

Study	Category	Age	Finding		
McCormick et al. (1981)	Accidental injuries	0–12mo	Requiring medical attention	8.6%	429
			Serious sequelae infrequent		4,989
			Independent mobility (e.g. walking) is major factor in risk of injury		

TABLE 4.10
(cont'd)

Reference	Series	Age of study population	Details	%	n	Population
McClelland and Heiple (1982)	Trauma Accidental (any fracture in 1st year of life)	0–12mo	24 patients with 55 fractures			15
			Skull fracture		8	15
			Extremities		7	15
			Other fractures		9	15
	NAHI		Skull fracture		13	19
			Extremities		12	19
			Other fractures		6	19
Rib fractures						
Sieben et al. (1971)	Falls from height	1–14yr	Rib fracture		1	60
		1–14yr	Clavicle		1	60
		(12 were <2y)	Rib fracture		≤1	12
		(1 <1yr; 11 1–2yr)	Clavicle		≤1	12
Bulloch et al. (2000)	All causes	≤12mo	Rib fractures		39	?
	Trauma (RTA, forceful blow, fall from height)		Rib fractures		3	39
	NAI		Rib fractures		32	39
	Birth		Rib fractures		1	32
	Bone fragility		Rib fractures		3	39
Feldman et al. (2001)	NAHI	≤36mo 0.6–16.8mo	Rib fractures/long bone fractures		20	66
	RTA, or other documented major trauma	9.1–29.0mo	Rib fractures/long bone fractures		1	39
	Indeterminate cause		Rib fractures/long bone fractures		1	12

178

Accidents in pre-mobile infants/falls ± bruises

Study	Injury type	Age	Finding	%	n	N
Warrington et al. (2001)	Accidents	≤6mo				11,466
	Falls		3357 falls in 2554 children	22%	2,554	11,466
			Bed/settee		1,779	11,466
			Arms/while carried		403	11,466
			Any visible injury		467	11,466
			Bruises seen		262	11,466
	HI (97% of falls)				3,256	11,466
	Concussion/fracture (<1% of those injured)				21	11,466
	Burns/scalds			1.50%	172	11,466

Skull fractures

Study	Injury type	Age	Finding	%	n	N
Berney et al. (1994)	Head trauma	0–3yo	Skull fracture		164	348
Gruskin and Schutzman (1999) (278 HI cases reviewed)	Head trauma	≤2yr	Skull fracture		39	278
			Intracranial injury		3	278
			Intracranial injury + skull fracture		9	278
			Minor injury		227	278
	Falls ≤1m (with no loss of consciousness, seizures, vomiting, scalp injury)	<12mo	Skull fracture		0	20
		<24mo	Skull fracture		0	31
Greenes and Schutzman (2001)	Assymptomatic head injury	0–24mo	Scalp abnormalities (parietal/temporal haematoma associated with skull #)			
			Large scalp haematoma + parietal haematoma associated with intracranial injury			
			Skull fracture	11%	45	422
			Intracranial injury	3%	13	422

Skin injuries in normal children

Study	Injury type	Age	Finding	%	n	N
Pascoe et al. (1979)	Patterns of skin injuries	0–18yr				47
	NAHI	<1yr	Lacerations			41
	Trauma (Emergency Room with soft tissue injury)		Lacerations (lesions generally over bony prominences, not on 'soft' sites)			7

TABLE 4.10
(cont'd)

Reference	Series	Age of study population	Details	%	n	Population
Carpenter (1999)	Skin bruises	6–12mo	32 bruises found in 22 babies	12%	22	177
			Only one bruise		15	177
			More than one bruise		7	177
			All bruises on front of body, over bony prominences			
			Association between number of bruises and mobility			
Sugar et al. (1999)	Bruises	0–36mo				973
		<6mo		0.6%	2	366
		<9mo		1.7%	8	473
			Not yet walking with support (cruising)	2.2%	11	511
			Cruising	17.8%		
			Walking	51.9%		
Labbe and Caouette (2001)	Recent skin injuries (i.e. bruises, abrasions, scratches, burns)	0–8mo	Mean number of lesions each = 1.3	11.4%	246	2,040
			Forehead	3.7%	9	246
			Chin	0.4%	1	246
			Cheeks	3.2%	8	246
			Ears	0.4%	1	246
			Others on head or face	5.7%	14	246
			Wrists	0.8%	2	246
			Thighs	0.8%	2	246
			Legs	0.4%	1	246
			No lesions of neck, thorax, abdo, pelvis, back, lumbar region upper arms, shoulders elbows, forearms, buttocks, knees, feet, ankles			
		9mo – 4yr	Bruises	1.2%		246
			Mean number of lesions each = 3.9		1012	

Abbreviations: ICH = intracerbral haemorrhage; HI = head injury; NAI = non-accidental injury; RTA = road traffic accident; SDH = subdural haemorrhage. Highlighted data have been used in summaries.

combination of clinical features, then this combination of clinical features indicates this specific medical condition. The relative likelihood that these symptoms or combinations of symptoms would be proof of a diagnosis of non-accidental injury could only be determined by statistical multivariant modelling in prospective studies that included both accidental and non-accidental injuries to children. As our own database does not include accidental injuries, we have used literature sources to assess this probability. Goldstein et al. (1993) in a prospective clinical study of all patients with a diagnosis of head injury (N = 40) found that in victims of child abuse the combination of any two of the following three factors was associated with inflicted head injury; an inconsistent history/physical examination; retinal haemorrhages; and parental risk factors (alcohol or drug abuse, previous social service intervention within the family, or a past history of child abuse or neglect).

A mean of any four components out of the following (inappropriate history, SDH, retinal haemorrhages, epileptic seizures, encephalopathy) were present in all the confessed cases from the database, although the addition of signs of malicious intent (malicious injury) with any one or none of the above indicates intent and the certainty of a non-accidental diagnosis. However, in a syndromic diagnosis of NAHI or shaken baby syndrome the variables are not all totally independent: only if they were would the probability that the above combinations were not due to non-accidental injury be extremely small.

It is stressed that the figures from this Scottish Database remain explorative and further surveillance of the Scottish population and modelling will be required.

Level of proof

It is accepted that the level of proof required for child protection proceedings, to ensure the child's place of safety, is on a balance of probability (greater than a 50% chance, i.e. $p > 0.5$). However, the burden of proof required for criminal conviction in Scotland is beyond 'reasonable doubt', which may be at the 0.1% level ($p < 0.001$) for capital crimes or at the 1% level ($p < 0.01$) for other cases. There is no formal definition in statistical terms for the level of proof required for legal or criminal proceedings. It has been recently re-stated in the Cornell Law Review 2000, quoting William Blackstone (1723–1780, Blackstone's Commentaries on the Laws of England, Vol. 4, Chapter 27) that "it is better that 10 guilty persons escape than that one innocent suffer" (or $p < 0.1$), while in the US Supreme Court Reports (Schlup v Delo, 1995), a quote from Thomas Starkie (1782–1849) was reiterated that "it is better that ninety-nine . . . offenders shall escape than that one innocent man be condemned" (i.e. $p < 0.01$).

Statistics from our database can provide a level of probability that the clinical features that are seen in any case, alone or in combination, are supportive of the diagnosis of non-accidental injury rather than, for example, "the child had fallen from a table." The level of proof is a changing and personal level in different contexts in different cases and in different criminal justice systems.

REFERENCES

Anteby II, Anteby EY, Chen B, Hamvas A, McAlister W, Tychsen L (2001) Retinal and intraventricular cerebral hemorrhages in the preterm infant born at or before 30 weeks' gestation. *J AAPOS* **5**: 90–94.

181

Aoki N, Masuzawa H (1984) Infantile acute subdural hematoma. Clinical analysis of 26 cases. *J Neurosurg* **61**: 273–280.

Asproudis IC, Andronikou SK, Hotoura EA, Kalogeropoulos CD, Kitsos GK, Psilas KE (2002) Retinopathy of prematurity and other ocular problems in premature infants weighing less than 1500g at birth. *Eur J Ophthalmol* **12**: 506–511.

Barlow KM, Minns RA (2000) Annual incidence of shaken impact syndrome in young children. *Lancet* **356**: 1571–1572.

Bergen R, Margolis S (1976) Retinal hemorrhages in the newborn. *Ann Ophthalmol* **8**: 53–56.

Berney J, Favier J, Froidevaux AC (1994a) Paediatric head trauma: influence of age and sex. I. Epidemiology. *Child's Nerv Syst* **10**: 509–516.

Berney J, Froidevaux AC, Favier J (1994b) Paediatric head trauma: influence of age and sex. II. Biomechanical and anatomo-clinical correlations. *Child's Nerv Syst* **10**: 517–523.

Besio R, Caballero C, Meerhoff E, Schwarcz R (1979) Neonatal retinal hemorrhages and influence of perinatal factors. *Am J Ophthalmol* **87**: 74–76.

Bhat BV, Kumar A, Oumachigui A (1994) Bone injuries during delivery. *Indian J Pediatr* **61**: 401–405.

Bulloch B, Schubert CJ, Brophy PD, Johnson N, Reed MH, Shapiro, RA (2000) Cause and clinical characteristics of rib fractures in infants. *Pediatrics* **105**: e48.

Buys YM, Levin AV, Enzenauer RW, Elder JE, Letourneau MA, Humphreys RP, Mian M, Morin JD (1992) Retinal findings after head trauma in infants and young children. *Ophthalmology* **99**: 1718–1723.

Carpenter RF (1999) The prevalence and distribution of bruising in babies. [Comment.] *Arch Dis Child* **80**: 363–366.

Chiaviello CT, Christoph RA, Bond GR (1994a) Infant walker-related injuries: a prospective study of severity and incidence. *Pediatrics* **93**: 974–976.

Chiaviello CT, Christoph RA, Bond GR (1994b) Stairway-related injuries in children. *Pediatrics* **94**: 679–681.

Christian CW, Taylor AA, Hertle RW, Duhaime AC (1999) Retinal hemorrhages caused by accidental household trauma. [Comment]. *J Pediatrics* **135**: 125–127.

Dashti SR, Decker DD, Razzaq A, Cohen AR (1999) Current patterns of inflicted head injury in children. *Pediatr Neurosurg* **31**: 302–306.

de Tezanos Pinto M, Fernandez J, Perez Bianco PR (1992) Update of 156 episodes of central nervous system bleeding in hemophiliacs. *Haemostasis* **22**: 259–267.

Dinakaran S, Chan TK, Rogers NK, Brosnahan DM (2002) Retinal hemorrhages in meningococcal septicemia. *J AAPOS* **6**: 221–223.

DiScala C, Sege R, Li G, Reece RM (2000) Child abuse and unintentional injuries: a 10-year retrospective. [Comment]. *Arch Pediatr Adolesc Med* **154**: 16–22.

Duhaime AC, Alario AJ, Lewander WJ, Schut L, Sutton LN, Seidl TS, Nudelman S, Budenz D, Hertle R, Tsiaras W (1992) Head injury in very young children: mechanisms, injury types, and ophthalmologic findings in 100 hospitalized patients younger than 2 years of age. *Pediatrics* **90**: 179–185.

Egge K, Lyng G, Maltau JM (1980) Retinal haemorrhages in the newborn. *Acta Ophthalmol* **58**: 231–236.

Elder JE, Taylor RG, Klug GL (1991) Retinal haemorrhage in accidental head trauma in childhood. *J Paediatr Child Health* **27**: 286–289.

Emerson MV, Pieramici DJ, Stoessel KM, Berreen JP, Gariano RF (2001) Incidence and rate of disappearance of retinal hemorrhage in newborns. *Ophthalmology* **108**: 36–39.

Ewing-Cobbs L, Kramer L, Prasad M, Canales DN, Louis PT, Fletcher JM, Vollero H, Landry SH, Cheung K (1998) Neuroimaging, physical, and developmental findings after inflicted and noninflicted traumatic brain injury in young children. *Pediatrics* **102**: 300–307.

Ewing-Cobbs L, Prasad M, Kramer L, Louis PT, Baumgartner J, Fletcher JM, Alpert B (2000) Acute neuro-radiologic findings in young children with inflicted or noninflicted traumatic brain injury. *Child's Nerv Syst* **16**: 25–33, discussion 34.

Feldman KW, Bethel R, Shugerman RP, Grossman DC, Grady MS, Ellenbogen RG (2001) The cause of infant and toddler subdural hemorrhage: a prospective study. *Pediatrics* **108**: 636–646.

Geddes JF, Tasker RC, Hackshaw AK, Nickols CD, Adams GG, Whitwell HL, Scheimberg I (2003) Dural haemorrhage in non-traumatic infant deaths: does it explain the bleeding in 'shaken baby syndrome'? *Neuropathol Appl Neurobiol* **29**: 14–22.

Gilliland MG, Luckenbach MW (1993) Are retinal hemorrhages found after resuscitation attempts? A study of the eyes of 169 children. *Am J Forensic Med Pathol* **14**: 187–192.

Gilliland MG, Luckenbach MW, Chenier TC (1994) Systemic and ocular findings in 169 prospectively studied child deaths: retinal hemorrhages usually mean child abuse. *Forensic Sci Int* **68**: 117–132.

Goldstein B, Kelly MM, Bruton D, Cox C (1993) Inflicted versus accidental head injury in critically injured children. *Crit Care Med* **21**: 1328–1332.

Gradnitzer E, Urlesberger B, Maurer U, Riccabona M, Muller W (2002) [Cerebral hemorrhage in term newborn infants—an analysis of 10 years (1989–1999).] *Wien Med Wochenschr* **152**: 9–13. (German.)

Greenes DS, Schutzman SA (2001) Clinical significance of scalp abnormalities in asymptomatic head-injured infants. *Pediatr Emerg Care* **17**: 88–92.

Greenes DS, Wigotsky M, Schutzman SA (2001) Gender differences in rates of unintentional head injury in the first 3 months of life *Ambul Pediatr* **1**: 178–180.

Gruskin KD, Schutzman SA (1999) Head trauma in children younger than 2 years: are there predictors for complications? *Arch Pediatr Adol Med* **153**: 15–20. [Erratum appears in *Arch Pediatr Adolesc Med* 1999 **153**: 453.]

Hayashi T, Hashimoto T, Fukuda S, Ohshima Y, Moritaka K (1987) Neonatal subdural hematoma secondary to birth injury. Clinical analysis of 48 survivors. *Child's Nerv Syst* 3: 23–29.

Helfer RE, Slovis TL, Black M (1977) Injuries resulting when small children fall out of bed. *Pediatrics* **60**: 533–535.

Hirsch W, Schobess A, Eichler G, Zumkeller W, Teichler H, Schluter A (2002) Severe head trauma in children: cranial computer tomography and clinical consequences. *Paediatr Anaesth* **12**: 337–344.

Hoskote A, Richards P, Anslow P, McShane T (2002) Subdural haematoma and non-accidental head injury in children. *Child's Nerv Syst* **18**: 311–317.

Jayawant S, Rawlinson A, Gibbon F, Price J, Schulte J, Sharples P, Sibert JR, Kemp AM (1998) Subdural haemorrhages in infants: population based study. [Comment]. *BMJ* **317**: 1558–1561.

Joffe M, Ludwig S (1988) Stairway injuries in children. *Pediatrics* **82**: 457–461.

Johanson RB, Menon BK (2000) Vacuum extraction versus forceps for assisted vaginal delivery. *Cochrane Database Syst Rev (2)*: CD000224.

Johnson DL, Braun D, Friendly D (1993) Accidental head trauma and retinal hemorrhage. *Neurosurgery* **33**: 231–234.

Kravitz H, Driessen G, Gomberg R, Korach A (1969) Accidental falls from elevated surfaces in infants from birth to one year of age. *Pediatrics* **44** (Suppl.): 869–876.

Labbe J, Caouette G (2001) Recent skin injuries in normal children. *Pediatrics* **108**: 271–276.

Levin S, Janive I, Mintz M, Kreisler C, Romem M, Klutznik A, Feingold M, Insler V (1980) Diagnostic and prognostic value of retinal hemorrhages in the neonate. *Obstet Gynecol* **55**: 309–314.

Liu X, Cheng G, Yang S, Ling Y, Ke P (1993) [Retinal hemorrhage in newborn infants.] *J Yan Ke Xue Bao* **9**: 200–202. (Chinese.)

Loh JK, Lin CL, Kwan AL, Howng SL (2002) Acute subdural hematoma in infancy. *Surg Neurol* **58**: 218–224.

Lyons TJ, Oates RK (1993) Falling out of bed: a relatively benign occurrence. *Pediatrics*, **92**: 125–127.

Maxeiner H (2001) [Evaluation of subdural hemorrhage in infants after alleged minor trauma.] *Unfallchirurg* **104**: 569–576. (German.)

McClelland CQ, Heiple KG (1982) Fractures in the first year of life. A diagnostic dilemma. *Am J Dis Child* **136**: 26–29.

McCormick MC, Shapiro S, Starfield BH (1981) Injury and its correlates among 1-year-old children. Study of children with both normal and low birth weights. *Am J Dis Child* **135**: 159–163.

Mei-Zahav M, Uziel Y, Raz J, Ginot N, Wolach B, Fainmesser P (2002) Convulsions and retinal haemorrhage: should we look further? *Arch Dis Child* **86**: 334–335.

Morris MW, Smith S, Cressman J, Ancheta J (2000) Evaluation of infants with subdural hematoma who lack external evidence of abuse. *Pediatrics* **105**: 549–553.

Nimityongskul P, Anderson LD (1987) The likelihood of injuries when children fall out of bed. *J Pediatr Orthoped* **7**: 184–186.

Odom A, Christ E, Kerr N, Byrd K, Cochran J, Barr F, Bugnitz M, Ring JC, Storgion S, Walling R, Stidham G, Quasney MW (1997) Prevalence of retinal hemorrhages in pediatric patients after in-hospital cardio-pulmonary resuscitation: a prospective study. *Pediatrics* **99**: E3.

Oi S, Yamada H, Sasaki K, Matsumoto S (1986) [Incidence and characteristics of cerebrovascular disorders in children—critical analysis of 120 cases experienced at a children's general hospital.] *No Shinkei Geka* **14**: 161–168. (Japanese.)

O'Leary JA, Ferrell RE, Randolph CR (1986) Retinal hemorrhage and vacuum extraction delivery. *J Perinat Med* **14**: 197–199.

Olumese PE, Adeyemo AA, Gbadegesin RA, Walker O (1997) Retinal haemorrhage in cerebral malaria. *East Afr Med J* **74**: 285–287.

Partington MD, Swanson JA, Meyer FB (1991) Head injury and the use of baby walkers: a continuing problem. *Ann Emerg Med* **20**: 652–654.

Pascoe JM, Hildebrandt HM, Tarrier A, Murphy M (1979) Patterns of skin injury in nonaccidental and accidental injury. *Pediatrics* **64**: 245–247.

Plunkett J (2001) Fatal pediatric head injuries caused by short-distance falls. [Comment]. *Am J Forens Med Pathol* **22**: 1–12.

Pollack JS, Tychsen L (1996) Prevalence of retinal hemorrhages in infants after extracorporeal membrane oxygenation. *Am J Ophthalmol* **121**: 297–303.

Reece RM, Sege R (2000) Childhood head injuries: accidental or inflicted? [Comment]. *Arch Pediatr Adol Med* **154**: 11–15.

Reed WF, Feldman KW, Weiss AH, Tencer AF (2002) Does soccer ball heading cause retinal bleeding? *Arch Pediatr Adol Med* **156**: 337–340.

Reiber GD (1993) Fatal falls in childhood. How far must children fall to sustain fatal head injury? Report of cases and review of the literature. *Am J Forensic Med Pathol* **14**: 201–207.

Saito A, Nakazawa T, Matsuda M, Handa J (1987) [Association of subdural hematoma and middle fossa arachnoid cyst: report of 3 cases and a review.] *No Shinkei Geka* **15**: 689–6893. [Japanese.]

Schloff S, Mullaney PB, Armstrong DC, Simantirakis E, Humphreys RP, Myseros JS, Buncic JR, Levin AV (2002) Retinal findings in children with intracranial hemorrhage. *Ophthalmology* **109**: 1472–1476.

Shugerman RP, Paez A, Grossman DC, Feldman KW, Grady MS (1996) Epidural hemorrhage: is it abuse? *Pediatrics* **97**: 664–668.

Sieben RL, Leavitt JD, French JH (1971) Falls as childhood accidents: an increasing urban risk. *Pediatrics* **47**: 886–892.

Stein JD, Jaeger EA, Jeffers JB (1999) Air bags and ocular injuries. *Trans Am Ophthalmol Soc* **97**: 59–82.

Stoffman JM, Bass MJ, Fox AM (1984) Head injuries related to the use of baby walkers. *Can Med Assoc J* **131**: 573–575.

Sugar NF, Taylor JA, Feldman KW (1999) Bruises in infants and toddlers: those who don't cruise rarely bruise. Puget Sound Pediatric Research Network. *Arch Pediatr Adolesc Med* **153**: 399–403.

Thomas SA, Rosenfield NS, Leventhal JM, Markowitz RI (1991) Long-bone fractures in young children: distinguishing accidental injuries from child abuse. *Pediatrics* **88**: 471–476.

Towner D, Castro MA, Eby-Wilkens E, Gilbert WM (1999) Effect of mode of delivery in nulliparous women on neonatal intracranial injury. [Comment]. *N Engl J Med* **341**: 1709–1714.

Tursz A, Lelong N, Crost M (1990) Home accidents to children under 2 years of age. *Paediatr Perinat Epidemiol* **4**: 408–421.

Tyagi AK, Scotcher S, Kozeis N, Willshaw HE (1998) Can convulsions alone cause retinal haemorrhages in infants? *Br J Ophthalmol* **82**: 659–660.

Tzioumi D, Oates RK (1998) Subdural hematomas in children under 2 years. Accidental or inflicted? A 10-year experience. [Comment]. *Child Abuse Negl* **22**: 1105–1112.

Varn MM, Donahue ML, Saunders RA, Baker JD, Smith CM, Wilson ME (1997) Retinal examinations in infants after extracorporeal membrane oxygenation. *J Pediatr Ophthalmol Strabismus* **34**: 182–185.

Vinchon M, Noule N, Soto-Ares G, Dhellemmes P (2001) Subduroperitoneal drainage for subdural hematomas in infants: results in 244 cases. *J Neurosurg* **95**: 249–255.

Vinchon M, Noizet O, Defoort-Dhellemmes S, Soto-Ares G, Dhellemmes P (2002) Infantile subdural hematomas due to traffic accidents. *Pediatr Neurosurg* **37**: 245–253.

Warrington SA, Wright CM, Team AS (2001) Accidents and resulting injuries in premobile infants: data from the ALSPAC study. *Arch Dis Child* **85**: 104–107.

Whitby EH, Paley MN, Rutter S, Ohadike P, Smith MF, Davies NP, Griffiths PD (2003) Do clinically silent subdural haemorrhages occur in the neonate? *Arch Dis Child* **88** (Suppl. 1): A5.

White VA, Lewallen S, Beare N, Kayira K, Carr RA, Taylor TE (2001) Correlation of retinal haemorrhages with brain haemorrhages in children dying of cerebral malaria in Malawi. *Trans R Soc Trop Med Hyg* **95**: 618–621.

Worlock P, Stower M (1986) Fracture patterns in Nottingham children. *J Pediatr Orthoped* **6**: 656–660.

Young TL, Quinn GE, Baumgart S, Petersen RA, Schaffer DB (1997) Extracorporeal membrane oxygenation causing asymmetric vasculopathy in neonatal infants. *J AAPOS* **1**: 235–240.

184

5
HAEMORRHAGIC RETINOPATHY OF SHAKING INJURY: CLINICAL AND PATHOLOGICAL ASPECTS

Kristina May, M Andrew Parsons and Robert Doran

Historical background

The association between eye signs and physical abuse had been recognized a number of years before the term 'whiplash–shaken infant syndrome' was proposed by Caffey (1972). Kiffney (1964) is said to have been the first to describe the occurrence of ocular injury in the setting of child abuse when he reported a case of bilateral traumatic retinal detachment in a 7-month-old infant. Gilkes and Mann (1967) were more specific in suggesting that intraocular haemorrhage may be indicative of physical abuse, while the association between subdural and retinal haemorrhage in infants was described as long ago as 1958 (Hollenhurst and Stein 1958).

Modern day perspective

It has become increasingly recognized that the ophthalmologist has an important contribution to make in the diagnosis or exclusion of shaken baby syndrome (SBS). Despite this, ophthalmic opinion is often sought late, if at all, in suspicious cases of infantile intracranial bleeding. In a retrospective study carried out on infants with subdural haemorrhages between 1993 and 1995, only 42% of cases were examined by an ophthalmologist. It was suggested that mandatory investigations in cases of subdural haemorrhage in infancy should include ocular examination by an ophthalmologist (Jayawant et al. 1998).

Presentation

In the context of SBS an ophthalmologist will rarely be the first clinician to be presented with the signs of abuse. Most cases in which a suspicion of SBS arises will present to paediatricians with intracranial haemorrhage in which the severity of injury is not compatible with the history given. They will then be referred for ophthalmic assessment. Ophthalmic input may also help in the diagnosis of infants presenting with nonspecific life-threatening symptoms even when intracranial haemorrhage has not been suspected. In 1995, New York ophthalmologists were asked to examine cases of "apparent life threatening events"; five out of 75 cases were found to be occult SBS (Altman et al. 1998).

Ophthalmologists are more likely to be the first to see the results of direct ocular trauma (Waterhouse et al. 1992). Abuse should be considered in the differential diagnosis of any child under the age of 3 years presenting with retinal detachment or dialysis (tearing of the retina at the extreme retinal periphery), cataract or subluxed lens, chorioretinal or macular scarring, or periorbital bruising. The Royal College of Ophthalmologists (1999) has published best practice guidelines detailing the procedures to be followed for ophthalmologists who may suspect child abuse.

Ophthalmic examination and documentation

It is not possible to examine the full extent of the infant fundus with a direct ophthalmoscope (i.e. instrumentation available to paediatricians). To fully examine the retina the pupils must be dilated and indirect ophthalmoscopy, with or without indentation, must be performed. It is essential that the periphery of the retina be visualized for retinal haemorrhages to be truly excluded. Furthermore, it has been suggested that retinal haemorrhages may be seen only at the periphery in mild cases of SBS (Green et al. 1996), although this has yet to be proven by clinical studies. If retinal haemorrhages are present, detailed documentation is vital (see below). This is possible only with the wide angle and three-dimensional fundal view that is available with an indirect ophthalmoscope. For these reasons we agree with Jayawant et al. (1998) who state that all cases of suspected shaken baby syndrome must be examined by an ophthalmologist.

Ophthalmic assessment

Ophthalmic assessment at presentation or subsequent reassessment should include the following.

- *Visual behaviour and function.* In the unsedated child it is important to assess visual behaviour. Most newborn infants should fix and follow a large, bright, interesting stimulus, while older infants will normally look at faces and hand-held toys. It should be remembered that there may be signs of ocular trauma even if there is no manifest change in visual behaviour. Visual function can be assessed by observing fixation ability with each eye. Visual acuity may be measured in a 3- to 12-month-old child using a preferential looking technique with grating targets (Chanda et al. 1988), or in a slightly older child using vanishing optotypes (Cardiff cards) (Woodhouse et al. 1992).

- *Pupil responses.* Pupil responses to light must be documented prior to dilatation. Several studies have confirmed that an impaired pupil response at the time of presentation is a poor prognostic finding as it usually indicates visual pathway, and therefore central nervous system damage (Greenwald et al. 1986, McCabe and Donahue 2000). Pupil dilatation (mydriasis) can be achieved in an infant with phenylephrine (2.5%) and cyclopentolate (0.5%) eye drops. When infants are undergoing neurological observations, the medical staff must be informed if the pupils are to be dilated.

- *Documentation.* It is essential that any fundal findings are described in detail. We recommend as a minimum both written and detailed diagrammatic documentation. The type of retinal haemorrhage (see below), their geographical location and distribution throughout the retina must be described. There are many different causes of 'retinal haemorrhages' in infants but the precise type and distribution of haemorrhage may differ between aetiologies, and therefore detailed documentation may have important medicolegal value. Fundus cameras, particularly digital cameras, are becoming increasingly available and easier to use. Fundus photographs of retinal haemorrhages are ideal for documentation and can be presented as evidence in court, provided of course that they are properly labelled, dated and annotated to denote which eye is being photographed (House of Lords Select Committee on Science and Technology 1999). A reference to any photographs taken should also be made in the patient's records.

Short-term management

Ophthalmic findings, positive or negative, should be discussed with the paediatricians. They may be of importance in establishing or refuting a diagnosis of non-accidental injury. Haemorrhages involving the macula or within the vitreous, obstructing the visual axis, may cause long-term visual impairment. Ophthalmic follow-up should be arranged in these cases.

The role of the ophthalmic or forensic pathologist

In all cases of infant death where non accidental injury is to be excluded it is essential that the eyes be removed. Even if the cause of death does not appear to be related to injury to the head or eyes, examination of the eyes may reveal signs of previous abuse. In such cases it is vital that the vitreous is not removed for electrolyte or toxicology assessment as this procedure may induce external or internal ocular artifacts, such as subscleral haemorrhage similar to that seen in strangulation (Di Maio 1985). If death has been rapid or has occurred at home the child may well not have been examined by an ophthalmologist and important clinical information may be missed if the eyes are not examined in detail.

After opening the cranial cavity and removing the brain, the roof of the orbit is removed, and the eye and orbital contents carefully dissected out en bloc. It is important that as much of the optic nerve is removed as possible to document the presence or absence of continuity between intracranial haemorrhage and optic nerve sheath haemorrhages immediately behind the eye. It is best to make the conjunctival incisions from the front, as this reduces the possibility of cosmetic eyelid damage. Once the orbital contents are removed the bony wall of the orbit can be examined for fractures. We recommend formalin fixation of all orbital contents en bloc before careful dissection to look for injuries such as muscle sheath and orbital apex haemorrhage (Levin 2000). At each stage of the dissection it is important to take high quality macroscopic photographs to document findings for subsequent legal proceedings.

Gilliland and Folberg (1992) recommend removing the cornea via a coronal section just anterior to the ora serrata, so that any photographs that are taken are equivalent to a clinician's view. However, in order to avoid disruption of continuity between the anterior and posterior segments of the eye (important if there is also blunt trauma), we now make conventional horizontal cuts through the eye (Fig. 5.1, top). We do not now make further cuts through the central clock of the eye (as seen in Fig. 5.1, bottom), for the same reason. Whichever practice is used, it is important to fully document the findings and to consider the possibility that unhelpful artifacts may have been produced (Parsons and Start 2001).

Clinical and pathological appearance of retinal haemorrhages seen in SBS

Retinal haemorrhages are reported in 75–90% of cases of shaken baby syndrome (American

187

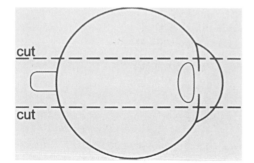

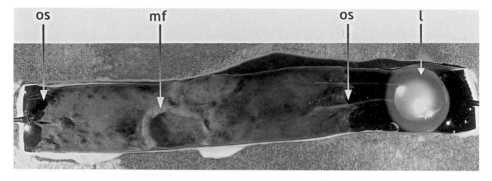

Fig. 5.1. Post-mortem examination of the eye.

    (Top) Standard cuts are made in the horizontal plane (avoiding the lens).

    (Bottom) The central block of this eye was cut through the pars plana of the ciliary body, revealing the ora serrata (os), the edge of a circular macular fold (mf), and the lens (l). Note that this second cut is for illustrative purposes only, and should not be used in a standard investigation (see text).

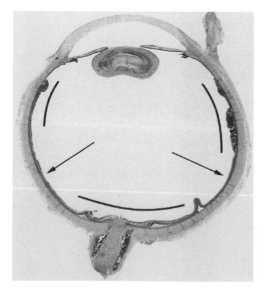

Fig. 5.2. Peripheral and posterior pole retinal haemorrhages (bars), with relative sparing of the equator (arrows) from the autopsy of a violently shaken infant.

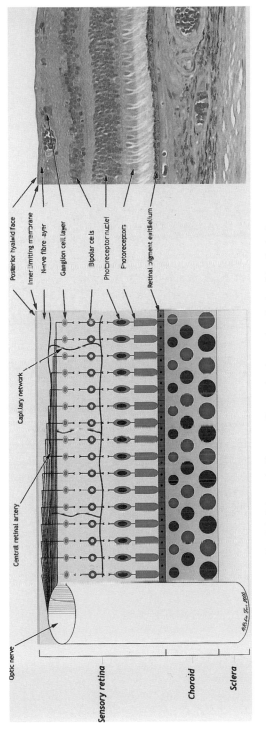

Optic nerve

Central retinal artery

Capillary network

Posterior hyaloid face
Inner limiting membrane
Nerve fibre layer
Ganglion cell layer

Bipolar cells

Photoreceptor nuclei

Photoreceptors

Retinal pigment epithelium

Sensory retina

Choroid

Sclera

Fig. 5.3. Schematic diagram of normal retina and equivalent histological appearance.

189

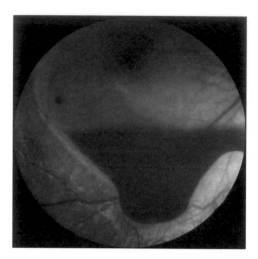

Fig. 5.4. Boat-shaped subhyaloid haemorrhage with fluid level.

Academy of Pediatrics 1993). Although they are usually bilateral, there is often marked asymmetry in severity, and unilateral retinal haemorrhages are well documented (Budenz et al. 1994, Tyagi et al. 1997).

It is important to note that (traumatic) retinal haemorrhages in the absence of intracranial injury may indicate direct trauma to the eye rather than shaking. This will be frequently, although not invariably, accompanied by anterior eye signs such as periorbital bruising, subconjunctival haemorrhage, hyphaema and/or a subluxed or dislocated lens.

DISTRIBUTION OF RETINAL HAEMORRHAGES IN SBS

To date there are no studies that conclusively demonstrate a characteristic distribution of retinal haemorrhages in survivors of SBS. A post-mortem morphometric study by Green et al. (1996) of eyes removed from infants who had died as a result of non-accidental head injury (shaking with or without additional impact) looked at the distribution of haemorrhages in their subjects. They found that in 10 cases "subhyaloid haemorrhage" and "retinal detachment" occurred with greater frequency at the periphery and posterior pole with relative sparing of the equator (Fig. 5.2). This has yet to be corroborated by clinical studies in surviving infants. [Note: The "retinal detachment" referred to in the paper by Green et al. is a pathological term to describe focal areas of haemorrhagic retinal detachment. Clinically, ophthalmologists would describe these lesions as 'subretinal haemorrhages'.]

CLASSIFICATION OF RETINAL HAEMORRHAGES

Retinal haemorrhages in SBS can involve any or all layers of the retina and are classified by anatomical location (Fig. 5.3).

Superficial retinal haemorrhage

Superficial retinal haemorrhages are dome-shaped accumulations of deep red blood that obscure the retinal vessels. With time and the effect of gravity they often develop a fluid

190

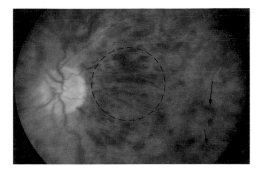

Fig. 5.5. Linear nerve fibre layer haemorrhages in the macular region (circled area) and peripheral intraretinal haemorrhages (arrows).

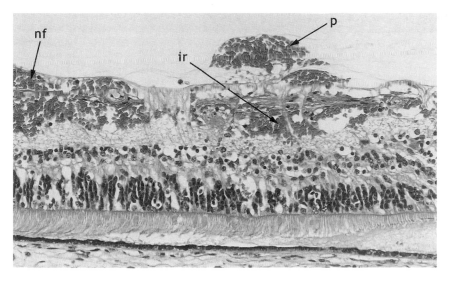

Fig. 5.6. Histology of the retina from a shaken baby, showing preretinal haemorrhage (p), nerve fibre layer (nf), and intraretinal haemorrhage (ir). (Haematoxylin–eosin stain.)

level (Fig. 5.4). These are often seen in cases of SBS in combination with intraretinal haemorrhages.

Superficial retinal haemorrhages may fall into two anatomical categories, although clinically they are indistinguishable. Subhyaloid (or preretinal) haemorrhages lie between the posterior hyaloid (vitreous) face and the inner limiting membrane (ILM). Similar collections of blood may be found lying between the ILM and nerve-fibre layer of the retina (sub-ILM haemorrhages).

Intraretinal haemorrhage
When situated within the nerve fibre layer, intraretinal haemorrhages have a streaked or 'flame-shaped' appearance. In the middle layers of the retina they have a more localized 'blot' appearance with or without a white centre (Figs. 5.5, 5.6). A white centre may be

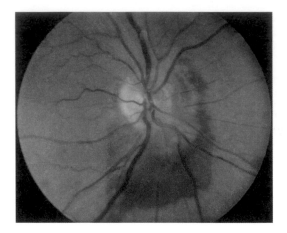

Fig. 5.7. Dark red geographical subretinal haemorrhage surrounding the optic disc.

caused by altered blood including platelet/fibrin aggregates, ischaemia and local exudates, or may be due to artifactual light reflection. Although white-centred intraretinal haemorrhages are commonly seen in SBS, they may also be present in other conditions such as birth-related haemorrhages; in SBS they have no prognostic significance (Kapoor et al. 1997).

Subretinal, subretinal pigment epithelial and choroidal haemorrhages
Subretinal haemorrhages lie between the photoreceptors and the retinal pigment epithelium and in pathological terms these are described as focal haemorrhagic retinal detachments. These haemorrhages are typically larger than intraretinal haemorrhages and irregular in shape (Fig. 5.7). Subretinal pigment epithelial and choroidal haemorrhages are darker as they are seen through the retinal pigment epithelium. Clinically, all three deeper types of haemorrhage are seen more frequently in direct trauma to the eye than in SBS.

Vitreous haemorrhage
Bleeding into the vitreous is thought to occur by extension from a large subhyaloid or sub-ILM haemorrhage. These haemorrhages can occur at the time of injury or they may develop some time after the appearance of other retinal haemorrhages (Greenwald et al. 1986). In SBS, Green et al. (1996) found that vitreous haemorrhages were seen in association with the more severe head injuries. The infant vitreous is more compact than the adult, and vitreous haemorrhage may persist for several months (Kaur and Taylor 1990).

Optic nerve sheath haemorrhages
Lambert et al. (1986) were the first to describe the pathological finding of optic nerve sheath haemorrhages in association with shaken baby syndrome (Fig. 5.8). These are believed to result from rupture of local vessels rather than from an extension of intracranial blood (Green et al. 1996). Their appearance at autopsy (they cannot be seen clinically) with retinal haemorrhages is highly suggestive of child abuse (either by shaking or with associated impact) and they have been reported in cases of SBS even in the absence of retinal

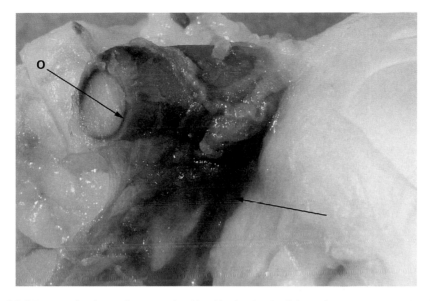

Fig. 5.8. Macroscopic picture demonstrating blood in the sheath of the optic nerve (o). Note the blood extending into the orbital fat (arrow). Infant death due to violent shaking.

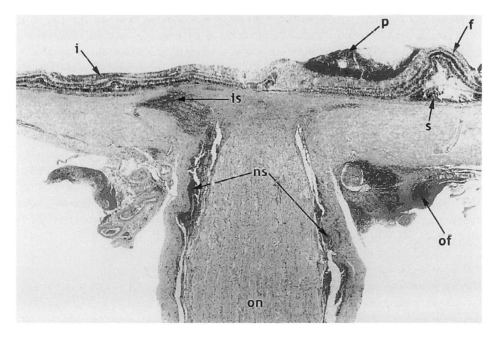

Fig. 5.9. Section through the optic nerve (on) and posterior pole (infant death due to violent shaking). There is a retinal fold (f) and preretinal (p), intraretinal (i), subretinal (s), intrascleral (is), optic nerve sheath (ns) and orbital fat (of) haemorrhages. (Haematoxylin–eosin staining.)

haemorrhage. Although they occur with greater frequency in cases of subdural haemorrhage secondary to SBS, they can occur in severe accidental head injury (Budenz et al. 1994).

At autopsy the possibility of direct extension of an intracranial haemorrhage into the optic nerve sheath should be considered.

Intrascleral haemorrhages

At autopsy of infants with SBS, intrascleral haemorrhages have been reported at the point of attachment of the optic nerve sheath to the sclera, usually in association with optic nerve sheath haemorrhages (Fig. 5.9). As with the perineural haemorrhages, they are strongly, but not invariably, associated with non-accidental head injury. It is believed that they are caused by tearing of local intrascleral ciliary vessels (Lin and Glasgow 1999).

Resolution of retinal haemorrhages and the ageing of intraocular injuries

In criminal or civil legal proceedings the timing of an injury is vitally important as different responsible adults may have had access to the injured child at different times.

In clinical practice it is not possible to determine the age of retinal haemorrhages with much accuracy. Not only is the colour of a retinal haemorrhage determined more by its thickness and position within the retina than by its age, but the background colour of the infant fundus is also highly variable depending on, among other things, the ethnic origin of the child. Different types of retinal haemorrhage also vary considerably in the time taken to resolve:

• superficial nerve fibre layer haemorrhages resolve within a few days
• intraretinal haemorrhages can take several weeks to resolve
• subhyaloid, sub-ILM and vitreous haemorrhages may persist for several months.

There is no evidence to suggest, in adults or children, that haemorrhages migrate through the retina, i.e. an intraretinal haemorrhage cannot become a nerve fibre layer haemorrhage.

In pathology practice, haemosiderin (a breakdown product of haemoglobin) can be identified histochemically from around 48 hours after injury. However, if haemosiderin is not identified it cannot be concluded that the injury in less than 48 hours old. Furthermore, if haemosiderin is identified within a haemorrhage it may be difficult to determine whether the haemorrhage arose from a single episode more than 48 hours before death, or from two separate episodes of injury with fresh haemorrhage over the site of an older haemorrhage (Gilliland et al. 1991). There is increasing use of immunohistochemistry to identify infiltrating macrophages, and to indicate glial cell activation, but these techniques are still in their infancy.

Relationship between the eye and brain in shaking injuries

There is good evidence that ocular and brain injury are linked in SBS, with a correlation between the severity of ocular injury and the severity of intracerebral injury (although this may be true only of fatally injured or more severely injured babies). Green et al. (1996) reviewed the eyes and brains of 23 children who had died from non-accidental injuries. They found that at the lowest level of trauma resulting in death, subdural haemorrhage was present. Progressively more trauma was required for subhyaloid, intraretinal haemorrhages and retinal detachment (subretinal haemorrhage). At the greatest levels of trauma, choroidal and vitreous haemorrhages were seen in association with additional cerebral lacerations, intracerebral and subarachnoid haemorrhages. In their clinicopathological review of 75 infants, Morad et al (2002) confirmed that the severity of retinal and intracranial injuries is correlated in SBS. In a clinical study, Wilkinson et al. (1989) reported a significant correlation between severity of retinal findings and acute neurological findings in infants who had been shaken. Kilvin et al (2000) also found that the patient's visual reaction and pupillary response on clinical presentation correlated highly with both survival and good final visual and neurological outcome.

In the clinical situation, a child with a combination of intracranial injury and retinal haemorrhages is likely to have suffered violent shaking. Note, however, that retinal haemorrhages secondary to SBS may precede CT-detectable intracranial haemorrhage by several hours or days (Giangiacomo et al. 1988). Therefore a child presenting with retinal haemorrhages, but no initial signs of intracranial injury, should remain under neurological observation including further neuroimaging, if SBS is suspected.

Ocular haemorrhages in the absence of intracranial trauma implies direct ocular trauma. Conversely, intracranial haemorrhage following child abuse in the absence of retinal haemorrhages suggests direct head trauma, although it should be noted that retinal haemorrhages may develop subsequently as a result of a rapid rise in intracranial pressure (see below).

MECHANISM

There are basically two suggested mechanisms responsible for eye injuries secondary to violent shaking: (i) vitreous traction on the underlying retina as the vitreous swirls within the eye; or (ii) raised venous pressure secondary to raised intracranial pressure and/or chest compression (if the infant is squeezed during shaking).

It is probable that both of these mechanisms play a part in the pathogenesis of ocular haemorrhages. For further discussion of pathogenic theories and mechanisms, see Lieberman et al. (1996), Ophthalmology Child Abuse Working Party (1999), Levin (2000) and Morad et al. (2002).

Differential diagnosis of intraocular haemorrhage

Retinal haemorrhages are not always synonymous with child abuse. There are many other causes of retinal haemorrhage in children. These must be considered and excluded before a diagnosis of SBS is made. Most of them, however, present with a distinct history and appearance and can be identified or excluded by appropriate investigation.

BIRTH-RELATED RETINAL HAEMORRHAGES

Retinal haemorrhages have been reported in from 2.6% to 59% of all newborn infants (Ophthalmology Child Abuse Working Party 1999). Such a broad range of frequency is a reflection of how soon infants are examined after birth, as many haemorrhages resolve within 24 hours (Giles 1960, Sezen 1970). They are seen following all modes of delivery, but occur with greater frequency following vacuum extraction, and less often following forceps

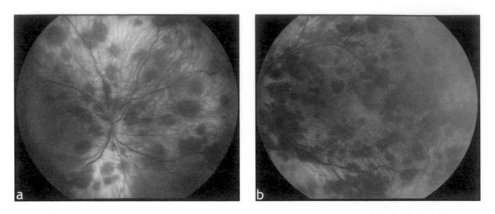

Fig. 5.10. (a) The right fundus of an infant delivered by vacuum extraction (at day 1). Image centred on the optic nerve.

(b) The left eye in the same infant (centred on the macula) with the optic disc on the left. Note the peripheral extension of the haemorrhages (far right) and the dense preretinal haemorrhages adjacent to the disc.

delivery and caesarian sections (emergency or elective). In one study, the frequency following vacuum extraction, normal vaginal delivery and forceps delivery was 50%, 41% and 16% respectively (Egge et al. 1981). There have been various studies of other factors that may affect incidence of birth-related retinal haemorrhages, such as maternal parity, birthweight and length of second stage of labour, but with few consistent results. It is postulated that compression of the fetal head leads to raised cephalic venous pressure resulting in retinal haemorrhage, and the relatively low incidence of retinal haemorrhages in preterm infants (who have smaller heads) supports this theory (Maltau et al. 1984). Others suggest that a combination of hypercapnia and hypoxia causes venous dilatation and raised intracranial pressure during delivery that impairs venous return, leading to rupture of retinal vessels (Ophthalmology Child Abuse Working Party 1999).

The accepted wisdom is that most birth-related retinal haemorrhages are mild, unilateral or bilateral, intraretinal, predominately at the posterior pole, and resolve within 3–4 weeks without long-term retinal sequelae. However, we have personal experience of extensive intra-retinal haemorrhages extending to the periphery in normal deliveries, and we have also seen superficial retinal haemorrhages (subhyaloid and sub-ILM) associated with vacuum extraction delivery (Fig. 5.10). In our experience the superficial retinal haemorrhages resolved by 8 weeks. We have also seen an intraretinal haemorrhage adjacent to the optic disc that persisted to 11 weeks. We would therefore be very concerned about the possibility of SBS if a child presents (i) 2 weeks after birth with extensive nerve fibre ('flame-shaped') haemorrhages, or (ii) 4 weeks after birth with extensive intraretinal ('blot') haemorrhages.

Vitreous haemorrhage rarely occurs following birth trauma, but if it does it is usually associated with a coagulopathy (Ferrone and De Juan 1994).

Most birth-related retinal haemorrhages appear to resolve without long-term visual sequelae. There have been a few reported cases of long-term visual impairment associated

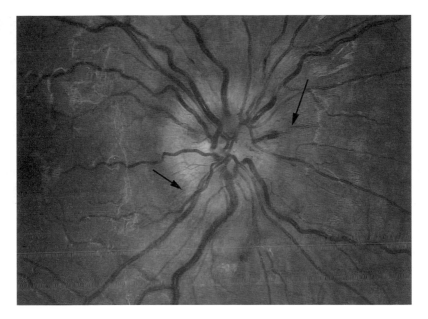

Fig. 5.11. Fine nerve fibre layer haemorrhages at the optic disc border in papilloedema (arrows).

with macular haemorrhages (Zwaan et al 1997). Another study, involving only five children, demonstrated no increased incidence of amblyopia or strabismus following macular neonatal haemorrhages (Von Noorden and Khoudadoust 1973). In addition, CT in 10 neonates with large retinal haemorrhages failed to demonstrate any correlation with intracranial pathology (Skalpe et al. 1982).

In Accidental Head Injury

Retinal haemorrhages are extremely rare in accidental head injury even when the injury is very severe, such as following a high speed road traffic accident (Alario et al. 1990, Buys et al. 1992, Duhaime et al. 1992, Gilliland et al. 1994). More recently, three cases of accidental household trauma in infants were reported with unilateral, posterior pole retinal haemorrhages (Christian et al. 1999). However, in these three cases the level of trauma was still major and included falling down 13 concrete steps in a baby walker, falling through a stair rail onto a concrete floor, and falling 30–60 cm while being swung

The retinal haemorrhages associated with accidental head injury are usually at the posterior pole. In an extensive review of literature on retinal haemorrhages and child abuse, Levin (2000) states that "retinal haemorrhages are reported in no greater than 3% of accidental head trauma victims and the nature of the head injury is, almost always, severe and life threatening, with an obvious mechanism that would not raise the suspicion of abuse." Trivial haemorrhages are common in the first 2 years of life, but the outcomes from such haemorrhages are almost always benign (Punt et al. 2004). This conclusion is supported by a large population study (Warrington et al. 2001), and by observations of children falling

197

from heights of 3–4 feet (100–125 cm) while in hospital (Helfer et al. 1977, Nimityongskul and Anderson 1987). The often quoted study by Plunkett (2001) did not demonstrate injuries of the kind seen in inflicted head injury in any of the 5 children of less than 2 years of age who died following falls from playground equipment.

Recently Geddes et al. (2001a,b; 2003) generated considerable controversy by suggesting that only very minor trauma might be required to cause the eye and brain changes that are attributed to abusive head injury. We consider, with Punt et al. (2004) that there are serious methodological flaws in these studies, and that their conclusions are not supported by the evidence, notwithstanding the published response by the authors to this criticism (Geddes et al. 2004). Indeed, under cross-examination in a recent court case, Geddes did admit to an error in the Geddes et al. (2003) paper (Dyer 2005; for further discussion see Chapter 9).

SECONDARY TO ACUTE RISE IN INTRACRANIAL PRESSURE
Acute papilloedema is associated with optic disc swelling and retinal haemorrhages, which are usually in the nerve fibre layer and lie within 1–2 disc diameters of the optic nerve head (Fig. 5.11). In adults with raised intracranial pressure secondary to conditions other than intracranial haemorrhage, there are a few reports of macular subhyaloid/sub-ILM haemorrhages (Morris and Sanders 1980), vitreous haemorrhage (Keane 1981) and peripheral retinal haemorrhages (Galvin and Sanders 1980). Such findings have not been described in children or infants, although in some cases of accidental and non-accidental head injury in infants (whether direct or indirect injury from shaking) an acute rise in intracranial pressure may cause this pattern of retinal haemorrhages.

ASPHYXIA AND RELATED MECHANISMS
Petechial haemorrhages affecting the eyelids and/or conjunctiva are not a feature of SBS. If they are present, however, even in small numbers, they should be carefully documented and photographed, because they may indicate an asphyxial mechanism such as due to smothering (Knight 1996). Retinal haemorrhages have been documented in traumatic asphyxia (Ravin and Meyer 1973) and Valsalva manoeuvre in adults (Duane 1972, Bourne et al. 1999), but their relationship to abusive asphyxia is very uncertain (Levin 2000).

CARDIOPULMONARY RESUSCITATION (CPR)
A few case reports have described retinal haemorrhages in association with CPR (Weedn et al. 1990). Gilliland and Luckenbach (1993) examined the eyes of 131 infants who had died after unsuccessful, prolonged (more than 30 minutes) CPR. They found a total of 61 cases with retinal haemorrhages but these were felt to be the result of events prior to CPR, such as sepsis, and not due to CPR itself. Another study examined the eyes of 54 consecutive children on whom CPR was performed. A single case with retinal haemorrhages was identified, but it was felt that these could have been caused by the concurrent arterial hypertension or trauma (Kanter 1986). Experimental studies in animals have not demonstrated retinal haemorrhages in association with CPR (Fackler et al. 1994). In short, "CPR alone is very unlikely to cause retinal haemorrhages, even if carried out by unskilled individuals" (Ophthalmology Child Abuse Working Party 1999).

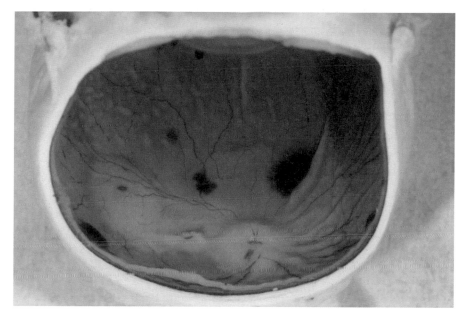

Fig. 5.12. Macroscopic photograph of retinal haemorrhages in an 8-year-old child who died of meningococcal meningitis.

SEIZURES

It has been postulated that retinal haemorrhages can occur following prolonged convulsions. A prospective study in Birmingham (England) looked at a total of 62 children with convulsions. No cases of retinal haemorrhages were found (Sandramouli et al. 1997, Tyagi et al. 1998). In conclusion, "convulsions in young children rarely, if ever, cause retinal haemorrhages" (Ophthalmology Child Abuse Working Party 1999).

MENINGITIS

Meningococcal bacterial meningitis has been associated with diffuse retinal haemorrhages (Fraser 1995). Our department has experience of diffuse intraretinal and subhyaloid/sub-ILM haemorrhages in several cases of meningococcal meningitis (Fig. 5.12).

BLOOD DYSCRASIAS

Various haematological abnormalities can be associated with retinal haemorrhages such as leukaemias and protein C deficiency. These can be excluded with appropriate clinical and haematological investigations.

INTRAOCULAR PATHOLOGY

Several eye conditions may present with retinal haemorrhages in infancy including retinopathy of prematurity, retinal vascular malformations and cytomegalovirus retinitis. Such conditions can usually be diagnosed by the clinical history and presentation.

EXTRA-CORPOREAL MEMBRANE OXYGENATION (ECMO)

There is evidence of increased vascular tortuosity with reports of retinal haemorrhages in association with ECMO. It was concluded that the changes were infrequent and deemed non-sight-threatening (Pollack and Tychsen 1996).

METABOLIC DISORDERS

Galactosaemia is more commonly associated with infantile cataracts, but Levy et al. (1996) have described five neonates with galactosaemia and vitreous haemorrhage. Glutaric aciduria is another rare autosomal disorder in which retinal haemorrhages have been described. The condition is associated with macrocephaly and basal ganglia lesions that eventually result in severe dystonia. The condition predisposes infants to subdural haemorrhage following mild trauma. The retinal haemorrhages described occur very rarely, are usually mild intra-retinal haemorrhages and are most likely secondary to a rapid rise in intracranial pressure (Hoffman and Naughten 1998, Levin 2000).

'TERSON SYNDROME' AND RETINAL HAEMORRHAGES SECONDARY TO
NON-TRAUMATIC INTRACRANIAL HAEMORRHAGES

In 1900 Dr Albert Terson described the case of a 60-year-old male who collapsed from a presumed, but not proven, intracerebral haemorrhage. On regaining consciousness, he was found to have a unilateral vitreous haemorrhage (Terson 1900). In the last few decades the eponym of 'Terson syndrome' has been used more widely to describe vitreous haemorrhage secondary to all forms of non-traumatic intracranial haemorrhage, usually following the rupture of an intracranial aneurysm. Other types of retinal haemorrhage (intraretinal and preretinal) have also been described in adult cases of non-traumatic intracranial haemorrhage (Fahmy 1973). It is postulated that the haemorrhages occur secondary to venous hypertension, rather than from direct spread of blood down the optic nerve sheath from the cranial cavity, as post-mortem examinations in fatal cases have shown discontinuity in optic nerve sheath haemorrhages (Weingeist et al. 1986).

Similar cases of intraocular haemorrhage secondary to non-traumatic intracranial bleeding have very rarely been reported in children. The possibility of child abuse does not appear to have been considered in the many reports of children described as having Terson syndrome. However, McLellan et al. (1986) report the case of a 6-week old infant found to have bilateral retinal haemorrhages, including a preretinal haemorrhage, secondary to a ruptured intracerebral arterial aneurysm.

In conclusion, there is little evidence to indicate that intraocular haemorrhages occur in children secondary to non-traumatic intracranial haemorrhage. If it does occur, it is very rare. In practice, retinal haemorrhages found in a child with intracranial haemorrhages are due to child abuse by violent shaking, until proven otherwise.

Other intraocular findings associated with SBS

TRAUMATIC RETINOSCHISIS

The term 'traumatic retinoschisis' in the setting of SBS was first used in 1986, when five cases of physical child abuse were reported in which blood-filled premacular 'cysts' were

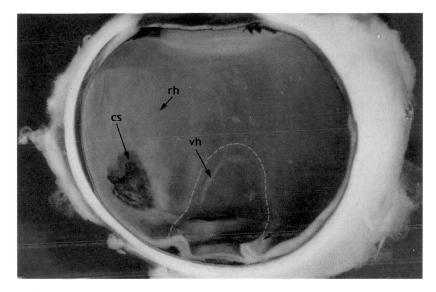

Fig. 5.13. Opened eye of a shaken infant, showing extensive retinal haemorrhage (rh), a crater-like posterior pole retinal fold (f) with domed posterior vitreous detachment (highlight) and related vitreous haemorrhage (vh). Note the black choreoretinal scar (cs) indicating old trauma.

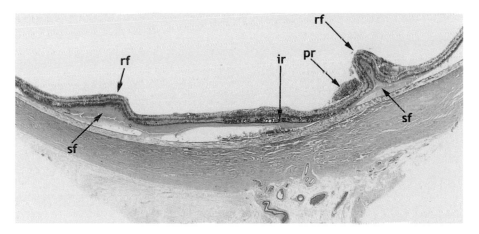

Fig. 5.14. Histology across the same retinal fold (rf) as seen in Fig. 5.13, with subretinal fluid (rf). Note the extensive preretinal (pr) and intraretinal (ir) haemorrhage.

described (Greenwald et al. 1986). Electroretinograms in these children consistently demonstrated loss or reduction of the b-wave with relative preservation of the a-wave indicating damage to the inner layers of the retina. It was postulated that vitreous traction (particularly in light of the firm vitreous to retinal attachments that are thought to exist in the young) was responsible for physically creating a split within the retina, characteristically at the posterior

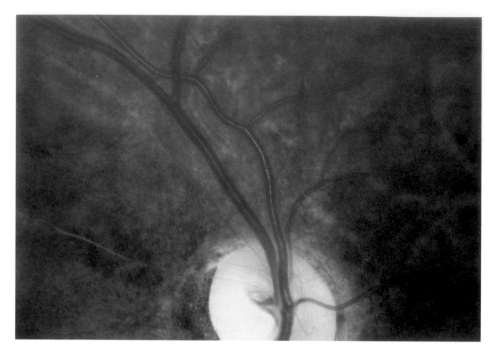

Fig. 5.15. Post-traumatic optic atrophy.

pole. As yet, traumatic retinoschisis has not been demonstrated in other conditions associated with retinal haemorrhages (Levin 2000).

RETINAL FOLDS

Retinal folds encircling the macular region may be seen in one or both eyes in association with more severe ocular damage following shaking (Gaynon et al. 1988) (Figs. 5.13, 5.14). They are more commonly seen in SBS but have been reported in adult cases of Terson syndrome (intraocular haemorrhage associated with intracranial haemorrhage) (Keithahn et al. 1993). Massicotte et al. (1991) found that histologically there was partial vitreous detachment except at the apices of the folds, confirming their belief that vitreous traction was the pathogenic mechanism.

RETINAL DETACHMENT OR DIALYSIS

Severe trauma to the head may result in retinal detachment or dialysis. In these cases it is often difficult to determine whether the ocular trauma is direct, or indirect via a shaking mechanism.

CHORIORETINAL ATROPHY AND RETINAL GLIOSIS

Areas of white chorioretinal scarring, often associated with areas of increased pigmentation,

202

are a sign of previous trauma (Harcourt and Hopkins 1973), which may be accidental or non-accidental (Fig. 5.13). Retinal gliosis (proliferation of retinal astrocytes) can also occur as a reaction to previous retinal damage.

Long-term visual prognosis and management

Infants who sustain head injuries due to abuse have a greater morbidity than equivalent children in whom the head injury is accidental (Haviland and Russell 1997). Permanent visual impairment is reported in 30–80% of children who have been physically abused (Han and Wilkinson 1990). Poor ocular prognostic indicators at presentation include pupil non-reaction to light (McCabe and Donahue 2000) and dense vitreous haemorrhage (Matthews and Das 1996). In view of these statistics it is important that these surviving children receive long-term follow-up from ophthalmic services. The effects of coincidental intellectual and physical disability may compound visual problems.

CORTICAL BLINDNESS AND OPTIC ATROPHY

Cortical blindness and optic atrophy secondary to neurological damage are the commonest causes of long-term visual impairment following SBS (Fig. 5.15). Infarction and atrophy of the cerebral cortex can be quite marked in affected infants, even if the acute intracranial haemorrhage is relatively minor. These children may need to be registered as partially sighted or blind. Follow-up will include long-term assessment of visual development and help with low visual aids.

VITREOUS HAEMORRHAGE

The primary concern in infants with vitreous haemorrhage is that of profound occlusive amblyopia. In addition, it has been demonstrated that visual deprivation before 1 year of age, in this case following vitreous haemorrhage, is associated with the development of axial myopia (short sightedness secondary to elongation of the eye). This is related to interruption of the visually dependent process of emmetropization in the developing eye (this is the process by which the eye develops to become neither long- nor short-sighted). In one study there was evidence of myopic shift even after 2 months of occlusion due to vitreous haemorrhage (Miller-Meeks and Bennett 1990). In children with occlusive vitreous haemorrhage, early vitrectomy is recommended (within 3–4 weeks after onset). This is to minimize the risk of sequelae, including amblyopia, tractional retinal detachment, epiretinal membrane formation and pigmentary retinopathy (Ferrone and De Juan 1994).

Note that dense vitreous haemorrhage in association with SBS has a poor visual prognosis, as it is frequently associated with retinal and cerebral cortex pathology. (Matthews and Das 1996). Gaynon et al. (1988) suggest that an ERG (electroretinogram) may help to exclude retinal dysfunction prior to vitrectomy.

MACULAR HAEMORRHAGE

In the past the only management of macular haemorrhage was observation and treatment of subsequent amblyopia and strabismus. Recently the use of intravitreal tPA (tissue plasminogen activator) and SF_6 (sulphur hexafluoride gas) has been recommended to promote clearing of premacular subhyaloid haemorrhage (Conway et al. 1999). The results from this single study are promising, with resolution of the haemorrhage within a week.

STRABISMUS AND AMBLYOPIA
Strabismus is most commonly secondary to sensory deprivation due to ocular damage, but it may result from intracranial damage causing VIth cranial nerve palsy.

Conclusion
Ophthalmic findings are only part of the clinical picture when assessing a suspected case of child abuse. In isolation they are insufficient to confirm the diagnosis of shaken baby syndrome; this requires multidisciplinary input from not only physicians but also social services and legal services. However, the ophthalmologist and ophthalmic pathologist have a real contribution to make in both the diagnosis of shaken baby syndrome and the continuing management of the affected surviving children and their siblings.

REFERENCES

Alario A, Duhaime A, Lewander W, Tsiaras W, Wallach M, O'Shea JS (1990) Do retinal hemorrhages occur with accidental head trauma in young children? *Am J Dis Child* **144**: 445 (abstract).
Altman RV, Kutscher ML, Brand DA (1998) The "shaken baby syndrome". *N Engl J Med* **339**: 1329–1330.
American Academy of Pediatrics (1993) Shaken baby syndrome: inflicted cerebral injury. *Pediatrics* **92**: 872–875.
Bourne RA, Talks SJ, Richards AB (1999) Treatment of pre-retinal Valsalva haemorrhages with neodymium:YAG laser. *Eye* **13**: 791–793.
Budenz DL, Farber MG, Mirchandani HG, Park H, Rorke LB (1994) Ocular and optic nerve hemorrhages in abused infants with intracranial injuries. *Ophthalmology* **101**: 559–565.
Buys YM, Levin AV, Enzenauer RW, Elder JE, Letoumeau MA, Humphreys RP, Mian M, Morin JD (1992) Retinal findings after head trauma in infants and young children. *Ophthalmology* **99**: 1718–1723.
Caffey J (1972) On the theory and practice of shaking infants. *Am J Dis Child* **124**: 161–169.
Chanda A, Pearson CM, Doran RML (1988) Preferential looking in clinical practice: a year's experience. *Eye* **2**: 488–495.
Christian CW, Taylor AA, Hertle RW, Duhaime AC (1999) Retinal hemorrhages caused by accidental household trauma. *J Pediatr* **135**: 125–127.
Conway MD, Peyman GA, Recasens M (1999) Intravitreal tPA and SF_6 promote clearing of premacular subhyaloid hemorrhages in shaken and battered baby syndrome. *Ophthalmic Surg Lasers* **30**: 435–441.
Di Maio VJ (1985) Subscleral hemorrhage. *Am J Forensic Med Pathol* **6**: 95.
Duane T (1972) Valsalva haemorrhagic retinopathy. *Trans Am Ophthalmol Soc* **70**: 298–313.
Duhaime AC, Alario AJ, Lewander WJ, Schut L, Sutton LN, Seidl TS, Nudelman S, Budenz D, Hertle R, Tsiaras W, Loporchio S (1992) Head injury in very young children: mechanisms, injury types, and ophthalmologic findings in 100 hospitalized patients younger than 2 years of age. *Pediatrics* **90**: 179–185.
Dyer C (2005) Court hears shaken baby cases. *BMJ* **330**: 1463.
Egge K, Lyng G, Maltau JM (1981) Effect of instrumental delivery on the frequency and severity of retinal hemorrhages in the newborn. *Acta Obstet Gynecol Scand* **60**: 153–155.
Fackler JC, Berkowitz ID, Green WR (1994) Retinal hemorrhages in newborn piglets following cardiopulmonary resuscitation. *Am J Dis Child* **146**: 1294–1296.
Fahmy J (1973) Fundal haemorrhages in ruptured intracranial aneurysms. I. Material, frequency and morphology. *Acta Ophthalmol* **51**: 289–298.
Ferrone P, De Juan E (1994) Vitreous haemorrhage in infants. *Arch Ophthalmol* **112**: 1185–1189.
Fraser S (1995) Retinal haemorrhage in meningitis. *Eye* **9**: 659–660.
Galvin R, Sanders M (1980) Peripheral retinal haemorrhages with papilloedema. *Br J Ophthalmol* **64**: 262–266.
Gaynon MW, Koh K, Marmor MF, Frankel LR (1988) Retinal folds in the shaken baby syndrome. *Am J Ophthalmol* **106**: 423–425.

Geddes JF, Hackshaw AK, Vowles GH, Nickols CD, Whitwell HL (2001a) Neuropathology of inflicted head injury in children. I. Patterns of brain damage. *Brain* **124**: 1290–1298.

Geddes JF, Vowles GH, Hackshaw AK, Nickols CD, Scott IS, Whitwell HL (2001b) Neuropathology of inflicted head injury in children. II. Microscopic brain injury in infants. *Brain* **124**: 1299–1306.

Geddes JF, Tasker RC, Hackshaw AK, Nickols CD, Adams GG, Whitwell HL, Scheimberg I (2003) Dural haemorrhage in non-traumatic infant deaths: does it explain the bleeding in 'shaken baby syndrome'? *Neuropathol Appl Neurobiol* **29**: 14-22. Erratum in: *Neuropathol Appl Neurobiol* 2003 **29**: 322.

Geddes JF, Tasker RC, Adams GG, Whitwell HL (2004) Violence is not necessary to produce subdural and retinal haemorrhage: a reply to Punt et al. *Pediatr Rehabil* **7**: 261–265.

Giangiacomo J, Khan J, Levine C, Thompson VM (1988) Sequential cranial computed tomography in infants with retinal haemorrhages. *Ophthalmology* **95**: 295–299.

Giles C (1960) Retinal haemorrhages in the newborn. *Am J Ophthalmol* **49**: 1005.

Gilkes M, Mann T (1967) Fundi of battered babies. *Lancet* **2**: 468–467.

Gilliland MG, Folberg R (1992) Retinal haemorrhages: Replicating the clinician's view of the eye. *Forensic Sci Int* **56**: 77–80.

Gilliland MG, Luckenbach MW (1993) Are retinal haemorrhages found after resuscitation attempts? *Am J Forensic Med Pathol* **14**: 187–192.

Gilliland MG, Luckenbach MW, Massicotte SJ, Folberg R (1991) The medicolegal implications of detecting hemosiderin in the eyes of children who are suspected of being abused. *Arch Ophthalmol* **109**: 321–322.

Gilliland MG, Luckenbach MW, Chenier TC (1994) Systemic and ocular findings in 169 prospectively studied child deaths: Retinal hemorrhages usually mean child abuse. *Forensic Sci Int* **68**: 117–132.

Green MA, Lieberman G, Milroy CM, Parsons MA (1996) Ocular and cerebral trauma in non-accidental injury in infancy: underlying mechanisms and implications for paediatric practice. *Br J Ophthalmol* **80**: 282–287.

Greenwald MJ, Weiss A, Oesterle CS, Friendly DS (1986) Traumatic retinoschisis in battered babies. *Ophthalmology* **93**: 618–625

Han D, Wilkinson W (1990) Late ophthalmic manifestations of the shaken baby syndrome. *J Paediatr Ophthalmol Strabismus* **27**: 299–303.

Harcourt B, Hopkins D (1973) Permanent chorioretinal lesions in childhood of suspected traumatic origin. *Trans Ophthalmol Soc UK* **93**: 199 205.

Haviland J, Russell R (1997) Outcome after severe non-accidental head injury. *Arch Dis Child* **77**: 504–507.

Helfer R, Slovis T, Black M (1977) Injuries resulting when small children fall out of bed. *Pediatrics* **60**: 533–535.

Hoffman G, Naughten E (1998) Abuse or metabolic disorder? *Arch Dis Child* **78**: 399–400.

Hollenhorst R, Stein H (1958) Ocular signs and prognosis in subdural and subarachnoid bleeding in young children. *Arch Ophthalmol* **60**: 187–192.

Jayawant S, Rawlinson A, Gibbon F, Price J, Schulte J, Sharples P, Sibert JR, Kemp AM (1998) Subdural haemorrhages in infants: population based study. *BMJ* **317**: 1558–1561.

Kanter RK (1986) Retinal hemorrhage after cardiopulmonary resuscitation or child abuse. *J Pediatr* **108**: 430–432.

Kapoor S, Schiffman J, Tang R, Kiang E, Li H, Woodward J (1997) The significance of white-centered retinal hemorrhages in the shaken baby syndrome. *Pediatr Emerg Care* **13**: 183–185.

Kaur B, Taylor D (1990) Retinal haemorrhages. *Arch Dis Child* **65**: 1369–1372.

Keane J (1981) Papilledema with unusual ocular haemorrhages. *Arch Ophthalmol* **99**: 262–263

Keithahn MA, Bennett SR, Cameron D, Mieter WF (1993) Retinal folds in Terson syndrome. *Ophthalmology* **100**: 1187–1190.

Kiffney G (1964) The eye of the battered child. *Arch Ophthalmol* **72**: 231–233.

Kivlin JD, Simons KB, Lazoritz S, Ruttum MS (2000) Shaken baby syndrome. *Ophthalmology*. **107**: 1246–1254.

Knight B (1996) Suffocation and asphyxia. In: *Forensic Pathology*. London: Arnold, pp. 345–360.

Lambert SR, Johnson TE, Hoyt CS (1986) Optic nerve sheath and retinal hemorrhages associated with the shaken baby syndrome. *Arch Ophthalmol* **104**: 1509–1512.

Levin A (2000) Retinal haemorrhages and child abuse. In: David TJ (Ed.) *Recent Advances in Paediatrics, Vol. 18*. Edinburgh: Churchill Livingstone, pp. 151–219.

Levy HL, Brown AE, Williams SE, de Juan E (1996) Vitreous hemorrhage as an ophthalmic complication of galactosemia. *J Pediatr* **129**: 922–925.

205

Lin KC, Glasgow BJ (1999) Bilateral periopticointrascleral hemorrhages associated with traumatic child abuse. *Am J Ophthalmol* **127**: 473–475.

Maltau JM, Egge K, Moe N (1984) Retinal haemorrhages in the preterm neonate. A prospective randomized study comparing the occurrence of hemorrhages after spontaneous versus forceps delivery. *Acta Obstet Gynecol Scand* **63**: 219–221.

Massicotte SJ, Folberg R, Torczynski E, Gilliland MG, Luckenbach (1991) Vitreoretinal traction and perimacular retinal folds in the eyes of deliberately traumatized children. *Ophthalmology* **98**: 1124–1127.

Matthews GP, Das A (1996) Dense vitreous hemorrhages predict poor visual and neurological prognosis in infants with shaken baby syndrome. *J Pediatr Ophthalmol Strabismus* **33**: 260–265.

McCabe C, Donahue S (2000) Prognostic indicators for vision and mortality in shaken baby syndrome. *Arch Ophthalmol* **118**: 373–377.

McLellan NJ, Prasad R, Punt J (1986) Spontaneous subhyaloid and retinal haemorrhages in an infant. *Arch Dis Child* **61**: 1130–1132.

Miller-Meeks M, Bennett S (1990) Myopia induced by vitreous hemorrhage. *Am J Ophthalmol* **109**: 199–203.

Morad Y, Kim YM, Armstrong DC, Huyer D, Mian M, Levin AV (2002) Correlation between retinal abnormalities and intracranial abnormalities in the shaken baby syndrome. *Am J Ophthalmol* **134**: 354–359.

Morris A, Sanders M (1980) Macular changes resulting from papilloedema. *Br J Ophthalmol* **64**: 211–216.

Nimityongskul P, Anderson LD (1987) The likelihood of injuries when children fall out of bed. *J Pediatr Orthop* **7**: 184–186.

Ophthalmology Child Abuse Working Party (1999) Child abuse and the eye. *Eye* **13**: 3–10.

Parsons M, Start R (2001) ACP Best Practice No. 164. Necropsy techniques in ophthalmic pathology. *J Clin Pathol* **54**: 417–427.

Plunkett J (2001) Fatal pediatric head injuries caused by short-distance falls. *Am J Forensic Med Pathol* **22**: 1–12.

Pollack J, Tychsen I (1996) The prevalence of retinal hemorrhages in infants after extra-corporeal membrane oxygenation. *Am J Ophthalmol* **121**: 297–303.

Punt J, Bonshek RE, Jaspan T, McConachie NS, Punt N, Ratcliffe JM (2004) The 'unified hypothesis' of Geddes et al. is not supported by the data. *Pediatr Rehabil* **7**: 173–184.

Ravin J, Meyer R (1973) Flourescein angiographic findings in a case of traumatic asphyxia. *Am J Ophthalmol* **75**: 643–647.

Royal College of Ophthalmologists (1999) Procedures for the Ophthalmologist Who Suspects Child Abuse. Child Abuse Working Party.

Sandramouli S, Robinson R, Tsaloumas M, Willshaw HE (1997) Retinal haemorrhages and convulsions. *Arch Dis Child* **76**: 449–451.

House of Lords Select Committee on Science and Technology (1999) Digital Images as Evidence. London: HMSO.

Sezen F (1970) Retinal haemorrhages in newborn infants. *Br J Ophthalmol* **55**: 248–253.

Skalpe IO, Egge K, Maltau JM (1982) Cerebral computed tomography in newborn children with large retinal hemorrhages. *Neuroradiology* **23**: 213–214.

Terson A (1900) De l'hemorrhagie dans le corps vitre au cours de l'hemorrhagie cerebrale. *Clin Ophtalmol* **22**: 309–312.

Tyagi AK, Willshaw HE, Ainsworth JR (1997) Unilateral retinal haemorrhages in non-accidental injury. *Lancet* **349**: 1224 (letter).

Tyagi AK, Scotcher S, Kozeis N, Willshaw HE (1998) Can convulsions alone cause retinal haemorrhages in infants? *Br J Ophthalmol* **82**: 659–660.

Von Noorden G, Khoudadoust A (1973) Retinal hemorrhage in newborns and organic amblyopia. *Arch Ophthalmol* **89**: 91–93.

Warrington SA, Wright CM, and the ALSPAC Study Team (2001) Accidents and resulting injuries in premobile infants: data from the ALSPAC study. *Arch Dis Child* **85**: 104–107.

Waterhouse W, Enzenauer RW, Parmley VC (1992) Inflammatory orbital tumor as an ocular sign of a battered child. *Am J Ophthalmol* **114**: 510–512.

Weedn VW, Mansour AM, Nichols MM (1990) Retinal hemorrhage in an infant after cardiopulmonary resuscitation. *Am J Forensic Med Pathol* **11**: 79–82.

Weingeist TA, Goldman EJ, Folk JC, Packer AJ, Ossoinig KC (1986) Terson's syndrome. Clinicopathologic correlations. *Ophthalmology* **93**: 1435–1442.

Wilkinson WS, Han DP, Rappley MD, Owings CL (1989) Retinal hemorrhage predicts neurologic injury in the shaken baby syndrome. *Arch Ophthalmol* **107**: 1472–1474.

Woodhouse JM, Adoh TO, Oduwaiye KA, Batchelor BG, Megji S, Unwin N, Jones N (1992) New acuity test for toddlers. *Ophthalmic Physiol Opt* **12**: 249–251.

Zwaan J, Cardenas R, O'Connor PS (1997) Long-term outcome of neonatal macular hemorrhage. *J Paediatr Ophthalmol Strabismus* **34**: 286–288.

6
ULTRASOUND AND COMPUTED TOMOGRAPHY IN THE DIAGNOSIS OF NON-ACCIDENTAL HEAD INJURY

Tim Jaspan

Non-accidental head injury (NAHI) is one of the most challenging and difficult areas of paediatric neuroimaging. Abusive head injury is the most common cause of traumatic death in infancy. The diagnosis of inflicted head injury carries important and far-reaching medical, social and legal consequences. Early detection and diagnosis of head injury permits appropriate management triage and may alert the attending physician(s) to the possibility of a non-accidental mechanism for the trauma. The removal of a child from a potentially abusive environment is vital to prevent further harm. The corollary to this is that an incorrect evaluation of the neuroimaging may result in a misdiagnosis of abuse and a spiralling sequence of events that may prove damaging to the infant, the primary carers and the complex social interactions and dynamics of the care network associated with nurturing a young infant.

The introduction of computed tomography (CT) in the 1970s provided a major advance in the diagnosis and management of neurological disorders generally and, specifically, intracranial injury in the context of suspected child abuse. Early reports, based upon first and second generation CT scanners, were hampered by technical and quality limitations (Svendsen 1976, Zimmerman et al. 1978, Bruce and Schut 1980, Tsai et al. 1980). Over the next two decades advances in CT technology resulted in a significant leap forward in the utility and availability of this modality. Cranial ultrasound (sonography) had a less well defined role over this period. Recent developments in ultrasound equipment and technique, and the advent of Doppler imaging, have revived interest in this modality and established its place in the evaluation of NAHI (Mercker et al. 1985, Jaspan et al. 1992, Jaspan 1998).

Over the past 15 years magnetic resonance imaging (MRI) has come to the fore in the evaluation of intracranial pathology and has become increasingly important in the imaging of craniocerebral trauma in infancy, particularly in the subacute and chronic phases (Sato et al. 1989). Although this chapter primarily addresses the role of ultrasound and CT in the evaluation of NAHI, the integral relationship between these modalities and MRI will also be considered.

The pathway to cranial imaging for an infant who has suffered NAHI may be broadly considered under the following categories:

- serendipitously in an infant undergoing cranial imaging as part of the investigation of a presumed non-traumatic illness or encephalopathy (e.g. meningoencephalitis), developmental delay or regression, focal neurological deficits, psychomotor retardation, seizures or increasing head size
- clinical concern regarding the possibility of inflicted injury in a child presenting with altered consciousness following apparently minor head injury, unusual bruising or suspicious skeletal injury, leading to a request for cranial imaging
- an overtly injured child presenting in extremis, requiring resuscitation, intensive medical support and/or neurosurgical intervention.

As infants who suffer NAHI may present with nonspecific clinical features and are often admitted to non-specialist units, cranial ultrasound may be employed as the initial or even only imaging modality. Inexpertly executed ultrasound scans not infrequently fail to detect subtle or even more gross intracranial pathology and thus run the risk of failing to make the diagnosis of intracranial injury. Excessive reliance upon ultrasound is thus to be deprecated. A falsely reassuring cranial ultrasound scan report may result in failure to detect potential NAHI and thus leave the infant open to discharge from hospital and a return to a potentially abusive environment. CT must be undertaken as early as possible to enable correct diagnosis, guide appropriate management, provide prognostic information and forensic evidence for subsequent care or criminal proceedings. The latter should not be underestimated. Identification of NAHI may prevent serial and progressively more damaging injury or enable implementation of social support mechanisms to alleviate the conditions that often give rise to child abuse.

Imaging protocol

A universally accepted protocol for NAHI has yet to be defined. Imaging protocols vary according to local availability of imaging modalities and expertise. Regrettably this frequently leads to variable quality and inconsistent imaging. The consequences of inadequate imaging can be far reaching, including misdiagnosis, ambiguous or inconclusive data for medicolegal purposes and the risk of further subsequent abuse (Alexander et al. 1990).

Kleinman (1998) proposed a protocol based upon the neurological presentation. For those children with a suspected acute presentation, CT is recommended, proceeding to MRI if positive or highly suspicious. The imaging of a suspected chronic presentation or high specificity skeletal injury is by MRI. Ultrasound is suggested as an optional or useful additional imaging tool.

Such a protocol assumes knowledge of the timing of the injury and correct clinical evaluation. Unfortunately, as there is often delay in bringing the child to medical attention and the presentation is frequently nonspecific, initial clinical evaluation is often incorrect or misleading, leading to delayed or inappropriate cranial imaging. Timing of the injury or injuries on clinical grounds is often problematic. In a prospective post-mortem study, Gilliland (1998) demonstrated that the interval between the time of inflicted injury and onset of symptoms in infants who subsequently died is variable. In over 25% of shaking impact or blunt impact injuries the interval was greater than 24 hours. However, other studies involving cases of fatal accidental head injury (Willman et al. 1997) and NAHI (Gilles and

Library
Education Centre
RLC (NHS) Trust, Alder Hey
Liverpool L12 2AP
0151-252-5476

Nelson 1998) indicate that a so-called lucid interval between the traumatic event and onset of altered consciousness or neurological abnormality is minimal or does not exist. In addition, some infants have often been subjected to more than one episode of abuse. A more comprehensive and robust imaging protocol for all head injury may improve the diagnostic accuracy, management and forensic evaluation of NAHI.

Legitimate concerns exist regarding the radiation dose associated with CT. The effective dose from a complete head examination in an infant, approximately 6 mSv, is not inconsiderable, being equivalent to exposure to 2 years of natural background radiation (Karellas and Raptopoulos 1998). More modern CT scanners, however, probably deliver a lower radiation dosage, in the order of 1.5–2 mSv. At this level, the lifetime risk of fatal cancer for a 1-year-old child is of the order of 1 in 4000. Recent research has also suggested that even relatively low doses of ionising radiation such as that arising from cranial CT to the infant brain may affect cognitive function in adulthood (Hall et al. 2004). However, failure to detect NAHI can have far-reaching and serious consequences. The risks of missing or incorrectly diagnosing NAHI (due to delayed scanning, lack of an interval scan or not scanning at all) thus outweigh these concerns and justify CT scanning in all suspected cases. An infant who has suffered suspicious skeletal injury harbours the potential for intracranial injury, and should undergo cranial imaging, even if clinically unsuspected.

In a study by Rubin et al. (2003), 19 (37%) of 51 children under 2 years of age at high risk of child abuse were found to have occult head injuries. Intracranial injuries were identified in 10 infants. Subdural haemorrhage or haemorrhagic contusions were present in nine infants and subcortical shear injuries in three. These results clearly demonstrate that serious brain injuries can be found in neurologically intact infants. However, 14 of these 19 infants had a skull fracture or fractures identified on skull radiographs obtained as part of a skeletal survey. Assuming that the presence of a skull fracture would have led to cross-sectional neuroimaging in these infants, five (10%) of the 51 infants would have had their head injury missed if CT/MRI had not been employed.

Ultrasound can detect subtle injuries and monitor the status of larger subdural collections and major parenchymal injury. However, this modality represents a blunt edged sword. If ultrasound is undertaken by inexperienced or inexpert sonographers (as is frequently the case in both tertiary and non-tertiary centres) as the first and only imaging investigation in an infant presenting with a nonspecific illness who has suffered occult NAHI, subtle and even in some cases gross abnormality can be and often is missed. MRI, discussed elsewhere in this book, has potentially the greatest value in the assessment of the acute but more especially subacute and chronic phases of NAHI.

Traumatic brain injury is a dynamic and potentially complex process that evolves over time. A single 'snap-shot' radiological examination of such an injury is thus fraught with diagnostic pitfalls. In addition the final outcome cannot be determined other than by long-term clinical (Bonnier et al. 1995) and radiological evaluation. In many centres, the imaging protocols lack consistency and often only a single cross-sectional scan is undertaken. Particularly with early scans, the well-established evolution of brain parenchymal injuries will be missed. A protocol for the investigation of an infant suspected of suffering physical abuse has been recently proposed (Jaspan et al. 2003) (Fig. 6.1).

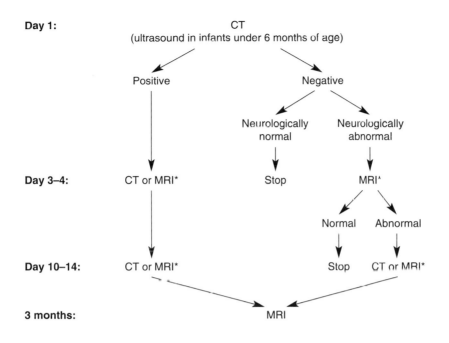

Imaging techniques

ULTRASOUND

Scanning should be undertaken employing good quality modern ultrasound equipment. The patient's identification, and the time and date of the examination (which may vary with changes in summer/winter time or recalibration following servicing of the machine), must be registered meticulously. One of the major advantages of the technique is its portability. Very ill or unstable infants do not tolerate handling well; these infants can be examined at the cot side with minimal disturbance.

Standard coronal and sagittal images are obtained through the anterior fontanelle, the area of connective tissue lying between the frontal and parietal bones where the coronal, sagittal and metopic sutures meet. A high frequency sector transducer (6–10 MHz) should be used in infants less than 3 months of age. Older infants may require a lower frequency transducer (3–5 MHz) to obtain sufficient depth penetration. Anatomical side marking must be displayed according to the standard neuroimaging convention; the right hemicranium on the left side of the image on coronal sections and anterior (face) on the left side of the image for sagittal sections. Supplementary high resolution scanning of the near field underlying the anterior fontanelle should be undertaken in all cases, employing a high frequency

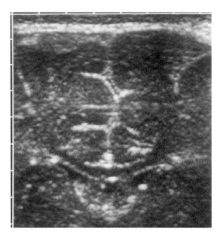

Fig. 6.2. Coronal high-resolution image demonstrating the echogenic scalp tissues of the anterior fontanelle, underlying hypoechoic normal brain, triangular superior sagittal sinus (arrows) and echogenic sulci.

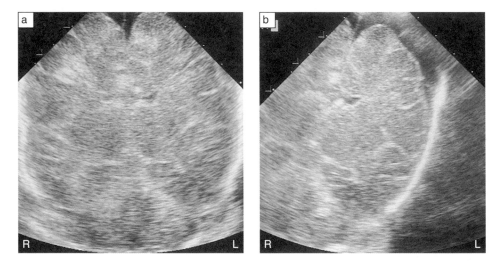

Fig. 6.3. (a) Coronal image of a 2-month-old infant with hypoechoic subdural haematomas over the surface of the brain. (b) Transducer angulation shows the lateral extension of the collection. Note the diffusely echogenic oedematous brain and compressed ventricles.

linear array transducer (7–10 MHz). Generous amounts of ultrasound coupling gel should be applied to the anterior fontanelle to enhance image quality. Meticulous attention must be paid to the time-gain curve (TGC) settings to optimize the near and far field spatial resolution. Thin subdural collections over the high cerebral convexity may be easily missed if the gain is not decreased in the near field. All too often the near field on poorly executed examinations is artificially hyperechogenic, resultiung in loss of anatomical detail.

A good quality high resolution scan should permit visualization of the superior surface of the brain and the superior sagittal sinus (Fig. 6.2). Angulation of the sector transducer

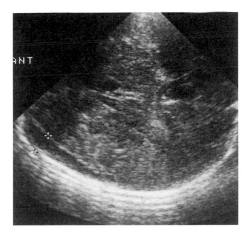

Fig. 6.4. Axial transcranial sonogram demonstrating a hypoechoic subdural haematoma (between the two cursors) over the lateral surface of the brain.

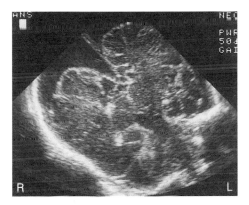

Fig. 6.5. Coronal transcranial image showing the extent of subdural collections over both cerebral hemispheres.

on the fontanelle enables fuller evaluation of laterally located subdural collections (Fig. 6.3). Trans-squamosal scanning in the axial (Fig. 6.4) and coronal planes (Fig. 6.5), employing a low frequency (2–3 MHz) transducer, can demonstrate the presence and extent of extra-axial collections over the contralateral cerebral hemisphere. The TGC settings must be adjusted so that the near field is not excessively obscured by acoustic damping from the temporal bone. More importantly, the far field should not appear too bright, which can result in a thin hyperechogenic collection blending with the overlying echogenic calvarium. Colour Doppler imaging assists in evaluating the integrity of the major cerebral arteries and the patency of the major venous sinuses, thereby allowing spectral Doppler studies to be undertaken much sooner.

The limitations of cranial ultrasonography must be clearly understood by the operator, the clinicians requesting the examination and, in cases in which the due process of law ensues, the legal authorities. Ultrasound examinations are all too frequently poorly executed. Spatial resolution decreases with increasing age; there is an insensitivity for laterally based extra-cerebral collections and posterior fossa pathology; and a lack of reproducibility. The role of cranial sonography should be considered as adjunctive to the less subjective and more universally accepted cross-sectional imaging tools represented by CT and MRI.

COMPUTED TOMOGRAPHY
A standard protocol for infant trauma scanning must be adopted. Scanning should employ a slice thickness of 8 mm or less in the supratentorial compartment and 5 mm or less through the posterior fossa. Our preference is to use 5 mm thick slices throughout the brain. The examination should be imaged using soft tissue settings appropriate for infants, with the window and levels set at 70–80 Hounsfield Units (HU) and 30–40 HU respectively. Bone window settings must be routinely obtained and imaged (e.g. window 3000 HU, level 400 HU). Intermediate settings (e.g. window 150 HU, level 50 HU) may be necessary to demonstrate subtle extra-axial fluid collections or parenchymal injury close to the skull, which may be obscured by the beam hardening effect. Administration of intravenous contrast medium is seldom indicated but may occasionally assist in demonstrating hyper-vascular subdural membranes, ischaemic lesions or focal vascular injury.

Injury patterns
Head injury resulting from physical abuse may be considered in terms of the immediate (primary), early subsequent (secondary) and late or end-stage (chronic) damage. The complex issues reated to the mechanism(s) of injury are discussed elsewhere in this book.

PRIMARY
Primary injury occurs as the immediate consequence of the absorption or dissipation of traumatic forces. Damage to the cerebral parenchyma is irreversible. The injuries may involve one or more of the following: (1) scalp soft tissues and skull; (2) meninges and vessels overlying the brain; (3) brain parenchyma and ventricles; (4) spine and spinal canal contents.

Scalp soft tissues and skull
Injury to the scalp and skull occurs as a consequence of direct impact forces. There may be clinical evidence of scalp injury in the form of an abrasion, bruise or focal swelling. A scalp injury may, however, evade detection if: (i) the volume of the lesion is small due to severe systemic hypotension, which may be detected only at autopsy (Duhaime et al. 1987); (ii) the scalp is inspected before the swelling has evolved; (iii) swelling has resolved by the time the child is brought to medical attention; or (iv) there is thick overlying hair (particularly in Afro-Caribbean infants).

Scalp injury may involve the subcutaneous (caput succedaneum), subgaleal or sub-periosteal (cephalhaematoma) space(s). Subgaleal haematomas are commonest, the bleeding occurring into the space below the galea aponeurotica and above the temporalis or occipito-frontalis muscle and periosteum of the skull. The haematoma may spread over a large area of the scalp, often distant from the site of impact, and may track over both sides of the head when there is a diastatic sutural fracture or a fracture extending across the midline (Fig. 6.6). It should be noted, however that a seriously injured child nursed in the recumbent position

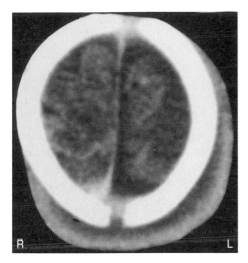

Fig. 6.6. CT demonstrating a large subgaleal haematoma in a 2-month-old infant with a diastased sagittal suture. The cerebral cortex and subcortical white matter are hypodense. Extensive intracranial injuries were present elsewhere.

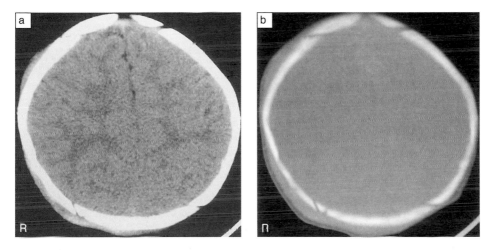

Fig. 6.7. (a) CT shows scalp swelling in a 6-month-old infant who fell from a first floor window. Note a right parietal fracture immediately anterior to the lambdoid suture. (b) Bone-window settings demonstrate more clearly the extent of the swelling. There was no intracranial injury.

in the intensive care unit or who has had intracranial pressure monitoring devices/external drainage catheters may develop scalp swelling. Scalp injury can be detected on skull radiographs employing a 'bright light' technique, particularly on over-exposed films, although small scalp injuries may evade detection. CT, with appropriate windowing, is well suited to detect these injuries (Fig. 6.7).

A cephalhaematoma is a collection of blood located between the outer periosteum and outer table of the skull, present below the temporalis muscle. It is seen classically in the newborn infant delivered by forceps or ventouse extraction, and rarely occurs outside of

215

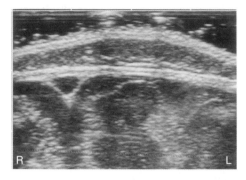

Fig. 6.8. High-resolution coronal ultrasound over the anterior fontanelle demonstrating a subgaleal haematoma. The superior sagittal sinus is clearly identified as a transonic triangular structure. Normal subarachnoid spaces overlie the surface of the brain.

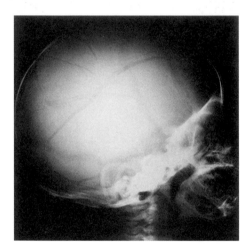

Fig. 6.9. Lateral skull radiograph in a fatally abused 4-month-old infant showing multiple wide skull vault fractures crossing diastased cranial sutures.

the newborn period. Most cephalhaematomas resorb within two weeks of life. Healing may be accompanied by incorporation into the diplöic space with consequent thickening of the outer table of the skull.

Demonstration of a scalp injury can provide corroborative evidence of the nature and timing of the injury. Ultrasound has been employed to detect scalp injuries and to assess the underlying calvarium and surface of the brain (Fig. 6.8); however, it adds little to the overall assessment of the injury when CT has been performed.

Skull injuries are evidence of an impact or blow to the head. Skull radiographs remain essential in their evaluation (Fig. 6.9). There is no one type of injury that is diagnostic of NAHI; however, certain features or patterns of skull fracture are more consistent with abuse, particularly multiple, bilateral, branching, comminuted, depressed, wide (>3 mm) and growing fractures, crossing sutures and occipito-parietal location (Hobbs 1984, Brown and Minns 1993). The history given, clinical features and presence and type of other skeletal, intraocular and intracranial injuries may provide important clues as to the aetiology. In a series of 89 children under the age of 2 who had suffered a skull fracture (Hobbs 1984), 60 were adjudged to have suffered accidental injury. None of these children had an associated

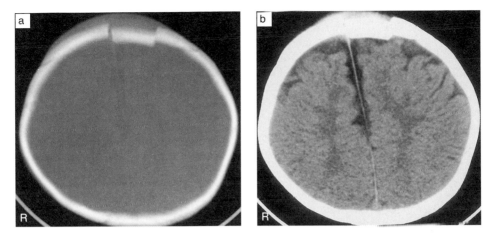

Fig. 6.10 (a) CT in a 3-month-old infant who had been struck with a hard toy. Bone settings show a depressed left frontal bone fracture. (b) Note absence of underlying intracranial injury.

subdural haematoma. Only one of the accidental group sustained a fracture after a fall from a height of less than 3 feet (1 metre).

The cranial sutures are relatively pliable or elastic structures made of dense fibrous connective tissue that form the joints between the membranous derived skull vault bony plates. Skull growth occurs along the sutural margins by osteoblastic activity. The sutures are usually patent in the first year of life, becoming fused at variable periods over the first two decades. The inner margins of the cranial sutures have a relatively well-defined and straight margin, whilst the outer table is interdigitated. Knowledge of the sutures is essential in the interpretation of skull vault injury. Interpretative pitfalls include wormian bones, squamo-parietal sutures and posterior skull base sutures, which may be mistaken for fractures. The synchondroses, composed of cartilaginous tissue, separate the skull base bones. Their presence in the posterior fossa may also lead to interpretative difficulties; however, their symmetrical appearance, location and lack of associated overlying soft tissue swelling helps to differentiate them from fractures. Skull base fractures are, however, uncommon in NAHI.

Evaluation of sutural widening can be difficult due to considerable biological variability. A sutural width in excess of 3 mm in the first year of life has been taken as indicative of diastasis (Schachenmayr and Friede 1978); however, retrospective analysis of serial skull radiographs or CT scans may be the only reliable method of determining whether the sutures are pathologically widened.

Approximately 50% of infants suffering intracranial NAHI have a skull fracture (Tsai et al. 1980, Merten and Osborne 1984). The reported incidence of skull fractures in all cases of child abuse varies from 10% to 35% (O'Neill et al. 1973, Tsai et al. 1980, Merten et al. 1984, Cohen et al. 1986, Duhaime et al. 1987, Loder and Bookout 1991). Serious intracranial injury may occur in the absence of a skull fracture, which may indeed have a protective effect in absorbing some or much of the imparted force following an impact injury (Fig. 6.10).

217

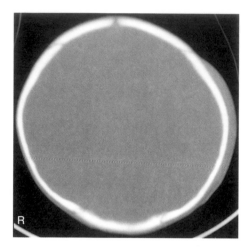

Fig. 6.11. CT in an infant whose plain skull radiograph demonstrated a thin left parietal fracture. The orientation of the fracture is parallel to the CT scan plane. The fracture cannot be detected, although overlying scalp swelling is readily identified.

Caution is required in interpreting skull fractures by CT alone. Linear fractures that have an orientation similar to that of the scan plane employed may be easily overlooked (Fig. 6.11). If skull radiographs are not available, the lateral pilot scan should be carefully scrutinized to exclude a simple linear convexity fracture.

Precise dating of skull fractures is impossible. Features consistent with a recent skull fracture are an overlying scalp haematoma, sharp fracture margins and, if present, associated acute intracranial injury. Serial scanning may demonstrate resolution of any scalp swelling and a progressive blunting or indistinctness of the fracture margins (Brown and Minns 1993). As there is no osteoblastic response in the membranous skull bones, linear undisplaced skull fractures heal without sclerosis. In the first year of life most disappear completely by 3–6 months or may simulate a vascular groove. In older children, fractures may take up to a year to heal.

Meninges and vessels overlying the brain
Understanding the anatomy of the linings investing the brain and skull is essential for the evaluation of intracranial injury. Figure 6.12 depicts the anatomy in the coronal plane and its relationship to subdural haematoma formation.

• *Dural injury.* The dura may be disrupted as a consequence of a skull fracture or traumatic sutural diastasis. The commonest sequel of a skull fracture is an underlying subdural haemorrhage, although an extradural haematoma (EDH) may occur. Extradural haematomas are located between the inner table of the skull and the outer (periosteal) dural layer. Unlike in older children and adults, EDH in infancy is more likely to be venous in origin. EDHs are, however, rare in NAHI (Merten et al. 1984, Kleinman 1998). Disruption of the dura underlying a fracture at the time of injury may lead to interposition of leptomeninges between the fracture margins with gradual widening of the fracture. A large defect, termed a growing fracture, may contain brain as well as the leptomeninges and CSF (see later).

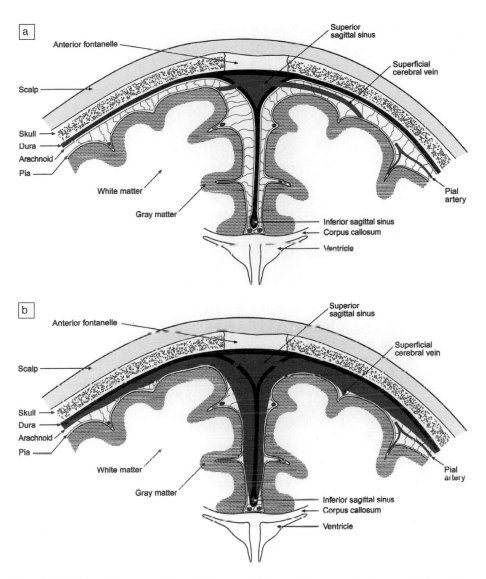

Fig. 6.12. (a) Schematic representation of the normal intracranial anatomy in the coronal plane. Note the bridging veins piercing the inner dural lining of the superior sagittal sinus. (b) Bilateral parafalcine subdural haematomas.

• *Subdural haematoma (SDH)*. The commonest intracranial abnormality in NAHI is SDH (Caffey 1974, Zimmerman et al. 1979, Calder et al. 1984). SDHs are present in 90–98% of fatal cases of NAHI (Duhaime et al. 1987, Gilles and Nelson 1998). Very thin films of SDH may not be detected by CT, probably accounting for the lower detection rate of 80–85% in non-fatal cases (Jenny et al. 1999). As some SDHs may be only in the order of 2–3 ml

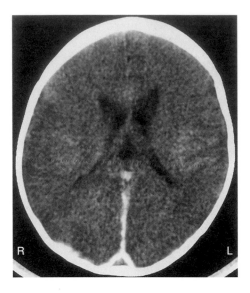

Fig. 6.13. CT in a 3-month-old infant with a severe shaking injury, showing typical posterior parafalcine SDH tracking over the posterior surface of the brain (the full extent of which was defined by MRI). Note diffuse cerebral oedema with grey and white matter hypodensity.

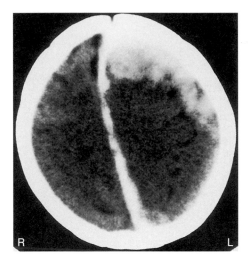

Fig. 6.14. CT showing acute parafalcine SDH extending over the surface of the left cerebral hemisphere. Note the ill-defined margin of the laterally located collection, due to a partial volume effect, the SDH being orientated in the same plane as the imaging plane, and coexisting subarachnoid haemorrhage.

in volume, they may evade detection at autopsy if the examination is not undertaken by an experienced paediatric neuropathologist or the subdural space is not carefully examined when the calvarium is being removed (Case et al. 2001).

SDHs are located between the inner dural layer and the arachnoid mater (Fig. 6.12). The typical site of SDH in NAHI, adjacent to the cerebral falx (parafalcine) and coating the adjacent surface of the cerebral hemispheres, corresponds to the location of the cortical veins that traverse the subarachnoid space as they pass towards the superior sagittal sinus (Zimmerman et al. 1979). Acceleration–deceleration forces generated by shaking are orientated in an anteroposterior direction, directed towards the vertex. The cerebral falx

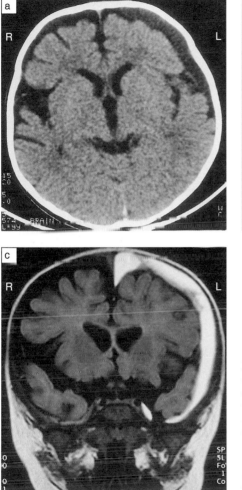

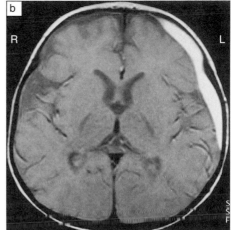

Fig. 6.15. Late subacute left-sided SDH. (a) CT shows a mildly hypodense left frontal convexity collection. The prominent extracerebral fluid over the right cerebral hemisphere is in the subarachnoid space. (b) Axial proton density MRI showing more clearly the left SDH and confirming that the right-sided fluid is CSF in the subarachnoid compartment. (c) Coronal T_1-weighted MRI demonstrating the subtemporal extension of the SDH, not appreciated on CT.

prevents dissipation of these forces across the midline, thus focusing the shear–strain forces in the region adjacent to the midline. As a result the delicate cortical bridging veins are stretched and torn. Additional shear–strain forces produced by lateral rotation increase the risk of disruption of these vessels and of the underlying brain. The point of fixation of the veins, where they pierce the arachnoid mater and inner dural layer to enter the venous sinus, thus represents a particularly vulnerable site. The resultant haemorrhage tracks along the potential subdural space alongside the cerebral falx and medial surface of the brain (Fig. 6.13).

Acute SDHs are often relatively small. In most cases the importance of an SDH is that it is a marker of the mechanism of the injury rather than as a space occupying mass lesion requiring intervention in its own right. The volume of the subdural blood is rarely of a

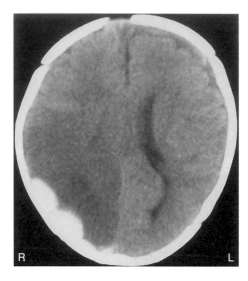

Fig. 6.16. Acute SDH in a 2-month-old infant suffering an impact injury. Note the unusual irregular contour of the SDH and the underlying cerebral oedema. The SDH was evacuated but the child was left with a hemiplegic cerebral palsy.

magnitude to produce significant elevation of the intracranial pressure. Larger collections extend out laterally over the surface of the brain (Fig. 6.14), spread over the superior tentorial surface or under the temporal lobe. Particularly if accompanied by underlying cerebral swelling or oedema, larger SDHs may elevate the intracranial pressure so that arterial blood supply to the brain is compromised due to vessel entrapment against rigid structures (e.g. the cerebral falx or tentorial margins) or venous pressure is raised to the extent that adequate cerebral perfusion is impeded.

The full extent of an SDH can easily be underestimated by CT and ultrasound and is best evaluated by MRI (Sato and Smith 1994, Zimmerman and Bilaniuk 1994), particularly in the subacute and chronic phases (Fig. 6.15). Subdural haematomas may be predominantly unilateral, either alongside the cerebral falx or over the lateral convexity. The latter may be associated with a direct impact injury and may be accompanied by a skull fracture or scalp swelling. Underlying acute cerebral oedema and swelling may be seen with laterally located SDHs (Fig. 6.16), which is associated with a poor outcome (Kleinman 1998).

Hypodense, anteriorly located SDHs commonly coexist with thin high-density parafalcine and/or posterior cerebral convexity SDHs (Fig. 6.17). The latter are frequently accompanied by a small posterior fossa SDH, typically located alongside the falx cerebelli and posterior surface of the cerebellum (Fig. 6.18). Such collections are often subtle, undetectable on ultrasound, easily missed on CT, and best visualized by MRI (Fig. 6.19). The importance of these collections is that they represent a completely separate anatomical compartment from supratentorial SDHs. Therefore rebleeding cannot be implicated in their aetiology, an issue of considerable importance when establishing the number and age of various intracranial episodes of injury.

Ageing of SDHs is fraught with difficulties. The attenuation of acute haemorrhage on CT is dependent upon the globin moiety of haemoglobin and clot retraction, and not the iron component (New and Aronow 1976). Acute clotted blood has an attenuation of

222

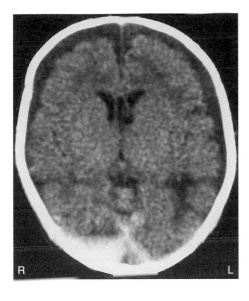

Fig. 6.17. Four-month-old infant who had a previously documented abusive head injury and increasing head circumference and was readmitted acutely ill. There are bilateral low density older anterior and acute posterior SDHs.

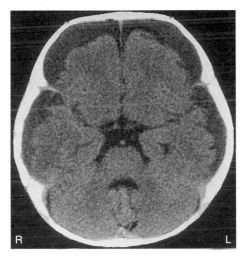

Fig. 6.18. Subtle posterior fossa acute SDH lying alongside the falx cerebelli (arrow), confirmed by MRI. Note the large chronic supratentorial SDHs.

60–80 HU. Normal grey matter has a value of 34–38 HU and white matter 28–34 HU (Bruce and Schut 1980). The maturing process of subdural clot formation involves initial hyperacute bleeding into the subdural space, the blood being in a liquid, unclotted form that may appear hypodense. As the blood clots, the aggregated globin complex results in a hyperdense appearance of the blood. The gradual breakdown of the globin complex by proteolysis results in a reduction in the CT density.

Early descriptions of the evolving appearance of SDH on CT were based on studies in adults (Scotti et al. 1977). In the initial (*acute*) phase, described as from the first few minutes to several days, the haematoma is of high density. A gradual reduction in the density of the

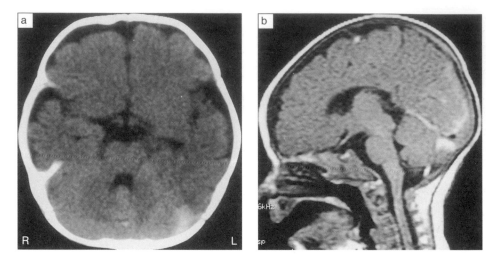

Fig. 6.19. Acute posterior fossa SDH. (a) CT demonstrating a small hyperdensity at the deep margin of the falx cerebelli and a small hyperdense collection over the posterior surface of the left cerebellar hemisphere. (b) Sagittal T_1-weighted MRI showing hyperintense SDH alongside the falx cerebelli, tentorium cerebelli and posterior surface of the occipital lobe.

SDH, approaching that of brain tissue (isodense) occurs after approximately 1 week and lasts variably until 10–14 days after the onset of the bleed (*subacute* phase). The final (*chronic*) phase is characterized thereafter by a progressive reduction of the density of blood, falling below the density of brain (hypodense). Older collections gradually take on the density of CSF, at which time they may be indistinguishable from subdural collections derived from CSF effusions of a variety of causes (subdural hygromas).

Contrary to this widely held dictum, the density of SDH in infants often increases progressively over the course of the first few days and may only reach its peak density 5–7 days post-haemorrhage. The reasons for this are probably multifactorial, including progressive clot retraction, relative hyperdensity if the adjacent brain tissue becomes ischaemic (low density), and possibly slow ongoing haemorrhage of blood with a higher haematocrit following transfusion (Fig. 6.20). Thereafter the blood gradually decreases in density, although this process may also be variable.

Acute SDH may show a heterogeneous appearance due to: (1) a pre-existing SDH; (2) actively bleeding unclotted blood mixing with organized clot; (3) a tear of the arachnoid mater allowing ingress of low density CSF mixing with subdural blood; (4) a hyperdense inner membrane associated with a pre-existing mature SDH.

The variable appearance of SDH, in the context of NAHI, is the subject of much diagnostic and forensic difficulty. Re-haemorrhage into a pre-existing subacute or chronic SDH, as a result of normal handling or trivial trauma, is often suggested. Whilst this scenario cannot be excluded, rebleeding into documented SDHs and collections of a known non-traumatic aetiology (e.g. post-surgical, post-inflammatory) or into chronic SDHs in infants who have been removed from a potentially harmful environment is uncommon. When re-

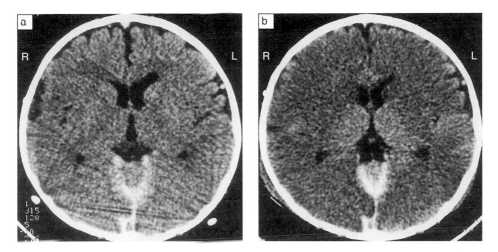

Fig. 6.20. Three-month-old infant presenting with a history of apnoea and subsequent cardiorespiratory arrest. (a) CT on admission demonstrates acute hyperdense subdural haematoma along the tentorial margin and posterior cerebral falx. (b) Repeat CT 6 days later, imaged at same window settings, demonstrates increased density of the subdural blood. Note diffuse oedema/ischaemia in both cerebral hemispheres with relative sparing of the thalami.

bleeding is seen in the context of routine follow-up scanning in infants known to have chronic SDHs of a non-inflicted cause (e.g. postoperative), fresh bleeding often occurs within the old collection. Such bleeding is not associated with any other known risk factors associated with NAHI (bruising, fractures, retinal haemorrhages, subarachnoid haemorrhage and parenchymal injuries). In addition, such re-haemorrhage into an older SDH is almost invariably asymptomatic and is not accompanied by an acute alteration of the child's neurological status unless it results in a large mass-producing collection. The latter, however, is rarely encountered.

It has become increasingly apparent that in some cases low density subdural collections may be acute in nature. In a series of 33 infants referred to a tertiary neurosurgical centre in Buffalo, New York, with a proven shaken impact syndrome, serial scanning by way of CT and MRI was undertaken (Dias et al. 1998). In one case, an initial CT scan obtained 2 hours 45 minutes following the alleged injury showed only a thin acute hyperdense SDH. A follow-up scan 17 hours later demonstrated new bilateral frontal and anterior temporal low density subdural collections described as being 'reminiscent' of chronic SDHs. In addition, in one infant an acute SDH evolved into a 'chronic' collection three days after the initial presentation scan, and in another infant the transformation occurred over seven days. This research concurs with the author's experience and may be why in some cases of infants presenting acutely there is a combination of anterior low density subdural collections and thin posterior high density SDHs. Tapping of these low density subdural collections reveals acute fresh blood in some cases (Fig. 6.21). Such a scenario may also underlie at least some of the described cases of infants presenting with a combination of

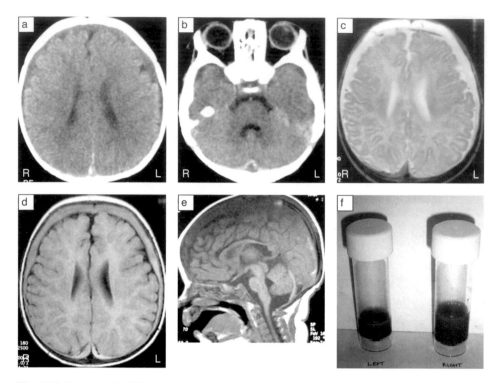

Fig. 6.21. Four-month-old baby girl allegedly hit on the head by her 2-year old brother. Admitted with vomiting, drowsiness and fitting. Bruises on the face and body were noted, along with multiple retinal haemorrhages. CT on the day of admission (a) demonstrates supratentorial low-density subdural collections over the lateral cerebral convexities anteriorly and thin high-density posterior parafalcine subdural blood, as well as acute infratentorial high-density SDH (b) alongside the falx cerebelli and related to the left tentorial leaf. Axial T_2-weighted (c), axial FLAIR (d) and sagittal T_1-weighted (e) images demonstrate subdural collections of mixed signal characteristics anteriorly and posteriorly in the supratentorial compartment and in the posterior fossa. (f) Photograph of the fluid aspirated from the anterior subdural collections via the anterior fontanelle on the same day as the CT and MRI examinations, demonstrating uniformly heavily blood-stained (red) fluid.

acute and chronic SDHs in other series (Cohen et al. 1986, Sinal and Ball 1987, Giangiacomo et al. 1988).

The forensic and medicolegal context of neuroimaging calls for caution when being asked to provide an opinion regarding the age of SDHs on the basis of their CT and MRI characteristics. The variable appearances of intracranial haemorrhage at the various stages of clot formation, maturation and resorbtion pose significant difficulties in estimating the age of the blood in such cases. When preparing medicolegal reports or witness statements, dogmatic opinions should be avoided. Wherever possible, supplementary information, be it clinical or imaging, should be sought to assist in determining the age of SDHs and correlated with the appearance or evolution of cerebral oedema and ischaemia. Additional information in the form of diagnostic or therapeutic tapping of SDHs can be crucial in this

226

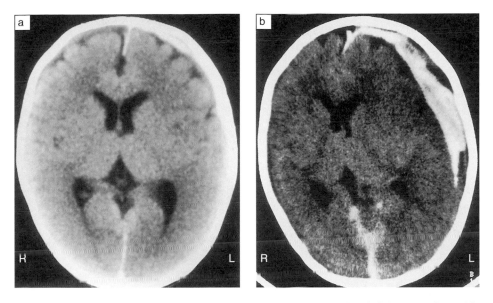

Fig. 6.22. Ten-month-old female. (a) CT on admission to the receiving hospital demonstrating a thin hyperdense subdural haematoma over the left cerebral convexity and cerebral falx. (b) CT 3 hours later (transferred to tertiary centre for deteriorating condition) shows rapid enlargement of the left-sided SDH, which is now heterogeneous with hyperacute unclotted blood appearing as a hypodense outer layer.

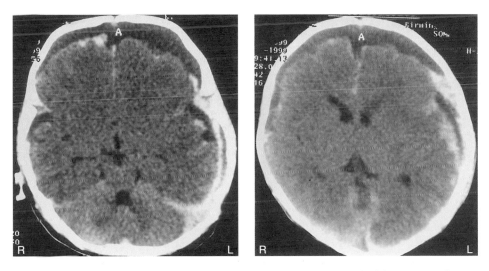

Fig. 6.23. Three-month-old infant presenting with an acute encephalopathy. Serial head circumference measurements had documented a progressive increase in the head size prior to the acute presentation. Axial CT images demonstrate thin acute SDHs in the posterior fossa. In the supratentorial compartment there are older low-density anterior SDHs containing fresh hyperdense haematoma layering out within the older collections. There is also acute subarachnoid haemorrhage and posterior parafalcine acute SDH.

227

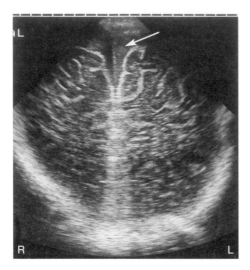

Fig. 6.24. Coronal ultrasound in a 2-month-old infant performed on the day of injury demonstrating acute hyperechogenic posterior parafalcine SDH on the left (arrow).

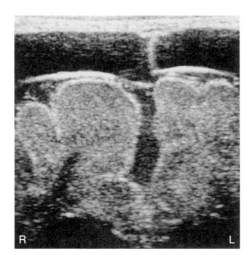

Fig. 6.25. High resolution near field coronal ultrasound of a 3-month-old infant two weeks after admission with severe acute injury. There are bilateral hypoechogenic SDHs with strongly echogenic inner membranes and prominent underlying subarachnoid spaces.

respect. A colour photograph of the aspirate should be obtained immediately after the subdural tap. It should be timed and dated, and securely placed in the clinical case records.

Heterogeneous or mixed density SDHs may represent either hyperacute evolving collections (Fig. 6.22), re-haemorrhage from a second significant and usually abusive injury (Fig. 6.23) or CSF admixture within an acute SDH. Associated clinical findings (encephalopathic presentation, anaemia, fresh or mixed age bruising, retinal haemorrhages), skeletal injuries, or scalp, skull or acute intracranial injuries may help to establish the diagnosis of re-injury. In addition acute SDHs are frequently located at sites anatomically remote from older collections and thus aetiologically consistent with a separate traumatic event.

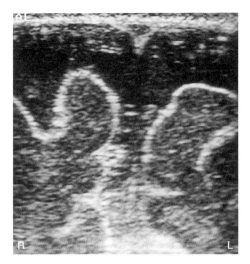

Fig. 6.26. Coronal ultrasound in a well 5-month old infant presenting with increasing head circumference measurements. There are prominent transonic subarachnoid fluid collections extending from the dural surface to the brain, widening the sulci, consistent with benign communicating hydrocephalus of infancy.

Cerebral swelling occurring after an acute injury may be of a sufficient magnitude that thin subacute or chronic SDHs may be compressed and evade detection on early CT. As the intracranial swelling subsides, the hypodense collections become evident and progressively expand on serial scanning. This may be due to evolving cerebral atrophy, cerebral shrinkage (for instance following mannitol infusion), an osmotic effect drawing in fluid, or tearing of the arachnoid mater leading to CSF ingress.

Repeated inflicted trauma may result in membrane formation within a subdural collection and layering of blood of variable density on CT. Residual intact cortical veins may be seen coursing through an older collection, often with clot adherent to the vessel.

There are relatively few reports on the value of ultrasound in the evaluation of traumatic extracerebral haematomas (Magnano et al. 1989, Jaspan 1998). Acute SDH is hyperechogenic (Fig. 6.24). Subacute and chronic SDHs are generally hypoechoic and are frequently associated with a strongly echogenic inner membrane. The surface of the brain may be flattened and compressed by larger subdural collections, the sulci becoming effaced (Fig. 6.25). These two features are helpful in distinguishing SDH from a subarachnoid effusion, a distinction that can be difficult on CT when the SDH is hypodense. In the latter case, prominent subarachnoid fluid collections extend from the calvarium down to the surface of the brain, filling and splaying the sulci (Fig. 6.26). In addition, normal vessels are easily identified on colour Doppler imaging, extending from the surface of the brain through the subarachnoid space to the superior sagittal sinus. With a large SDH, the pial vessels and bridging cortical veins are compressed and underlie the collection. Colour Doppler imaging may, however, show residual intact cortical veins passing through the collection and extending towards the superior sagittal sinus.

• *Subarachnoid haemorrhage (SAH)*. SAH is a common occurrence in NAHI, as determined by the frequent finding of blood stained CSF at lumbar puncture in acutely injured infants.

229

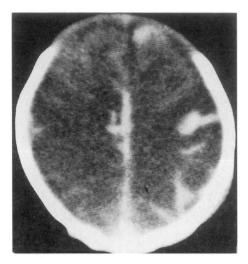

Fig. 6.27. Acute SAH alongside the cerebral falx filling the sulci. Probable haemorrhagic cortical contusions are present in the left frontal and parietal regions.

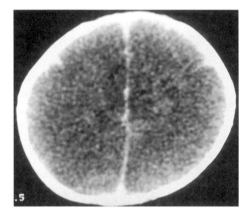

Fig. 6.28. Irregular hyperdensity along the cerebral falx in keeping with acute SAH. Further SAH over the cerebral convexities is partially obscured by the hyperdense halo adjacent to the calvarium that is common particularly with older generation scanners.

SAH is present in virtually all cases at autopsy, occurring as a thin film or in patches over the cerebral hemispheres, particularly the parasagittal convexities (Case et al. 2001).

However, detection of SAH by the various imaging modalities is variable, with a reported incidence of between 10% and 73% (Zimmerman et al. 1979, Cohen et al. 1986, Sato and Smith 1991, Cheah et al. 1994). CT readily detects acute SAH as hyperdense material smearing the surface of the brain, filling in sulci and producing a fluffy, irregular margin alongside the cerebral falx (Fig. 6.27). The frequent coexistence of SDH(s) may mask the presence of SAH. In these cases, the subarachnoid blood can be detected as delicate inter-digitating hyperdensity within the sulci lying in intimate relationship to the more linear thin streak-like hyperdensity of the typical acute parafalcine SDH. In addition, partial voluming effects from the adjacent calvarium, particularly on slices close to the vertex, may lead to difficulties in detecting a small volume of SAH on acute CT scanning (Fig. 6.28). MRI, particularly applying sequences sensitive to the detection of blood (FLAIR, T_2-weighted

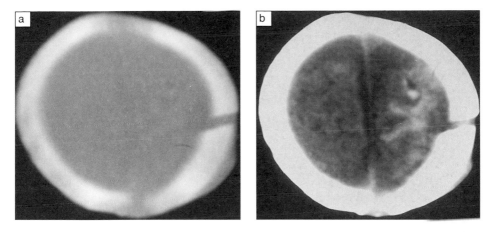

Fig. 6.29. CT in a 4-month-old infant who had suffered a severe impact-shaking trauma with extensive intracranial injuries. (a) Bone-window setting showing a 4 mm wide left parietal fracture. (b) Soft-tissue setting demonstrating an underlying (coup) haemorrhagic cortical contusion.

gradient echo), can be helpful in clarifying the precise anatomical compartment within which the surface blood lies. SAH usually resolves within a few days of injury.

Acute SAH can be difficult to identify by sonography, particularly when associated with acute SDH, which it invariably is. The SAH appears hyperechogenic with mobile particulate debris easily seen on dynamic scanning, and may be seen underlying a subdural collection of different echogenicity. As the SAH resolves, the subarachnoid fluid becomes transonic and the underlying subarachnoid space may expand.

Brain parenchyma and ventricles
Acute primary parenchymal injury can be divided into: (1) haemorrhagic or non-haemorrhagic cortical contusions; (2) subcortical shearing contusional tears; (3) diffuse axonal injury; (4) cerebral lacerations; (5) bursting lobar or hemispheric injury.

• *Cortical contusion.* A blow to the head may impart forces that lead to disruption of the surface of the brain or deeper structures. An impact injury of a magnitude sufficient to focally deform or fracture the skull and sutures may produce an injury to the underlying cerebral cortex, a *coup* injury (Fig 6.29), or remote cortical injury due to transmission of forces through the brain to a site opposite the impact point, resulting in the brain striking rigid calvarial or dural structures, a *contra coup* injury. The typical site of a major impact injury is the parieto-occipital region. Transmission of the inertial forces through the blancmange-like immature brain results in the surface of the brain impacting against the hard surface of the anterior and/or middle cranial fossa floor, accounting for the characteristic location of contra coup contusions in the midline basal and orbital regions of the frontal lobe (Fig. 6.30) and the anterior pole of the temporal lobes. Superficial cortical contusions are said to be rare in infants less than 5 months of age due to the smoothness of the inside of the

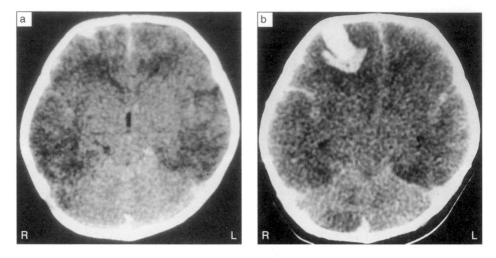

Fig. 6.30. CT in a 2-month-old infant with a right frontal contra coup haemorrhagic cortical contusion. (a) Scan 1 hour after admission demonstrating a small hyperdense cortical lesion and early parenchymal hypodensity in the temporal lobes. (b) Scan 3 hours later showing rapid evolution of the cortical contusion and global cerebral oedema. Note SAH filling the sylvian fissures and posterior fossa SDH.

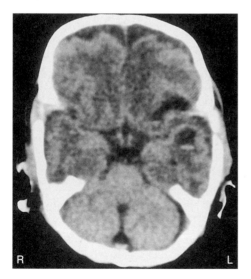

Fig. 6.31. CT in a 5-week-old infant, born preterm, showing predominantly hypodense contusions in the left frontal and temporal basal regions, with a small amount of hyperdense blood layering in the temporal lobe lesion.

skull, shifting the forces from the surface of the brain to the underlying white matter (Calder et al. 1984, Vowles et al. 1987, Hadley et al. 1989). However, in the author's experience and in other reports (Mercker et al. 1985, Sato et al. 1989), cortical contusions occur not infrequently in very young infants subjected to impact forces. These lesions have variable appearances on CT, dependent upon whether they are haemorrhagic (hyperdense) or filled with CSF or unclotted blood (hypodense) (Fig. 6.31).

232

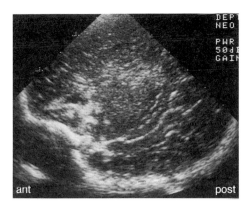

Fig. 6.32. Sagittal ultrasound demonstrating a mixed echogenicity contusion in the right frontobasal region and a small contusion in the temporal pole.

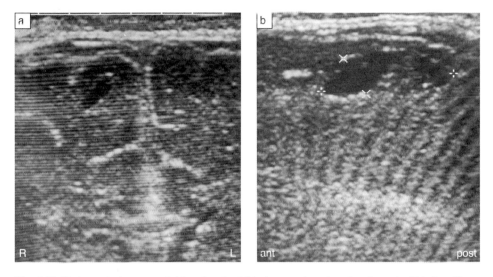

Fig. 6.33. High-resolution coronal (a) and sagittal (b) ultrasound sections in a 6-week-old infant. There is a discrete transonic cleft-like lesion at the corticomedullary junction. The sagittal image shows a small amount of echogenic blood within the lesion.

Ultrasound appearances parallel the CT findings with lesions that are predominantly either echogenic or transonic but not infrequently are of mixed echogenicity (Fig. 6.32) and occur in predictably vulnerable surfaces of the brain (Mercker et al. 1985).

• *Subcortical shearing contusional tears*. A specific pattern of injury is seen in infants involving white matter tears or clefts in the subcortical regions, first described by Lindenberg and Freytag (1969). The water content of the neonatal and early infant white matter is significantly higher (~90%) than in older infants (~70%). The junction between the compact six cell layered cortex and the subcortical white matter represents a vulnerable zone due to their differential physical properties. The shear stresses associated with shaking or blunt

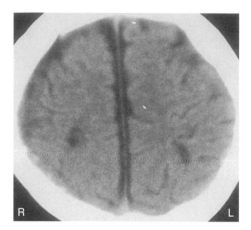

Fig. 6.34. Axial CT demonstrating symmetrical small hypodense contusional tears. The scan was performed 2 weeks after injury. There is a fracture extending through the right coronal suture and a residual thin hypodense underlying SDH.

impact result in splitting or separation at this transitional zone. The typical location of these lesions is in the frontal and parietal lobes, particularly adjacent to the midline, and the temporal lobes (Calder et al. 1984, Vowles et al. 1987, Jaspan et al. 1992). The lesions are orientated parallel to the cortical surface, are often small, and may be filled with blood or CSF (Fig. 6.33). Most are non-haemorrhagic and therefore difficult to detect by CT, although the first report of such lesions was paradoxically using this modality (Ordia et al. 1981). However, the late stage of their evolution may be detected as small discrete hypodensities (Fig. 6.34). Ultrasound has been shown to have a high sensitivity for their detection (Hausdorf and Helmke 1984, Jaspan et al. 1992). The high spatial resolution and sensitivity of certain pulse sequences to the detection of blood products in these lesions makes MRI the most useful modality in identifying contusional tears.

• *Diffuse axonal injury*. Damage to white matter due to high velocity rotational or accelera-tion–deceleration forces associated with impact or shaking results in a pattern of damage termed diffuse axonal injury (DAI). The typical sites of these lesions are the superficial and deep lobar white matter (Fig. 6.35), the corpus callosum (Fig. 6.36), basal ganglia (Fig. 6.37), internal capsule and dorsolateral brainstem. The subcortical white matter contusional tears described above probably represent a continuum of the DAI spectrum of abnormalities. The consequent damage is almost invariably coma inducing and results in a profound neurological injury. Autopsy reveals extensive axonal disruption with axonal swelling and retraction balls.

However, in a large autopsy series of infants who had succumbed to acknowledged inflicted head injury, Geddes et al. (2001) found that DAI was uncommon, occurring in only two out of 37 infants less than 1 year in age. In addition, contusional tears were also infrequently found (4/37). The authors questioned the true incidence of DAI reported in older post-mortem based research and proposed that most, if not all, of the neuronal damage seen histologically was due to hypoxia–ischaemia. The authors did, however, find evidence of focal neuronal injury involving the corticospinal tracts in the lower brainstem or upper

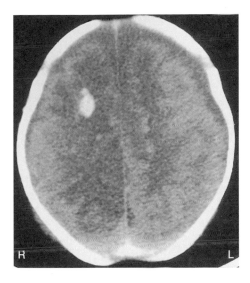

Fig. 6.35. Axial CT through the central semiovale showing a haemorrhagic lesion with a second smaller lesion immediately posteriorly. Note older hypodense anterior SDHs.

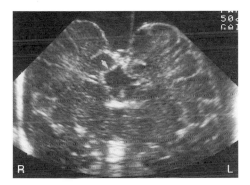

Fig. 6.36. Coronal ultrasound showing a large transonic lesion in the body of the corpus callosum (arrow). Hypoechoic subdural haematomas overlie both cerebral hemispheres.

cervical cord (11 out of 37 infants), which they ascribed to focal stretch injury. Such injury, the authors speculated, could be the cause of the global hypoxic–ischaemic injury seen in NAHI. However, of 13 cases in their series with evidence of a neck injury, nine had skull fractures and ten had severe bruising or skeletal or skull fractures present, including an infant who had sustained a ruptured liver. None of these injuries are compatible with minor levels of trauma. In contradistinction, this group appears to have suffered more severe levels of injury. It is thus counterintuitive to suggest that these infants have suffered anything other than violent or major injury. On this issue, the authors speculatively contend that "it may not be necessary to shake an infant very violently to produce stretch injury to its neuraxis".

The research undertaken by Geddes and coworkers, while being observationally important, has raised significant concerns regarding the methodology of their study and, maybe more importantly, interpretation of their data, which is addressed in Chapter 9. In the present author's experience, both contusional tears and DAI are uncommon. However, they are encountered in a not insignificant number of cases in vivo. The research by Geddes

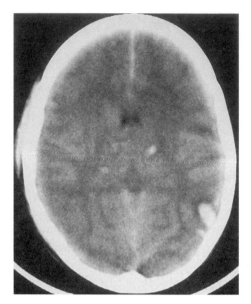

Fig. 6.37. Eight-month-old infant admitted in a comatose state. Axial CT demonstrating small haemorrhagic foci in the thalami. Note a haemorrhagic cortical contusion in the left parietal region and a thin parafalcine SDH. There is diffuse cerebral swelling, compressing the ventricles and basal cisterns.

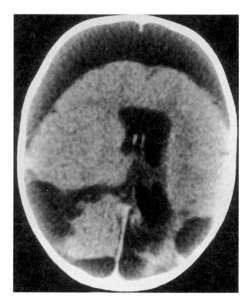

Fig. 6.38. Axial CT in an ex-preterm 6-week-old infant, undertaken two weeks after admission. There is a transparenchymal laceration in the right parietal region extending into the adjacent lateral ventricle. There are large hypodense SDHs overlying both cerebral hemispheres anteriorly and smaller loculated SDHs posteriorly. Note disruption of the septi pellucidi and medial left occipital encephalomalacia.

and her coworkers was based entirely upon post-mortem material. As only a small proportion (approximately 10%) of infants suffering trauma in the first year of life die as a result of their injuries, the authors are therefore dealing with a highly selected subset of cases of abusive head injury. In addition, in this author's experience, pre-mortem ultrasound as well as ultrasound examination of the intact fixed brain can reveal contusional injuries that were

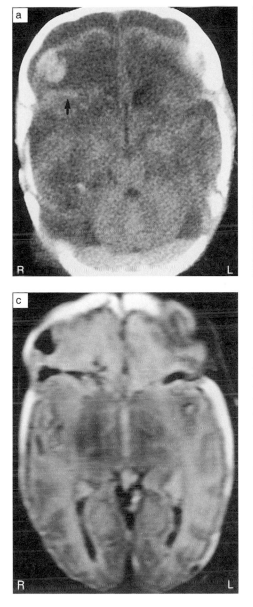

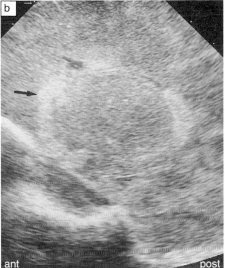

Fig. 6.39. Five-week-old ex-preterm infant admitted unconscious. Skull radiographs demonstrated multiple fractures. (a) CT scan showing a right frontal contra coup haemorrhagic contusion and an ill-defined mildly hyperdense transparenchymal lesion in the right frontal lobe (arrow). There is a posterior fossa SDH. (b) Sagittal ultrasound showing a poorly defined hyperechogenic lesion extending from the surface of the brain deep to the frontal horn of the left lateral ventricle (arrow). There is a small transonic contusional lesion in the deep white matter adjacent to the ventricle. (c) Axial T$_2$-weighted image showing the right frontal lobe cortical contusion and bilateral transcerebral lacerations extending to the frontal horns of the lateral ventricle, identified by hypointense blood. Note the presence of blood in the lateral ventricles.

undetected macroscopically by an experienced neuropathologist, and can guide the pathologist to examine the appropriate segment of the brain (Jaspan et al. 1992). Post-mortem examination of an extremely swollen brain can prove, at best, challenging to the pathologist. As a not insignificant proportion of autopsies in this group of infants are undertaken by pathologists without specific expertise in the field of paediatric pathology or neuropathology, it is likely that interpretive errors may occur.

The post-mortem interpretation of delicate parenchymal injuries can be difficult in the context of a grossly swollen brain. The decision as to whether lesions are due to post-mortem fixation artefact or pre-mortem injury has been based in some cases on the reported findings of the pre-mortem imaging. If this interpretation is incorrect, there is a real risk that the pathologist will be adversely influenced in his or her interpretation of the pathological findings.

The lesions in DAI are often small. Approximately 30% are haemorrhagic (Murray et al. 1996). CT thus often fails to detect or underestimates the extent of damage, which is best evaluated by MRI. Subarachnoid and intraventricular haemorrhage frequently accompanies DAI, which should alert the radiologist to this possibility.

• *Cerebral lacerations*. Very young infants and those born preterm appear to have a predilection to major transparenchymal lacerating injuries of the brain. These injuries occur as a consequence of impact trauma and are typically seen in the temporal and frontal lobes adjacent to the skull base. The lesions often extend from the brain surface deep to the adjacent ventricle (Fig. 6.38). The lacerations may be filled with blood (traumatic intracerebral haematomas) or CSF. Being large, cerebral lacerations are readily detected by all the major imaging modalities, although MRI undoubtedly shows the lesions to maximum advantage (Fig. 6.39). Surviving infants will demonstrate areas of cystic encephalomalacia on subsequent neuroimaging, best appreciated on MRI.

• *Bursting lobar or hemispheric injury*. Gross disruption of the brain may occur as a consequence of high velocity impact injuries to the head. Complex skull fractures are frequently associated with these injuries, which are usually life threatening. Large areas of brain are affected with disruption of the cerebral architecture, acute oedema, cerebral swelling, haemorrhagic contusions and lacerations (Fig. 6.40). Ultrasound examination reveals mixed echogenicity abnormality with loss of visualization of normal landmarks.

CT demonstrates diffuse low attenuation and swelling with patchy or larger foci of hyperdense parenchymal haemorrhage (Fig. 6.41). Herniation of brain tissue may occur through a skull vault defect. Although relatively unusual in infants, transtentorial or subfalcine herniation can occur, with secondary compromise of major cerebral arterial pedicles and brainstem injury.

Disruption of delicate subependymal veins may lead to intraventricular haemorrhage (IVH). Extension of a haemorrhagic laceration into a ventricle may also result in IVH (Fig. 6.39). The volume of IVH is often small and may be difficult to detect on CT and ultrasound. Coexisting cerebral swelling and oedema may compress the ventricles in the acute phase of the injury, masking the presence of the IVH. As the swelling subsides and the ventricles re-expand, the intraventricular blood may become apparent as a hyperdense fluid–fluid layer in the dependent occipital horns of the lateral ventricles. IVH is most sensitively detected by MRI, particularly employing a T_2* gradient echo sequence. The demonstration of IVH is forensically important insomuch as it is a marker of a major injury.

Disruption of deep structures such as the septi pellucidi may occasionally be identified following major abusive head injury (Fig. 6.38).

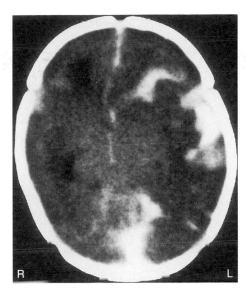

Fig. 6.40. CT obtained within 45 minutes of admission in a 2-month old ex-preterm infant found in a moribund state by his parents. There are haemorrhagic transcerebral lacerations and parenchymal haematomas, SDHs, subarachnoid haemorrhage, diffuse early post-traumatic cerebral oedema and intraventricular haemorrhage.

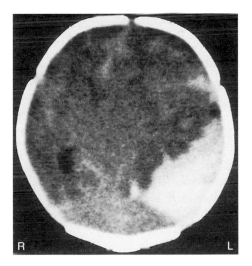

Fig. 6.41. Axial CT in a 1-month-old ex-preterm infant suffering a fatal shaking-impact injury showing a large temporo-occipital haemorrhagic lesion and diffuse cerebral oedema.

SECONDARY

Secondary injury occurs as the consequence of acute traumatic head injury. The secondary effects may affect (1) the brain, or (2) CSF pathways.

Secondary brain injury

When present, it is likely that secondary brain damage commences immediately after the primary injury with the initiation of a cascade of reactive events, probably chemically mediated metabolic derangements (Haseler et al. 1997). Physical disruption of the brain

239

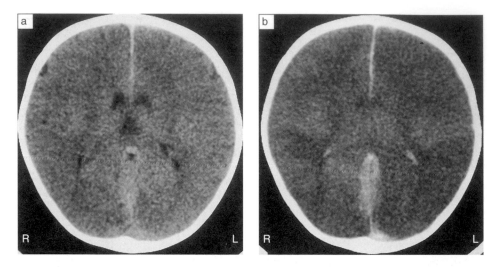

Fig. 6.42. (a) CT obtained 70 minutes after admission in a 4-month-old infant presenting with a history of prolonged apnoea requiring resuscitation by the child's carer. There is subtle but diffuse hypodensity in both cerebral hemispheres. (b) CT 6 hours later demonstrates progressive reduction in attenuation of the brain apart from an equatorial band of preserved brain density. Note compression of the ventricles and increased density of parafalcine SDH.

may play a significant role or contribute to the secondary changes. The pattern of damage seen is highly variable and may manifest different stages in the evolution or regression of brain swelling, oedema, ischaemia and infarction. The major patterns of damage are as follows.

• *Cerebral swelling and oedema.* The earliest changes that occur following acute injury are focal or global cerebral swelling and oedema, which may be coma inducing. The aetiology of this process is not fully known. Loss of cerebral vascular autoregulation, transient hyperaemia followed by hypoperfusion, vasogenic oedema, cerebral contusion and axonal injury have all been implicated. Cerebral swelling may result in early cortical vascular congestion. Although potentially reversible, there is a 50% reported incidence of mortality (Aldrich et al. 1992). The imaging correlate on CT is a subtle increase in density of the cortex. In reality, this finding is at best variable. This period may then be followed by the onset of cerebral oedema. The latter may be focal, conform to a vascular territory or territories, or be generalized in distribution.

The pattern of oedema associated with an acute unilateral compressive SDH is different from that seen with the more patchy or diffuse distribution occurring as a consequence of cerebral hypoperfusion and/or hypoxia. Early and aggressive oedema may be identified by marked hypodensity underlying the collection (Hanigan et al. 1987). The mass effect is often profound and carries a poor prognosis.

The aetiology of the early low-density change seen on CT is ill understood and probably multifactorial; discussion of it is beyond the scope of this chapter. The onset may occur within the first 1–2 hours following injury (Willman et al. 1997, Dias et al. 1998), or may

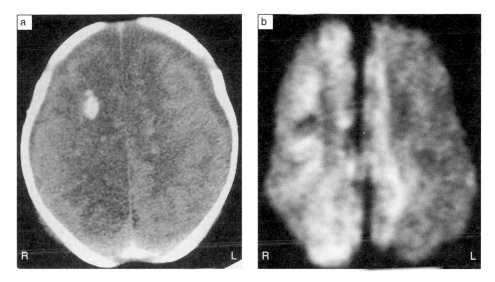

Fig. 6.43. (a) CT of a 6-month-old infant obtained 90 minutes after admission (same case as Fig. 6.33), following resuscitation. There is subtle low density in the medial right cerebral hemisphere with loss of grey–white matter differentiation. (b) Diffusion weighted image 1 hour later shows extensive high signal in both cerebral hemispheres.

be delayed for up to 24–48 hours (Kleinman 1998). The earliest manifestations are a subtle reduction of the normal density of the brain and ill-definition of the grey–white matter junction (Fig. 6.42). The oedema may be patchy and focal or diffuse. CT is often more sensitive and informative than MRI in the detection of early cerebral oedema, particularly in very young infants and in those born preterm (who normally have a high water content). Differentiation of normal brain from cerebral oedema can therefore be difficult to appreciate employing routine T_2-weighted sequences; diffusion weighted MRI may be of greater value in this respect (Fig. 6.43). Global cerebral oedema results in homogeneous low attenuation, the deep nuclear structures being equally affected. The presence of diffuse oedema carries a poor prognosis with high risk of global cerebral necrosis and death, particularly when there is accompanying cerebellar oedema (Fig. 6.44). In surviving infants, global cerebral atrophy and encephalomalacia are usual. The thalami may appear small and hyperdense secondary to microcalcifications.

Treatment, such as controlling the intracranial pressure and cooling, is aimed at maximizing the potential for recovery, although it is likely that some degree of permanent structural damage occurs in the affected areas of the brain. A tendency to involve the posterior halves of the brain has been documented (Bruce and Schut 1980, Jaspan 1998), with progression to infarction and gliosis in the affected areas. Oedema may, however, be evanescent, clearing rapidly. Timing of CT and lack of appropriate follow-up examinations may thus lead to a failure to detect these early changes in some cases.

Ultrasound may demonstrate focal or diffuse hyperechogenicity and loss of normal anatomical landmarks (Fig. 6.45). Extra-axial CSF spaces are effaced or obliterated, and

241

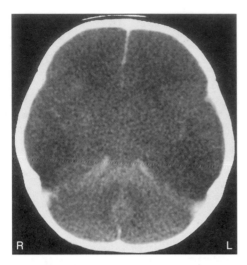

Fig. 6.44. CT in a 7-month-old infant admitted in a moribund state requiring cardiopulmonary resuscitation, obtained 80 minutes after admission. There is generalized oedema of the cerebral hemispheres including the deep grey matter. There is early low density in the right cerebellar hemisphere. Note posterior fossa and anterior parafalcine SDHs. The infant died shortly after the scan.

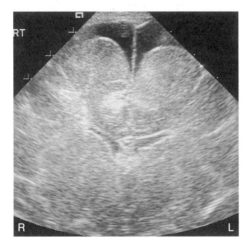

Fig. 6.45. Coronal ultrasound image in a 3-month-old infant obtained shortly after admission showing diffuse increased echogenicity of the brain indicative of oedema, compressed ventricles and poor definition of anatomical landmarks. There are low density SDHs over the cerebral convexity due to an older injury.

the ventricles are compressed and slit-like. Intracranial arterial vessel pulsations may be damped. Resistive index (RI) measurement may demonstrate an early increase, probably reflecting transient hyperaemia; however, with progressive cerebral swelling the RI falls. In more severe cases, as the cerebral perfusion pressure falls and intracranial pressure rises, the diastolic flow may progressively fall. Reversal of flow in diastole is indicative of severe irreversible brain damage incompatible with life (Fig. 6.46) (Jaspan 1998).

• *Hypoxic–ischaemic injury.* The transition from oedema to hypoxic–ischaemic injury is not clearly defined on the basis of ultrasound or CT. The underlying causes are complex. Much of the literature is notable for the interchangeable use of the terms oedema and hypoxia–ischaemia to describe the CT scan appearances arising from both processes. The

242

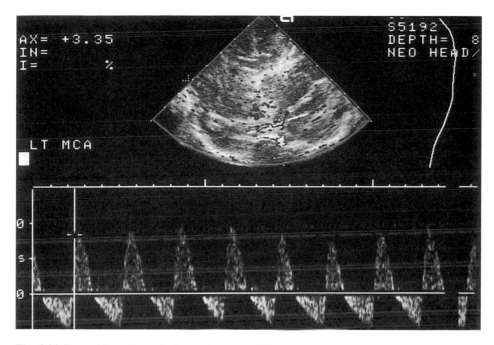

Fig. 6.46. Spectral Doppler analysis in a 2-month-old infant demonstrating reversed diastolic flow in the left middle cerebral artery. Ancillary tests confirmed brainstem death.

more seriously injured infants may sustain a period of shock, hypoventilation, hypoxia or prolonged apnoea following trauma (Johnson et al. 1995). By its nature, NAHI is usually unwitnessed and the mechanism of injury is thus often speculative in the absence of features of major impact trauma. However, a consistent theme is evident from the history provided by the carer(s) of an infant who has been subjected to severe NAHI. The infant is often described as having been apnoeic (leading to attempted resuscitation), limp, pale, unresponsive, cold or cyanosed. There is increasing speculation as to whether severe shaking may have more profound effects upon the rostral spinal cord and/or brainstem. The pivotal point during a violent shaking is located at the craniocervical junction. The proportionately large infant head swings violently backwards and forwards upon the cervical spine. The weak neck muscles in an infant provide no protection or damping of the forces generated. There is thus the potential for stretching of the craniocervical region and axonal shearing injury to these critical areas (Geddes et al. 2001). Petechial haemorrhage may be identified in the brainstem and cerebellum at post-mortem examination (Han et al. 1989). Damage to the reticular activating system and cardiac and respiratory centres may result in profound cardiorespiratory depression and coma.

Hypoxic–ischaemic injury, seen on CT as focal or diffuse low-density abnormality, evolves over time. The changes may be reversible to a greater or lesser extent. Diffuse low density of the cortex and/or white matter with preservation of or apparent mild increased attenuation of the basal ganglia, thalami and brainstem is a striking finding first described

243

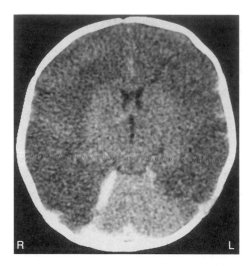

Fig. 6.47. 'Reversal sign'. There is cortical and white matter low density with preservation of normal deep grey matter attenuation. Acute SDH is present along the incisural margin and in the posterior fossa. The cerebellum retains a normal density.

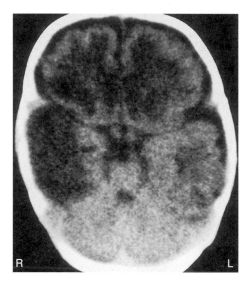

Fig. 6.48. 'White cerebellum sign'. Diffuse cerebral hypodensity contrasts with the apparently bright but normal cerebellum.

as the cerebral reversal sign by Cohen et al. (1986) and further elucidated by Han et al. (1989). Confusion has arisen around the term 'cerebral reversal sign'. This may stem from the initial description of the reversal sign as (i) a diffuse reduction of the density of the cortical grey and white matter, or (ii) reversal of the normal grey/white matter densities (the cortex being hypodense and white matter mildly hyperdense), both being accompanied by relatively increased density of the thalami, brainstem and cerebellum (Fig. 6.47). The reversal sign is associated with a poor prognosis. The preservation of the normal attenuation of the cerebellum in contrast to the hypodense cerebral hemispheres (Fig. 6.48) has also been described as the white cerebellum sign (Harwood-Nash 1992).

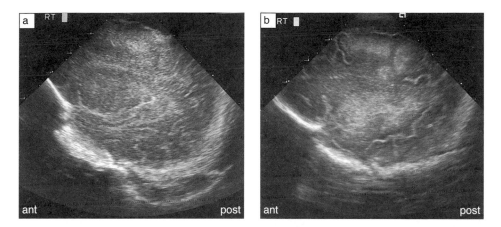

Fig. 6.49. Parasagittal ultrasound on the day of admission (a) showing subtle hyperechogenicity in the right posterior frontal white matter. (b) Follow-up examination 6 days later shows established hyperechogenic infarction.

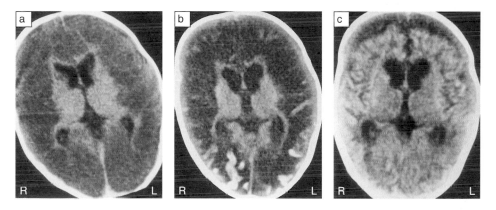

Fig. 6.50. (a) CT on the day of admission demonstrating the reversal sign. (b) CT 8 days later demonstrates mainly posterior cortical hyperdensity probably representing haemorrhagic laminar cortical infarction/ necrosis. (c) CT scan 12 days later shows resolution of the cortical hyperdensity and evolving cerebral atrophy with low density SDHs anteriorly.

Ultrasound examination may show evolution of focal or diffuse cortical or subcortical hyperechogenicity (Fig. 6.49).

• *Cerebral infarction*. Various patterns of cerebral infarction are associated with NAHI including selective neuronal necrosis with focal or widespread cortical infarction, subcortical laminar necrosis, and infarction conforming to a vascular territory or territories.

Hyperdensity may develop in the subcortical white matter 7–10 days after the acute injury. Kleinman (1998) ascribes the hyperdensity of the cortex to mineralization, particularly calcification. In the present author's experience this appearance is more suggestive of

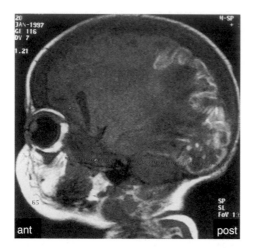

Fig. 6.51. Sagittal T_1-weighted MRI 10 days after admission showing posteriorly located gyriform cortical/subcortical hyperintensity probably representing haemorrhagic cortical necrosis/infarction.

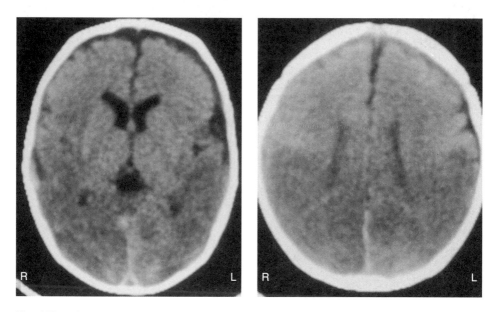

Fig. 6.52. Axial CT demonstrating posteriorly located hypoxic–ischaemic injury affecting both cerebral hemispheres, not conforming to vascular territories.

haemorrhagic transformation, as evidenced by transient hyperdensity that lasts for 1–2 weeks and then rapidly resolves (Fig. 6.50). The MRI correlate is extensive transient delicate gyriform hyperintensity on T_1-weighted images (Fig. 6.51) and hypointensity on T_2*-weighted gradient echo images. These changes have a predilection for the parietal, occipital and temporal regions but may extend into the frontal lobes. The involved areas of the brain, in general, do not conform to a specific vascular territory. The pathophysiology of this process

246

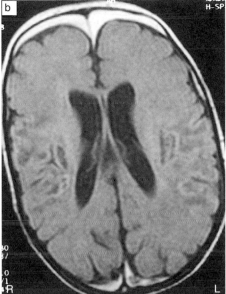

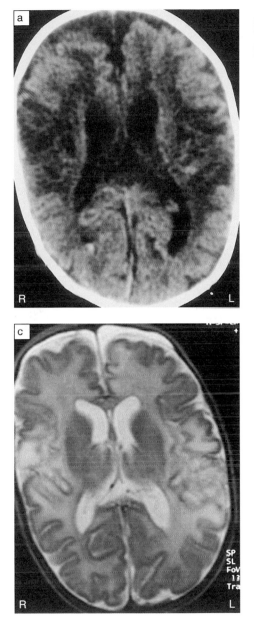

Fig. 6.53. (a) Bilateral middle cerebral artery (MCA) territory infarcts seen as low density on CT. Note blood in right lateral ventricle, and posterior parafalcine SDH. (b) Axial T_1-weighted MRI shows ill-defined hypointensity and subtle cortical hyperintensity. Note better visualization of the anterior and posterior SDHs. (c) Axial T_2-weighted MRI shows the bilateral MCA infarction as symmetrical hyperintense abnormality with loss of the normal hypointense cortical ribbon.

remains uncertain. While the subcortical white matter may represent a vulnerable watershed territory, the predominantly posterior involvement of the brain may indicate other mechanisms as yet to be determined.

A tendency for infarction of the posterior halves of the cerebral hemispheres has been noted, extending beyond the territories of any one major cerebral artery (Fig. 6.52). Infarction

247

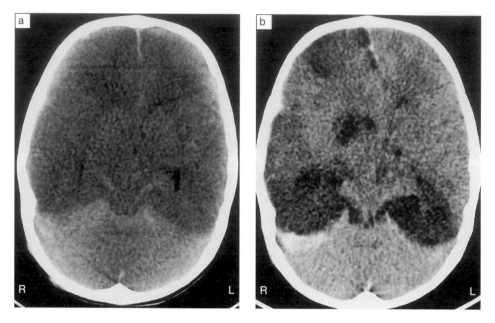

Fig. 6.54. (a) CT of a 4-month-old infant obtained on the day of admission demonstrating acute global cerebral oedema with obliteration of the basal cisterns and compression of the ventricles. (b) Repeat examination 3 days later shows infarction in the posterior cerebral artery territories posteriorly, the right thalamo-capsular region and a right frontal lobe infarct conforming to the anterior cerebral artery territory.

occurring within a vascular territory may result, however, from damage to a major vessel, such as dissection or compression of the common carotid artery in the neck by strangulation (Fig. 6.53), dissection of an intracranial major vessel, embolic occlusion of a vessel consequent upon extracranial arterial trauma or vascular compression secondary to intracranial herniation. This last typically occurs in the territory of the posterior cerebral artery, the vessel being compressed against the incisural margin following transtentorial herniation (Fig. 6.54). Subfalcine herniation may lead to compression of the anterior cerebral artery producing parasagittal infarction.

The late consequences of widespread cortical infarction or subcortical laminar necrosis are gliosis, encephalomalacia and atrophy.

CSF pathway abnormalities
Traumatic subarachnoid haemorrhage, disruption of cortical veins and dural venous sinuses, and intraventricular haemorrhage may individually or in combination lead to impaired CSF circulation and absorption (Orrison et al. 1978, Kapila et al. 1982). Progressive expansion of the subarachnoid spaces and enlargement of the ventricular system not infrequently follows acute intracranial injury. However, the distinction between hydrocephalus secondary to CSF resorption block and cerebral atrophy may be difficult. In addition, the two processes may occur concurrently leading to further diagnostic difficulties. Serial head circumference

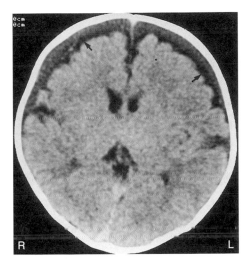

Fig. 6.55. Axial CT demonstrating mildly hypo-dense anterior SDHs and underlying subarachnoid fluid of CSF density (arrows).

measurements are essential for the interpretation of abnormalities of the ventricular system and extra-axial spaces. Clinicians should be educated in the need for recording such data on the request form for cranial imaging.

High resolution ultrasound is well suited to assess extra-axial spaces and abnormal fluid collections in the young infant. Prominence of the subarachnoid fluid space separated from hypoechoic subdural haematoma by an echogenic membrane, often coupled with mild ventricular enlargement, is one of the hallmark features of post-traumatic communicating hydrocephalus (see Fig. 6.26).

Similar appearances may be seen with CT with low density subarachnoid fluid under-lying subdural collections (Fig. 6.55). The ease of identification of these subarachnoid effusions is heavily dependent upon the age, size and appearance of the overlying SDH. Chronic low density post-traumatic subdural collections may exhibit attenuation values very similar to CSF, from which they may be indistinguishable. Differentiating features include visualization of the CSF filling and widening the sulci over the cerebral hemispheres, unlike chronic SDHs that tend to flatten the sulci and surface of the brain.

As with benign communicating hydrocephalus of infancy (external hydrocephalus), post-traumatic hydrocephalus tends to follow a self-limiting course. The hydrocephalus may, however, progress to the extent that external CSF drainage is required.

CHRONIC

The late or tertiary effects arising from NAHI can be detected by scanning only after a suitable interval, ideally at least three months after the primary injury. Due to the continued growth and maturation of the brain and skull, a more complete evaluation may be possible only later in childhood. The major sequelae are (i) atrophy, (ii) encephalomalacia, (iii) hydro-cephalus, (iv) chronic SDH, (v) growing fracture (leptomeningeal cyst), (vi) calcification, and (vii) skull deformity.

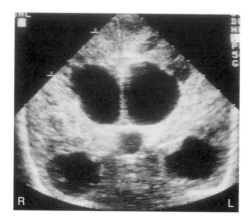

Fig. 6.56. Coronal ultrasound in a 3-month-old infant 2 weeks after an asphyxial injury, showing diffuse hyperechogenicity of the cortex and white matter indicative of gliosis/infarction. There is some early cystic change in the deep left periventricular white matter.

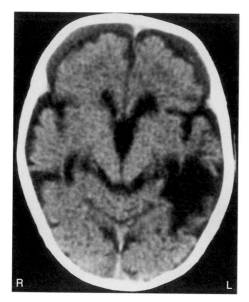

Fig. 6.57. Focal encephalomalacia in the left temporal lobe at a site of a previous cortical contusion. Note evolving cerebral atrophy.

Atrophy

Atrophy represents the common endpoint of loss of brain substance due to destruction by a variety of causes (infarction, contusion, diffuse axonal injury). The pattern of atrophy may be focal or generalized, dependent upon the cause of the brain damage (Tsai et al. 1980). Loss of cerebral volume results in widening of cortical sulci, basal cisterns and focal expansion of an adjacent part(s) of the ventricular system filling the space created by the deficient cerebral tissue (so-called ex-vacuo ventricular dilatation). Gliosis and encephalomalacia frequently accompany atrophy, which can be well seen on ultrasound (Fig. 6.56).

Damage to the corticospinal tracts results in neuronal atrophy, evident as loss of deep white matter and hypoplasia of the brainstem (Wallerian degeneration). Global cerebral atrophy

250

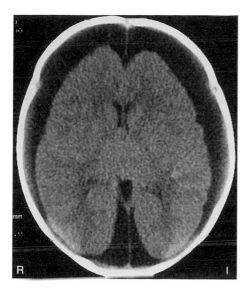

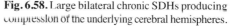
Fig. 6.58. Large bilateral chronic SDHs producing compression of the underlying cerebral hemispheres.

leads to decelerating brain growth. As the skull grows under the stimulation of growth of the underlying brain, the end-stage consequence in severe cases may be microcephaly. Predominantly unilateral damage may produce hemicranial failure of growth.

Encephalomalacia
Focal destruction of brain tissue may result in a discreet area of low (CSF) density on CT (Fig. 6.57) or a transonic cavity on ultrasound. Such lesions are particularly associated with large areas of lobar haemorrhagic contusion or disruption.

Hydrocephalus
As described above, CSF absorption may be disrupted following acute trauma. This may be secondary to SAH impairing the function of the arachnoid (pacchonian) granulations, basal cistern adhesions and inflammatory change. Less commonly, intraventricular clot may obstruct the cerebral aqueduct. Communicating hydrocephalus is frequently transient; however, it may lead to persisting ventricular dilatation. Long-standing hydrocephalus is more likely to be the result of a combination of impaired CSF absorption and basal cisternal obstruction.

Chronic SDH
Large chronic SDHs may be the first manifestation of NAHI, presenting as macrocephaly and non-specific systemic or neurological signs and symptoms (Fig. 6.58). In children who have suffered an acute injury leading to admission, serial scanning may demonstrate progressive enlargement of initially small SDHs. Large SDHs can pose major management problems, requiring decompression by either repeated transfontanellar tapping or, in more resistant cases, external drainage (subduro-peritoneal shunting). The subdural collections

251

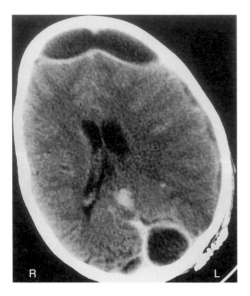

Fig. 6.59. Enhanced axial CT demonstrating secondary infection of bilateral SDHs, which required frequent tapping. There is strong enhancement of the inner membranes of the loculated SDHs.

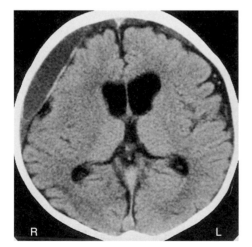

Fig. 6.60. Axial CT showing a loculated right-sided chronic SDH with a thickened inner membrane. There is mild ventricular dilatation and widening of the subarachnoid spaces secondary to communicating hydrocephalus (enlarging head circumference recorded on serial measurements).

may become secondarily infected (Fig. 6.59), thick walled and encapsulated (Fig. 6.60), or calcified.

End-stage brain damage may produce large subdural collections, which fill the vacuum left by the loss of brain substance. In such cases there may be little or no enlargement of the head circumference (Fig. 6.61).

Growing fracture (leptomeningeal cyst)
Complex or diastatic skull fractures have a greater propensity for tearing of the dura at the time of injury, particularly with fractures >3 mm in width. Protrusion of arachnoid and CSF

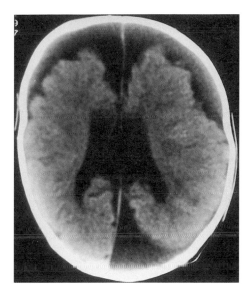

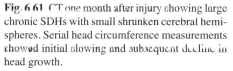

Fig. 6.61 CT one month after injury showing large chronic SDHs with small shrunken cerebral hemispheres. Serial head circumference measurements showed initial slowing and subsequent decline in head growth.

and, in more severe cases, brain tissue, through the defect allows transmission of continuous brain and CSF pulsations. In this way healing of the fracture margins is inhibited with gradual 'growth' of the fracture and development of a post-traumatic leptomeningeal cyst or encephalocele in the defect (Gugliantini et al. 1980, Muhonen et al. 1995). The underlying brain is frequently atrophic and may be tethered to the fracture site (Fig. 6.62). In rare instances, the brain may herniate through a defect in a subdural haematoma membrane (Ceccherini and Jaspan 1999).

Calcification
Dystrophic calcification may develop in areas of brain damage, either at the site of primary haemorrhagic brain injury or at sites of hypoxic–ischaemic injury.

Skull deformity
Severe brain damage resulting in failure of brain growth may, as stated above, result in microcephaly due to the loss of stimulation for calvarial bone growth. Extensive unilateral brain damage may similarly result in asymmetric brain growth and a small hemicranium. Fractures involving sutures may also result in impaired, premature or asymmetric sutural fusion with consequent local areas of skull deformity. Deeply depressed or incompletely elevated fractures may also produce focal defects or step-like irregularity of the skull. Growing skull fractures have been discussed above.

Pitfalls of imaging
Drawbacks to ultrasound examination include the following:
• age dependent – spatial resolution is increasingly poor beyond 6 months of age
• highly dependent on size of anterior fontanelle

253

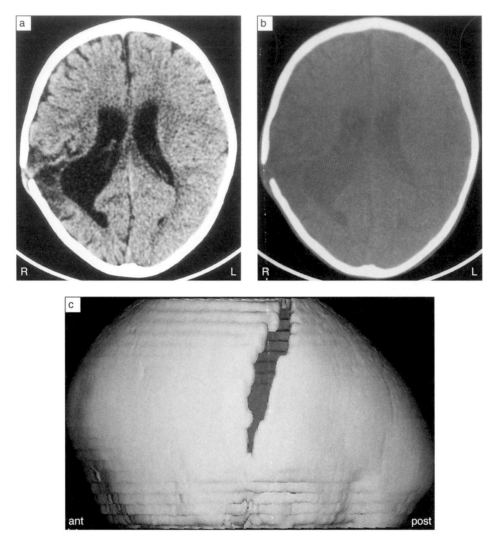

Fig. 6.62. Growing fracture (leptomeningeal cyst). Axial CT scan (a) demonstrating encephalomalacia in the right parietal lobe associated with a wide fracture seen on bone window settings (b). Surface reconstructed image (c) clearly demonstrates the wide parietal fracture.

- highly operator and machine dependent
- the recording medium is variable; poor quality of reproduction especially on paper
- images are not easily comparable as slice orientation is at the operator's discretion
- relatively insensitive to subarachnoid haemorrhage compared with CT/MRI
- blind spots, particularly high lateral cerebral convexities and the posterior fossa
- less easily understood by non-specialists, especially non-medical personnel, such as the legal community.

254

Drawbacks of computed tomography include:

- artefacts, particularly 'beam hardening' in the posterior fossa and 'partial voluming' adjacent to the calvarium
- relatively poor sensitivity to posterior fossa and upper cervical extra-axial haematomas compared with MRI
- anatomical compartments and localization not as well appreciated as by MRI
- relative insensitivity to small non-haemorrhagic parenchymal injuries compared with ultrasound and MRI
- relative insensitivity to very early ischaemia compared with diffusion weighted MRI
- radiation dose not insignificant, especially if numerous follow up investigations are required.

Differential diagnosis

SUBDURAL HAEMATOMA

The primary differential diagnosis centres upon the issue of causation of SDHs. The causes of SDH in infants have been summarized by Kemp (2002) as follows:

- intentional injury
- non-intentional injury
- neurosurgical complications
- perinatal – in utero causes, traumatic labour
- cranial malformation – aneurysms, arachnoid cyst
- cerebral infections – meningitis
- coagulation and haematological disorders – leukaemia, sickle cell anaemia, disseminated intravascular coagulation, haemophilia, Von Willibrand's disease, haemorrhagic disease of the newborn, idiopathic thrombocytopaenic purpura
- metabolic disorders – glutaric aciduria type 1, galactosaemia
- biochemical disorders – hypernatraemia

This list is not exhaustive; there are many other rare causes of SDH in infants. There are few medical conditions that fully mimic all the features of NAHI. However, all reasonable alternative causes of SDH should be considered in every case. An open mind should be given when posed with the problem of an infant found to have an SDH on neuroimaging. However, the speculative inclusion of vanishingly rare conditions (e.g. vitamin C deficiency) by some experts in an adversarial medicolegal context results in wastage of time and resources for the legal system and should be deprecated. It must always be borne in mind that the role of the expert is first and foremost to consider the well being of the infant. Whilst every effort should be made to exclude alternative pathology, it should always be remembered that trauma is by far the commonest cause of SDH in infants.

In the context of traumatic SDH, it is worth noting that SDH is uncommon following verifiable accidental head trauma, and is much more common following NAI (Billmire and Myers 1985, Dashti et al. 1999, Ewing-Cobbs et al. 2000).

Many of the alternative causes of SDH can be excluded by routine biochemical, haematological and metabolic analysis of samples of the appropriate biological material. In addition, some of these conditions are associated with highly characteristic findings on neuroimaging that clearly indicate the cause of the SDH. For instance, the rare SDHs that occur in glutaric aciduria type 1 are always accompanied by characteristic imaging findings of this condition, such as frontotemporal atrophy and expanded CSF spaces, and striatal and white matter lesions (Morris et al. 1999).

The possibility of a coagulation disorder as a cause of SDHs is frequently raised in cases of suspected NAHI. It should be noted, however, that even in children with coagulopathies, intracranial haemorrhage is very unusual following head trauma. In a group of 123 children with congenital coagulopathies studied by Dietrich et al. (1994), all of whom had sustained a head injury including falls from heights, simple falls at play and during rough play, only two were demonstrated to have SDHs. In one of these cases, the infant had sustained a skull fracture following a fall down five stairs; the other infant had sustained intracranial bleeding including SDH following a traumatic birth.

Birth related trauma is a particularly difficult issue when considering SDH in the neonate. Recent research has demonstrated that the incidence of SDH following normal vaginal delivery is very low (Whitby et al. 2004). While SDHs do occur following difficult deliveries, particularly when associated with the use of mechanical extraction devices such as forceps or ventouse suction caps, most such SDHs are thin and clear completely by 4 weeks. As some infants present acutely within the first month of life following discharge from the maternity unit setting, the finding of an SDH in these children needs to be interpreted with caution. The possibility that the bleeding dated back to birth should be considered in all cases, and it may indeed be impossible to differentiate birth trauma from other non-birth-related postnatal causes on imaging grounds. In this scenario, the clinical presentation and additional neuroimaging findings such as primary or secondary brain damage may assist in determining the causation and timing of the SDHs.

BRAIN INJURY

Hypoxic–ischaemic brain injury may occur in association with infection (viral or overwhelming bacterial infection), metabolic disorders (e.g. mitochondrial cytopathies, Alpers disease), intentional or unintentional asphyxiation, and strangulation, drowning or drug-induced coma. The absence of intracranial haemorrhage, specifically SDH, and the appropriate clinical and laboratory findings will usually indicate the underlying cause.

Gastro-oesophageal reflux and laryngospasm associated with aspiration of milk or stomach contents have recently been propounded in the context of criminal proceedings as the cause of hypoxic–ischaemic injury leading to subsequent intracranial and retinal haemorrhages. Elevation of the cerebral venous pressure has been proposed as the aetiological agent resulting in hypoxic brain injury, subdural haemorrhage and retinal haemorrhages.

In a review of 50 paediatric cases aged up to 5 months (including 17 intrauterine deaths and three spontaneous abortions), Geddes et al. (2003) observed intradural haemorrhage in 36 cases. However, in only one case in their series was there evidence of macroscopic SDH, that being a 25-week-old fetus which died from severe sepsis and disseminated intravascular coagulation. Severe hypoxia was present in 27 of these 36 cases. Based on this study and their earlier research, Geddes and her colleagues hypothesize that severe brain swelling with venous congestion produces widespread 'oozing' from leaky hypoxic dural

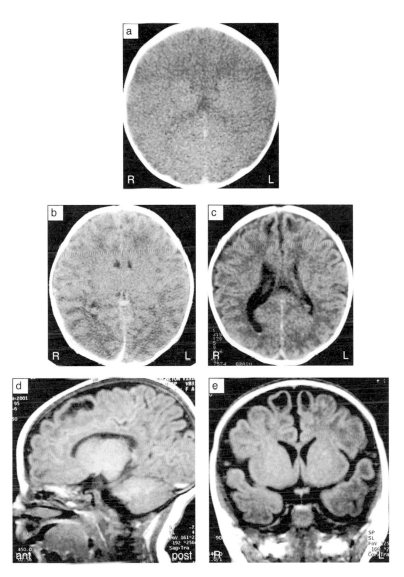

Fig. 6.63. SIDS versus NAHI. (a) Three-month-old male infant admitted immediately following an acute life-threatening event at home. No physical stigmata of injury or evidence of retinal haemorrhage were identified on admission to hospital. Axial CT scan undertaken 90 minutes following admission shows global hypodense, swollen brain but no SDH. The baby was declared dead shortly afterwards. No intracranial haemorrhage, ocular or skeletal abnormalities were identified at autopsy.

(b) Three-month-old male infant admitted following an unexplained collapse at home. Extensive bilateral retinal haemorrhages, facial and body bruising, and rib and metaphyseal limb fractures were found. Axial CT scan 2 hours after admission shows acute parafalcine and convexity SDH, early cerebral oedema and subtle frontal shearing contusions. Axial CT 9 days later (c) shows maturing frontal parasagittal contusions, residual thin posterior parafalcine SDH, a small amount of intraventricular haemorrhage and developing atrophy. Sagittal (d) and coronal (e) T_1-weighted MR images show the mature frontal contusional tears. The father admitted to subjecting the baby to severe shaking.

257

veins, possibly with a contribution from similarly leaky bridging veins, which would account for the thin film of subdural blood seen in NAHI. It should be noted, however, that none of these 50 cases shared the causative or clinical features of traumatically injured neonates and infants.

Geddes et al. also make the assumption that "Most infants with inflicted head injury have severe hypoxic brain damage and rapidly develop grossly raised ICP from secondary brain damage." However, the majority of infants who survive inflicted trauma do not have severe brain swelling or evidence of grossly elevated ICP. The typical presentation is that of an infant with thin posterior parasagittal SDHs, retinal haemorrhages and little or no evidence of brain oedema or hypoxic brain damage on either early or late cross-sectional brain imaging. In those infants who do develop brain swelling and hypoxic–ischaemic brain damage, the volume of SDH is frequently similar to that seen in those who do not, and the amount of SDH does not increase on serial scanning.

In contradistinction, sudden infant death syndrome (SIDS) is not associated with the typical imaging appearances seen in NAHI: subdural and retinal haemorrhages are rarely seen in SIDS cases (Fig. 6.63). Autopsy alone often cannot differentiate SIDS from acute asphyxiation (Kairys 2002). Asphyxiation involves an acute, global, and by definition severe hypoxic insult to the brain, and is the underlying process proposed by Geddes et al. as the cause of subdural and retinal haemorrhages. The model employed by the Geddes group to explain the cause of SDH in NAHI requires further critical analysis. The conclusions drawn by those authors bear little relationship to the experience of radiologists and clinicians dealing with the large majority of infants who survive both intentional and non-intentional head injury.

Conclusion

Appropriately targeted and timely imaging plays a vital role in the assessment and management of craniocerebral NAHI. The potential risks of failing to consider the diagnosis may be profound, particularly in those infants who survive a first or sentinel episode of abuse and go on to suffer serial abuse. The radiologist must play a full and active role in the diagnostic process. A heightened level of awareness of the possibility of child abuse is necessary in view of the protean clinical and radiological manifestations of NAHI. Some of the injuries sustained are subtle, particularly in the very acute phase. The need for a standardized protocol to evaluate NAHI is emphasized, as is the dynamic nature of any secondary brain injury. Cranial CT clearly has a pivotal role in this process. In combination with the newer MR techniques, it is hoped that some of the more complex patterns of injury encountered will be better understood and therapeutic interventions developed to assist in the management of these unfortunate children.

REFERENCES

Aldrich EF, Eisenberg HM, Saydjari C, Luerssen TG, Loulkes MA, Jane JA, Marshall LF, Marmarou A, Young HF (1992) Diffuse brain swelling in severely head injured children. *J Neurosurg* **76**: 450–454.
Alexander R, Crabbe L, Sato Y, Smith W, Bennett T (1990) Serial abuse in children who are shaken. *Am J Dis Child* **144**: 58–60.
Billmire ME, Myers PA (1985) Serious head injury in infants: accident or abuse? *Pediatrics* **75**: 340–342.

Bonnier C, Nassogne MC, Evrard P (1995) Outcome and prognosis of whiplash shaken infant syndrome: late consequences after a symptom-free interval. *Dev Med Child Neurol* **37**: 943–956.

Brown JK, Minns RA (1993) Non-accidental head injury, with particular reference to whiplash shaking injury and medico-legal aspects. *Dev Med Child Neurol* **35**: 849–869.

Bruce DA, Schut L (1980) The value of CAT scanning following pediatric head injury. *Clin Pediatr* **19**: 719–725.

Cheah IG, Kasim MS, Shafie HM, Khoo TH (1994) Intracranial haemorrhage and child abuse. *Ann Trop Paediatr* **14**: 325–328.

Caffey J (1974) The whiplash shaken infant syndrome: manual shaking by the extremities with whiplash-induced intracranial and intraocular bleedings, linked with residual permanent brain damage and mental retardation. *Pediatrics* **54**: 396–403.

Calder IM, Hill I, Scholtz CL (1984) Primary brain trauma in non-accidental injury. *J Clin Pathol* **37**: 1095–1100.

Case ME, Graham MA, Handy TC, Jentzen JM, Monteleone JA; National Association of Medical Examiners Ad Hoc Committee on Shaken Baby Syndrome (2001) 'Position paper on fatal head injuries in infants and young children. *Am J Forensic Med Pathol* **22**: 112–122.

Ceccherini AF, Jaspan T (1999) Cerebral herniation through a subdural membrane defect following non-accidental injury. *Clin Radiol* **54**: 550–552.

Cohen RA, Kaufman RA, Myers PA, Towbin RB (1986) Cranial computed tomography in the abused child with head injury. *AJNR* **6**: 883–888.

Dashti SR, Decker D, Razzaq A, Cohen AR (1999) Current patterns of inflicted head injury in children. *Pediatr Neurosurg* **31**: 302–306.

Dias MS, Backstrom J, Falk M, Li V (1998) Serial radiography in the infant shaken impact syndrome. *Pediatr Neurosurg* **29**: 77–85.

Dietrich AM, James CD, King DR, Ginn-Pease ME, Cecalupo AJ (1994) Head trauma in children with congenital coagulation disorders. *J Pediatr Surg* **29**: 28–32.

Duhaime AC, Gennarelli TA, Thibault LE, Bruce DA, Margulies SS, Wiser R (1987) The shaken baby syndrome: a clinical, pathological, and biomechanical study. *J Neurosurg* **66**: 409–415

Ewing-Cobbs L, Prasad M, Kramer L, Louis PT, Baumgartner J, Fletcher JM, Alpert B (2000) Acute neuro radiological findings in young children with inflicted or non-inflicted traumatic brain injury. *Child's Nerv Syst* **16**: 25–34.

Geddes JF, Vowles GH, Hackshaw AK, Nickols CD, Scott IS, Whitwell HL (2001) Neuropathology of inflicted head injury in children. II. Microscopic brain injury in infants. *Brain* **124**: 1299–1306.

Geddes JF, Tasker RC, Hackshaw AK, Nickols CD, Adams GGW, Whitwell HL, Scheimberg I (2003) Dural haemorrhage in non-traumatic infant deaths: does it explain the bleeding in 'shaken baby syndrome'? *Neuropathol Appl Neurobiol* **29**: 14–22. [Erratum in: *Neuropathol Appl Neurobiol* 2003 **29**: 322.]

Giangiacomo J, Khan JA, Levine C, Thompson VM (1988) Sequential cranial computed tomography in infants with retinal hemorrhages. *Ophthalmology* **59**: 295–299.

Gilles EE, Nelson MD (1998) Cerebral complications of nonaccidental head injury in childhood. *Pediatr Neurol* **19**: 119–128.

Gilliland MG (1998) Interval duration between injury and severe symptoms in nonaccidental head trauma in infants and young children. *J Forensic Sci* **43**: 723–725.

Gugliantini P, Caione P, Fariello G, Rivosecchi M (1980) Posttraumatic leptomeningeal cysts in infancy. *Pediatr Radiol* **9**: 11–14.

Hadley MN, Sonntag VK, Rekate HL, Murphy A (1989) The infant whiplash-shake injury syndrome: a clinical and pathological study. *Neurosurgery* **24**: 536–540.

Hall P, Adami H-O, Trichopoulos D, Pedersen NL, Lagiou P, Ekbom A, Ingvar M, Lundell M, Granath F (2004) Effect of low doses of ionising radiation in infancy on cognitive function in adulthood: Swedish population based cohort study. *BMJ* **328**: 19–21.

Han BK, Towbin RB, De Courten-Myers G, McLaurin RL, Ball WS (1989) Reversal sign on CT: Effect of anoxic/ischaemic cerebral injury in children. *AJNR* **10**: 1191–1197.

Hanigan WC, Peterson RA, Njus G (1987) Tin ear syndrome: rotational acceleration in pediatric head injuries. *Pediatrics* **80**: 616–622.

Harwood-Nash DC (1992) Abuse to the pediatric central nervous system. *AJNR* **13**: 569–575.

Haseler LJ, Arcinue E, Danielsen ER, Bluml S, Ross BD (1997) Evidence from proton magnetic resonance spectroscopy for a metabolic cascade of neuronal damage in shaken baby syndrome. *Pediatrics* **99**: 4–14.

Hausdorf G, Heimke K (1984) Sonographic demonstration of contusional white matter clefts in an infant. *Neuropediatrics* **15**: 110–112.

Hobbs CJ (1984) Skull fracture and the diagnosis of abuse. *Arch Dis Child* **59**: 246–252.

Jaspan T (1998) Cranial ultrasound in non-accidental injury. *Br Med Ultrasound Bull* **6**: 29–38.

Jaspan T, Narborough G, Punt JAG, Lowe J (1992) Cerebral contusional tears as a marker of child abuse – detection by cranial sonography. *Paediatr Radiol* **22**, 237–245.

Jaspan T, Griffiths PD, McConachie NS, Punt JA (2003) Neuroimaging for non-accidental head injury in childhood: a proposed protocol. *Clin Radiol* **58**: 44–53.

Jenny C, Hymel KP, Ritzen A, Reinert SE, Hay TC (1999) Analysis of missed cases of abusive head trauma. *JAMA* **281**: 621–626.

Johnson DL, Boal D, Baule R (1995) Role of apnea in nonaccidental head injury. *Pediatr Neurosurg* **23**: 305–310.

Kairys S (2002) Distinguishing sudden infant death syndrome from child abuse fatalities. *Ann Emerg Med* **40**: 126–127.

Kapila A, Trice J, Spies WG, Siegel BA, Gado MH (1982) Enlarged cerebrospinal fluid spaces in infants with subdural hematomas. *Radiology* **142**: 669–672.

Karellas A, Raptopoulos V (1980) Imaging technologies: physical principles and radiation safety considerations. In: Kleinman PK, editor. *Diagnostic Imaging of Child Abuse*. St Louis: Mosby, p 392–401.

Kemp AM (2002) Investigating subdural haemorrhage in infants. *Arch Dis Child* **86**: 98–102.

Kleinman PK (1998) Head trauma. In: Kleinman PK, editor. *Diagnostic Imaging of Child Abuse*. St Louis: Mosby, p 285–342.

Lindenberg R, Freytag E (1969) Morphology of brain lesions from blunt trauma in early infancy. *Arch Pathol* **87**: 298–305.

Loder RT, Bookout C (1991) Fracture patterns in battered children. *J Orthop Trauma* **5**, 428–433.

Magnano GM, Dell'Acqua A, Taccone A, Toma P (1989) [Ultrasonics in the study of periencephalic post-traumatic effusions in the newborn and suckling infants.] *Radiol Med* **78**: 492–495 [Italian].

Mercker JM, Blumhagen JD, Brewer DK (1985) Sonography of a hemorrhagic cerebral contusion. *AJNR* **6**: 115–116.

Merten DF, Osborne DR, Radkowski MA, Leonidas JC (1984) Craniocerebral trauma in the child abuse syndrome: radiological observations. *Pediatr Radiol* **14**: 272–277.

Morris AAM, Hoffman GF, Naughten ER, Monavari AA, Collins JE, Leonard JV (1999) Glutaric aciduria and suspected child abuse. *Arch Dis Child* **80**: 404–405.

Muhonen MG, Piper JG, Menezes AH (1995) Pathogenesis and treatment of growing skull fractures. *Surg Neurol* **43**: 367–373.

Murray JG, Gean AD, Evans SJ (1996) Imaging of acute head injury. *Semin Ultrasound CT MR* **17**: 185–205.

New PF, Aronow S (1976) Attenuation measurements of whole blood and blood fractions in computed tomography. *Radiology* **121**: 635–640.

O'Neill JA, Meacham WF, Griffin JP, Sawyers JL (1973) Patterns of injury in the battered child syndrome. *J Trauma* **13**: 332–339.

Ordia IJ, Strand R, Giles F, Welch K (1981) Computerized tomography of contusional clefts in the white matter in infants. Report of two cases. *J Neurosurg* **54**: 696–698.

Orrison WW, Robertson WC, Sackett JF (1978) Computerized tomography in chronic subdural hematomas (effusions) of infancy. *Neuroradiology* **16**: 79–81.

Rubin DM, Christian CW, Bilaniuk LT, Zazyczny KA, Durbin DR (2003) Occult head injury in high-risk abused children. *Pediatrics* **111**: 1382–1386.

Sato Y, Smith WL (1994) Head injury in child abuse. *Neuroimaging Clin N Am* **1**: 475–491.

Sato Y, Yuh WT, Smith WL, Alexander RC, Kao SC, Ellerbroek CJ (1989) Head injury in child abuse: evaluation with MR imaging. *Radiology* **173**: 653–657.

Schachenmayr W, Friede RL (1978) The origin of subdural neomembranes. I. Fine structure of the dura–arachnoid interface in man. *Am J Pathol* **92**: 53–68.

Scotti G, Terbrugge K, Melancon D, Belanger G (1977) Evaluation of the age of subdural hematomas by computerized tomography. *J Neurosurg* **47**: 311–315.

Sinal SH, Ball MR (1987) Head trauma due to child abuse: serial computerized tomography in diagnosis and management. *South Med J* **80**: 1505–1512.

Svendsen P (1976) Computer tomography of traumatic extracerebral lesions. *Br J Radiol* **49**: 1004–1012.

Tsai FY, Zee C-S, Apthorp JS, Dixon GH (1980) Computed tomography in child abuse head trauma. *J Comput Tomogr* **4**: 277–286.

Willman KY, Bank DE, Senac M, Chadwick DL (1997) Restricting the time of injury in fatal inflicted head injuries. *Child Abuse Negl* **21**: 929–940.

Vowles GH, Scholtz CL, Cameron JM (1987) Diffuse axonal injury in early infancy. *J Clin Pathol* **40**: 185–189.

Whitby EH, Griffiths PD, Rutter S, Smith MF, Sprigg A, Ohadike P, Davies NP, Rigby AS, Paley MN (2004) Frequency and natural history of subdural haemorrhages in babies and relation to obstetric factors. *Lancet* **363**: 846–851.

Zimmerman RA, Bilaniuk LT (1994) Pediatric head trauma. *Neuroimaging Clin N Am* **4**: 349–366.

Zimmerman RA, Bilaniuk LT, Bruce D, Schut L, Uzzel B, Goldberg HI (1978) Interhemispheric acute subdural hematoma: a computed tomographic manifestation of child abuse by shaking. *Neuroradiology* **16**: 39–40.

Zimmerman RA, Bilaniuk LT, Bruce D, Schut L, Uzzell B, Goldberg HI (1979) Computed tomography of craniocerebral injury in the abused child. *Radiology* **130**: 687–690.

7
INITIAL AND SEQUENTIAL MRI IN NON-ACCIDENTAL HEAD INJURY

Maeve McPhillips

The use of magnetic resonance imaging (MRI) as a standard imaging tool in the investigation of non-accidental head injury in children is increasing. This is mainly due to its identification of intracerebral injury and hypoxic–ischaemic damage at an earlier stage than achieved by either computerized tomography (CT) or ultrasound.

New sequences, such as fluid attenuated inversion recovery (FLAIR), allow small quantities of subdural blood to be recognized. Diffusion weighted imaging (DWI) is very sensitive to cell damage, even in the acute phase. The advent of faster acquisition times and of open format magnets has increased the availability of anaesthesia in the MR suite.

Subdural haemorrhage

Subdural haemorrhage is a hallmark of non-accidental head injury. The haemorrhage is seen at presentation and is usually bilateral. The multiplanar capabilities of MRI, together with the lack of bony artefact, show that the subdural blood is normally a continuous collection, visible over the convexity and in the subtemporal and subfrontal regions (Figs 7.1a,b). Blood can be seen in the interhemispheric fissure, along the falx, a site well recognized on CT. Blood can also be recognized along the tentorium, with posterior fossa subdural blood occasionally identified, particularly on sagittal imaging (see Figs. 7.1a, 7.2a) (Barlow *et al.* 1999)

Most subdural haemorrhage is associated with widening of the subdural space. While acute haemorrhage may be isointense with brain or of low intensity on T_1-weighted images, acute or subacute blood is more likely to be moderately hyperintense on these sequences. T_2-weighted sequences also show high intensity, although this may be difficult to separate from the adjacent high signal in normal cerebrospinal fluid (CSF) (Figs. 7.3a,b,c). The FLAIR sequence suppresses the signal from normal CSF, allowing the high signal haemorrhage to be visualized (Noguchi *et al.* 1995). This sequence is, therefore, a useful tool in the identification of haemorrhage which has spread as a thin smear over the surface of the cerebral hemispheres, without any widening of the subdural space (Sato *et al.* 1989).

Blood in the extraaxial spaces seems to behave differently to intracerebral haemorrhage (Bradley 1993) in its temporal evolution. This may be due to layering in the dilated subdural space (Fig. 7.4b), dilution by CSF, or because of higher oxygen concentration in the surrounding fluid (Kleinman and Barnes 1998). Whatever the cause, the changes in subdural haemorrhage are not predictable, and do not follow a standard pattern. Caution should be

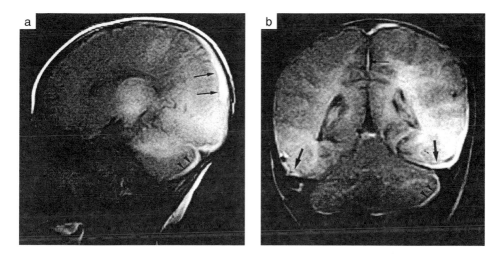

Fig. 7.1. Ten-week-old baby who presented with seizures. MRI obtained 2 days after admission. (a) T_1 sagittal, field echo (FE) 3D 35/13, flip angle (FA) 40° showing high intensity subdural haemorrhage over the convexity posteriorly (arrows) and in the posterior fossa (arrowheads). (b) FLAIR coronal, inversion recovery spin echo (IRSE) 3567(1600)/120, FA 90° showing high intensity over the convexity, along the falx (arrow), in the sub temporal region (thick arrows) and in the posterior fossa (arrowheads).

exercised in the use of MRI alone to estimate the age of the haemorrhage. CT may still have a role in this context.

The initial appearances of subdural haemorrhage are usually of a uniform intensity in the subdural space. There is usually widening of this space, but this may not be apparent in the seriously ill child with cerebral oedema, or in other cases may not yet have developed. The blood is hyperintense on all T_1- and T_2-weighted sequences, and on the FLAIR sequence.

The evolution of such a collection may show great variability (Figs. 7.3d,e), with increasing intensity from anterior to posterior due to layering of blood products. There may be a difference in intensity from one side of the falx to the other. There may be apparent loculation with septation, or the formation of presumed fibrinous stranding. These are particularly troublesome where there has been diagnostic or therapeutic aspiration, but can also be seen in collections where there has been no intervention. These appearances have been observed where the initial examinations show unequivocal uniform intensity, and where there has been no question of repeated injury. It is therefore foolhardy to ascribe the presence of a subdural collection of mixed intensities to repeated episodes of trauma. However, the presence on initial imaging of collections of uniform, symmetric intensity strongly suggests that there has been only one episode of trauma.

Acute subdural haemorrhage may eventually progress to form a collection that is of CSF intensity on all sequences, a chronic subdural collection. This is uncommon, but may be observed when there has been significant atrophy. The majority of subdural bleeds associated with non-accidental head injury seem to resolve by 4 months after injury (Fig. 7.2f).

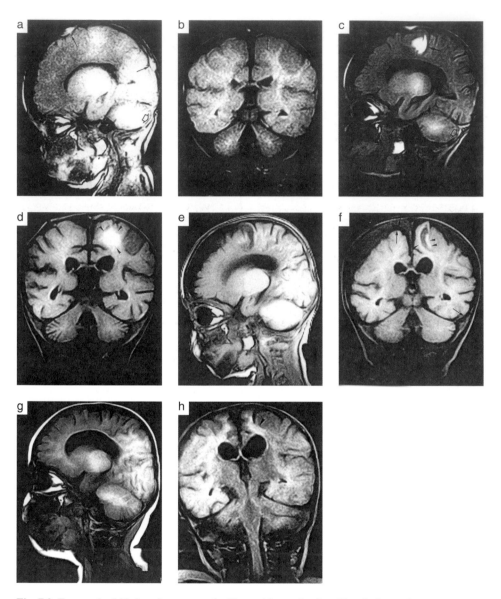

Fig. 7.2. Ten-week-old baby who presented with vomiting and reduced level of consciousness

Initial MRI obtained 3 days after presentation. (a) T$_1$ sagittal, FE 3D 35/13, FA 40° showing a high intensity posterior fossa subdural haemorrhage (open arrow), and two areas of high intensity within widened subdural spaces (arrows). (b) FLAIR coronal, IRSE 3567(1600)/120, FA 90° showing widened subdural spaces and an ill-defined area of high intensity over the left convexity (arrow).

Nine days after presentation. (c) T$_1$ sagittal, FE 3D 35/13, FA 40° showing a small persistent high signal posterior fossa subdural (open arrow) and a widened subdural space in the frontal region. The high intensity over the convexity is smaller, but well defined. There is a subcortical tear in the anterior parietal region (short arrow) which is high intensity. (d) FLAIR coronal, IRSE 3567(1600)/120, FA 90°

(cont'd opposite)↗

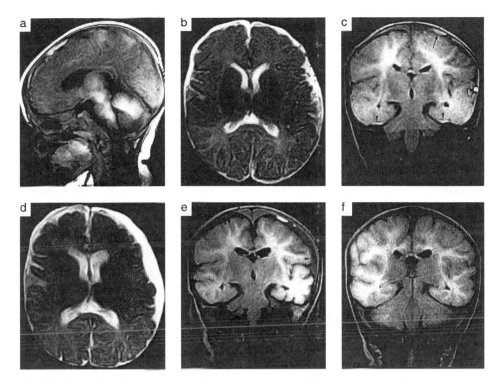

Fig. 7.3. Ten-week-old boy, born 9 weeks preterm, admitted with a suspicion of shaking injury.

Initial MRI on day of presentation. (a) T_1 sagittal, FE 3D 35/13, FA 40° showing moderately high intensity bilateral subdural haemorrhage, highest intensity over the parieto-occipital cortex, slightly less intense in the occipital region. (b) T_2 axial, SE 3400/200 showing a difference in signal between the subarachnoid space (between arrowheads) and the subdural space. (c) FLAIR coronal, IRSE 3567(1600)/120, FA 90° showing the low intensity CSF in the subarachnoid space, higher intensity haemorrhage in the subdural space and focal areas of high intensity in the subtemporal regions (arrowheads), in the left temporal region (open arrow) and over the fronto-parietal convexity (arrow).

Four weeks later. (d) T_2 axial, SE 3400/200 showing ventricular dilatation, increase in depth of the left subdural space and widening of the right subarachnoid space. (e) FLAIR coronal, IRSE 3564(1600)/120 showing that the signal from the subdural space is of varying intensities, lower laterally (arrowheads). The prominent right subarachnoid space is again visible.

Three months after presentation (f) FLAIR coronal, IRSE 3567(1600)/120, FA 90° showing that the subdural space has returned to normal.

⊾ the subcortical tear (arrowheads) is high intensity, in keeping with haemorrhage. There is now prominence of sulci and ventricles indicating either atrophy or hydrocephalus.

Three weeks after presentation. (e) T_1 sagittal, FE 3D 35/13, FA 40°. The posterior fossa subdural space is no longer high intensity. The subcortical tear is of low intensity, indicating cystic change. (f) FLAIR coronal, IRSE 3567(1600)/120, FA 90° the cystic change in the subcortical tear is again visible as low intensity. There is a surrounding rim of high signal (arrowheads) indicating gliotic change. The subdural collections are of a slightly higher intensity than the clear low intensity subarachnoid space (arrows).

Images 13 months after presentation. (g) T_1 sagittal, FE 3D 35/13, FA 40° showing no focal abnormality. (h) FLAIR coronal, IRSE 3567(1600)/120, FA 90°. The subdural spaces are normal. The ventricles are dilated. The subcortical tear is not visible except as a subtle area of white matter atrophy and high intensity gliosis (arrowheads).

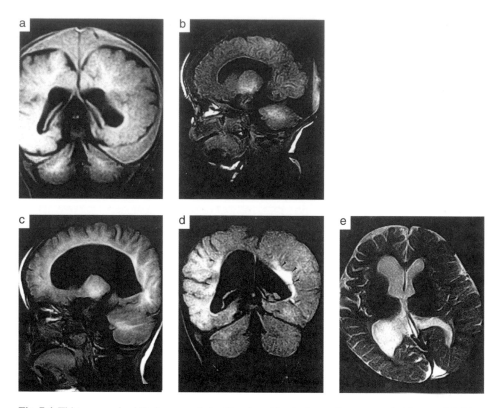

Fig. 7.4. Thirteen-week-old baby presented with reduced level of consciousness and a history of shaking injury.

MRI on day of presentation. (a) FLAIR coronal, IRSE 3567(1600)/120, FA 90°. Bilateral subdural collections of high intensity, with low intensity subarachnoid space and prominent ventricles. (b) T_1 sagittal, FE 3D 35/13, FA 40°. The subdural space is of high intensity, with a fluid–fluid level posteriorly, due to layering of blood products.

13 months later. (c) T_1 sagittal, FE 3D 35/13, FA 40°. Dilated lateral ventricle. Normal subdural space. (d) FLAIR coronal, IRSE 3567(1600)/120, FA 90°. Asymmetry of cerebral hemispheres and hemicranium. The right lateral ventricle is larger than the left. High signal in the periventricular region (arrowheads), more marked on the left, in keeping with gliosis. (e) T_2 transverse, FSE 5100/80. FA 90°. Marked asymmetry with a dilated lateral ventricle and prominent sulci on the right, a small left hemicranium and deviation of the midline. There is marked loss of white matter bilaterally, with high signal on the left indicating gliosis (arrows).

Direct intracerebral injury

Intracerebral haemorrhage can be due to impact of the head against a firm surface, to impaction of the cerebrum against the hard internal surface of the calvarium, or to shearing injury caused by acceleration–deceleration and associated rotational forces.

While skull fractures are not often directly visible on MRI, the associated soft tissue swelling and haemorrhage may be identified. Injury due to external impact often shows as a cortical contusion at the site of impact, with associated abnormality on the opposite aspect of the brain, the so-called 'contre-coup' injury. Contusions due to internal impact are most common on the antero-lateral and inferior surfaces of the frontal and temporal lobes (Figs. 7.5a,b).

Large contusions may be visible at presentation, while smaller areas of injury become more evident with time. Contusions are likely to be at their most prominent 2 weeks after presentation, but remain visible for several months. Cyst formation may be seen within the areas of haemorrhage, and may persist indefinitely (Figs. 7.5g,h,i).

Shearing injury is seen at junctions between tissue densities, typically at the grey- and white-matter interface. It is frequently petechial and may or may not be haemorrhagic. Haemorrhagic injury, when acute or subacute, is seen as increased intensity on T_1-weighted images, or low intensity on T_2-weighted images. FLAIR images, however, may reveal non-haemorrhagic injury as high-intensity lesions. Petechial injury is often widespread. When it is seen in the corpus callosum, internal capsule and brainstem, it may be termed diffuse axonal injury (DAI). Occasionally shearing injuries may be larger and haemorrhagic. These may be evident at presentation. Petechial injury may only be visible quite transiently at presentation, while some may be briefly evident at about 2 weeks after presentation.

White-matter tears are a particular manifestation of shearing injury, which are occasionally transient. They are found in the anterior parietal or the frontal lobes, and rarely extend to the cortex (Figs. 7.2c,d) (Sato et al. 1989, Jaspan et al. 1992). They may be non-haemorrhagic, although haemorrhage is more common. Internal fluid–fluid levels may be identified during the evolution of white-matter tears. Healing is often by cyst formation (Figs. 7.2e,f) The cyst may persist indefinitely or collapse with the appearance of focal atrophy (Figs. 7.2g,h).

SECONDARY INJURY
Secondary injury to the brain is an indirect result of head trauma. This may be seen as acute brain swelling, cerebral oedema, or the full range of changes associated with hypoxia and ischaemia.

Diffuse brain swelling may be seen acutely. It is thought to be due to an increase in blood volume of the affected area, not to an increase in water content. The mechanism is unclear. Although it is a diffuse process, it is often unilateral. It is seen as compression of the lateral ventricles with associated loss of the CSF spaces. There is little change in intensity, as there is no increase in water content (Bruce et al. 1981).

Cerebral oedema may follow acute brain swelling, or be due to hypoxia–ischaemia. Focal oedema can also be associated with areas of contusion or shearing injury. In oedema there is increased water content with loss of the differentiation between grey and white matter. This is manifest as a reduction in intensity of the affected area on T_1-weighted imaging and an increase in intensity on T_2-weighted imaging. This signal change may be seen more extensively than anticipated. It can become apparent as early as 5 days after presentation, but more usually within 1 to 2 weeks. Areas of injury may be identifiable earlier, even at presentation, if DWI is used.

These areas of signal change may resolve. Alternatively, they may progress to cystic encephalomalacia where the intensity changes are similar to those of oedema, being low

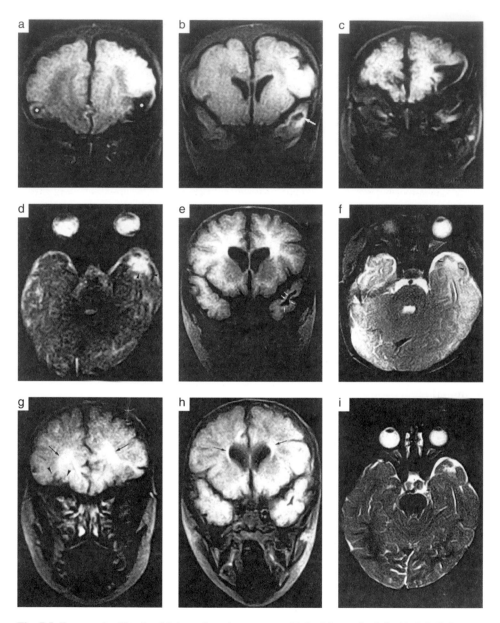

Fig. 7.5. Four-week-old twin girl, born 5 weeks preterm, with bruising and a left-sided skull fracture seen on skull X-ray.

First MRI, 5 days after presentation. (a) FLAIR coronal, IRSE 3564(1600)/120 showing bilateral high intensity subdural haemorrhage, with higher intensity underlying the skull fracture. There is also widening of the subarachnoid space. Low-intensity cyst formation is visible in the inferior frontal lobes bilaterally (white stars) suggesting injury prior to the presenting episode. (b) FLAIR coronal, IRSE 3564(1600)/120 through the temporal lobes, showing further cystic change, now visible in the left temporal lobe (white arrow).

(cont'd opposite)↗

268

intensity on T_1 and FLAIR images and high intensity on T_2 images. There may be considerable loss of detail of the cerebral structure, but the ghost-like appearance of the involved brain is usually visible. Less commonly, porencephalic cyst formation is seen with well-defined cysts of CSF intensity replacing white matter. There may be communication between the porencephalic cyst and the lateral ventricle. Gliotic change may become visible following marked hypoxic–ischaemic damage. This is seen as areas of high intensity on the T_2-weighted and FLAIR sequences (Figs. 7.4d,e; 7.5h).

After several weeks, but sometimes as early as 1 week after presentation, a pattern of sub-cortical hyperintensity may be seen on T_1-weighted images, the area being hypointense on T_2-weighted images. This finding is thought to be due to haemorrhage following ischaemia, with haemosiderin deposition accounting for the signal change. (Sener 1983, Close and Carty 1991, Jaspan and Stevens 1999).

Following non-accidental head injury, prominence of sulci and ventricles can become apparent quite quickly (Figs. 7.2d,f). This may occasionally be associated with an increasing head circumference, which may indicate the development of communicating hydrocephalus. Usually the head does not enlarge, and those appearances then indicate the development of atrophy. The subdural space may remain widened, causing confusion with a chronic subdural collection. The subarachnoid space also becomes prominent, allowing widening of the sulci. There is associated ventricular dilatation. The atrophy may be focal, involving an area of significant damage. It is occasionally unilateral, when a small hemicranium might also be noted (Figs. 7.4d,c).

Summary

MR imaging is a sensitive tool in the search for evidence of non-accidental head injury. It can identify subdural haemorrhage and monitor its progress. A uniform intensity of the subdural space on an early scan is useful in supporting an assertion of a single episode of shaking.

Early MR examination, within the first week, may reveal cerebral oedema, intracerebral contusion or transient petechial haemorrhage. Within 2–4 weeks encephalomalacia may be apparent and even early atrophy. Contusions and tears are at their most prominent at this time.

By 2 to 3 months atrophy is well established. Areas of contusion and hypoxia–ischaemia have evolved into cysts. Subdural haemorrhages should be clearing

---

◁ *Four weeks after presentation.* (c) FLAIR coronal, IRSE 3564(1600)/120 shows bilateral frontal cyst formation. (d) T_2 axial, SE 3400/200 shows the left temporal cyst visible as an ill-defined area of high intensity (arrowhead).

Five months after presentation. (e) FLAIR coronal, IRSE 3564(1600)/120 showing the left temporal lobe cyst as smaller and better defined (white arrows). (f) T_2 axial, FSE 5100/80, FA 90° again shows improved definition of the left temporal cyst (arrowhead).

Seventeen months after presentation. (g) FLAIR coronal, IRSE 3564(1600)/120 showing focal atrophy in the right inferior frontal area (arrowheads) and high signal gliosis bilaterally (arrows). (h) FLAIR coronal, IRSE 3564(1600)/120 shows that the left temporal cyst is again visible. Periventricular gliosis is present bilaterally, more marked on the left (arrows). (i) T_2 axial, FSE 5100/80, FA 90° again showing the left temporal cyst.

Any recovery in appearance will have commenced by 6 months. Later scans may be helpful for further prognosis and planning for support, care and education.

REFERENCES

Barlow KM, Gibson RJ, McPhillips M, Minns RA (1999) Magnetic resonance imaging in acute non-accidental head injury. *Acta Paediatr* **88:** 734–740.

Bradley W (1993) MR appearance of hemorrhage in the brain. *Radiology* **189:** 15–26.

Bruce DA, Alavi A, Bilaniuk L, Dolinskas C, Obrist W, Uzzell B (1981) Diffuse cerebral swelling following head injuries in children: the syndrome of "malignant brain edema". *J Neurosurg* **54:** 170–178.

Close PJ, Carty HM (1991) Transient gyriform brightness on non-contrast enhanced computed tomography (CT) brain scan of seven infants. *Pediatr Radiol* **21:** 189–192.

Jaspan T, Narborough G, Punt JAG, Lowe J (1992) Cerebral contusional tears as a marker of child abuse – detection by cranial sonography. *Pediatr Radiol* 22: 237–245.

Jaspan T, Stevens KJ (1999) Radiological imaging of craniocerebral non-accidental imaging in infancy. *RAD Magazine* **288:** 66–69.

Kleinman PK, Barnes PD (1998) Head trauma. *In:* Kleinman PK, ed. *Diagnostic Imaging of Child Abuse, 2nd edn.* St. Louis: Mosby, pp. 296–325.

Noguchi K, Ogawa T, Inugami A, Toyoshima H, Sugawara S, Hatazawa J, Fujita H, Shimosegawa E, Kanno I, Okudera T, Uemura K, Yasui N (1995) Acute subarachnoid hemorrhage: MR imaging with fluid-attenuated inversion recovery pulse sequences. *Radiology* **196:** 773–777.

Sato Y, Yuh WTC, Smith WL, Alexander RC, Kao SCS, Ellerbroek CJ (1989) Head injury in child abuse – evaluation with MR imaging. *Radiology* **173:** 653–657.

Sener RN (1993) Gyral calcifications detected on the 45th day after cerebral infarction. *Pediatr Radiol* **23:** 570–571.

8
SKELETAL INJURIES

Stephanie Mackenzie

Any bone anywhere can be fractured due to non-accidental injury (NAI). However, there are particular sites and types of fractures that are specifically associated with the shaken baby syndrome and are rarely encountered in other circumstances. These are rib and meta-physeal fractures which are mostly found before the age of 1 year (Magid and Glass 1990). Diaphyseal fractures, although numerically more common than metaphyseal and rib fractures, are less specific for NAI (King et al. 1991). Any fracture without a history of appropriate trauma must arouse suspicion of NAI especially in infants.

The discovery of fractures on X-rays taken for other clinical indications can be the pointer towards abuse and lead to the discovery of a subdural haematoma and vice versa. Often it is the presence of fractures – single, multiple, recent or healing – that confirms the suspicion of NAI and allows protective measures to be put in place. Dating of the fractures, inexact as this is, can help to time the insult and therefore help identify the perpetrator. As fractures can be subtle, especially in the early stages, the skeletal survey, the mainstay of investigation, must be of a very high standard.

Imaging
X-RAYS
Below the age of 2 years the accepted practice in the case of suspected NAI is to X-ray the entire skeleton. This involves a substantial radiation burden and should be requested only by senior staff who have evaluated the infant from a NAI perspective. There should be a hospital policy in place with clear lines of communication. A single view of the baby on one film is inadequate. Localized views of the entire skeleton including hands and feet are essential, using high-resolution film screen combination and a small focal spot. However, the future of the X-ray department is to become digitalized. Digital images currently have poorer resolution by a factor of approximately four but compensate by possessing inherently improved contrast. Kleinman et al. (2002) assessed the diagnostic performance of digital radiography in the detection of rib fractures using autopsy specimens of normal and fractured ribs from an abused infant aged 10 months. Despite the lower spatial resolution, the images were diagnostically comparable and the conclusion was that digital radiography has the potential to replace film screen imaging in NAI.

Recent publications have highlighted variability in the quality and completeness of skeletal coverage in the routine skeletal survey obtained in different centres (James et al. 2003, Offiah and Hall 2003). Commenting on these papers, Carty (2003) has stressed the

TABLE 8.1
Skeletal survey for non-accidental injury*

Skull: AP and lateral, plus Towne's view if occipital injury suspected
Body: AP/frontal chest (including clavicles)
Oblique views of the ribs (left and right)
AP abdomen with pelvis and hips
Spine: lateral, cervical and thoracolumbar
Limbs:
    AP humeri, AP forearms
    AP femurs, AP lower legs
    PA hands, AP feet

*Adapted from British Society of Paediatric Neurology draft guidelines
(http://www.bspr.org.uk).
AP = anteroposterior; PA – posteroanterior.

need for best practice and conformity and recommends following the British Society of Paediatric Radiology (BSPR) draft guidelines (Table 8.1).

The skeletal survey films must be checked by the radiologist before the infant leaves the department, and supplementary views of any area of concern, in particular wrists, knees and ankles, obtained as necessary for elucidation. Follow-up X-ray of the chest and of other doubtful areas may be extremely helpful 10–14 days later when callus can reveal healing fractures. Indeed, Kleinman (1998) recommends that the whole skeleton examination be repeated after 2 weeks.

NUCLEAR MEDICINE
Isotope bone scan has been used to identify fractures and can be positive within 24 hours of injury. The isotope bone scan has been shown to be more sensitive in the detection of fractures. In one study, 88% of fractures were detected by isotope bone scan but only 52% by skeletal survey (Jaudes 1984). However, in the metaphyses the increase in activity due to fractures can be subtle and can be confused with the normal increase in activity in the epiphyseal plates, especially if the fractures are symmetrical. Dating is not possible on an isotope bone scan. At present the isotope bone scan is not obtained routinely but can be used selectively if more proof of bony injury is required.

ULTRASOUND
Ultrasound can demonstrate both soft tissue injuries and fractures. Ultrasound is particularly useful to show cartilage damage, especially fractures of ribs at the costocartilage junction (Smeets et al. 1990) and epiphyseal injuries in infants before the epiphyses are ossified (Kleinman 1998).

COMPUTERIZED TOMOGRAPHY (CT)
CT is not used routinely (except for examining the head), but if obtained for other reasons, usually to evaluate trauma to intra-abdominal organs, the images should be carefully

272

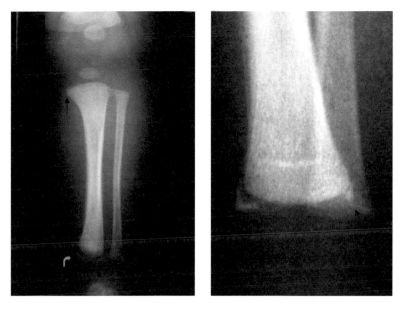

Fig. 8.1. Classic metaphyseal fracture of the distal tibia. On the anteroposterior view (left) this distal tibial metaphyseal fracture has a 'bucket handle' appearance (curved arrow) but on the lateral film (right) it looks more like two corner fractures (arrow head). The straight arrow points to a possible metaphyseal fracture of the proximal tibia. (Courtesy of Dr M McPhillips.)

scrutinized using bony window settings when unsuspected rib, vertebral and pelvic fractures may be identified.

MAGNETIC RESONANCE IMAGING (MRI)
MRI is very sensitive to bone bruising and the detection of fractures but is not used for bone survey purposes at present. However, the orthopaedic team may request MRI to further clarify fractures especially of unossified epiphyses.

Metaphyseal fracture or classic metaphyseal lesion
The nature of the injury to the metaphysis has been elucidated by Kleinman and coworkers, who published their findings in an award winning paper in 1986. By pathological analysis of the metaphyseal regions of infants who had died from NAI they established that the fracture occurs across the weakest layer of the metaphysis, the primary spongiosa. Repetitive movements cause microfractures across this layer. These microfractures coalesce to form a fracture traversing the metaphysis. At the cortex the fracture moves further away from the epiphysis and thus undercuts a subperiosteal collar of bone, which is thin centrally and thicker peripherally. This is why this fracture can appear as an isolated corner fracture or give the 'bucket handle' appearance depending on the position in which the X-ray is taken (Kleinman et al. 1986) (Fig. 8.1).

Good quality images are essential if these fractures are to be reliably identified.

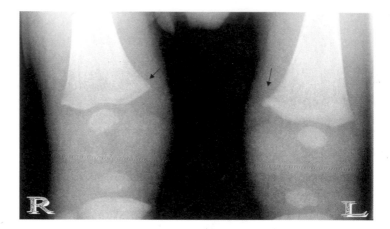

Fig. 8.2. Bilateral classic metaphyseal fractures of the distal femora. The right manifests as a trans-metaphyseal lucency, the left as a medial corner fracture.

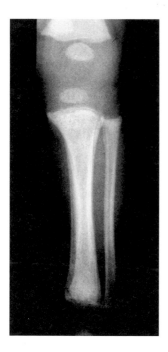

Fig. 8.3. Same patient as Figure 8.1. Healing distal and proximal tibial fractures. The callus formation surrounds the whole bone. There is also a healing fracture of the proximal fibula. The proximal metaphyseal fractures have become more apparent in the healing phase. (Courtesy of Dr M McPhillips.)

Metaphyseal fractures may heal without periosteal reaction as the periosteum is tightly adherent to the cortex in this region, and the X-ray appearances can then be very subtle with a submetaphyseal lucency and minimal irregularity of the lateral margin (Fig. 8.2). If the injury has been more extensive the periosteum can be ruptured, producing a large sub-periosteal haematoma with subsequent exuberant callus formation (Carty 1993) (Fig. 8.3).

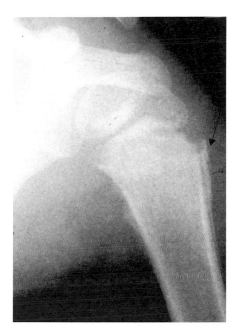

Fig. 8.4. Healing classic metaphyseal lesion of the proximal humerus.

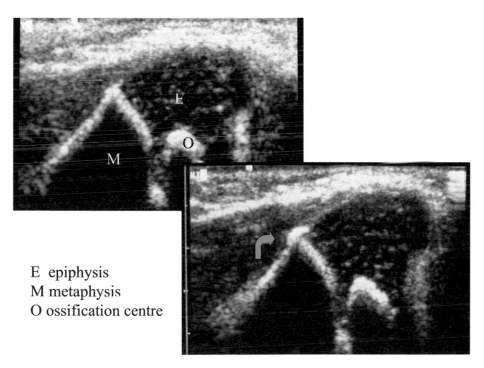

E epiphysis
M metaphysis
O ossification centre

Fig. 8.5. Ultrasound of the distal femora of an infant aged 1 month: (top) normal (straight arrow); (bottom) thickened perichondral ring confirming a healing metaphyseal fracture (curved arrow).

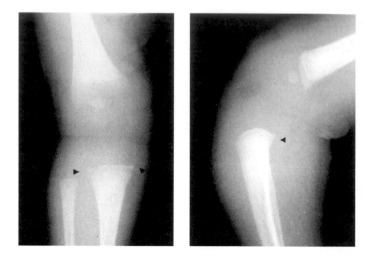

Fig. 8.6. Metaphyseal fracture of the proximal tibia. This is a baby a few days old with a fixed flexion deformity of the knee who developed bruising after too vigorous physiotherapy. As in every case the importance of the full clinical history cannot be overemphasized.

Metaphyseal fractures occur because of shearing forces associated with rapid acceleration and deceleration from violent shaking or twisting traction on a solitary limb. Shaking injuries are likely to produce bilateral similar fractures whereas twisting a limb may result in a solitary fracture or asymmetrical injuries. Metaphyseal fractures most commonly affect both ends of the tibia, distal femur and proximal humerus (Kleinman et al. 1995) (Fig. 8.4). Healing occurs in 4–8 weeks but the fractures are difficult to date.

The Salter–Harris type of epiphyseal–metaphyseal injury is rare in abused infants.

The metaphysis in a normal infant may have a spur-like appearance. Careful scrutiny of the cortical margin as it blends into the spur will show that this cortical line is intact in a normal child. A gap or blurred area of the cortex may signal trauma to the perichondral ring. Ultrasound can be used to show subtle displacement or irregularity of the perichondral ring and so may help to clarify indeterminate X-rays (Markowitz et al. 1993) (Fig. 8.5).

Metaphyseal lesions are seen in Schimdt-type metaphyseal chondrodysplasia, and these can look identical to the metaphyseal fracture of NAI. However, the skeletal survey will show other dysplastic features, and unlike fractures, the lesions in this dysplasia will not disappear with time.

Metaphyseal fractures, however, are not exclusive to NAI. They have been described in osteogenesis imperfecta, but in all cases the bones were grossly abnormal and had obvious osteoporosis so that the diagnosis of osteogenesis imperfecta was easily made radiologically (Astley 1979). Grayev et al. (2001) reported 8 infants with clubfeet who incurred metaphyseal fractures during physiotherapy (Fig. 8.6).

Rib fractures

Almost never seen in infants outside the context of NAI, rib fractures were not mentioned

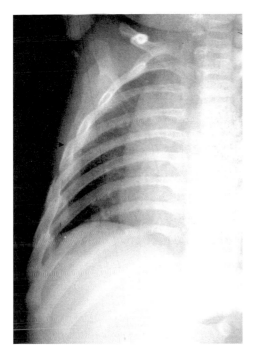

Fig. 8.7. Acute rib fractures. The anteroposterior chest view of this 5-week-old infant looked normal. However, the right oblique view showed acute fractures of the anterolateral aspect of the right 4th and 5th ribs with overlying soft tissue swelling.

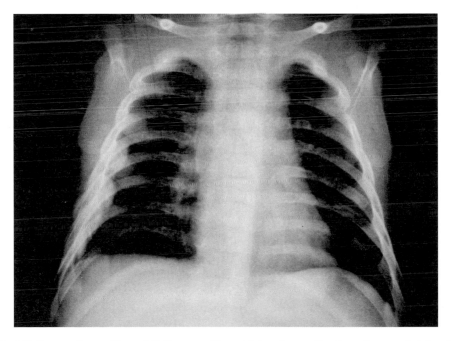

Fig. 8.8. Same patient as Figure 8.7. On repeat X-ray 14 days later, callus formation revealed that the right 3rd to 8th ribs had all been fractured.

277

in the original descriptions of the whiplash shaken infant syndrome by Caffey (1946, 1972, 1974). However, rib fractures and metaphyseal injuries are common bony manifestations of the shaken baby and are highly specific for this. Rib fractures account for up to a third of detected fractures in children who live, but 51% at post-mortem examination (Kleinman et al. 1995). This suggests that many fractures are missed on the initial chest film. Therefore the initial skeletal survey should include both oblique views of the ribs. The oblique view is positioned to project the posterior aspect of the ribs away from the transverse processes and so increase recognition of posterior rib fractures (Fig. 8.7). A follow-up film in 10–14 days can become dramatically positive as callus formation reveals the injuries not visible on the original films (Fig. 8.8).

Even one rib fracture found incidentally on a chest film has a high probability of being due to NAI and justifies a full skeletal survey (Carty and Pierce 2002).

Difficulties in the visualization of rib fractures can be due to a number of factors such as the fracture line crossing at an obliquity to the incident beam; the fracture not being displaced as the periosteum often stays intact; superimposition of other structures especially posteriorly where the transverse processes can overlie the rib fracture site; and poor radiography (Ng and Hall 1998). Fractures involving the costochondral junctions are especially difficult to see, and ultrasound may reveal costochondral dislocation and associated soft tissue changes not demonstrated on the chest X-ray (Smeets et al. 1990).

Fractures can occur at any site, with the majority involving the posterior aspect. They are usually bilateral and multiple, and often symmetrical but not necessarily so. Increasingly the accepted mechanism of injury is anteroposterior compression by encircling hands, which also limit the lateral movement of the chest wall. Fractures of the posterior ribs occur at the articulation of the rib head with the costal facet of the vertebral body and where the rib tubercle articulates with the transverse process. With anteroposterior compression the transverse processes act as the fulcrum fracturing the posterior aspect of the ribs as they are levered over the transverse processes. This requires the spine to move anteriorly with respect to the posterior ribs. Shaking rabbits in the laboratory reproduced this pattern of injuries (Kleinman and Schlesinger 1997). These posterior rib fractures did not occur when anteroposterior compression was applied with the rabbit lying supine on a flat surface mimicking the position for cardiopulmonary resuscitation. Slamming the infant face down could also produce the conditions in which posterior rib fractures occur.

The chest X-ray may initially look normal or show a widespread abnormality, localized abnormality of the lateral rib contour, soft tissue thickening, pleural reaction, malalignment of fractured ends, surgical emphysema, fracture of different ages, pneumothorax or pneumo-mediastinum (Fig. 8.9).

Isotope bone scan is more sensitive than radiographs in the detection of acute rib fractures (Cadzow and Armstrong 2000).

Ultrasound can be used to identify fractures of the ribs and associated soft tissue trauma. A linear probe with a small footprint and high frequency around 10MHz is best. Even with a great deal of patience and time the experienced operator can have difficulty numbering the rib on which a fracture has been demonstrated. However, ultrasound can be used to identify injury in a child with a negative initial X-ray and can direct follow-up films. Both bone

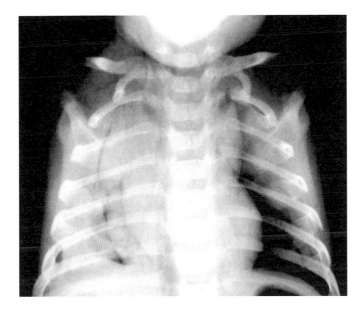

Fig. 8.9. Chest X-ray showing pneumothorax, pneumomediastinum, chest wall emphysema and bilateral acute rib fractures.

fractures and fractures of the costal cartilages can be identified, as can pleural haemorrhage (Figs. 8.10–8.12).

Rib fractures can show evidence on X-ray of healing 7–10 days after injury, and the amount of callus formation will depend on the disruption caused by the original injury (Figs. 8.13, 8.14). The fracture line may become apparent but often does not. Increased density and rib expansion occur initially with ill-defined margins then these become sharper as the callus becomes organized and lamellar bone is formed. Resorption of the fracture ends coupled with callus formation can give the appearance of a hole in a rib (Magid and Glass 1990).

Cardiopulmonary resuscitation (CPR) of the baby is often given as a mechanism for producing rib fractures. One review of infants surviving CPR for medical conditions did not identify any cases (Feldman and Brewer 1984). A more recent series of post-mortem examinations of 211 children who died despite CPR found only one infant of 3 months with bilateral rib fractures (Bush et al 1996). However, there is a recent report of rib fractures following physiotherapy in 5 infants hospitalized with bronchiolitis (4) or pneumonia (1): a fracture rate of 1 in 1000 (Chalumeau et al. 2002). This French paper suggests that the fractures might have been a local problem due to insufficient training in the physiotherapy technique used.

Long bones
A single diaphyseal fracture is the most common presenting skeletal manifestation of NAI and occurs four times more often than metaphyseal fractures (King et al. 1988, Merten and

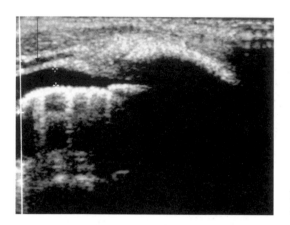

Fig. 8.10. Ultrasound of pleural haemorrhage associated with lateral rib fractures.

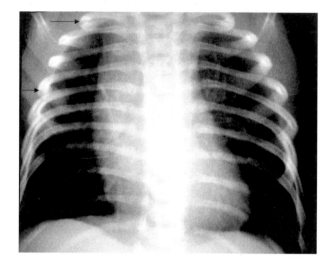

Fig. 8.11. Chest film of same child shows angulation of the left 4th and 5th ribs due to fractures and associated pleural reaction. The right 1st and 4th ribs have clearly shown fracture lines. This plus the appearance of the callus on follow-up films indicated two episodes of abuse.

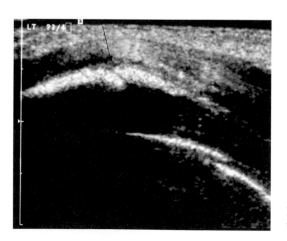

Fig. 8.12. Ultrasound showing a fracture of the posterolateral aspect of a rib.

280

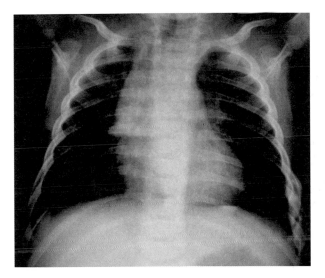

Fig. 8.13. This 7-week-old boy had a skeletal survey because his twin sister had bilateral parietal skull fractures, subdural haematomas and healing rib fractures. The chest film shows left 7th–9th rib fractures unsuspected clinically

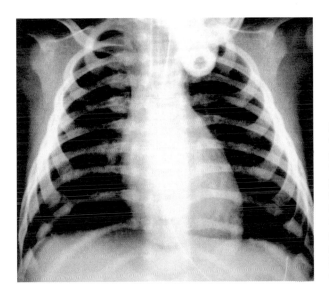

Fig. 8.14. Chest X-ray of an infant who presented in a collapsed state and required resuscitation and ventilation. Film taken to show position of the endotracheal tube shows healing posterior 3rd–7th rib fractures on the right, and fractures of the costochondral junctions of the 4th–7th ribs bilaterally that also showed signs of healing. This is indicative of abuse prior to the episode leading to admission.

Carpenter 1990). However, Kleinman et al. (1995) have suggested that rib fractures are more common than long bone fractures in infants. Several studies have tried to define a pattern of accidental versus non-accidental injury (Beals and Tufts 1983, Worlock et al. 1986, King et al. 1988, Blakemore et al. 1996, Scherl et al. 2000).

The challenge is different in the pre-mobile infant than in the mobile child. Falls in infants and children are common but injury occurs seldom and is usually mild.

Warrington et al. (2001) reported the results of a postal questionnaire collecting information in falls in pre-mobile infants. Out of 2554 children (3357 falls) under the age

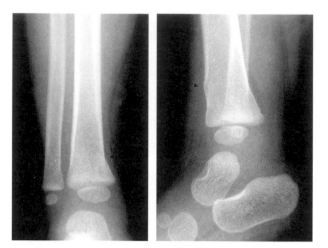

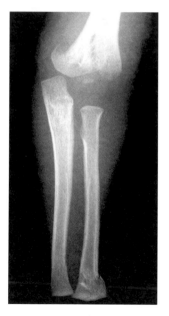

Fig. 8.15. Buckle fracture of the distal tibia.

Fig. 8.16. Displaced supracondylar fracture of the distal humerus and greenstick fractures of the distal shafts of radius and ulna due to NAI.

This is an example of fractures often seen as a result of an accidental fall onto an outstretched hand and both these fractures are at the junction of the diaphysis and metaphysis and can occur simultaneously. However, in this 15-month-old these and multiple other fractures were due to abuse.

of 6 months less than 1% resulted in concussion or fracture. Serious injury was due to complex accidents.

A typical impact fracture in accidental injury is the buckle fracture that occurs at the junction of the diaphysis and the metaphysis and is a frequent positive finding in the casualty reporting pile (Figs. 8.15, 8.16). This fracture can also be found in the abused child thrust onto the foot with force.

The undisplaced spiral fracture of the tibia, the so-called toddlers' fracture, is a well-recognized accidental injury in the child who is beginning to walk, falls frequently, and is

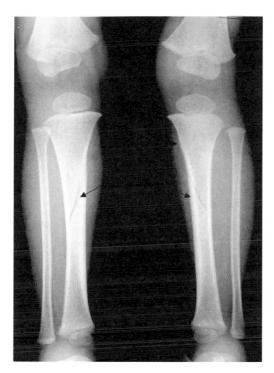

Fig. 8.17. Along with other fractures due to abuse this child has bilateral spiral fractures of the tibia (arrows) and a buckle fracture of the left proximal tibia (arrow head)

brought to casualty with the history of refusing to weight bear (Fig. 8.17). This should not be confused with abuse.

Subperiosteal new bone without a fracture can occur following a gripping or twisting force, as the periosteum is loose along the diaphysis. Confusion with physiological periosteal reaction can occur. However, physiological periosteal reaction is bilateral, symmetrical and subtle in infants aged 6 weeks to 6 months, and should be able to be excluded on those grounds. Isotope bone scan can discriminate by showing increased uptake in a subperiosteal haematoma but not in physiological periosteal reaction (Rao and Carty 1999).

Diaphyseal fractures may be either spiral, oblique or transverse. In abuse the femur, humerus and tibia are the most often affected. All types of fractures can occur, with spiral being more frequent in some series (Worlock et al. 1986). A more recent paper found an equal incidence of spiral and transverse fractures of the femur in abuse (Scherl et al. 2000). In one study of children below 1 year of age, 65% of femoral fractures were due to abuse (Gross and Stranger 1983). However, above the age of a year, the incidence of isolated fracture of the femur due to abuse has been found to be low (Blakemore et al. 1996). As always the history is vitally important.

Apart from a supracondylar fracture, any fracture of the humerus is highly specific for NAI in a child less than 3 years old (Thomas et al. 1991).

In the daily casualty reporting pile, greenstick and buckle fractures are common, whereas transverse fractures are rare especially in infants (Fig. 8.18).

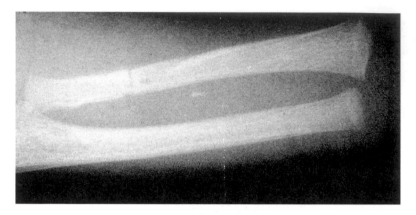

Fig. 8.18. Transverse fracture of the radius in an infant who presented acutely having collapsed at home. There is faint periosteal reaction around the fracture indicating an injury at least 5 days old. This was therefore a separate insult from the acute subdural haemorrhage that prompted the collapse.

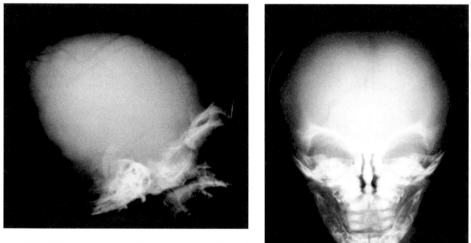

Fig. 8.19. Bilateral parietal skull fractures. Metaphyseal and rib fractures were also present.

Skull fractures

Single linear parietal fractures are relatively common injuries in infants due to accidental falls. Fractures that are branching, diastatic and bilateral are more likely to be due to NAI (Fig. 8.19). Dating of skull fractures is not possible. However, the association with soft tissue swelling with the maximum depth at the cortical break can narrow the timing to 2–12 days in some instances. The time to resolve depends on the initial size of the haematoma (Rao and Carty 1999).

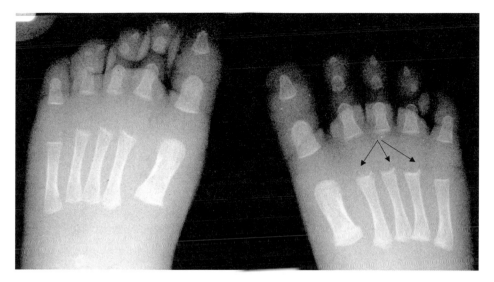

Fig. 8.20. Metaphyseal fractures of the 2nd–4th metatarsal bones on the right.

Other fractures

Other fractures that occur rarely but which are also highly specific for NAI include fractures of the scapula, outer end of the clavicle, vertebrae, hands and feet. Hence there is the requirement to perform a high quality skeletal survey and then give careful scrutiny.

SPINE

Spinal injuries in NAI are uncommon but must be identified. Crush fractures from hyper-flexion or forcing the child into a sitting position occur more often than spinal cord injuries. Hangman's fracture, that is a vertical fracture of the pedicles of C2 with anterior subluxation of C2 on C3, due to NAI has been reported in the literature (Kleinman and Shelton 1997, Rooks et al. 1998). These fractures are rare but may be asymptomatic, and the X-ray appearances can be confused with primary spondylolysis. Thin-slice CT should help to differentiate (Parisi et al. 1991). Kleinman and Shelton (1997) attributed the injury to a hyperextension injury with shaking.

Compression fractures in a preterm infant following a lumbar puncture have been reported (Halbert and Haller 2000).

PELVIC FRACTURES

These are rare but have been reported in both infants and older children and can represent both physical and sexual abuse (Ablin et al. 1992) (Fig. 8.21).

STERNAL INJURIES

Although reported in the literature as highly specific for child abuse especially in the under-twos, these injuries are rare and recognized more commonly following accidental trauma

285

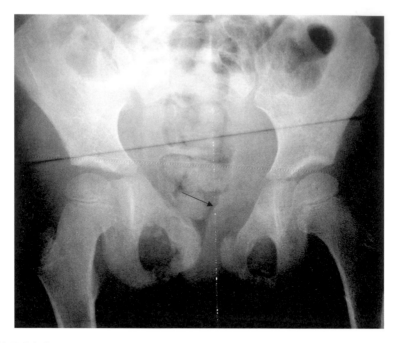

Fig. 8.21. Pelvic fractures. Bilateral superior and inferior pubic rami fractures and widening of the right sacroiliac joint are present with deformity of the contour of the pelvis. Periosteal reaction seen below the right superior ramus indicates a healing fracture, whereas the deviation of the obturator fat line on the left denotes a fresh haematoma (arrow) and therefore at least two episodes of abuse.

usually due to either a direct force or hyperflexion (Hechter et al. 2002). None of the fractures in this series of 12 children occurred under the age of 1 year. Of the four fractures in the 1–2 year age group, only one was definitely due to NAI, another a possibility. Trampoline accidents have been responsible for a few sternal fractures in young children attending our hospital.

CLAVICLE
Fractures of the lateral aspect are said to be highly specific, but fractures of the mid-shaft are more common and overall the clavicle is not a common site of injury in abuse.

Dating of injuries
This is plagued by imprecision, heavily affected by the quality of X-rays, confused by repetition of injury and dependent on the severity of injury. The more severe the injury, the longer the soft tissues changes and callus take to resolve.

Factors used to date fractures are:
• Soft tissue swelling. Soft tissue thickening and blurring of tissue planes due to haemorrage and inflammation can disappear within 2 days or persist up to 3 weeks. Most swelling disappears by 4–5 days.

TABLE 8.3
Differential diagnosis*

Birth injury
Osteogenesis imperfecta
Copper deficiency
Menkes syndrome
Ostemyelitis
Congenital syphilis
Rickets
Scurvey
Hypervitaminosis A
Congenital insensitivity to pain
Paraplegia
Metaphyseal dysplasia
Prostaglandin E therapy

*Compiled from Shaw (1988), Ablin et al. (1990), Smith (1995), and Carty (1997, 1998).

- Periosteal new bone formation. On good quality radiographs this can be identified as early as 4 days in infants, but 7–10 days for faint reaction to be visible is more common.
- Fracture line definition. Resorption of bone results in widening of the line and ill-definition during the 2nd to 3rd week post-injury.
- Soft callus formation. The calcification of osteoid follows after periosteal reaction and results in increased density around the fracture line 2–3 weeks after injury.
- Hard callus formation. Laying down of lamellar bone usually occurs one week after osteoid calcification, and the outline of the bridging density becomes sharper and the fracture line disappears. This happens at between 3 and 6 weeks.
- Remodelling. This is the most variable of all the factors: in infants it can occur very rapidly, whereas in older children residual deformity may persist beyond a year. As the site of the fracture moves away from the epiphyseal plate the remodelling process becomes more inefficient.

Differential diagnosis

There is a long list of possible differential diagnoses for some of the fractures (Table 8.3), even those reported to be more specific for NAI, and indeed there is no type of fracture that has not been reported in other circumstances.

A careful clinical history of the infant and of the extended family combined with appropriate biochemistry should eliminate or identify the majority of these conditions.

Osteogenesis imperfecta types I and IV have caused the most controversy, but even in this complex area a thorough clinical and radiological examination by experienced specialists should leave few cases in which the diagnosis is in doubt (Lachman et al. 1998).

However, it must be borne in mind that none of these conditions preclude NAI and that two diagnoses can coexist (Duncan and Chandy 1993).

A full discussion of the differential dignoses and especially of the recent controversies with type IV ostegenesis imperfecta is provided by Kleinman (1998).

Conclusion

Fractures of the skeleton provide confirmatory evidence that the head injury has been due to NAI. Fractures that are found incidentally or are multiple especially of different ages are easier to assign to NAI than a single diaphyseal fracture. However, even one subtle fracture can provide the proof of abuse. The skeletal survey must be of a very high standard or fractures will be missed. The skeletal survey must be reported with the knowledge of the full clinical history and possible differential diagnosis. The harm to a family mistakenly accused of NAI should not be underestimated. However, if not protected, the infant is left vulnerable to repeated acts of abuse with permanent consequences.

REFERENCES

Ablin DS, Greenspan A, Reinhart M, Grix A (1990) Differentiation of child abuse from osteogenesis imperfecta. *AJR* **154**: 1035–1046.
Ablin DS, Greenspan A, Reinhart MA (1992) Pelvic injuries in child abuse. *Pediatr Radiol* **22**: 454–457.
Astley R (1979) Metaphyseal fractures in osteogenesis imperfecta. *Br J Radiol* **52**: 441–443.
Beals RK, Tufts T (1983) Fractured femur in infancy: the role of child abuse. *J Pediatr Orthoped* **3**: 583–586.
Blakemore LC, Loder RT, Hensinger RN (1996) Role of intentional abuse in children 1 to 5 years old with isolated femoral shaft fractures. *J Pediatr Orthoped* **15**: 585–588.
Bush CM, Jones JS, Cohle SD, Johnson H (1996) Pediatric injuries from cardiopulmonary resuscitation. *Ann Emerg Med* **28**: 40–44.
Cadzow SP, Armstrong LL (2000) Rib fractures in infants: red alert! The clinical features, investigations and child protection outcomes. *J Paediatr Child Health* **4**: 322–326.
Caffey J (1946) Multiple fractures in the long bones of infants suffering from chronic subdural hematoma. *Am J Roentgenol Radium Ther* **56**: 163–167.
Caffey J (1972) On the theory and practice of shaking infants. *Am J Dis Child* **124**: 161–169.
Caffey J (1974) The whiplash shaken infant syndrome: manual shaking by the extremities with whiplash-induced intracranial and intraocular bleedings, linked with residual permanent brain damage and mental retardation. *Pediatrics* **54**: 396–403.
Carty H (1997) Non-accidental injury: Review of the radiology. *Eur Radiol* **9**: 1365–1376.
Carty H (1998) Brittle or battered? *Arch Dis Child* **63**: 350–352.
Carty H (2003) Commentary on: A survey of non-accidental injury imaging in England, Scotland and Wales and observational study of skeletal surveys in suspected non-accidental injury. *Clin Radiol* **58**: 694–695.
Carty H, Pierce A (2002) Non-accidental injury: a retrospective analysis of a large cohort. *Eur Radiol* **12**: 2919–2915.
Carty HM (1993) Fractures caused by child abuse. *J Bone Joint Surg Br* **75**: 849–857.
Chalumeau M, Foix-L'Helias L, Scheinmann P, Zuani P, Gendrel D, Ducou-le-Pointe H (2002) Rib fractures after chest physiotherapy for bronchiolitis or pneumonia in infants. *Pediatr Radiol* **32**: 644–647.
Duncan AA, Chandy J (1993) Case report: Multiple neonatal fractures— dietary or deliberate? *Clin Radiol* **48**: 137–139.
Feldman KW, Brewer DK (1984) Child abuse, cardiopulmonary resuscitation, and rib fractures. *Pediatrics* **73**: 339–342.
Grayev AM, Boal DK, Wallach DM, Segal LS (2001) Metaphyseal fractures mimicking abuse during treatment for clubfoot. *Paediatr Radiol* **31**: 559–563.
Gross RH, Stranger M (1983) Causative factors responsible for femoral fractures in infants and young children. *J Paediatr Orthop* **3**: 341–343.
Halbert J, Haller JO (2000) Iatrogenic vertebral body compression fracture in a premature infant caused by extreme flexion during positioning for a lumbar puncture. *Pediatr Radiol* **30**: 410–411.

Hechter H, Huyer D, Manson D (2002) Sternal fractures as a manifestation of abusive injury in children. *Pediatr Radiol* **32**: 902–906.

James SLJ, Halliday K, Somers J, Broderick N (2003) A survey of non-accidental injury imaging in England, Scotland and Wales. *Clin Radiol* **58**: 696–701.

Jaudes PK (1984) Comparison of radiography and radionuclide bone scanning in the detection of child abuse. *Paediatrics* **73**: 166–168.

King J, Diefendorf D, Apthorp J, Negrete VF, Carlson M (1988) Analysis of 429 fractures in 189 battered children. *J Pediatr Orthop* **8**: 586–589.

Kleinman PK, Marks SC, Blackbourne B (1986) The metaphyseal lesion in abused infants: a radiologic–histopathologic study. *AJR* **146**: 895–905.

Kleinman PK, Marks SC, Richmond JM, Blackbourne BD (1995) Inflicted skeletal injury: a postmortem radiologic–histopathologic study in 31 infants. *AJR* **165**: 647–650.

Kleinman PK, Schlesinger AE (1997) Mechanical factors associated with posterior rib fractures: laboratory and case studies. *Pediatr Radiol* **27**: 87–91.

Kleinman PK, Shelton YA (1997) Hangman's fracture in an abused infant: imaging features. *Pediatr Radiol* **27**: 776–777.

Kleinman PK (1998) *Diagnostic Imaging of Child Abuse. 2nd edn.* St Louis: Mosby.

Kleinman PK, O'Conner B, Mimkin K, Rayder SM, Spevak MR, Belanger PL, Getty DJ, Karellas A (2002) Detection of rib fractures in an abused infant using digital radiography: a laboratory study. *Paediatr Radiol* **32**: 896–901.

Magid N, Glass T (1990) A "hole in a rib" as a sign of child abuse. *Paediatr Radiol* **20**: 334–336.

Markowitz RI, Hubbard AM, Harty MP, Bellah RD, Kessler A, Meyer JS (1993) Sonography of the knee in normal and abused infants. *Pediatr Radiol* **23**: 264–267.

Merten DF, Carpenter BLM (1990) Radiologic imaging of inflicted injury in the child abuse syndrome. *Pediatr Clin N Am* **37**: 815–837

Ng CS, Hall CM (1998) Costochondral junction fractures and intra-abdominal trauma in non-accidental injury (child abuse). *Pediatric Radiol* **28**: 671–676.

Offiah AC, Hall CM (2003) Observational study of skeletal surveys in suspected non-accidental injury. *Clin Radiol* **58**: 702–705.

Parisi M, Lieberson R, Shatsky S (1991) Hangman's fracture or primary spondylosis: a patient and a brief review. *Pediatr Radiol* **21**: 367–368.

Rao P, Carty H (1999) Non-accidental injury: Review of the radiology. *Clin Radiol* **54**: 11–24.

Rooks VJ, Sisler C, Burton B (1998) Cervical spine injury in child abuse: report of two cases. *Pediatr Radiol* **28**: 193–195.

Scherl SS, Miller L, Lively N, Russinoff S, Sullivan CM, Tornetta P (2000) Accidental and nonaccidental femur fractures in children. *Clin Orthop* **376**: 96–105.

Shaw JCL (1988) Copper deficiency and non-accidental injury. *Arch Dis Child* **63**: 448–455.

Smeets AJ, Robben SG, Meradji M (1990) Sonographically detected costo-chondral dislocation in an abused child. *Paediatr Radiol* **20**: 566–567.

Smith R (1995) Osteogenesis imperfecta, non-accidental injury, and temporary brittle bone disease. *Arch Dis Child* **72**: 169–176.

Thomas SA, Rosenfield NS, Leventhal JM, Markowitz RI (1991) Long bone fractures in young children: distinguishing accidental fractures from child abuse. *Pediatrics* **88**: 471–476.

Worlock P, Stower M, Barbor P (1986) Patterns of fractures in accidental and non-accidental injury in children: a comparative study. *BMJ (Clin Res Ed)* **293**: 100–102.

Warrington SA, Wright CM, Team AS (2001) Accidents and resulting injuries in premobile infants: data from the ALSR. *Arch Dis Child* **85**: 104–107.

9
MECHANISMS AND MANAGEMENT OF SUBDURAL HAEMORRHAGE

Jonathan Punt

Subdural haemorrhage (SDH) has long been identified as one of the sentinel lesions of inflicted head injury in babies and infants (Weston 1968, Guthkelch 1971, Caffey 1972). A population-based study in south Wales and south west England detected an incidence of SDH of 12.8/100,000/year in children aged less than 2 years, and a higher incidence of 21/100,000/year in infants aged less than 1 year (Jayawant *et al.* 1998). There are many reported causes of SDH (Table 9.1), some of which may represent associations rather than true causal relationships. For practical purposes, the list in infants is substantially shorter (Kemp 2002). Over 80% of SDHs encountered in children in the first 2 years of life are the consequence of inflicted injury (Jayawant *et al.* 1998).

Although in the past it has more often been extracranial manifestations that have led to suspicion and diagnosis of physical abuse, the more widespread application of cranial imaging to babies and infants under investigation, and to their infant siblings, will inevitably uncover more incidents of SDH because of the occult nature of some cases. In this regard, the relative infrequency of other abnormalities associated with abuse, such as extracranial bruising or skeletal injuries, is noteworthy, as found in one large institutional series of patients encountered in a regional paediatric neuroscience service (Table 9.2) (partially reported by Stevens *et al.* 1998a,b). The broad similarity of the features between the large institutional series and the much smaller but tighter epidemiological series suggests that the findings in the former are indeed representative (Table 9.3).

A clear corollary of these observations is that, increasingly, the diagnosis of inflicted injury in cases of SDH will have to be considered upon the neurological aspects alone, although the finding of other stigmata may be supportive.

Another feature of SDH is that its presence spans the entire clinical spectrum of neurological disturbance, with presentations ranging from progressive macrocephaly (10%) in a well child to fatal cardiorespiratory collapse (2%) (Tables 9.4, 9.5). Of 53 fatal cases of inflicted head injury in children, 84% of infants aged less than 1 year, and 75% of those aged 1 year or more than 1 year, had SDHs (Geddes *et al.* 2001a). This chapter will address the subject from a practical angle, reflecting current views and controversies. Unless otherwise stated explicitly, the remarks relate to children in the first 2 years of life.

Classification and definitions
A traditional classification of traumatic SDHs is that devised over 40 years ago by McKissock

290

TABLE 9.1
Reported causes and associations of subdural haemorrhage in individuals of all ages

Prenatal and perinatal
Intrauterine trauma, accidental or intentional
Intrauterine isoimmune thrombocytopaenia
Pre-eclampsia
Idiopathic intrauterine SDH
Cerebral infarction
Delivery
    Spontaneous normal vaginal delivery
    Instrumental, forceps or ventouse assisted
    Caesarean, without or with preceding labour
    Traumatic

Developmental
Middle fossa arachnoid cysts (+ trauma)
Benign infantile hydrocephalus

Genetically determined diseases
Alagille syndrome
Autosomal dominant polycystic kidneys
Ehlers–Danlos syndrome
Menkes disease
Osteogenesis imperfecta

Inborn metabolic disorders
Galactosaemia
Glutaric aciduria types I & II
Pyruvate carboxylase deficiency

Haematological disorders
Haemophilia A and B
Factor V deficiency
Factor XII deficiency
Thrombocytopaenic purpura
Haemorrhagic disease of the newborn
Hermansky–Pudlak syndrome
Disseminated intravascular coagulation
Hepatic cirrhosis
Plasma clotting factor inhibition
Sickle cell disease

Vascular malformations and processes
Arteriovenous malformations
Arterial aneurysms
Moya moya disease
Atherosclerosis

Toxic and metabolic
Hypernatraemia
Lead poisoning
Cocaine abuse
Gingko biloba poisoning

Malignant disease
Leukaemia
Primary CNS lymphoma
Disseminated meningeal malignancy
Primary parenchymal CNS tumours
Haemophagocytic lymphohistiocytosis

Infectious diseases
Intracranial infections
    Bacterial meningitis – Haemophilus influenzae,
      Streptococcus pneumoniae, other
    Viral meningo-encephalitis – Herpes simplex
      virus, possibly other
    Congenital toxoplasmosis
    Chronic otitis media
Systemic infections
    Kawasaki disease
    Malaria
    Bacterial endocarditis with mycotic intracranial
      aneurysm

Inflammatory
Lupus erythematosus
Wegener granulomatosis

Iatrogenic
Medications
    Anticoagulants
    Drug-induced thrombocytopaenia
    Tamoxifen
Intracranial procedures
    External ventricular drainage
    Ventricular shunt
    Craniotomy
Extracranial procedures
    Cardiac bypass surgery
    Extracorporeal membrane oxygenation
    Bone marrow transplantation
    Haemodialysis
    Lumbar puncture
    Lumbar myelography
    Spinal anaesthesia

Trauma
Accidental impact injury
Traumatic intracranial aneurysm
Activity-related
    Roller coaster rides
    Break dancing
    Head banging to music
Inflicted head injury

TABLE 9.2

Findings in 120 cases of suspected inflicted head injury encountered in a regional paediatric neuroscience service*

Subdural haemorrhage	98%
Signs of head trauma	
External signs	35%
Soft tissue scalp swelling on skull X-ray	41%
Skull fracture	20%
Retinal haemorrhages (in 97 cases examined)	57%
Bruising elsewhere on body	29%
Extracranial fractures (in 99 cases examined)	
Fractures characteristic of abuse	46%
Rib fractures	23%
Upper-limb fractures	14%
Lower-limb fractures	20%

*Stevens et al. (1998a,b), with additional unpublished data.

TABLE 9.3

Comparison of findings between an epidemiological (A) and an institutional (B) series of childhood subdural haemorrhages*

	A (N=33)	B (N=120)
Median age	3 months	14 weeks
Subdural haemorrhage	33	98%
Ophthalmic examination	27	81%
Retinal haemorrhage	19/27	55%
Skeletal survey	27	83%
Skull fracture(s)	5/27	20%
Other fracture(s)	16/27	46%
Extracranial soft tissue injury	13	29%
Anaemia <10g/dl	16	70%
Previously seen at hospital	6	52%
Dead on arrival	4	3%
Major disability	15	55%
Died	9	8%

*A = Jayawant et al. (1998); B = Stevens et al. (1998a,b), with additional unpublished data.

et al. (1960). This created a temporal definition that related the time of presentation to the time of injury, such that 'acute' indicated an interval of less than 72 hours; 'chronic', an interval greater than 21 days; and 'subacute', an interval of 72 hours to 21 days. This definition, and similar variations, was valuable at the time, and served well for many years, providing a uniform basis for purposes of epidemiology, clinical description, management guidelines, and comparative outcomes. In the context of babies and infants, these time-honoured classifications have limitations due to the following factors:

• they presuppose that there is accurate and reliable knowledge of the time of trauma
• they are derived principally from adult data

TABLE 9.4
Clinical presentation in 120 children with suspected inflicted head injury (of whom 98% had subdural haemorrhage)

Seizures	42%
Non-specific – vomiting, fever	31%
Apnoea/breathing difficulties	23%
Trauma	23%
Increasing head circumference	10%
Cardiorespiratory arrest	2%
Dead on arrival	3%

Stevens et al. (1998a).

TABLE 9.5
Clinical findings in 120 children with suspected inflicted head injury (of whom 98% had subdural haemorrhages or haematomas)

Bulging fontanelle	43%
External head trauma	35%
Bruising over body	29%
Decreased consciousness	24%
Crying / miserable / irritable	18%
Abnormal tone	17%
Seizures	17%
Completely well	6%

Stevens et al. (1998a).

- such a rigid temporal time frame is inappropriate to the medical and forensic requirements of the management of SDHs in babies and infants.
- they do not fully take into account the range of appearances that may be seen on computerized tomography (CT) and magnetic resonance imaging (MRI), and the wider confidence limits in terms of timing that flow from those appearances with increasing experience of neuroimaging in infants (Kleinman 1998) and less reliance on data derived from adults (Scotti et al. 1977)
- the terms always require their own definition for non-medical audiences
- the terms may hold slightly, but significantly, different meanings for different medical disciplines
- even practitioners within one discipline, for example neuroradiology or neurosurgery, may not work to quite the same definition
- the macroscopic appearances and consistency of subdural haematomas of all ages, as found at time of evacuation, are frequently very different in babies and infants to those found in adults.

The *Oxford English Dictionary* (2002) describes the words 'acute' and 'chronic' when employed as descriptors of disease as follows:

Acute: coming sharply to a point or crisis of severity; opposed to chronic.

Chronic: lasting a long time, long continued, lingering, inveterate; opposed to acute.

These are clear meanings that have been in English usage in connection with disease since the 17th century. It seems to the present writer that a terminology is required that encompasses both subdural haemorrhage (the event), and subdural haematoma (the mass lesion); the clinical markers of timing; the imaging criteria of ageing; and the appearances found at surgical drainage. The ideal nomenclature would therefore link with events that can be known or discovered with some certainty even at an interval, such as changes in health status of the child and dates of diagnosis. These events would inter-relate with each other, which would correlate data from different sources and disciplines. This, in turn, would allow precision when such was appropriate, and approximation when that was all that could be achieved. The terms suggested are 'recent' and 'old'. These terms will be employed throughout this chapter, except when there are direct quotes from other sources and previously published work.

Another area that requires clarification and greater uniformity is in the description of abnormalities that are found in the subdural space on imaging, at operation, and at autopsy. Terms that are currently employed are: (1) haemorrhage; (2) haematoma; (3) collection; (4) effusion; (5) hygroma.

'Haemorrhage' refers to the event of bleeding, and does not imply any particular volume of residual blood. Indeed, often the greatest significance of such a finding lies in the detection of very small amounts of recently shed blood in the context of a severe encephalopathy, as seen on CT in the parafalcine area, or as described as thin layer subdural blood found at autopsy. Such lesions do not constitute important mass lesions, and therefore hardly justify the use of the term haematoma. The latter implies mass, and is used to describe both solid and liquid lesions resulting from haemorrhage and constituting some bulk or volume. The terms collection, effusion and hygroma describe liquid lesions that have mass, but that are not necessarily the result of haemorrhage. A volume of proteinaceous liquid over the brain resulting from meningitis or from rupture of cerebrospinal fluid (CSF) into the subdural space can be described as both a collection and an effusion, but neither would have had their origins in haemorrhage. Hygroma implies that the principal component is derived from CSF.

A collection or an effusion that is derived from bleeding can also be described as a haematoma. The importance of making a clear distinction between lesions of haemorrhagic and non-haemorrhagic origin is that bleeding has only two broad causations – natural (otherwise known as spontaneous), and traumatic. If, in a particular case, there is no natural cause for haemorrhage, then the causation must be trauma, either accidental or inflicted. It would therefore be preferable for haemorrhage to be used only to describe an event; haematoma could continue to describe solid or liquid mass lesions derived from blood products following a haemorrhage; collection and effusion should always be qualified as haemorrhagic or non-haemorrhagic, so as to distinguish between those arising from haemorrhage, traumatic or spontaneous, and those resulting from infection or other event. The importance of identifying that there has been subdural haemorrhage is often central to the recognition of the true origins of an infant's illness. The failure to identify a thin layer of parafalcine blood on the CT of an encephalopathic infant may result in the death or serious injury of that child or of a sibling in a subsequent episode of abuse.

Mechanisms of subdural haemorrhage

In the context of trauma, the following mechanisms are generally, if not universally, accepted as causes of SDH: (1) impact; (2) shaking; (3) penetration.

There is no scope for dispute that impact head trauma, and the very rarely encountered penetrating injuries, can cause SDH in infants. The principal current controversies are whether shaking, and in particular shaking alone, can cause SDH; and how much force is required to produce SDH by any means, with or without producing any traumatic brain injury.

IMPACT INJURY

The absence of external signs of head injury, skull fracture, or soft tissue scalp swelling in many cases of SDH (see Tables 9.2 and 9.3) probably results in the role of impact injury being underestimated. Certainly the incidence of identifiable impact injury increases in fatal cases where autopsy is carried out. Thus in one large series of 53 fatal cases, 81% of which had SDH, the overall incidence of impact injury, as evidenced by subscalp bruising, was 77%, even though only 36% had skull fractures. Of the 16 children aged 1 year or over, all had subscalp bruising, but only 3 had skull fractures. However, of the 37 children aged less than 1 year, only 27 had subscalp bruising and 16 had skull fractures (Geddes *et al.* 2001a). What is of greater interest is that of 30 fatal cases in infants aged less than 1 year (median age 73 days) who had recent subdural haemorrhage, only 12 had skull fractures; in 6 fatal cases without recent SDH, 4 had skull fractures, which were bilateral in 2 cases; in only 2 of the 30 infants with recent subdural haemorrhage was the lesion of sufficient size to be regarded as a space occupying lesion – neither of these infants had skull fractures (Geddes *et al.* 2001b).

Impact injury, as demonstrated by skull fracture, in those aged less than 1 year would therefore appear to be of greater relevance to the generation of fatal brain injury than to the production of SDH.

In a neuroradiological study of 14 infants sustaining serious brain injury resulting in cerebral infarction or death, all of whom had recent SDH, only 8 had unequivocal evidence of impact injury, and only 2 had skull fractures (Gilles and Nelson 1998). The paediatric neurosurgeon will not be surprised by the variable nature of externally detectable scalp swelling and bruising, as this is a very individual matter after surgical trauma. The layered structure of the scalp contributes to the occult nature of scalp bruising. CT on modern machinery with soft tissue settings optimized to babies and infants may be more successful at demonstrating evidence of impact injury (Jaspan *et al.* 2003).

SHAKING INJURY

Infants with enlarging old subdural haematomas, no skull fractures, and no or minimal encephalopathy, are very much more frequently encountered than those with thin layer recent SDHs and severe encephalopathy. Put together with the foregoing data, this provides further reason for looking beyond impact injury to the role of shaking in the genesis of SDH, as first propounded by Guthkelch (1971).

It is frequently stated that there is no proof that shaking produces the clinical, radiological and pathological findings that are attributed to it (David 1999). In pure experimental terms, this is a correct statement. Despite very natural reservations regarding confessions, most specialist medical, and no doubt some legal, practitioners have acquired experience of acknowledgements of shaking obtained in non-adversarial settings. However, in most cases such an acknowledgement is not forthcoming (Ludwig and Warman 1984); the same absence of history can also be true for impact injury. There is no perception of there being any clinical, radiological or pathological features that distinguish those cases in which there is an acknowledgement from those in which there is not. In many cases a carer will describe handling of a less-than-violent nature that is akin to shaking or to trivial impact. A study of 48 infants aged 1 month to 2 years (mean 7.85 months) who had experienced inflicted head injury, all of whom had subdural or subarachnoid haemorrhage, showed that 18 had no evidence of blunt impact injury to the head (Duhaime *et al.* 1987). All of 13 fatal cases

295

had SDH, and all of this subset had evidence of impact injury at autopsy, although such had only been apparent on initial clinical examination in 5 of them. Interestingly, the skull fractures found in 12 of the 48 cases from the whole series were predominantly occipital or occipito-parietal in location. Of the 38 cases for whom a history was available, there had been some shaking in 11, but in only 1 of these was shaking the sole insult. The investigators proceeded to investigate the forces thought to be generated by shaking by employing an age-appropriate model. The outcome of the physical experiments was that shaking produced angular accelerations below those produced by impact, leading to the conclusion that shaking alone was an improbable cause of the features found in infants thought to have experienced an inflicted shaking injury "at least in its most severe form".

A similarly cautious conclusion was that death was "not likely to occur from the shaking that occurs during play, feeding, or in a swing" (Duhaime *et al*. 1987). These measured remarks fall short of the assertion that is still sometimes made that this research demonstrated that shaking alone could not produce serious intracranial consequences. It has been central to the view that both shaking and impact are required, hence the introduction of the term shaking–impact injury (Bruce and Zimmerman 1989). The absence of readily discernible external signs of impact is explained by dissipation of force when the head strikes a soft surface, such as a mattress, yet the brain and its blood vessels undergo sudden angular deceleration resulting in SDH and a varying degree of cerebral dysfunction (Duhaime *et al*. 1998). Despite the near-obsessional emphasis that is placed on the role of models in the study of head injury, a recent review (Ommaya *et al*. 2002) leads the present writer to the conclusion that biomechanical models have failed to answer the questions that are posed by inflicted head injury in infants. The reverse engineering approach proposed, whereby after a head injury has been sustained the biomechanics are reconstructed and integrated with the biomedical data, may well be useful in the sphere of motor vehicle crashes, but is unlikely to be feasible in many cases of suspected inflicted head injury in infants. An interesting application of that approach was the demonstration that the forceful bouncing in a rocker of a 2-month old baby, who developed encephalopathy with subdural and retinal haemorrhages, was at a level that could only have represented an abusive act (San Lazaro *et al*. 2003).

In terms of child protection, a pragmatic approach is that the precise mechanism is only of importance if an innocent, accidental explanation for the medical findings is proposed by the carers. In the absence of any such explanation – such as the fall from the bed, the sudden deceleration of the motor vehicle carrying the child, the blow from the tail of the family dog, or the resuscitative shake – it may not be too important to identify precisely the method of mishandling that has caused the injuries, although it may acquire importance in forensic issues of intent. In terms of prevention, parents in the UK are now given the general advice never to shake a baby. It is self-evident, and a matter of common knowledge, that to deliberately cause an impact injury can only have the intention to cause pain and distress, and has the capacity to produce serious harm.

FORCE
The level of force required, however caused, remains the subject of debate and controversy.

A study of the neuropathology of 37 cases of fatal inflicted head injury in infants, 30 of whom had recent SDH, discovered that whereas diffuse traumatic axonal injury was very rare, being found in only two cases, 11 cases showed focal traumatic axonal damage in the cervico-medullary region (Geddes *et al.* 2001b). This led to the authors' supposition that "it may not be necessary to shake an infant very violently to produce stretch injury to its neuraxis", and that "the conditions that produce these [subdural and retinal] haemorrhages in infants . . . require fresh examination." Predictably this has been seized upon as evidence that non-abusive, normal handling can have serious or fatal consequences.

Close examination of the study reveals that there are no data within it to support these contentions, and in fact there are copious data to the contrary (Punt et al. 2004). Despite "full documentation, including clinical histories and witness statements" being available for all cases (Geddes et al. 2001a) the authors could not advance a single case in which a less than violent act had led to a fatal injury. There was ample evidence of injuries that are strongly associated with violence, in that 16/37 had skull fractures and 15/37 had serious injuries to other body parts. Those infants with neural lesions in the cervico-medullary region had a greater burden of other traumatic lesions (10/13) compared to the larger number of infants who did not have the cervico-medullary lesions (11/22). This can only imply that the focal cervico-medullary lesions are actually a marker for a greater, not lesser, degree of force having been visited upon these infants, contrary to the authors' supposition. Despite the lead author having acknowledged that the manner of handling that she envisaged was such that an onlooker witnessing the act would think, "My God, what are they doing to that child? Stop." (*R* v *Mark Andrew Cordice* 2001), this work is still cited as evidence that less-than-severe trauma is required in some cases (Geddes 2003). As it stands, there is no evidence that the application of any force that would be regarded as proper by a reasonable, responsible, average carer in the course of everyday childcare might produce SDH. This is appropriately expressed in a current international textbook of paediatric neurosurgery: namely, that "while controversy still exists as to the exact mechanism, most authors now agree that the forces necessary to cause this type of injury are far from trivial and in fact are considerable", and that "this sort of injury is unlikely to be inflicted 'accidentally' by well-meaning caretakers who do not know that their behavior can be injurious" (Duhaime and Christian 1999).

Further evidence regarding the forces required to produce SDH comes from a study of 100 consecutive cases of children aged less than 25 months who were admitted to hospital following head injury (Duhaime *et al.* 1992). Of these children, 24% had experienced inflicted head injury according to strict criteria, and a further 32% were suspicious. Of the 16% who had SDH, most (13/16) had sustained inflicted injury, and the only cases of accidental injury were children who had been involved in high-speed motor vehicle incidents. Another study of 66 children aged less than 37 months, all of whom had experienced SDH, distinguished between those children who had had abusive head injury (39/66), and those who had experienced head injury of accidental (15/66) or indeterminate (12/66) causation (Feldman *et al.* 2001). All of the cases of SDH associated with accidental injury had experienced identifiable trauma involving major forces.

It is frequently averred that the minimum force required to produce serious intracranial consequences is not known. Although in pure physical measurement terms this rather trite statement is correct, it is a matter of common knowledge, not restricted to those with medical qualifications, that there is a level of handling of babies and infants that has evolved in most cultures, such that the gentle handling of young children is intuitive, particularly if they are perceived to be unwell.

It has also been demonstrated in a large population-based study that the trivial domestic accidents that occur in even the best regulated households have benign outcomes (Warrington et al. 2001). Of a population of 11,466 infants aged less than 7 months, there were 3357 events in 2554 children: of these, 3202 falls led to 375 head injuries, 21 of which were associated with concussion or skull fracture. There were no serious consequences from head injuries involving minor forces. Of particular relevance was the finding that 1782 falls from beds or settees resulted in no head injuries, the only fracture of any type being that of a clavicle in one case. The data in this study are all the more powerful for being derived from the self-reporting of the carers.

A study of children aged less than 5 years who had fallen out of bed revealed that two of 176 episodes in the home, and one of 57 incidents in hospital, resulted in skull fracture, but none were associated with intracranial haemorrhage (Helfer et al. 1977). When children fall down stairs they rarely sustain intracranial injury: seven of 363 children sustained skull fractures, but none had intracranial haemorrhage or cerebral contusions (Joffe and Ludwig 1988). Five of 69 children aged less than 5 years (7%) experienced skull fractures, but only one developed a subdural haematoma (Chiavello et al. 1994). Of 61 children who fell from heights of not less than one storey, 17 (28%) had skull fractures but only one child developed a subdural haematoma (Barlow et al. 1983).

Interestingly, extradural haematomas in infants and toddlers typically result from minor impacts and very low-level falls, but are very seldom encountered in the context of inflicted head injury in this age group, despite the frequent suggestion by carers of children who have sustained SDHs and traumatic encephalopathy that there have been minor accidental impact injuries. None of 40 infants aged less than 2 years seen in a large French paediatric neurosurgical service on account of extradural haematoma had experienced inflicted injury (Leggate et al. 1989). Only two of 34 children aged 3 years or less (median age 15 months) with extradural haematomas, seen at a North American level-1 regional trauma centre, were diagnosed as having experienced abuse; this is contrasted with 28 of 59 children of the same age who were seen in the same 7-year time period with SDH who were diagnosed as having experienced abuse (Shugerman et al. 1996). The authors concluded that these findings were consistent with the concept that extradural haematomas were caused by brief linear contact forces, whereas SDHs were produced by high energy rotational acceleration/deceleration forces.

These studies, along with the common experiences of parents, belie the false, and more than faintly ludicrous, assertion of some pathologists that "nobody really knows how babies are injured" (Geddes et al. 2001b).

Two papers are regularly cited as evidence that low-level accidental falls in children may produce subdural and retinal haemorrhage with fatal (Plunkett 2001) or non-fatal consequences (Christian et al. 1999). Accurate reading of these papers does not support this application of the reported findings. One paper concerns fatal cases of head injury following falls from playground equipment (Plunkett 2001). Of 18 cases, only 5 were aged

TABLE 9.6
Summary of data in five fatal falls from playground equipment

Age (mo)	Injuries	Distance fallen (m)
12	Massive skull fracture + SDH	1.8
14	Severe brain swelling	0.5
17	Large SDH	1.5
20	Depressed skull fracture + SDH + RH	1.1
23	Large SDH + RH	0.7

SDH = subdural haemorrhage; RH = retinal haemorrhage.

less than 2 years, the youngest being 12 months. The author acknowledged that a weakness of the study was that not all cases were independently verified as being accidental: only one of the accidents in children aged less than 2 years was independently witnessed. Autopsies were not performed or were 'limited' in 3 of the 5 youngest children.

The findings in the 5 youngest children are summarized in Table 9.6, from which it is clear that the intracranial injuries sustained were not of a pattern generally seen in inflicted head injury in the first 2 years of life, with the possible exception of the youngest child who had sustained very extensive skull fractures.

The other paper (Christian *et al.* 1999) described 3 infants aged 7 to 13 months who all sustained unilateral retinal haemorrhages and ipsilateral SDHs in domestic accidents. The histories given indicate that all three infants had sustained substantial impacts.

It is a frank misrepresentation of these papers to imply that they support a notion that minor trauma or normal handling can produce SDH in babies and infants.

SHAKING AND THE OLDER CHILD
Although SDH associated with inflicted shaking–impact injury is seen most frequently in children in the first 2 years of life, it is occasionally encountered in older children. The case of an adult male of weight 44.3 kg and height 151 cm who experienced fatal brain swelling, diffuse axonal injury associated with an SDH and retinal haemorrhages as a consequence of repeated shaking at the hands of interrogators has been fully reported (Pounder 1997). The victim was shaken 12 times over the course of as many hours, in a way that left his head and neck free to move. On 10 occasions his clothes were gripped; on two occasions he was held by the shoulders. There was no evidence of neck injury, but there was extensive pectoral bruising.

As well as providing evidence that it must be possible to cause serious intracranial injury by shaking an older child, this case casts light on the absence of rib fractures or marks on the trunk in many younger children; it may be that some are gripped by their clothes.

REBLEEDING
Apart from fresh haemorrhage precipitated by transfontanelle taps or shunt insertion, many experienced paediatric neuroradiologists and neurosurgeons have encountered rebleeding. This writer's personal experience is that whenever rebleeding has been found, it has been in the context of very large, pre-existing older subdural haematomas that are being followed

by surveillance imaging. The rebleeding has always been within the cavity of the older haematoma; the more recent haemorrhage has not been large; the finding has not been associated with new neurological features; the child has been in a place of safety: there has been no trauma. There is no evidence that rebleeding causes encephalopathy (Showers 1999). It must be the case that if rebleeding can occur spontaneously it can also occur with minor, accidental trauma and normal activities.

It is of interest that when encephalopathy leads to the finding of recent SDH in the presence of older subdural haematomas, usually in a hitherto undiagnosed setting, the recent haemorrhages are frequently multiple and may be at sites other than the older haematomas, and are anatomically separate from those sites. This strongly suggests that this pattern of rebleeding is a different phenomenon and has a different causation, namely a further injury.

The source of the recent haemorrhage in cases of rebleeding is thought to be vascular subdural membranes (Uscinski 2002). It is often suggested that clinically silent SDH related to birth and delivery might generate subdural haematomas, which might be discovered at a later date and be mistakenly attributed to the consequences of inflicted injury; and that membranes arising from such haematomas might result in rebleeding that could be wrongly attributed to a further inflicted injury (Uscinski 2002). It is clear that for such an argument to be plausible the recent haemorrhage would necessarily need to be at the same site as the older subdural haematoma, and a subdural membrane would have to be present. MRI, if used appropriately and at the right time, has the capability to demonstrate the presence or absence of such subdural membranes (Jaspan *et al.* 2003). Clinical manifestations of encephalopathy, or the finding of recent, evolving cerebral contusions or multifocal recent SDHs on imaging, would go against a rebleeding phenomenon in the individual case.

The incidence of SDH related to birth is not known precisely. A large retrospective study of 583,340 live-born, singleton, first-born infants reported incidences of subdural or cerebral haemorrhage ranging from 2.9 per 10,000 infants born by spontaneous vaginal delivery to 7.3 per 10,000 infants born vaginally by use of both forceps and ventouse. For babies born by caesarean section the incidences ranged from 4.1 per 10,000 infants when there had been no prior labour, to 25.7 per 10,000 infants for caesarean delivery during labour following failed vaginal delivery (Towner *et al.* 1999).

The difficulties in projecting these findings to the setting of a case of putative, asymptomatic birth-related SDH are that the method of ascertainment employed codes from the *International Classification of Diseases, 9th Revision* (ICD-9), that did not permit distinction between subdural and intracerebral haemorrhage, and that all cases were diagnosed before the babies left hospital, suggesting that many, if not all, were in fact symptomatic. A more recent study of over 305,391 deliveries found incidences of SDH ranging from 1 per 10,000 for spontaneous vaginal deliveries to 7 per 10,000 for forceps- or ventouse-assisted deliveries (Wen *et al.* 2001).

A pilot study of 8 normally developing babies born to primigravida mothers, by uncomplicated spontaneous vaginal delivery at term, employed MRI during the first 4 days of life: 3 babies had small, supratentorial, parafalcine SDHs, and 1 baby had a tentorial notch haemorrhage (Holden *et al.* 1999). No baby had a convexity or parenchymal haemorrhage. Follow-up was achieved in 7 cases at an average of 3.9 years; normal growth and development were reported. The small size of the study, and the absence of any follow-up imaging, prohibits anything but the most general comments. However, the study provides justification for a larger prospective study with radiological and clinical follow-up. The pertinent question will be not so much the incidence of asymptomatic birth-related SDH, but more the location and outcome of any such haemorrhages.

It seems probable that the incidence will prove to be higher than had hitherto been held to be the case; if the haemorrhages resolve without issue, then the possibility of such haemorrhages being causative of future abnormalities can be disposed of once and for all.

THE DOUBTFUL ROLE OF PRE-EXISTING EXTRACEREBRAL CSF COLLECTIONS
Arachnoid cysts
It is well recognized that middle cranial fossa arachnoid cysts can infrequently be complicated by the development of cerebral convexity subdural CSF effusions (hygromas) and old subdural haematomas; it is exceptional for arachnoid cysts at other intracranial sites to be complicated in this way in the absence of surgical intervention. Typically such complications arise as a result of a relatively minor, but identifiable, impact injury to the head or even to the face. Any subdural haematoma is nearly always unilateral, and ipsilateral to the middle fossa arachnoid cyst. A subdural hygroma is a much more usual finding than a subdural haematoma.

A measure of how rare SDH must be as a complication of intracranial arachnoid cyst at any site is that a multicentre collaborative study of 285 children aged from birth to 15 years, encountered between 1980 and 1988 in 17 institutions spread across nine different European countries, reported no case of subdural haematoma (Oberbauer *et al.* 1992).

It is also noteworthy that the mean age of onset of symptoms was 6 years, which is substantially older than the age at which subdural haemorrhage and haematoma is usually encountered in childhood; although there was a peak in the first 2 years of life, this was due to cysts producing obstructive hydrocephalus. Two other single institution paediatric series of about the same era, one of 67 cases from Spain (Pascual-Castroviejo *et al.* 1991), and another of 40 cases from North America (Ciricillo *et al.* 1991) included no cases of SDH; presentation was at age less than 1 year in 55% in the former, and at a median age of 2 years in the latter. Looked at from another perspective, a series of 658 mixed paediatric and adult cases of subdural haematoma or hygroma contained 16 cases of middle fossa arachnoid cyst (2.4%), indicating that this is a rare underlying cause of SDH at any age. Furthermore, only two individuals of 89 (2.2%) with untreated cases of middle fossa arachnoid cyst who underwent a total of 94 MRI examinations showed any sign of haemorrhage on imaging (Parsch *et al.* 1997).

External hydrocephalus
The condition known as benign communicating infantile hydrocephalus is occasionally advanced as a factor that might predispose to SDH with minor trauma or normal handling, usually on the basis that the existence of such a state would render superficial bridging veins more likely to rupture in the event of trauma. However, there is no generally acknowledged agreement that this is indeed the case, either in recent child abuse literature (Kemp 2002)

or in current textbooks of paediatric neurology (Aicardi 1992) or neonatal neurology and neurosurgery (Whitelaw 2001). A lengthy analysis in a current textbook of paediatric neurosurgery does not lend great support to the view (Winston and Arnholz 1999).

In his own clinical practice, the present writer regularly followed infants with benign communicating hydrocephalus until the age of 12 months or even 2 years. Such children were followed clinically and by imaging up until the time that the anterior fontanelle closed. A very small number of infants were seen who had both enlarged subarachnoid spaces and fluid in the subdural space; on surgical exploration, the subdural fluid was invariably CSF. The only case that was encountered in which SDH developed was an infant who had sustained a well-documented fall from a substantial height, producing substantial soft tissue injury to the scalp and face. Case reports continue to appear purporting to describe subdural haematomas complicating benign communicating hydrocephalus, but frequently the collections have not been drained, or descriptions of the findings are incomplete, thus making it difficult to know whether the cases were ones of subdural haematoma or of hygroma (Ravid and Maytal 2003).

On present best evidence, opinions that rely upon pre-existing, asymptomatic, birth-related SDHs or arachnoid cysts, must be regarded as outside the mainstream of conventional wisdom. For any of these hypotheses to be applicable to a particular case, there will have to be evidence that the putative causative lesion was present prior to the development of the symptomatic subdural haematomas. In the case of arachnoid cysts and hydrocephalus this should be relatively simple to confirm or negate with certainty on the basis of correct interpretation of imaging and head circumference measurements.

With respect to perinatal SDH, the results of ongoing prospective studies are eagerly awaited, and, for the present, indirect evidence, such as appearances on imaging, the time course of changes in rate of head growth, the presence or absence of subdural membranes, the anatomical relation between recent haemorrhages and old haematomas, and clinical and radiological features of encephalopathy, will have to suffice.

THE EVEN MORE DOUBTFUL ROLE OF HYPOXIA

Babies and infants who undergo inflicted traumatic insults at the more severe end of the spectrum sustain parenchymal brain damage that is categorized variously as hypoxic, ischaemic or hypoxic–ischaemic. This is clear from clinical (Johnson *et al*. 1995), radiological (Gilles and Nelson 1998; Stevens *et al*. 1998a,b; Jaspan *et al*. 2003) and neuropathological studies (Geddes *et al*. 2001a,b), and from a correlative study (Kemp *et al*. 2003).

It has been suggested that the hypoxia could be the causative factor in the generation of SDHs and retinal haemorrhages (Geddes *et al*. 2003). The proposition is that a traumatic cervicomedullary lesion produces respiratory abnormalities that, in turn, produce global cerebral hypoxia and brain swelling. Hypoxia, brain swelling and raised central venous pressure then lead to leakage of blood from dural veins.

It is further suggested that, in combination with earlier work that demonstrated traumatic axonal damage at the cervicomedullary level (Geddes *et al*. 2001b), this would amount to a "unified hypothesis" (Geddes *et al*. 2003).

This "physiological" (Geddes *et al*. 2003) explanation is also advanced to suggest that infants with brain swelling, thin layer SDHs, and retinal haemorrhages, and no other evidence of trauma, may not have experienced injury at all, but have sustained a primary hypoxic event for which no cause can be identified. The difficulty with accepting this 'unified hypothesis' is that it is simply not supported by the facts contained in the studies concerned (Geddes *et al*. 2001b, 2003). In particular, the fetal/neonatal experimental model employed was inappropriate; the three cases of fatal inflicted head injury studied did not have the traumatic cervicomedullary lesions described in the earlier study; and brain swelling was present in only 5% of the fetal/neonatal models; the claim that the study provides a "physiological rather than a traumatic mechanism" for SDH is untenable, as no data of a physiological nature were acquired; there are no ophthalmological data. The 'unified hypothesis', as it stands, relies upon an unbroken chain that, on the authors' own data, simply does not exist, as argued by Punt et al. (2004). In an incomplete response to this critique, Geddes et al. (2004) further suggested that apnoea due to laryngeal spasm and gastro-oesophageal reflux, producing raised intrathoracic and central venous pressure, "would fit" their hypothesis. This assertion denies the experience of those caring for children in life. Babies born preterm may develop gastro-oesophageal reflux of a severity that requires surgical correction. The same population of babies frequently undergo concomitant neurosurgical surveillance, including neuroimaging, on account of post-haemorrhagic hydrocephalus, yet do not develop fatal brain swelling associated with subdural and retinal haemorrhages.

The scientific debate arising from this extension of the 'unified hypothesis' has inevitably been contested in legal proceedings, where it has been acknowledged by another neuro-pathologist that there is no evidence to support the contention (Squier 2004). Further, in a review of 297 cases of alleged infant homicide, the UK's Attorney-General did "not think it unfair to say that the Geddes theory has not been proven" (Attorney-General 2004). Subsequently, in the UK Court of Appeal, Geddes has "admitted under cross-examination that there was an error, previously unacknowledged, in her third paper [Geddes et al 2003]" (Dyer 2005). This saga has relevance to the whole interface between medical and legal practice that pervades the subject matter of this book. It is arguable that "retreat into non-disprovable hypotheses" (Kennedy 2005) is to enter the realm of the "fanciful" (Judge 2004) so far as to breach the strictures that should properly inhibit the medical expert tempted to "push a theory from the far end of the medical spectrum" (Royal College of Pathologists and Royal College of Paediatrics and Child Health 2004).

Management of subdural haemorrhage and haematoma
DIAGNOSIS AND PITFALLS
Management commences with diagnosis based upon imaging. Clinical presentations have been addressed in detail elsewhere (see Chapter 1), as have the intricacies of neuroimaging (Chapter 6), and will not be reiterated. However, it is appropriate to be reminded of the frequency with which an opportunity for earlier diagnosis is missed, and to explore some of the reasons for error.

In a population-based study (Jayawant *et al*. 1998), 4 of 33 infants had experienced previous physical abuse; all of these children died. In the same study, siblings of 6 of 17 infants with SDHs had been previously abused, and two had been concurrently abused.

Concurrent or serial abuse in twins has been frequently encountered in this writer's practice (personal observations, unpublished). In an institutional series (Stevens *et al*. 1998a,b) of 120 children with suspected inflicted head injury, 98% of whom had subdural haemorrhages or haematomas, 62 (52%) had been seen previously at a hospital; of these, 37 (60%) had displayed similar symptoms at the first presentation as at the occasion upon which the diagnosis was made, of whom 17 had shown evidence of trauma at the first presentation.

A frequent cause of diagnostic error is the nonspecific nature of the presentation with symptoms that are understandably mistaken for any of the incidental, infective illnesses to which babies and infants are prone. This is exacerbated by the transient, self-limiting evolution of the more mild cases. A particular source of error is the baby who presents in a fashion suggestive of bacterial meningitis, and who undergoes lumbar puncture that reveals a CSF that excludes that diagnosis, but which is bloodstained. There is a tendency to assume that the blood staining is spurious; when the baby improves, as is often the case, the matter is taken no further; the baby is discharged and thereby is exposed to the real risk of further injury with more serious consequences. In one study (Stevens *et al*. 1998a,b) of 120 children, 26 of 34 who had undergone lumbar puncture had bloodstained CSF that was sterile on culture, and a further 4 had xanthochromic CSF.

It is crucial that such children should undergo urgent radiological investigation by CT, looking specifically for recent SDH (Jaspan *et al*. 2003), and also competent fundoscopy by an ophthalmologist, even if the child's clinical state is improving. It is essentially illogical to conduct one test (lumbar puncture) to exclude a potentially damaging or fatal disease of the brain; to find that test to be negative, but possibly indicative of another disease of the brain with at least the same potential for disabling or lethal outcome; and then not to proceed to the test (CT) required to explore that alternative.

A further, and eminently avoidable, source of error lies in the use and abuse of imaging. Unfortunately a combination of factors continues to impede timely diagnosis, at least in the UK, dependent as it is on mostly non-specialist paediatric services.

The most common mistakes in respect of imaging are: (1) incomplete clinical information (e.g. the radiology request that states only "*?*fit"); (2) failure to ask the appropriate question (e.g. the radiology request that states only "*?*hydrocephalus"); (3) selection of inappropriate imaging modality (e.g. ultrasound instead of CT); (4) failure to image on an urgent basis; (5) incorrect interpretation of imaging (e.g. ultrasound performed by non-radiologists; CT or MRI reported by general radiologists).

The writer has encountered all of the above mistakes, and has known cases in which such errors have led to avoidable further injury, resultant disability, and death, either in the child or in a sibling, including cases of twins.

NEUROSURGICAL MANAGEMENT
Recent subdural haemorrhages
These are nearly always thin, and do not constitute mass lesions for which surgical evacuation is required. Management will be dictated by the severity of any associated encephalopathy, and will be directed at whatever medical measures are required to support vital functions, to control intracranial hypertension, and to halt traumatic seizures. The objective is to

minimize secondary brain insults. These matters are discussed in depth elsewhere (see Chapter 9). Many of these children will fulfil criteria that mandate discussion with a neuro-surgeon (Royal College of Surgeons 1999), and transfer to a children's intensive care unit with on-site neurosurgery (Royal College of Paediatrics and Child Health 2001). Such transfer will require the participation of a specialist paediatric transfer team (Royal College of Surgeons and British Orthopaedic Association 2000). Although the operative management of cranial trauma is often seen as falling within the remit of all neurosurgeons (Society of British Neurological Surgeons 2001), the totality of the special requirements of these very young children, and the need for age-appropriate multidisciplinary management (Royal College of Surgeons 1999), are more likely to be met by transfer to a specialist children's neuroscience service.

Only rarely will surgical evacuation be required. In the face of a baby with a rapidly deteriorating state due to cerebral compression from a recent subdural haematoma, it is some times possible to afford some relief as an interim measure by drainage through a subdural needle passed through the anterior fontanelle, or even through a diastased suture (Brill *et al.* 1985, Macdonald *et al.* 1994) as very often even a recent haematoma is part solid and part liquid. Formal evacuation and control of any active bleeding will require craniotomy undertaken by a team that is fully equipped, in every sense of the word, to manage a small child who is in an unstable physiological state (Westman and Davis 1999).

The role of invasive intracranial pressure monitoring and very aggressive measures to control intracranial hypertension, such as decompressive craniotomy (Cho *et al.* 1996), remains unclear, and there is no strong evidence base upon which to make management decisions. Seizure control can be difficult.

Old subdural haematomas
Many older subdural haematomas discovered by imaging will not be of a size that requires drainage, and can be followed clinically by neurodevelopmental reviews and serial measurements of head circumference, complemented by imaging by ultrasound, CT or MRI. Of these, 75% or more may never require operative intervention (Oi and Matsumoto 1988). There is, however, a strong argument in favour of removing some subdural fluid for diagnostic purposes. This is the approach favoured by the present writer in all but the smallest haematomas. By sampling the fluid and sending it for biochemical and microbiological examination, it will be possible to be more certain of its nature.

Even with modern imaging it may not be easy to distinguish between an old subdural haematoma and an effusion of non haemorrhagic origin. Such distinction is of great importance when considering any social or forensic investigation that may follow.

Diagnostic drainage can be performed satisfactorily in most cases via the anterior fontanelle employing either a special subdural needle or an 18 gauge lumbar puncture needle. The baby need not be sedated or anaesthetized for the procedure and is simply swaddled and held firmly by an assistant. The procedure can be performed in a side room with the same aseptic precautions that are employed for lumbar puncture. A point that is preferably at least 1.5 cm from the midline is selected so as to avoid the superior sagittal sinus. The needle is passed at an oblique angle through the scalp, and then, after a pause

TABLE 9.7
Results of operative treatment in 76 infants with old subdural haematomas or effusions*

| | n | Intelligence | | Died |
		Normal	Impaired	
Craniotomy	42	28	11	3
Subpleural shunt	34	29	4	1

*Till (1968).

to allow the baby to stop crying, onward through the tissue of the anterior fontanelle, which is moderately resistant. Subdural fluid is then drained passively until the flow ceases or until the baby becomes pale or unduly subdued. It is unwise to aspirate because of the danger of damaging brain tissue or a vein drawn into the needle. Most babies will tolerate drainage of up to 50 ml. It is not unusual for some CSF to emerge towards the end of the procedure because the arachnoid has been breached by the needle or by the original trauma. Most babies with an old subdural haematoma will have a degree of communicating hydrocephalus and a widened subarachnoid space.

If, as is usual, the haematoma is bilateral, both sides should be sampled and specimens sent to the laboratory for separate analysis. At the end of the procedure the needle is withdrawn, and the puncture site closed with a suture to prevent external leakage.

The indications for therapeutic, as opposed to diagnostic, drainage are empirical, but can be decided on an individual basis usually determined by features of raised intracranial pressure, macrocephaly, or sheer size on imaging. The simplest method of therapeutic drainage is by regular transfontanelle taps. Following the initial diagnostic needling, subdural taps are performed on a daily basis with drainage of the maximum volumes that the baby will tolerate. In the case of bilateral haematomas, alternate sides are tapped on alternate days. Evacuation can be encouraged by gentle digital pressure on the anterior fontanelle. Samples are sent to the microbiology laboratory on each occasion. Taps are continued until less than 10 ml is obtained on two successive days. The disadvantage of this regime is that it does involve some discomfort and distress for the child, and can be unnecessarily protracted. In the days before the development of CT it was recognized that if there was a depth of more than 1.5 cm between the frontal lobe and the inner table of the skull, then the haematoma was too great for definitive treatment by tapping (Till 1975). This simple guide, based upon CT or MRI still applies. There are also risks of infection and haemorrhage. The advantage is that the child avoids having an implanted device.

A reasonable balance is to employ subdural taps in order to provide prompt relief of symptomatic intracranial hypertension, and thereby allow the baby's general condition to improve; to allow heavily bloodstained fluid to become clearer and more suitable for shunting; and if after approximately 10 days the haematomas are not resolving, then to insert an implanted drain.

Some neurosurgeons prefer burr hole drainage. This has the advantage that a more extensive evacuation can be performed; the presence of any subdural membranes can be determined; and there may be less danger of iatrogenic haemorrhage. However, if there is marked macrocephaly due to very large haematomas, it is improbable that a shunt will be avoided. An intermediate approach is to insert an external subdural drain, and in one series of 16 infants thus treated, only 7 required an implanted shunt (Gaskill *et al*. 1991). Percutaneous placement of an external subdural drain via a Tuohy needle has been described as a prelude to insertion of a definitive implanted shunt (Ersahin and Mutluer 1995).

In those children for whom these temporary methods fail, a more definitive procedure will be required. In one series of 103 children managed initially by observation, percutaneous taps, burr hole drainage, or external subdural drainage, 73% ultimately required insertion of an implanted subdural–peritoneal shunt (Litofsky *et al*. 1993), and this remains the option preferred by most paediatric neurosurgeons. Up to the 1960s, and even into the 1970s, many surgeons performed wide craniotomies, open drainage, and also excised any subdural membranes. This was, however, major surgery, and was associated with morbidity and even mortality.

The rationale was dubious, and the procedure was replaced by insertion of internalized shunts, which initially comprised simple, non-valved, wide-bore, red rubber catheters inserted through bilateral posterior parietal burr holes, brought down via an intermediate incision in the nape of the neck, and inserted into the pleural cavity via a single incision on the posterior aspect of the trunk. The drains were removed after 6–12 weeks (Till 1975). A comparative study demonstrated clear advantages of this method over craniotomy (Table 9.7) (Till 1968).

The fine-bore silastic tubing used for ventricular shunts is now generally preferred, and, coincident with the move from ventriculo-atrial to ventriculo-peritoneal shunting for hydro-cephalus, the peritoneal cavity has replaced the pleural cavity. Another procedure that was introduced for resistant cases of subdural haematoma was lowering and advancement of the superior sagittal sinus. It has also passed into obscurity; of 16 children thus treated, 8 had normal intellectual development, 5 had learning difficulties; and 3 were borderline (Gutierrez et al. 1979).

The most commonly employed technique in current use by paediatric neurosurgeons is unilateral placement of a non-valved silastic shunt catheter inserted between the subdural space and the peritoneal cavity. A cranial reservoir is not generally employed. A cranial entry point is selected that is well away from a site that might be needed for insertion of any ventricular shunt that might be required in the future to treat hydrocephalus. It is best to create a small scalp flap rather than to have a linear incision overlying the shunt

Careful anchoring is required to reduce the risk of shunt migration. Postoperatively the child is followed clinically, with regular measurements of head circumference. At an interval of 6 months to 1 year, MRI is performed to confirm resolution of the haematomas, and the shunt is then removed to reduce the risk of late complications (see below).

Several authors have published results remarking on the effectiveness of unilateral shunting for bilateral subdural haematomas (Litofsky *et al*. 1993) despite apparent lack of communication on imaging (Aoki and Mauzawa 1988). Resolution of subdural haematomas has been observed as early as 1 month from shunt insertion, and is associated with expansion of the convexity subarachnoid space (Morota *et al*. 1995). In a large series of 168 cases of children undergoing subdural–peritoneal shunting for various reasons, complete resolution was observed at 3 months in 52%, and at 6 months in 95% (Sakka *et al.* 1997).

Reported complications of subdural–peritoneal shunting include proximal migration into the layers of the scalp (Pang and Wilberger 1980), or even intracranially (Todorow *et al.* 1982); infection necessitating early removal (Korinth *et al.* 2000); intracranial granuloma formation, with (Ono *et al.* 1983) or without (Korosue *et al.* 1981) infection; and bilateral subdural empyema with faecal flora implying large bowel perforation (Dan and Spiegelmann 1986). A major French paediatric neurosurgical service reported that revisional shunt surgery was required in 23% of 168 cases on account of either proximal catheter obstruction (14%) or malfunction related to surgical complication (9%) (Sakka *et al.* 1997).

In a North American series, 38 (51%) of 75 patients with subdural shunts did not have the device removed, and no adverse consequences were observed. On this basis the authors advised that elective removal of redundant shunts was not necessary (Litofsky *et al.* 1993). The Paris experience was that shunt removal was associated with minor complications in 7 (4%) of 168 cases, and more serious complications in 3 (1.7%) of 168 cases; the latter necessitated craniotomy for intracerebral haematoma in 1 case, and drainage of recurrent pericerebral collections in the other 2 cases (Sakka *et al.* 1997). The authors' observation that rigorous technique would reduce complications carried the implication that some adverse events could have been avoided.

A comparative retrospective study (Tolias *et al.* 2001) of 47 infants showed that 5 of 12 children undergoing taps as the initial treatment required some further alternative treatment, and 3/12 developed subdural infection. Alternatively, only 4 of 18 infants treated by burr hole drainage required further treatment, and 3/18 developed subdural infection. Those children treated by subdural–peritoneal shunting at any stage required no further treatment, and experienced no infections. Interestingly, only 3 out of 12 infants who underwent observational management required drainage. Although the high rate of infection among patients treated by taps or burr hole drainage indicates a failure of technique, there is an implication that when a shunt is likely to be needed, it is preferable to proceed rather than to prevaricate with taps.

General management

Inflicted head injury is a condition of such complexity that only a multidisciplinary team approach is appropriate. Unfortunately the child is at risk of falling between two stools, especially when there is transfer between hospitals in order to access specialist services. This is an area in which it is particularly important that all those specialists who treat children, fully understand and accept that they have wider responsibilities. Apart from the neurosurgical management of subdural haemorrhages and haematomas, and medical management of any encephalopathy, these children need full investigation to detect any causative natural disease process, and to exclude or confirm a diagnosis of inflicted head injury. Such investigation should be conducted according to a clear protocol (Kemp 2002), which should include: structured neuroimaging (Jaspan *et al.* 2003); radiographic skeletal survey; ophthalmic examination of the fundi by an ophthalmologist following pharmacological dilatation of the pupils; careful physical examination and full documentation of any external signs of

TABLE 9.8
Essential documents for preparation of medico-legal reports in cases of suspected inflicted head injury in children

Medical records from all hospitals attended
Nursing records from all hospitals attended
General practitioner records
Health visitor records
Personal child health record
Obstetric and birth records
NHS direct records
Ambulance records
Clinical, and where appropriate, autopsy photographs
Imaging*
Pathology material*
Witness statements
Transcripts of police interviews
Other medical reports

*Where relevant to speciality.

injury, and haematological and biochemical laboratory tests. These investigations will need to progress in concert with any therapeutic manoeuvres. Every effort should be made to obtain neuroimaging and skilled fundoscopy as soon as possible after admission, and before there has been any invasive neurosurgical intervention. This is particularly important in order to minimize the value of findings being vitiated by the effects of intervention or mounting intracranial hypertension. The child who is admitted on a Friday or over a public holiday should not have to wait upon the convenience of the hospital or the doctors.

Forensic aspects of subdural haemorrhages and haematomas
The possible forensic significance of these cases demands particularly fastidious attention to detail, including record keeping by all involved. The omission of investigations on the oft-pleaded basis that they are "not needed to treat the patient" is unacceptable, as an incomplete contemporary exploration may create considerable problems for the child and for the family, as well as impeding any independent experts who may be required to prepare reports and opinions for agencies and for the courts. It is in the character of the condition that it will initially present to a non-specialist who, in the less severe cases, may take on the total burden of investigation, yet the evidence is nearly always of a nature that requires specialist analysis and interpretation. Failure to involve the appropriate specialists can result in over-diagnosis of inflicted head injury as well as under-recognition.

The critical points at issue are: (1) natural disease versus trauma; (2) accidental trauma versus inflicted trauma; (3) mechanism; (4) force; (5) timing.

Except for the last, these have already been addressed under the heading of mechanisms (see above). In determining the often central matter of timing, it is useful to remember that it is most improbable that an event that produced SDH at any time after birth would not be associated with some disturbance of brain function that would be reflected in at least some

309

transient change in the child's behaviour, such as would be apparent to a carer or other person who knew the child in health, even if that person did not know what had befallen the child. The nature, extent and duration of such change would be at some point on a spectrum that would reflect the severity of brain dysfunction. Careful histories from all those who have had contact with the child is required. This should be complemented by a systematic review of all available records. These may be extensive (Table 9.8) and held in a variety of sites, but may well reveal highly pertinent data of a positive or negative nature. Agencies seeking such documents should also remember that all original laboratory and radiology reports may not necessarily be filed within the clinical notes, especially if the child has been transferred between hospitals, or has died. It may be necessary to request that a search be made of laboratory computers and radiology department files to ensure complete discovery. Some UK hospitals file Emergency Department records separately from the main notes. Newborn records may be found either in the mother's obstetric notes, or in a separate folder in the name of the baby. The family name of the child may not match that of the mother, or the name given at birth. Review of these documents may identify points in time at which the child was probably in an injured, or uninjured, state, as demonstrated by patterns of behaviour.

Retrieval of head circumference measurements from original sources and construction of growth curves may be a guide to the development of old subdural haematomas. It is preferable to reconstruct the curves rather than to rely upon those made by others, so as to ensure precision, uniformity and appropriate adjustments for preterm or post-term birth.

The principles of preparing medical reports for the courts can be summarized as follows: (1) thorough review of documents; (2) explain technical terms; (3) remain within area of expertise; (4) objectivity; (5) consideration of alternative facts; (6) reference to established evidence; (7) effects of new hypotheses; (8) awareness of the standard of proof that applies to the proceedings; (9) rules of privilege and disclosure; (10) consistency; (11) independence.

Rehabilitation

The high incidence of long-term sequelae is such that a secure arrangement for prolonged neurodevelopmental surveillance is essential. There are very real dangers that the infant who appears to have made a good physical recovery will be dropped from follow-up, and that the late neuropsychological sequelae will go unrecognized; the subsequent learning difficulties and behavioural problems may be wrongly attributed, with serious consequences for the child, the carers, and probably society, at a later date.

By 2–3 months atrophy is well established. Areas of contusion and hypoxia–ischaemia have evolved into cysts. Subdural haemorrhages should be clearing.

Any recovery in appearance will have commenced by 6 months. Later scans may be helpful for further prognosis and planning for support, care and education.

REFERENCES

Aicardi J (1992) Non-traumatic pericerebral collections. In: *Diseases of the Nervous System in Childhood*. London: Mac Keith Press, pp. 319–320.

Aoki N, Masuzawa H (1988) Bilateral chronic subdural hematomas without communication between the hematoma cavities: treatment with unilateral subdural-peritoneal shunt. *Neurosurgery* **22:** 911–913.

Attorney General (2004) The review of infant death cases following the Court of Appeal decision in the case of *R v Cannings*. The Legal Secretariat to the Law Officers. (online at: http://www.lslo.gov.uk).

Barlow B, Niemirska M, Gandhi RP, Leblanc W (1983) Ten years of experience with falls from a height in children. *J Pediatric Surg* **18:** 509–511.

Brill CB, Jarath V, Black P (1985) Occipital interhemispheric acute subdural hematoma treated by lambdoid suture tap. *Neurosurgery* **16:** 247–251.

Bruce DA, Zimmerman RA (1989) Shaken impact syndrome. *Pediatr Ann* **18:** 482–484.

Caffey J (1972) On the theory and practice of shaking infants. Its potential residual effects of permanent brain damage and mental retardation. *Am J Dis Child* **124:** 161–169.

Chiavello CT, Christoph RA, Randall Bond G (1994) Stairway related injuries in children. *Pediatrics* 94: 679–681.

Cho D, Wang Y, Chi C (1996) Decompressive craniotomy for acute shaken/impact baby syndrome. *Pediatr Neurosurg* **23:** 192–198.

Christian CW, Taylor AA, Hertle RW, Duhaime A-C (1999) Retinal hemorrhages caused by accidental household trauma. *J Pediatr* **135:** 125–127.

Ciricillo SF, Cogen PH, Harsh GR, Edwards MS (1991) Intracranial arachnoid cysts in children. A comparison of the effects of fenestration and shunting. *J Neurosurg* **74:** 230–235.

Dan M, Spiegelmann R (1986) Mixed bacterial subdural empyema complicating subdural peritoneal shunt. *Acta Neurochir* **81:** 77–78.

David TJ (1999) Shaken baby (shaken impact) syndrome: non-accidental head injury in infancy. *J R Soc Med* **92:** 556–561.

de San Lazaro C, Harvey R, Ogden, A (2003) Shaking infant trauma induced by misuse of a baby chair. *Arch Dis Child* **88:** 632–634.

Duhaime A-C, Christian C (1999) Nonaccidental trauma. In: Choux M, Di Rocco C, Hockley A, Walker M, editors, *Pediatric Neurosurgery*. London: Churchill Livingstone, pp. 373–379.

Duhaime A-C, Gennarelli TA, Thibault LE, Bruce DA, Margulies SS, Wiser R (1987) The shaken baby syndrome. A clinical, pathological, and biochemical study. *J Neurosurg* **66:** 409–415.

Duhaime AC, Alario AJ, Lewander WJ, Schut L, Sutton LN, Seidi TS, Nudelman S, Budenz D, Hertle R, Tsiaras W, Loporchio S (1992) Head injury in very young children: mechanisms, injury types, and ophthalmologic findings in 100 hospitalized patients younger than 2 years of age. *Pediatrics* **90:** 179–185.

Duhaime A-C, Christian CW, Rorke LB, Zimmerman RA (1998) Nonaccidental head injury in infants – the "shaken-baby syndrome". *N Eng J Med* **338:** 1822–1829.

Dyer C (2005) Court hears shaken baby cases. *BMJ* **330:** 1463.

Ersahin Y, Mutluer S (1995) A method for continuous external drainage in the management of infantile subdural collections. *Child's Nerv Syst* **11:** 418–420.

Feldman KW, Bethel R, Shugerman RP, Grossman DC, Grady MS, Ellenbogen RC (2001) The cause of infant and toddler subdural hemorrhage: a prospective study. *Pediatrics* **108:** 636–646.

Gaskill SJ, Oakes WJ, Marlin AE (1991) Continuous external drainage in the treatment of subdural hematomas of infancy. *Pediatr Neurosurgery* **17:** 121–123.

Geddes JF (2003) Commentary to Kemp AM, Stoodley N, Cobley C, Coles L, Kemp KW. Apnoea and brain swelling in non-accidental head injury. *Arch Dis Child* **88:** 472–476.

Geddes JF, Hackshaw AK, Vowles GH, Nickols CD, Whitwell HL (2001a) Neuropathology of inflicted head injury in children I. Patterns of brain damage. *Brain* 124: 1290–1298.

Geddes JF, Vowles GH, Hackshaw AK, Nickols CD, Scott IS, Whitwell HL (2001b) Neuropathology of inflicted head injury in children II. Microscopic brain injury in infants. *Brain* **124:** 1299–1306.

Geddes JF, Tasker RC, Hackshaw AK, Nickols CD, Adams GGW, Whitwell HL, Scheimberg I (2003) Dural haemorrhage in non-traumatic infant deaths: does it explain the bleeding in 'shaken baby syndrome'? *Neuropathol Appl Neurobiol* **29:** 14–22.

Geddes JF, Tasker RC, Adams GGW, Whitwell HL (2004) Violence is not necessary to produce subdural and retinal haemorrhage: a reply to Punt et al. *Pediatr Rehabil* **7:** 261-265.

Gilles EE, Nelson MD (1998) Cerebral complications of nonaccidental head injury in childhood. *Pediatr Neurol* **19:** 119–128.

Guthkelch AN (1971) Infantile subdural haematoma and its relationship to whiplash injuries. *BMJ* 2: 430–431.

Gutierrez FA, McLone DG, Raimondi AJ (1979) Physiopathology and a new treatment of chronic subdural hematoma in children. *Child's Brain* **5:** 216–232.

Helfer RE, Slovis TL, Black M (1977) Injuries resulting when small children fall out of bed. *Pediatrics* **60:** 533–535.

Holden KR, Titus O, Van Tassel P (1999) Cranial magnetic resonance imaging examination of normal term neonates: a pilot study. *J Child Neurol* **14:** 708–710.

Jaspan T, Griffiths PD, McConachie NS, Punt J (2003) Neuroimaging for non-accidental head injury in childhood: a proposed protocol. *Clin Radiol* **58:** 44–53.

Jayawant S, Rawlinson A, Gibbon F, Price J, Schulte J, Sharples P, Sibert JR, Kemp AM (1998) Subdural haemorrhages in infants: population based study. *BMJ* **317:** 1558–1561.

Joffe MD, Ludwig S (1988) Stairway injuries in children. *Pediatrics* **82:** 457–461.

Johnson DL, Boal D, Baule R (1995) The role of apnea in nonaccidental head injury. *Pediatr Neurosurg* **23:** 305–310.

Judge LJ (2004) *R v Cannings* EWCA Crim 1 [2004] 1 WLR 2607.

Kemp AM (2002) Investigating subdural haemorrhages in infants. *Arch Dis Child* **86:** 98–102.

Kemp AM, Stoodley N, Cobley C, Coles L, Kemp KW (2003) Apnoea and brain swelling in non-accidental head injury. *Arch Dis Child* **88:** 472–476.

Kennedy C (2005) Inflicted head injury in infancy and the wisdom of King Solomon. *Dev Med Child Neurol* **47**: 3 (editorial).

Kleinman PK (1998) Head trauma. In: Kleinman PK, ed. *Diagnostic Imaging of Child Abuse 2nd edn.* St Louis: Mosby, pp. 285–342.

Korinth MC, Lippitz B, Mayfrank L, Gilsbach JM (2000) Sub-atrial and subdural–peritoneal shunting in infants with chronic subdural fluid collections. *J Pediatr Surg* **35:** 1339–1343.

Korosue K, Tamaki N, Matsumoto S, Ohi Y (1981) Intracranial granuloma as an unusual complication of subdural peritoneal shunt. Case report. *J Neurosurg* **55:** 136–138.

Leggate JS, Lopez-Ramos N, Genitori L, Lena G, Choux M (1989) Extradural haematoma in infants. *Br J Neurosurg* **3:** 533–540.

Litofsky NS, Raffel C, McComb JG (1993) Management of symptomatic chronic extra-axial fluid collections in pediatric patients. *Neurosurgery* **31:** 445–450.

Ludwig S, Warman M (1984) Shaken baby syndrome: a review of 20 cases. *Ann Emerg Med* **13:** 104–107.

Macdonald RL, Hoffman HJ, Kestle JR, Rutka JT, Weinstein G (1994) Needle aspiration of acute subdural hematomas in infancy. *Pediatr Neurosurg* **20:** 73–77.

McKissock W, Richardson A, Bloom WH (1960) Subdural haematoma. A review of 389 cases. *Lancet* **i:** 1365–1369.

Morota N, Sakamoto K, Kobayashi N, Kitazawa K, Kobayashi S (1995) Infantile subdural fluid collection: diagnosis and postoperative course. *Child's Nerv Syst* **11:** 459–466.

Oberbauer RW, Haase J, Pucher R (1992) Arachnoid cysts in children: a European co-operative study. *Child's Nerv Syst* **8:** 281–285.

Oi S, Matsumoto S (1988) Natural history of subdural effusion in infants. *J Pediatr Neurosci* **4:** 15–24.

Ommaya AK, Goldsmith W, Thibault L (2002) Biomechanics and neuropathology of adult and paediatric head injury. *Br J Neurosurg* **16:** 220–242.

Ono J, Mimaki T, Okada S, Yamanishi Y, Morimoto K, Shimada N, Yabuuchi H (1983) Bilateral intracranial granulomas as a complication of infected subdural peritoneal shunt. *Brain Dev* **5:** 499–503.

Oxford English Dictionary, 2nd edn. (2002) CD-ROM. Version 3.0. Oxford: Oxford University Press.

Pang D, Wilberger JE (1980) Upward migration of peritoneal tubing. *Surg Neurol* **14:** 363–364.

Parsch CS, Krauss J, Hofmann E, Meixensberger J, Roosen K (1997) Arachnoid cysts associated with subdural hematomas and hygromas: analysis of 16 cases, long-term follow-up, and review of the literature. *Neurosurgery* **40:** 483–490.

Pascual-Castroviejo I, Roche MC, Martinez Bermejo A, Arcas J, Garcia Blazquez M (1991) Primary intracranial arachnoidal cysts. A study of 67 childhood cases. *Child's Nerv Syst* **7:** 257–263.

Plunkett J (2001) Fatal pediatric head injuries caused by short-distance falls. *Am J Forensic Med Pathol* **22:** 1012.

Pounder DJMP (1997) Shaken adult syndrome. *Am J Forensic Med Pathol* **18:** 321–324.

Punt J, Bonshek RE, Jaspan T, McConachie NS, Punt N Ratcliffe JM (2004) The 'unified hypothesis' of Geddes et al. is not supported by the data. *Pediatr Rehabil* **7:** 173-184.

R v Mark Andrew Cordice (2001) Heard in the Crown Court at Leeds, UK in March 2001 before the Honourable Mr Justice Owen: Summing-up and Verdict.

Ravid S, Maytal J (2003) External hydrocephalus: a probable cause for subdural hematoma in infancy. *Pediatr Neurol* **28:** 139–141.

Royal College of Pathologists and Royal College of Paediatrics and Child Health (2004) Sudden unexpected death in infancy. A multi-agency protocol for care and investigation. London: Royal College of Pathologists. (online at: http://www.rcpath.org and www.rcpath.org and http://www.rcpch.ac.uk.

Royal College of Paediatrics and Child Health (2001) *Guidelines for Good Practice. Early Management of Patients with a Head Injury.* London: Royal College of Paediatrics and Child Health.

Royal College of Surgeons (1999) *Report of the Working Party on the Management of Patients with Head Injuries.* London: Royal College of Surgeons of England.

Royal College of Surgeons and British Orthopaedic Association (2000) *Better Care for the Severely Injured. A Joint Report from the Royal College of Surgeons of England and the British Orthopaedic Association.* London: Royal College of Surgeons of England.

Sakka L, Cinalli G, Sainte-Rose C, Renier D, Zerah M, Pierre-Kahn A (1997) Subduro-peritoneal shunting in children. *Child's Nerv Syst* **13:** 487.

Scotti G, Terbrugge K, Melancon D, Belanger G (1977) Evaluation of the age of subdural hematomas by computerized tomography. *J Neurosurg* **47:** 311–315.

Showers J (1999) Never never never shake a baby. The challenge of shaken baby syndrome. In: Proceedings of the Second National Conference on Shaken Baby Syndrome, September 1998, Salt Lake City, Utah. Alexandria, VA: National Association of Children's Hospitals and Related Institutions, p. 22.

Shugerman RP, Paez A, Grossman DC, Feldman KW, Grady MS (1996) Epidural hemorrhage: is it abuse? *Pediatrics* **97:** 664–668.

Society of British Neurological Surgeons (2001) *Safe Paediatric Neurosurgery 2001.* Dundee: Society of British Neurological Surgeons.

Squier W (2004) In *R v Mark Douglas Latta.* Heard in the Crown Court at Winchester, UK in March-April 2004 before the Honourable Mr. Justice Grigson.

Stevens K, Jaspan T, Holt JC, Bagnall MJC, Punt JAG (1998a) Social, clinical and medicolegal aspects of cranial trauma in cases of suspected non-accidental injury. *Child's Nerv Syst* **14:** 679. (Abstract).

Stevens K, Jaspan T, Holt JC, Bagnall MJC, Punt JAG (1998b) Neuro-imaging of non-accidental injury. *Child's Nerv Syst* **14:** 679–680. (Abstract).

Till K (1968) Subdural haematoma and effusion in infancy. *BMJ* **3:** 400–402.

Till K (1975) *Paediatric Neurosurgery.* Oxford: Blackwell.

Todorow S, Happe M, Petersen D (1982) Migration of a subdural-peritoneal shunt into the interhemispheric space. Case report. *Neurosurgical Review* **5:** 25–26.

Tolias C, Sgouros S, Walsh AR, Hockley AD (2001) Outcome of surgical treatment for subdural fluid collections in infants. *Pediatr Neurosurg* **33:** 194–197.

Towner D, Castro MA, Eby-Wilkens E, Gilbert WM (1999) Effect of mode of delivery in nulliparous women on neonatal intracranial injury. *N Eng J Med* **341:** 1709–1714.

Uscinski R (2002) Shaken baby syndrome: fundamental questions. *Br J Neurosurg* **16:** 217–219.

Warrington SA, Wright CM, ALSPAC Study Team (2001) Accidents and resulting injuries in premobile infants: data from the ALSPAC study. *Arch Dis Child* **85:** 104–107.

Wen SW, Liu S, Kramer MS, Marcoux S, Ohlsson A, Sauve R, Liston R (2001) Comparison of maternal and infant outcomes between vacuum extraction and forceps delivery. *Am J Epidemiology* **153:** 103–107.

Westman HR, Davis PJ (1999) Anesthesia for neurosurgery. In: Albright AL, Pollack IF, Adelson PD, eds. *Principles and Practice of Pediatric Neurosurgery,* New York: Thieme, pp. 1249–1274.

Weston JT (1968) The pathology of child abuse. In: Heifer RE, Kempe CH, eds. *The Battered Child.* Chicago: University of Chicago Press, pp. 77–100.

Whitelaw A (2001) Neonatal hydrocephalus – clinical assessment and non surgical treatment. In: Levene MI, Chervenak FA, Whittle MJ, eds. *Fetal and Neonatal Neurology and Neurosurgery.* London: Churchill Livingstone, p. 741.

Winston KR, Arnholz D (1999) Extracerebral fluid collections. In: Albright AL, Pollack IF, Adelson PD, editors. *Principles and Practice of Pediatric Neurosurgery.* New York: Thieme, pp. 261–269.

313

10
NON-SURGICAL TREATMENT OF ACUTE ENCEPHALOPATHIES

K Kamath Tallur, Robert A Minns and J Keith Brown

The infant or child with a non-accidental head injury (NAHI) may present to the emergency department as a very sick child and it may not even be obvious that the pathology is in the head. Absence of a history and external signs of trauma means that the presentation may be of a nonspecific acute encephalopathy. The diagnosis may seem obvious after imaging, but differential diagnoses of threatened cot death, meningitis, septicaemia, encephalitis or metabolic disease may all seem possible.

The neurointensive management regime is independent of aetiology, as one does not know the cause when the child presents initially. In the management of the critically ill child the diagnosis and treatment need to run concurrently.

A well-sequenced, methodical approach to the emergency care of the seriously ill or injured infant (e.g. Advanced Paediatric Life Support, Mackway-Jones et al. 2001) will go a long way to preventing secondary brain damage from hypoxia or ischaemia, hypoglycaemia, sepsis, and raised intracranial pressure (ICP) (Fig. 10.1).

Supportive treatment
The first thing to be considered is what is often termed 'vital life supportive treatment', e.g. maintenance of airway, treatment of shock (circulatory support), control of fits, reduction of raised ICP, reversal of hypoglycaemia and secondary homeostatic defects (e.g. renal support), and provision of 'comfort care' (e.g. sedation, feeding). The second consideration is to arrive at a diagnosis regarding the cause of the acute encephalopathy. This is essential in order that specific treatment may be instituted, as in bacterial meningitis, diabetes, herpes simplex encephalitis, poisoning, or metabolic disease. The exact diagnosis may need several days or weeks to be confirmed and in the meantime the child may have recovered.

Nursing the unconscious patient
Regular changes of position are important to avoid pressure sores and positional deformity. Thus, physiotherapy is essential in the acute stage. Positional deformities in permanent brain damage may become more serious than those caused by spasticity. Pressure sores over the occiput and bilateral fixed equinus do not speak of good care.

No food must be attempted orally in any child with impaired consciousness level. In the initial stages a nasogastric tube is passed and the stomach emptied. H_2-receptor antagonists such as ranitidine or sucralfate or proton pump inhibitors such as omeprazole are required

Airway	Open and maintain airway
Breathing	Assess breathing. Administer high-flow (15 l/min) oxygen if breathing spontaneously, then assess work of breathing, efficacy of breathing, effect of respiratory failure on other physiology
	Intubate and ventilate under the following circumstances: 1. Inadequate/ ineffective breathing; 2. Absent airway protective reflex (cough or gag reflex); 3. Unresponsive child (e.g.GCS <8 = P on AVPU scale, see below); 4. Clinical signs of impending herniation
Circulation	Assess heart rate, pulse volume and perfusion (capillary refill and skin temperature), blood pressure. Establish intravenous or intraosseous access, bloods for FBC, clotting, glucose; cross-match if injury suspected; blood culture if sepsis suspected. Treat shock
Disability	Assess consciousness level (AVPU): A – Alert
	V – responds to Voice
	P – responds to Pain
	U – Unresponsive
	Assess posturing; check pupillary response; check blood sugar. Treat hypoglycaemia with 5 ml/kg 10% dextrose (<3mmol/l)
Exposure	Temperature, rash, injuries, signs of cardiac failure. (Weight is estimated pre-arrival of the child. Arterial blod gas / cap blood gas / lactate.)

History and examination (e.g. history of traumatic event, epilepsy, drugs, travel, social issues, etc.)

Investigation for diagnosis of a nonspecific encephalopathy

Imaging: Initially, CT of brain (trauma, tumour, infection, oedema); later, MRI

Infection:

Blood: White cell count, ESR, CRP, bacterial, viral, fungal cultures, PCR (e.g. meningococcal), request for – rickettsia, mycoplasma, toxoplasma, mycobacteria, protozoa, leptospira, listeria, etc, store serum for paired titres, antigen/antibody titres (e.g. latex agglutination, Elisa, immunofluorescence)

CSF: Leukocytes with differential, protein and glucose, gram stain and culture (bacterial and viral), viral PCR (e.g. herpes simplex), agglutination tests, oligoclonal antibodies. Mantoux for tuberculosis

Toxicity:

Exogenous: e.g. urinary toxicology screen
Endogenous: glucose (e.g. hypoglycaemia in hyperinsulinism, glycogen storage disorders, hyperglycaemia in diabetic ketoacidosis) metabolic screen (e.g. lactate, ammonia, organic and amino acids, CSF lactate and glycine), hepatic function (hepatic encephalopathy)

Hypoxia–ischaemia:

Trauma and evidence of multiorgan failure (e.g. requirement of inotropic support for myocardial dysfunction – ECG/echo, renal dysfunction – renal function, urinary electrolytes)

Supportive investigations and monitoring the coma

Bedside: Blood gas, sugar, fluid balance

Haematology: Full blood count, coagulation screen, blood group and type

Biochemistry: Urea + electrolytes, sugar, calcium, magnesium, antiepileptic drug levels

Cerebral: EEG/CFAM, Doppler cerebral blood flow

Urine: Output (catheterize), electrolytes, osmolality, culture

Monitor:

Monitoring to prevent secondary insult
Raised ICP, critical cerebral perfusion pressure, AVDO₂, hypotension/hypertension, pyrexia, hypoxia, maintenance of homeostasis, chest X-ray, ECG, CVP±Wedge

Medicolegal investigations *(if relevant)*:

Skeletal survey, clinical photographs, retinal photographs, etc.

Management of homeostatic abnormalities

Specific management of meningitis, seizures, subdural haemorrhage, etc.

Figure 10.1. Binary approach to management of acute encephalopathy.

before enteral feeding is established or if blood is aspirated (Yang and Lewis 2003). Nutrition should be commenced early and maintained, otherwise the resultant metabolic upset will further aggravate the child's condition. Care must be taken that the nasogastric tube is not in the trachea or oesophagus. Large bolus feeding must be avoided, and nasojejunal tubes may be tolerated where nasogastric feeds fail. Care must be taken with parenteral nutrition as certain very high glycine containing amino acid preparations may cause an encephalopathy. Fat preparations must be used cautiously in the presence of acidosis and coagulopathy, otherwise hyperviscosity and haemorrhagic infarction may result.

Regular oral hygiene and eye care should be practised. Artificial tear solutions or gelprem are required to prevent corneal drying in paralysed patients. Attention should also be paid to the presence of abdominal distension due to ileus (treated with a prokinetic, e.g. domperidone or low-dose erythromycin), severe constipation (treated with lactulose, senna, phosphate enema and fibre feeds), gastro-intestinal bleeding or violent injury to the viscera.

Innate neurocompensatory mechanisms

The brain has a whole series of compensatory mechanisms to protect itself and in acute encephalopathies will:

- Hyperventilate to reduce the pCO_2
- Secrete antidiuretic hormone to reduce brain water
- Produce adenosine to reduce cellular metabolism
- Produce corticotropin (ACTH) and adenosine, both of which have an anticonvulsant action
- Increase cerebral perfusion pressure – Cushing response
- Increase blood glucose as substrate for anaerobic metabolism.

Practical treatment principles

Treatment is in large part enhancement of these natural compensatory mechanisms. The treatment of acute encephalopathies is based on the maxim 'treat what is treatable', that is:

- Treat infection
- Treat raised ICP
- Control seizures
- Maintain cerebral perfusion
- Maintain oxygenation
- Maintain cerebral metabolism
- Maintain homeostasis
- Other specific treatments.

Treatment of infection

This is not considered in detail in this chapter – only some general principles relating to therapy will be considered here. The treatment of meningitis is the treatment of an acute encephalopathy, not simply the choice of antibiotic. It is usual practice in the early stages of management of any acute encephalopathy of uncertain origin to cover with a third generation cephalosporin and acyclovir. So, the initial therapy is now modified into ceftriaxone

316

(100 mg/kg/b.d.) or cefotaxime (300 mg/kg/day). Acyclovir is given in a dose of 7.0–10.0 mg/kg 8 hourly (30 mg/kg/day) in adults; 500 mg/m^2/dose hourly in infants and children; and 20 mg/kg/dose up to 8 hourly depending on the gestation in the newborn infant for 5 days on suspicion while investigations continue: if Herpes encephalitis is confirmed then at least 3 weeks' therapy is indicated. Penicillin (100,000 to 400,000 IU/kg/day) is still of value as an adjuvant for group B streptococcal and pneumococcal meningitis in Europe but not in Africa. In areas with known resistant strains vancomycin is indicated. The death rate and disability rate in pneumococcal meningitis leave no room for complacency or for differences of opinion between clinicians and microbiologists as to antibiotic policy. The oft-quoted antagonism between bactericidal and bacteristatic antibiotics does not seem to be a problem in clinical practice, when for 30 years a combination of penicillin and chloramphenicol was the most commonly prescribed and a successful therapy. Although effective if they penetrate into the cerebrospinal fluid (CSF), the cephalosporins do not penetrate in all cases. Like penicillin, they penetrate best in inflamed meninges, and concentrations can vary from 3–30 μg on the same dose. Brain abscess is often due to more than one organism but it should always be assumed to include anaerobes such as microaerophilic streptococci or bacteroides and should include metronidazole in the antibiotic cocktail.

These new cephalosporin derivatives have overcome the need for intrathecal therapy in the common meningitides although it is still needed in some cases of subdural empyemas, gram negative ventricultis, coagulase negative *Staphylococcus epidermidis* ventriculitis after shunt surgery and ventriculitis with methicillin-resistant *Staphylococcus aureus* (MRSA), when a CSF reservoir inserted into the lateral ventricles is then necessary. Intraventricular antibiotics include flucloxacillin. This is cell-wall active and therefore blocked by the bacterium discarding the cell wall (L forms). It may not penetrate mucoid colonies. Beta-lactamase production will inhibit many of the penicillins. In combination with gentamicin, which acts on cell protein synthesis, we did not have a single fatality in over 100 cases of *Staphylococcus epidermidis* ventricultis. Vancomycin has largely replaced them as first choice, but reliance on sensitivities from bacteriology is still essential.

Failure is nearly always due to use of the wrong antibiotic, wrong dose, by the wrong route, or given too late. Penetration into the CSF and brain must achieve concentration above the minimal lethal dose (MLD) concentration for that organism. This can be very different from the concentration necessary to inhibit the growth of the organism, i.e. the minimum inhibitory concentration (MIC). MLD may be more than tenfold greater than MIC for organisms such as *E. coli*. Many antibiotics used in treatment of gram-negative meningitis, such as ampicillin or the aminoglycosides, show very poor CSF penetration and are of limited use unless they are given by a ventriculosotomy reservoir. Penicillins penetrate best when the meninges are inflamed, and penetration lessens as the inflammatory response settles, hence the relapses at 2–3 weeks previously seen with ampicillin. Metronidazole, chloramphenicol, rifampicin and trimethoprim show good penetration. The dose may need to be monitored closely by measuring CSF levels, particularly if hydrocephalus is present producing a dilutional effect. The organism can be kept in culture and serial dilutions of CSF put against it to see if effective bactericidal levels have been achieved. There may be a wide gap between the MIC and MLD, so that relapse is then a risk if adequate concentrations are not achieved.

317

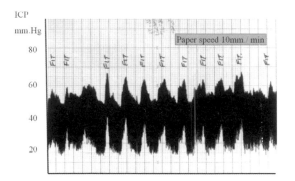

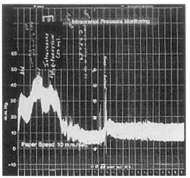

Fig. 10.2. Very high pulse pressure from loss of auto-regulation and effect of individual's fits on the intracranial pressure in an infant with non-accidental shaking injury.

Fig. 10.3. Effect of seizures on raising intracranial pressure and the effect of controlling seizures by intravenous phenytoin lowering the intracranial pressure to normal values.

Careful monitoring of CSF is required to look for persistent growth and cellular response. With modern antibiotic therapy one should not have any continued growth of organisms on culture after 24 hours. If there is evidence of continuing infection then antibiotic dosage may need to be increased, or the drug regimen altered. Polymorphonuclear, lymphocytic and eosinophilic preponderance in cellular response on cyto-centrifugation means that the infection is usually still active; while an increasing proportion of macrophages may indicate that the patient is responding to the therapy. Macrophages are the subarachnoid 'vacuum cleaners' and remove debris and fibrin; there may be an elevated cell count in the CSF for a week or more after the infection is controlled. However, macrophages containing visible organisms may reactivate, so the CSF should not be considered sterile, and therapy should not be stopped, nor should a shunt be inserted.

Treatment of raised intracranial pressure

Factors known to exacerbate raised ICP should first be avoided (Minns 1991). The airways should be carefully maintained, secretions aspirated, blood gases checked, and pCO_2 must be kept within the normal range. Compensatory hyperventilation is common in children with raised ICP, so pCO_2 may be in the region of 4 kPa. The child should be nursed head up, and care must be taken that head position does not occlude the veins. The transient increases in ICP in response to tracheal intubation and pharyngeal suction can be reduced to a minimum by hand ventilation, adequate analgesia and sedation, but are not necessarily abolished by neuromuscular blockade. Close monitoring for clinical and electrical seizures is important as seizures can cause raised ICP and treating the seizures promptly will lower the ICP (Figs. 10.2, 10.3).

Methods of reducing ICP are:
• Removal of CSF
• Hyperosmolar agents

318

TABLE 10.1
Treatment of raised intracranial pressure

Moderately raised intracranial pressure: more than 20mmHg for 5 minutes	*Severely raised intracranial pressure: more than 30mmHg for 15 minutes*
Check blood gases for raised pCO_2	Perform CT/MRI to detect for clot, oedema,
Check sedation and analgesia – asleep, not	hydrocephalus
paralysed and awake, not in pain, e.g. fractures.	Insert jugular bulb catheter and if oxygen
Maintain central venous pressure (CVP) at	saturation is low then commence thiopentone
8–10mmHg. Treat hypovolaemia	infusion
Cool if pyrexial to normothermia	
Check whether or not having seizures (EEG)	*Treatment*
Check not related to suction, physiotherapy,	Remove CSF
insertion lines	Fluid volume replacement
	Dopamine (or noradrenaline) to maintain CPP
Treatment	Mild to moderate hypothermia (to not less than
Hypothermia	34°C)
Hyperventilate to decrease pCO_2 (not less than	Craniectomy or subtemporal decompression
4kPa)	
Mannitol = 0.25–0.5g/kg over 15 mins (if serum	
osmolality <320) or 3% saline, 5–10ml/kg bolus	
over 10–15 mins	
Watch CVP and follow with 5.0ml/kg of 4.5%	
human albumin solution (plasma protein	
solution) over 15 mins	
Furosemide 0.25–1.0mg/kg intravenously	
Remove CSF if there is access	

- Hyperventilation
- Steroids
- Barbiturates
- Hypothermia
- Surgical – craniectomy.

A protocol for management of moderate to severely raised ICP is seen in Table 10.1.

REMOVAL OF CSF

The most effective method of reducing ICP in an emergency situation is to remove CSF or any source of space occupation e.g. pus, subdural haematoma, etc. These causes of raised ICP will not be helped by other methods of treatment until more space is made. Sufficiently large ventricles will be necessary on imaging, and a decision can be made regarding insertion of a ventriculostomy reservoir or ventricular tapping. Establishing a reservoir allows safe pressure monitoring and drainage if necessary (Minns 1977). Hydrocephalus is a frequent complication of acute encephalopathy due to intracranial haemorrhage or meningitis and these children eventually will require a definitive shunt procedure. The site of CSF removal will depend on whether the method of measurement will allow CSF removal, e.g. subdural, ventricular or subarachnoid space.

Displacement methods measuring CSF pressure are less valuable than using a miniature transducer directly on to the lumbar puncture (LP) needle or ventricular catheter. Displacement

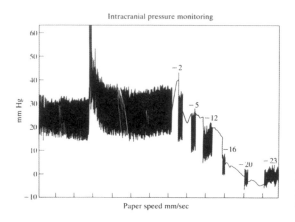

Fig. 10.4. Effects on intracranial and pulse pressure of removal of sequential aliquots of CSF.

allows a run-off of the CSF into the manometer, which may be sufficient to reduce the pressure and non-displacement methods are preferred. No child with impaired conscious level should ever have a LP without first undergoing computerized tomography (CT) or magnetic resonance imaging (MRI) to show that the basal cisterns are patent and there is no intracranial mass lesion. Very high pressure, e.g. over 50 mmHg, may be unexpectedly recorded at the time LP is carried out in order to diagnose meningitis. The LP needle should be left in situ and the stilette replaced. Panic removal of the needle allows CSF under pressure to escape into the extradural space and track upwards and along the intercostal nerves. A fatal coning can then result. Mannitol should be given over 20 minutes and the pressure recorded. If this does not bring the pressure down, furosemide (Lasix) should be given intravenously. The child should have a urinary catheter in situ and be adequately sedated. In most cases the pressure will return to normal, and the child's neck stiffness and drowsiness may disappear, even though the infection is not treated, and a sample of CSF can then be safely taken. A volume of CSF can also be removed to prevent the return of raised ICP (Fig. 10.4). Although this may be due to brain swelling, in many cases it appears to be due to arachnoiditis, as part of the meningitis, with failure of CSF absorption. Cerebral oedema should have been picked up on the scan and LP not performed.

HYPEROSMOLAR AGENTS

These agents act by inducing hyperosmolar dehydration provided that strict control of fluid balance is achieved to avoid subsequent overhydration and reduce the risk of rebound oedema. Even small amounts of hypo-osmolar fluid, e.g. water given by mouth, will be sufficient to induce this rebound oedema. Although plasma volume may at first be increased, many agents subsequently induce a diuresis, and plasma volume and central venous pressure may than fall requiring plasma expansion with colloid.

The most widely used drug is mannitol (Macdonald and Uden 1982). It improves the microcirculation, is a free radical scavenger and induces controlled hyperosmolar dehydration. It remains within the vascular compartment, increasing plasma osmolality and leading to 'brain dehydration' and brisk diuresis. Mannitol promotes diuresis within 20 minutes in

320

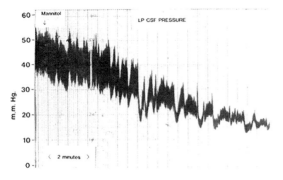

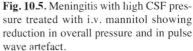

Fig. 10.5. Meningitis with high CSF pressure treated with i.v. mannitol showing reduction in overall pressure and in pulse wave artefact.

normally developing children, accompanied by increased excretion of sodium, potassium, chloride and calcium. Catheterization is routine in the unconscious patient, and will also allow an accurate record of output. During mannitol therapy, blood urea and electrolytes and osmolality should be checked regularly. Accurate weighing is a good guide to hydration, especially in younger infants, but is impractical in the paediatric intensive care unit (PICU). There is a theoretical risk of exacerbating oedema due to unwanted escape of mannitol across the damaged blood–brain barrier, e.g. into an infarcted area of the brain. Mannitol is contra-indicated in the presence of severe dehydration, renal failure or gross hyperosmolality, otherwise hypertension and severe pulmonary oedema may occur

The usual regimen is to administer in doses ranging from 0.25 g/kg over 20 minutes, up to 2.5 g/kg total in 24 hours (Fig. 10.5). High doses will reduce renal perfusion and cause an increase in blood urea. This policy is aimed at inducing a hyperosmolar state in plasma and then only slowly allowing the osmolality to fall, together with promoting a diuresis. In the presence of normal renal function it is unusual for plasma osmolality to rise above 320 mOsm and in many children not above 300 mOsm. In the presence of a CSF reservoir or ventricular cannula, estimation of blood and CSF osmolality provides a good guide to the rate at which fluid intake can be increased.

In the past, urea and glycerol were used as an alternative osmolar agent but there was difficulty in the preparation of appropriate sterile solutions of glycerol; however, there is now some renewed interest in its use. It has the advantage over mannitol in that it is metabolized in the liver and does not induce an osmotic diuresis, and therefore can be used in the presence of renal failure and is less likely to lead to hypovolaemia. Glycerol is given in a dose of 1–1.5 g/kg by nasogastric tube or intravenously in 0.45% or 0.9% saline, no faster than 1.5 ml (3.3 mOsm) per minute. Urea used as the initial hyperosmolar unit is now seldom given.

Hypertonic saline (7.2%) has recently regained interest and does not appear to induce dangerous hypernatraemia in adults. Munar et al. (2000) showed that the administration of 7.2% hypertonic saline in 14 patients with traumatic brain injury significantly reduced ICP without significant changes in relative global cerebral blood flow. In children, continuous infusion of 3% hypertonic saline reduces the ICP spikes and increases the CPP, and shortens the PICU stay. Its use is supported by most guidelines.

321

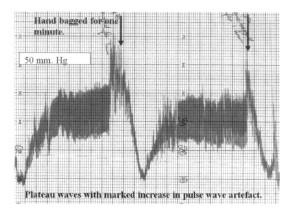

Fig. 10.6. Dramatic reduction in intracranial pressure which occurs with hyperventilation from hand bagging.

HYPERVENTILATION

Hypoxia and CO_2 retention are potent cerebral vasodilators leading to increased cerebral blood flow and cerebral blood volume with exacerbation of intracranial hypertension (Harcourt and Hopkins 1971, Miller 1979). The compensatory hyperventilation of many children with acute encephalopathies in response to raised ICP will dramatically reduce cerebral blood flow and there is always concern that overzealous therapeutic hyperventilation may actually reduce cerebral perfusion to ischaemic levels (Bruce 1984). Hyperventilation results in a significant decrease in saturation of jugular vein oxygen and an increase in arteriovenous difference in oxygen concentration ($AVDO_2$). Hypocapnia followed by mannitol administration led to a further decrease in jugular venous oxygen saturation and an increase in $AVDO_2$.

Another problem is that in the presence of severe brain damage, autoregulation and vascular reactivity to CO_2 may be lost, so that failure of hyperventilation to reduce raised ICP, in the absence of hydrocephalus and space occupation, is usually a very poor prognostic sign. However, for controlling ICP in children with brain swelling from cerebral oedema or cerebral congestion, controlled hyperventilation maintaining pCO_2 in the region of 4 kPa is a very effective short-term measure (Fig. 10.6). Unfortunately, after several hours, equilibration to the new level of pCO_2 and escape of ICP may occur. Any degree of respiratory failure necessitates controlled ventilation.

Controlled hyperventilation is of value when other methods such as mannitol and removal of CSF have failed. Controlled hyperventilation can be performed reducing pCO_2 to 4 kPa (20–27 mmHg) and keeping this constant, or bringing the mentioned ICP down and then gradually allowing pCO_2 to rise and noting the degree of hyperventilation required to keep the ICP within acceptable limits. The latter method has the advantage that a further crisis can be met with added hyperventilation.

The current policy in the Royal Hospital for Sick Children, Edinburgh, is to hyperventilate and attempt to maintain the pCO_2 as closely as possible at the level of 4.0–4.5 kPa

322

(23–34 mmHg). Short-term hyperventilation to lower levels is possible to reduce an acute plateau. Sudden swings in pCO_2 should be avoided since they lead to gross swings in CSF acid base status with the resultant severe disequilibrium and CSF acidosis, the so-called Posner encephalopathy (Posner and Plum 1967). Also, they may be followed by acute fluid retention and aggravation of inappropriate ADH secretion. Periods of high intrathoracic pressure, e.g. with coughing or tracheal suction, should be minimized as far as possible, e.g. by neuromuscular blockade and sedation. If the child is straining, coughing, struggling and out of synchrony with the ventilator then that unit should not be attempting neurointensive care.

The use of transcutaneous pO_2 and pCO_2 monitoring has allowed more accurate minute-to-minute variations to be monitored. Blood gases are still repeated should a problem arise.

STEROIDS

Although glucocorticoids are effective in reducing raised ICP both experimentally and clinically, their mode of action is incompletely understood (Wiles 1982). Steroids are known to reduce brain water, endothelial permeability, leukocyte diapedesis, and CSF formation. The effect of steroids on brain water is maintained over many weeks as shown by the apparent severe cerebral atrophy on CT scanning of children with leukaemia or infantile spasms. Sudden cessation of therapy will lead to rebound oedema and pseudotumour cerebri.

Steroids are most effective for the control of vasogenic oedema, especially surrounding subacute or chronic focal lesion such as a tumour. There is early improvement within hours of vascular responsiveness and regional blood flow (Miller 1979). However, they are less effective in cytotoxic oedema, e.g. hypoxic ischaemic encephalopathy or water intoxication. In severe shock states, steroids should be given in doses 10 times that required for the control of cerebral oedema to induce vasodilatation and open up the microcirculation. Steroids may therefore have many different actions, which has caused a resurgence in their use in acute *Haemophilus* meningitis:

• Our practice is still sometimes known to use 16-alpha methyl-9 fluoro-prednisolone (dexamethasone) in the management of children with acute hypoxic–ischaemic encephalo-pathy, Reye syndrome, tumour, acute meningitis (especially *H. influenzae*) with evidence of brain swelling, severe status epilepticus, burns and scalds encephalopathy, and some forms of toxic encephalopathies. The recognition of the deleterious effects of cytokines produced in pneumococcal, meningococcal and group B streptococcal meningitis means that steroids are now used more routinely in order to try and suppress cytokine release induced by antibiotics.

• In herpes simplex encephalitis with raised ICP and clinical deterioration, steroids may sometimes prove to be dramatically effective. Steroids are avoided in children with proven or suspected varicella zoster.

• Dexamethasone is usually given in a dose of 1.5 mg/kg stat. (adult max. 10 mg), followed by 0.25 mg/kg 4–6 hourly. Typical doses are 2 mg in infants, 4 mg in young children, and 10 mg by the age of 12 years, repeated 6 hourly. Therapy is continued according to the clinical response and then withdrawn gradually over several days. High-dose regimes of 1 mg/kg or more should not be continued for more than 48 hours.

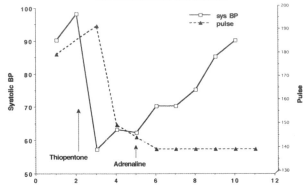

Status Epilepticus with poor prognosis.

Fig. 10.7. Effect of thiopentone in reducing cerebral perfusion pressure and increasing risk of hypoxic–ischaemic brain damage in status epilepticus. The child subsequently had severe learning disabilities and cerebral palsy.

BARBITURATES

Barbiturates, such as thiopentone, are used to stop seizures, and to reduce both ICP and cerebral metabolic demands. Cerebral metabolic rate and cerebral blood flow, it is claimed, are reduced in parallel with increasing barbiturate dosage (Pierce et al. 1962). If cerebral blood flow is reduced before fits are stopped and the metabolic demands of the brain for oxygen reduced, further damage could ensue (Fig. 10.7). There is little evidence base for barbiturates reducing ICP other than by reducing perfusion pressure. Barbiturates are used when there is increased cerebral metabolism demonstrated on jugular venous saturations (high ICP, which is resistant to osmotic diuresis and hyperventilation). A test dose of 4 mg/kg thiopentone is given first to detect sensitivity of ICP to barbiturates. If it induces a fall in ICP without a proportionate fall in blood pressure, this can be maintained by a thiopentone infusion (1–5 mg/hour) or by longer-acting barbiturates, e.g. pentobarbitone at 4 mg/kg. Inotropes and fluid boluses may be used for a fall in blood pressure. A protocol for the use of barbiturates is shown in Table 10.2.

Barbiturates should not be used empirically outside of specialist centres and full supportive care. These precautions include facilities for ventilation, full intensive care unit monitoring, EEG monitoring (to maintain a burst–suppression pattern), and access to regular assays of serum barbiturate levels; careful monitoring of cerebral perfusion pressure together with $AVDO_2$ measurement is also needed to prevent a perfusion to metabolism mismatch, thus causing brain damage. If blood pressure falls, dopamine or noradrenaline may be used to raise it in order to maintain perfusion. Barbiturates are effective in near-drowning, Reye syndrome, and head injuries.

HYPOTHERMIA

Hypothermia is achieved with a water-cooled blanket in the PICU. The patient needs to be fully sedated and paralysed so that shivering does not occur. Modern cooling blankets use

TABLE 10.2
Barbiturate for reduction of raised ICP

Thiopentone 2.0–5.0mg/kg stat. bolus injection (titrated to
 EEG/cerebral function analysing monitor (CFAM) response)
Continuous infusion 1.0–1.5mg/kg/hour – burst suppression
EEG control: Fast beta appears when awake, large amplitude
 asynchronous slow with onset of sleep, burst suppression in
 anaesthetic plane, flat less than $10\mu V/cm$ on overdose

a core temperature probe to regulate to requirements. Recent studies have shown hypothermia to be deleterious, and the Cochrane data show there is no evidence of efficacy. Mori et al. (1999) studied therapeutic hypothermia in head injury. Their results suggest that hypothermia may cause vasoconstriction and "misery perfusion" in the brain. This potential risk of relative ischaemia can be avoided by combination with vasopressor administration.

In experimental animals, prolonged hypothermia brings about a reduction in infarct size and oedema, and protects against hypoxia–ischaemia by reducing both apoptosis and necrosis after brain insults, and certainly protects *prior to* global ischaemia. This is made use of routinely during surgery. The recent vogue for head cooling in neonatal asphyxia still lacks convincing clinical proof of minimizing hypoxic brain damage (Michenfelder and Theyre 1968, Ohmura et al. 2005).

INDOMETHACIN

Bundgaard et al. (1997) reported on the use of indomethacin. Twenty individuals who underwent craniotomy for supratentorial cerebral tumours were randomized to intravenous indomethacin 50mg or placebo administered after exposure of the dura. A significant decrease in ICP from 6.5 to 1.5 mmHg (medians) was found after indomethacin administration. This decrease was caused by a significant decrease in cerebral blood flow associated with a significant increase in $AVDO_2$. Indomethacin did not affect cerebral oxygen uptake, arterio-venous difference in lactate, or the lactate–oxygen index, suggesting that indomethacin did not provoke global cerebral ischaemia. It is currently not recommended.

SUBTEMPORAL CRANIECTOMY

In some children with severe traumatic brain injury, the raised ICP can be refractory to medical management, and the course can be further complicated by side-effects. There has been a renewed interest in decompressive craniectomy to maintain adequate cerebral blood flow and oxygenation. A recent pilot study in children with traumatic head injury who were treated with decompressive craniectomy has shown encouraging results (Ruf et al. 2003).

Control of seizures

Seizures may be clinically obvious or may only show on EEG (Fig. 10.8). A single fit in an acute encephalopathic illness represents an acute cerebral dysrhythmia (not epilepsy) and is an indication for immediate termination of the fits but only short-term prophylactic anticonvulsant therapy, and in most cases this may be discontinued after a few weeks.

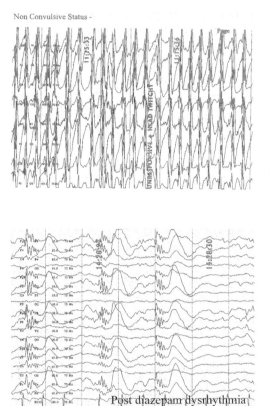

Fig. 10.8. The unexpected finding of continuous status epilepticus on EEG monitoring.

Fig. 10.9. Paradoxical response to diazepam, producing a polyspike wave discharge.

However, the role of continued prophylactic anticonvulsant therapy in the absence of clinical seizures and epileptiform EEG activity in not proven. Treatment of status epilepticus is independent of long-term medication.

BENZODIAZEPINES

Benzodiazepines form the bedrock of emergency care and can be given in several ways: intravenous diazepam, lorazepam, midazolam or clonazepam; rectal diazepam; intramuscular midazolam; sublingual lorazepam; or nasal or buccal midazolam.

DIAZEPAM

Primary care of fits is to give diazepam, but not intravenously unless the doctor is recently experienced in giving intravenous injections to small children; otherwise rectal diazepam solution (not suppositories)should be used, in a dose of 0.25–0.5 mg/kg. Rectal diazepam will give blood levels at 2 minutes equal to twice the dose intramuscularly at 30 minutes. It can also be used by parents and teachers of children known to have epilepsy. Older children are embarrassed by the administration of rectal diazepam and our preference is for rectal diazepam under 5 years and nasal midazolam over 5 years.

If the child arrives in hospital still having a seizure, lorazepam or diazepam given intravenously is first choice. Diazepam should not be injected near an artery, especially if the child is having a clonic fit at that time, as the limb may be jeopardized. It should not be mixed with other drugs and should be injected slowly at the rate of about 1 mg/min. Very rapid injection or overdose will cause apnoea, laryngeal spasm and hypotension. Very occasionally a paradoxical response occurs (Fig. 10.9), and diazepam actually causes fits so should not be repeated, with risk of hypotension and respiratory depression, if there is not an immediate response to intravenous injection (within 5 minutes). It may be repeated if fits stop and restart. If diazepam is given under EEG control, there is usually abolition of all spike activity and the appearance of fast beta activity. Peak brain levels occur about 1 minute after a diazepam injection, but it leaves the brain as rapidly as it enters and fits may return after 20 minutes. The dose of diazepam is generally 0.25–0.5 mg/kg, but in an emergency situation it is easy to consider the initial dose equals the age in years plus 1, e.g. 4 mg for a 3-year old child. As it is fixed in tissues and blood levels fall so rapidly, an intravenous infusion of diazepam is suitable for children who are diazepam sensitive. However, diazepam is very rapidly fixed onto plastic tubing, so one is never sure of the dose being administered. Diazepam plasma levels are not easy to estimate and are not usually available in most laboratories. Other benzodiazepines like clonazepam are more likely to cause hypotension and bronchorrhoea. Large doses produce hypotonia, ataxia and drowsiness.

If fits continue following initial intravenous benzodiazepine, the dose may be repeated, provided pupils have not dilated, blood pressure has not dropped, and the child is not known to be 'diazepam resistant'.

MIDAZOLAM

Intramuscular midazolam is likely to become more popular in the future. It is well absorbed intramuscularly compared to diazepam (bioavailability 90%) and is not absorbed onto plastic syringes. Its mean half life is 2 hours. Midazolam hydrochloride (Hypnovel) is an imidazobenzodiazepine, which has anticonvulsant, anxiolytic, hypnotic and muscle relaxant properties. The dose ranges from 0.07 to 0.2 mg/kg body weight for intravenous administration and 0.2 mg/kg body weight intranasally. Side-effects are a drop in blood pressure and cardiac output, and respiratory depression. Care must be taken with concomitant barbiturates. Midazolam has now replaced both diazepam and lorazepam for management in paediatric intensive care as it is used as part of basal anaesthesia in larger doses of up to 0.5 mg/kg followed by 2.0 μg/kg/min along with fentanyl or morphine infusion and muscle relaxant (vecuronium). It is used therefore as a continuous infusion in the management of seizures after the immediate intravenous bolus of benzodiazepine and phenytoin. Like other benzodiazepines it should abolish spike activity and produce fast beta in all areas of the normally developing brain.

LORAZEPAM

Reports over the last several years have demonstrated important advantages of lorazepam (Ativan) in the treatment of status epilepticus. It has the benefit of rapid onset of action like diazepam, stopping seizure activity within 2–3 minutes in 80–100% of patients. Furthermore,

327

unlike diazepam it controls seizures for 24–48 hours. Therefore, the risk of respiratory depression is low since it is not necessary to add other drugs such as phenobarbitone to maintain seizure control within the first 24–48 hours. It is effective in treating both partial (90%) and generalized tonic–clonic status. It should be given intravenously (0.05–0.2 mg/kg, maximum 4 mg) over 1–2 minutes. It may be repeated at 10- to 15-minute intervals, but its effectiveness decreases with successive doses (Shields 1989). Due to the lower dose schedule its use should be policy for all units in a hospital as otherwise confusion with other benzodiazepines raises the risk of overdosage.

PHENYTOIN

Although intravenous phenytoin is the drug of choice in some centres, it is used as a second choice in most UK centres, or as a back-up to diazepam where its slower onset of action takes over as the effects of the initial dose of diazepam begin to wear off. Phenytoin dosage is difficult to gauge and a high initial 'epanutinization' regime similar to digitalis is required. After this the maintenance dose may range from 2 to 25 mg/kg/day, so that blood levels must be monitored.

Phenytoin given intramuscularly is not absorbed but crystallizes in the muscle, causing focal haemorrhagic necrosis. Phenytoin needs to be given intravenously for rapid termination of fits; given too rapidly it can cause cardiac arrythmias. It is also very liable to cause tissue necrosis if extravasated. Rapid epanutinization consists of 18 mg/kg intravenously over 20 minutes (maximum 50 mg/min), followed by 10.0 mg/kg in divided doses over the next 24 hours (4-, 6-, then 8-hourly intervals). Blood level should be measured daily; the dose is usually between 2.0 and 8.0 mg/kg/day to maintain therapeutic plasma levels of phenytoin.

Enzyme induction vastly increases the dose necessary to achieve therapeutic blood levels. Up to 40 mg/kg/day may be needed, especially after thiopentone infusion. Blood level should be monitored as it is rapidly toxic and will then cause fits or marked choreiform movements which are not infrequently confused as continuing fits.

Failure to control seizures with acute encephalopathic illness is most likely caused by failure to achieve adequate plasma concentrations of the phenytoin. If the wrong route is used, the intramuscular injection crystallizes out and causes muscle necrosis. If too much phenytoin is used it causes seizures at concentrations over $150\,\mu$mol that are benzodiazepine- and paraldehyde-resistant. Too little leads to an enzyme induction from prolonged thiopentone or chlormethiazole infusion. Wrong spacing of doses with a large initial dose, which is absorbed into fat, means that it needs to be repeated in 1 hour.

Phenytoin should preferably be given under EEG and ECG control because it can cause cardiac arrythmias; the more rapidly acting phosphenytoin is quickly absorbed into the myocardium with risk of death from cardiac arrythmias and should not be used in children. As intravenous phenytoin is distributed rapidly into fat, blood levels fall rapidly if a second dose is not given 1 hour later.

PARALDEHYDE

This is a safe drug when given intramuscularly; it is often thought of as an old-fashioned drug and some centres never use it, yet it is a highly effective anticonvulsant. Its smell is probably its main disadvantage. It is one of the few drugs that can be given intramuscularly in an emergency situation. It can be given in the modern plastic syringes without the syringes disintegrating if it is given within 20 minutes. In young children, the buttocks should be avoided as one can never be sure of the position of the sciatic nerve. The lateral side of the thigh is preferred. Paraldehyde should be given deeply, otherwise if given subcutaneously, will lead to sterile abscess formation. The dose by intramuscular injection is 0.05 ml/kg or 1 ml per year of age. Its half-life is on average 6 hours. Paraldehyde induces sleep and appears on the breath 15 minutes after intramuscular injection. Paraldehyde is also useful if given rectally as 10% solution with normal saline or mixed with equal quantities of olive oil. The dose of the 10% solution is 0.5 ml/kg. This is very effective in children with intractable grouping of seizures going on for many days, and respiration is not compromised. The doses can be repeated every 2–4 hours if necessary. Occasionally in critical situations (e.g. epidural abscess or overdose of intrathecal drugs), paraldehyde may be given intravenously (but only by those with experience of its use) in a dose of 200 mg/kg followed by an infusion of 20 mg/kg/hour to attain a steady serum level of $200 \mu g/ml$ (Bostrom 1982). The dose should be reduced in the presence of hepatic or pulmonary disease. Intravenous injection, if not properly diluted, can lead to serious hepatic necrosis and pulmonary haemorrhage. Estimation of blood levels of paraldehyde can be performed in certain laboratories, and is helpful in management with a therapeutic range of $300–400 \mu g/ml$ (Curless et al. 1983).

THIOPENTONE

Thiopentone may be used to induce anaesthesia to control intractable seizures, for cerebral protection or to treat raised ICP. In using thiopentone to control fits only the dose needed to suppress seizures is required and this requires an EEG to see when spike activity is suppressed rather than dropping perfusion pressure or depressing ventilation. After prolonged convulsive status epilepticus the electrical abnormalities may persist as electrical status and later show evolution of resultant convulsive hypoxic–ischaemic damage (Figs. 10.10–10.12). A cannula rather than needle should be used as, although a needle may be placed in a vein, the fit may cause it to be replaced in an artery. Pentothal 1.0 g should be dissolved in 500 ml normal saline (not glucose or it precipitates out). Start with 5.0 ml/kg intravenously, then run to keep the child awake but with no fits showing on the EEG. The idea is not to produce continuous anaesthesia. Observe the fits and titrate until the dose is down to 15 drops per minute, then reduce concentration to 0.5 g and then 0.25 g per 500 ml. Wean the child off when they have been free from fits for 24 hours and put them on adequate background anticonvulsants. Apnoea, hypotension and laryngospasm may result if it is given too fast. Use only in an intensive care unit. Monitor blood pressure continuously, ECG and blood gases. Continuous EEG monitoring is essential for proper standard of care.

Intravenous sodium valproate

Sodium valproate can be given as a suppository when oral continuation therapy is not possible in an individual known to have epilepsy. It can be given as an intravenous starter bolus when initiating valproate therapy. Intravenous sodium valproate can now be considered in patients with intractable seizures from cerebral irritative lesions such as subdural empyema

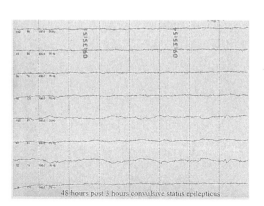

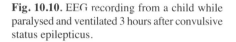

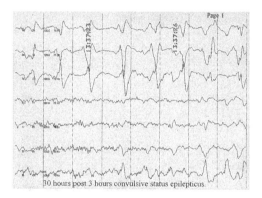

Fig. 10.10. EEG recording from a child while paralysed and ventilated 3 hours after convulsive status epilepticus.

Fig. 10.11. Continuing epileptic activity in the same patient although nothing is visible clinically. Cortical damage is evident on the right side.

Fig. 10.12. EEG of the same child 48 hours post status epilepticus with a flat EEG and severe postconvulsive hypoxic–ischaemic damage.

or cortical thrombophlebitis when phenytoin, midazolam infusion, or paraldehyde have not worked. Sodium valproate may take a long time to take full action in some children because only one of the three metabolites is an active anticonvulsant. It is a mitochondrial toxin and should never be used in mitochondrial or urea cycle abnormalities with hyperammonaemia. Valproic acid is related to octanoic acid and inhibits the enzyme succinic semialdehyde

330

dehydrogenase. It may act more quickly at high blood levels when given by bolus injection followed by an infusion rather than orally. A 400 mg ampoule is diluted with saline, and an initial 20 mg/kg is given followed by maintenance at 1 mg/kg/hour. There is not extensive experience with this method of administration in children but it is claimed to work in 30 minutes and to suppress epileptic activity on the EEG (Dutta et al. 2003).

CHLORMETHIAZOLE EDISYLATE (HEMINEVRIN)
This is of proven value in eclampsia and alcohol withdrawal seizures (Harvey et al. 1975). Some centres use heminevrin to control seizures, especially after cardiac bypass surgery. Our own experience in Edinburgh has not been as successful as other centres in that it has been of only occasional value. If given too slowly it can increase the number of seizures. It is provided in a solution of 8 mg/ml, in a slow or fast regime.

It may cause tingling in the nose, sneezing, headache, conjunctival irritation and a mild superficial phlebitis as common side-effects (Lingam et al. 1980). Heminevrin has the advantage that there is only a very mild drop in blood pressure with the fast regime and respiratory depression occurs only when the patient is comatose. If the drug is continued for more than 48–72 hours, hepatomegaly may appear.

LIGNOCAINE
Lignocaine must be given carefully as it will occasionally aggravate seizures. It has a depressant effect upon the myocardium so blood pressure and ECG must be monitored. Lignocaine has been used to treat status epilepticus since 1958. When given as a bolus dose of 1–2 mg/kg intravenously, it is effective within 20–30 seconds. However, the action is not sustained and an infusion of 2 mg/kg/hour is then required. Seizures can occur as a side-effect when lignocaine is used to treat cardiac arrhythmias. Brain uptake increases with the increased cerebral blood flow and impaired blood–brain barrier, so toxicity from the drug maintaining the seizure disorder is a possibility. It is used only as a tertiary treatment in intensive care units, when standard drugs have failed.

PYRIDOXINE
Almost a third of neonatal cases of pyridoxine dependency present with apparent hypoxic–ischaemic encephalopathy. All children with early onset intractable seizures or status should receive a trial of pyridoxine, whatever the suspected cause (Baxter 1999).

The pathway illustrated in Fig. 10.13 is used in Edinburgh to treat status epilepticus.

Maintenance of cerebral perfusion, oxygenation and metabolism
Cerebral perfusion pressure (CPP) is a better guide than intracranial pressure to eventual neurological outcome and the critical CPPs for different ages are shown in Table 10.3 (Chambers et al. 2005). In clinical practice, there may be a difficulty in balance between overhydration risking brain oedema and underhydration risking hyperviscosity and sludging.

PLASMA VISCOSITY
There are several parameters that should be monitored and maintained. A low haematocrit

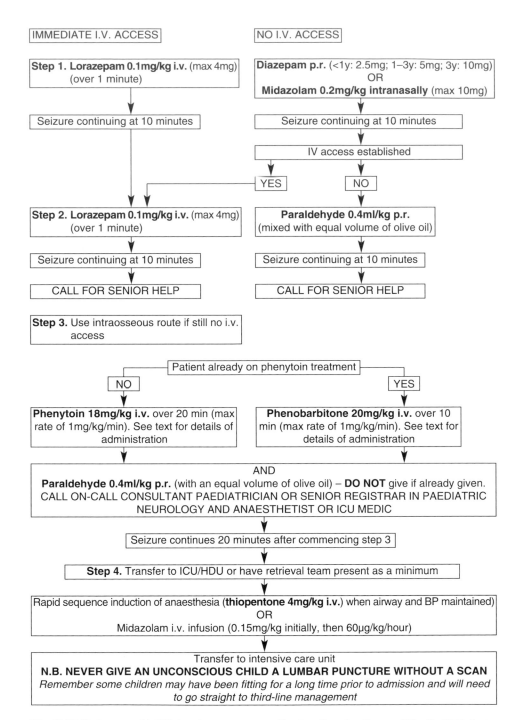

Step 1. Lorazepam 0.1mg/kg i.v. (max 4mg) (over 1 minute)

Diazepam p.r. (<1y: 2.5mg; 1–3y: 5mg; 3y: 10mg)
OR
Midazolam 0.2mg/kg intranasally (max 10mg)

Seizure continuing at 10 minutes

Seizure continuing at 10 minutes

IV access established

YES

NO

Step 2. Lorazepam 0.1mg/kg i.v. (max 4mg) (over 1 minute)

Paraldehyde 0.4ml/kg p.r. (mixed with equal volume of olive oil)

Seizure continuing at 10 minutes

Seizure continuing at 10 minutes

CALL FOR SENIOR HELP

CALL FOR SENIOR HELP

Step 3. Use intraosseous route if still no i.v. access

Patient already on phenytoin treatment

NO

YES

Phenytoin 18mg/kg i.v. over 20 min (max rate of 1mg/kg/min). See text for details of administration

Phenobarbitone 20mg/kg i.v. over 10 min (max rate of 1mg/kg/min). See text for details of administration

AND
Paraldehyde 0.4ml/kg p.r. (with an equal volume of olive oil) – **DO NOT** give if already given.
CALL ON-CALL CONSULTANT PAEDIATRICIAN OR SENIOR REGISTRAR IN PAEDIATRIC
NEUROLOGY AND ANAESTHETIST OR ICU MEDIC

Seizure continues 20 minutes after commencing step 3

Step 4. Transfer to ICU/HDU or have retrieval team present as a minimum

Rapid sequence induction of anaesthesia (**thiopentone 4mg/kg i.v.**) when airway and BP maintained)
OR
Midazolam i.v. infusion (0.15mg/kg initially, then 60µg/kg/hour)

Transfer to intensive care unit
N.B. NEVER GIVE AN UNCONSCIOUS CHILD A LUMBAR PUNCTURE WITHOUT A SCAN
Remember some children may have been fitting for a long time prior to admission and will need to go straight to third-line management

Fig. 10.13. Pathway used in Edinburgh to treat status epilepticus (based on Scott and Neville 1999, Status Epilepticus Working Party 2000).

TABLE 10.3
Critical cerebral perfusion pressure (CPP)

Age	Mean CPP threshold
2–6 yrs	≤48mmHg
7–10 yrs	≤54mmHg
11–16 yrs	≤58mmHg

is beneficial in maintaining the microcirculation, preventing sludging and infarct enlargement. It improves survival in experimental head injury. An haematocrit in the region of 35 will be ideal. There is no need to use low molecular dextran or hydroxyethyl starch with venesection routinely. Mannitol has been proved to be valuable experimentally in causing haemodilution and so improving the microcirculation (Little 1978, Morawski et al. 2003). Any acid base disturbance should be corrected because metabolic acidosis will exacerbate hyperviscosity increasing the risk of sludging.

Aly Hassan et al. (1997) studied normovolaemic haemodilution in children: 16 patients (1–8 years) scheduled for major general surgery were chosen for the study. They were divided into two groups according to the replacement solution used for haemodilution (HD): 6% middle molecular weight hydroxyethyl starch (HES), or 6% dextran 40. Isovolaemic haemodilution (haematocrit approximately 17%) is well tolerated by young children undergoing major elective surgery; global tissue oxygenation was preserved throughout the procedure and both solutions used for haemodilution were equally effective. There is insufficient evidence as yet for the use of haemodilution as a standard procedure for management of acute encephalopathy in children.

BLOOD PRESSURE
Hypotension
It is probably no understatement to say that, after ABC (airway, breathing, circulation), the single most important parameter to monitor and treat in any acute encephalopathy is blood pressure. The aim is to maintain a CPP at approximately the normal diastolic blood pressure. Central venous pressure monitoring is desirable in all cases to determine fluid status. There are three main problems to be considered: (1) reduced plasma volume; (2) reduced vasomotor tone, and (3) reduced cardiac output from myocardial failure.

Hypovolaemia may follow the use of mannitol with diuretics if plasma volume has not previously been expanded with crystalloid. An infusion of 5–20 ml/kg of isotonic fluid is needed in many children with acute encephalopathy even without plasma or fluid loss from the disease. A fluid push as with normal saline can be tried if one is in doubt as to the cause of hypotension, and one does not want to cause a fluid overload. Colloids increase and prolong the efficacy of crystalloid solutions in haemorrhagic shock. Dextran appeared to be the superior colloid compared to HES, particularly during the first hour after initiation of treatment, although direct proof of an improved long-term outcome has not been demonstrated.

Following correction of any hypovolaemia, if there is refractory hypotension in the presence of a healthy myocardium, it is more likely to be due to inappropriate vasomotor tone for a normal

333

or increased blood volume, i.e. vasoparalytic shock. Pressor agents may then be tried. Inotropes may be started while the child is normotensive to promote adequate CPP.

Noradrenaline following cardiac arrest increases myocardial contractility and maintains cerebral and coronary perfusion, but it has several disadvantages, namely induction of tachyarrhythmias or ventricular fibrillation (in susceptible children), reduction of renal blood flow (unless a vasodilator is used concurrently), and production of metabolic acidosis secondary to gut and tissue ischaemia. Noradrenaline may need to be added to dopamine if perfusion pressure cannot be maintained. It is thought to be helpful in the presence of low systemic resistance and a normal cardiac output as in 'septic shock' or 'liver disease'. Myburgh et al. (1998) showed that norepinephrine and epinephrine had no significant effects on ICP, cerebral blood flow (CBF), AVDO$_2$ or cerebral oxygen utilization at infusions of 0–60 μg/min. Infusions of dopamine up to 60 μg/kg/min, much higher than those used in routine clinical management (10 μg/kg/min), resulted in statistically significant increases in ICP. Experimentally induced hypertension by epinephrine and norepinephrine is not associated with global changes in CBF, ICP or CO$_2$, which remain constant. At equivalent doses, dopamine causes cerebral hyperaemia, increased ICP, and increased global cerebral oxygen utilization.

In spite of the experimental data, dopamine is a widely used sympathomimetic agent in children. It has beta 1 agonist stimulant effects at low doses and alpha stimulant effects (i.e. vasoconstrictive effects) at high doses (Goldberg 1974). It increases myocardial contractility and does not reduce renal blood flow, and is thought to increase renal and mesenteric flow at doses of 1–5 μg/kg/min. It may cause natreuresis at low dose with loss of sodium from an effect on renal tubules. It is used most often to maintain CPP after head injury and in status epilepticus when polypharmacy may decapitate the perfusion pressure. Dopamine is given in doses determined by continuous blood pressure monitoring. Its half-life is 3 minutes so it can only be given by monitored continuous infusion. The starting dose is 5–10 μg/kg/min. Doses above 20 μg/kg/min are contraindicated as they will impair renal and mesenteric blood flow. It is common practice to maintain acute head injuries mildly hypertensive with dopamine in order to maintain CPP.

Hypertension
Hypertension as high as 260/160 mmHg may occur due to several factors. It may be an acute Cushing's response due to raised ICP; or compounded by fluid overload, e.g. after mannitol, in the presence of impaired renal function; or occur during prolonged steroid therapy; or be paroxysmal, resembling a pheochromocytoma (Fig. 10.14). Hypertension may occur as part of the disease in acute nephritis or haemolytic–uraemic syndrome, or occasionally in tricyclic antidepressant poisoning. There is another type of hypertension seen in children with destructive lesions of the brainstem when the baroreceptor input to autonomic centres is blocked so that blood pressure control is inappropriate for the volume and tonicity of the circulation (vasoconstrictive hypertension, i.e. the opposite to vasoparalytic shock) (Eden et al. 1977).

Careful regulation of fluid and electrolytes is the most important measure. All may cause neurological deterioration with retinal haemorrhages and fits. Nitroprusside (i.v. infusion) causes cerebral vasodilatation and may cause a rise in ICP. In sympathetic overdrive use

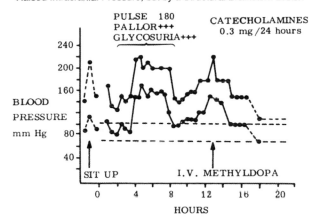

Postural Hypertension and Acute Hypertensive Crises not Caused by
Raised Intracranial Pressure, but by a Structural Brainstem Lesion

Fig. 10.14. Effect of encephalopathy on blood pressure that is not related to intracranial pressure (Cushing's response). Its paroxysmal pattern resembles hypertension in pheochromocytoma.

of beta blockers such as labetalol (i.v. infusion) is safer than diazoxide. Sublingual nifedipine is also used to control hypertension. If blood pressure is brought down too rapidly it may cause optic nerve ischaemia and blindness. Hypertension due to compensatory Cushing's response should not be reduced as this is the body's attempt to try to maintain cerebral perfusion. The main aim in this situation is to reduce the raised ICP. The use of nitroprusside, nitrites or clonidine in order to decrease cerebral vasospasm in an attempt to improve cerebral blood flow (e.g. when due to vasospasm following subarachnoid haemorrhage) is not of proven value in children and may be hazardous.

CEREBRAL PROTECTION
The concept of neuroprotection by pharmacological agents following global injury has received wide publicity but in practice has proved disappointing. These measures were designed to ameliorate the effects of brain damage after various brain insults, particularly cardiorespiratory arrest. This introduced the concept of 'brain-oriented' 'cardiopulmonary cerebral resuscitation'.

Endogenous cerebral protection
• *ACTH*. The normal body's response to stress is by producing corticosteroids, endorphins, adrenaline and sympathetic stimulation, and thus the heart rate increases, blood pressure increases and blood sugar rises in preparation for action – 'fight and flight'. The hypothalamic stress response is possibly also protective. Exogenously administered ACTH reduces the amplitude of the EEG to less than 10μV thus reducing the energy required by the brain to generate the EEG potentials; this is potentially a way of reducing energy demands in hypoxia or hypoglycaemia.

335

• *Adenosine*. Adenosine is an even more important natural substance that reduces cerebral metabolism and increases blood flow, i.e. produces luxury perfusion. Adenosine concentration rises before a fit terminates and after any hypoxic–ischaemic episode. It also flattens the EEG causing an energy switch-off. Kochanek et al. (1997) showed that adenosine may contribute delayed cerebral swelling after severe traumatic brain injury in humans. Adenosine stimulates a concurrent reduction in cerebral metabolic rate and an increase in CBF. CSF adenosine concentration was negatively associated with $AVDO_2$ and strongly associated with death (both $p<0.05$) (Clark et al. 1997).

Exogenous cerebral protection
• *Hypothermia*. Although hypothermia has been proved to be effective in improving the outcome when cerebral metabolism is reduced pre-insult, its effectiveness post-insult is not valid. The theoretical reduction of cerebral metabolic demand by hypothermia is difficult to organize and care must be exercised by concomitant use of barbiturates as a drop in CPP may exceed the protection and actually cause cerebral ischaemia. It should be remembered that the scalp receives blood from the external carotid and so if the scalp is cooled the brain still receives hot blood from the internal carotid and whole body cooling is necessary.

Furthermore, uncontrolled hypothermia in young infants may be dangerous as it may increase rather than decrease oxygen demands. There is also the possibility of cold injury leading to acidaemia, hypoglycaemia and disseminated intravascular coagulation (see above in hypothermia for raised ICP). There are case reports indicating mild hypothermia in combination with steroids or anticytokine agents may have beneficial effects in influenza encephalopathy (Kimura et al. 2000, Munakata et al. 2000, Ohtsuki et al. 2000).

• *Barbiturates*. Barbiturates have been proved to reduce cerebral metabolic demands and so brain damage and improve survival in experimental animals when given before an hypoxic–ischaemic insult. When given post-insult, the outcome is improved in focal ischaemia. Usually they are given in a dose to hold the monitored EEG at burst suppression level reducing cerebral metabolic demands to an optimum degree. Further doses are needed to maintain this EEG pattern, and serum levels should be checked regularly to prevent drug accumulation. However, these massive doses should only be given in specialized centres with appropriate monitoring facilities. If one reduces CPP without reducing cerebral metabolism the situation is worsened not improved.

• *Calcium channel blockers*. Calcium channel blockers have been tried using various animal models as well as newborn infants (Sopala et al. 2002). Calcium ion entry into the compromised cell triggers a cascade of biochemical events that can cripple or kill the cell. Phospholipase A2 is activated (Siesjo 1981), which leads to accumulation of arachidonic acid within the cell. Following reperfusion, the arachidonic acid is metabolized to vasoactive prostaglandins (Moncada and Vane 1978), leading to platelet activation and arteriolar vasoconstriction. These mechanisms best explain the repeatedly observed phenomenon of secondary cerebral hypoperfusion following hypoxic–ischaemic injury. Calcium channel blockers have been found to prevent or modify secondary cerebral insults through at least thrce potentially important actions: protection of the neurons from the effect of calcium ion entry; prevention of post-ischaemic cerebral arteriolar vasoconstriction; and improvement of myocardial function (Newberg et al. 1984). However, although calcium channel blockers reduce morbidity and mortality in adults with cerebrovascular accidents, in neonates with severe asphyxia they are followed by systemic hypotension and their use for asphyxiated human newborn infants must be undertaken only with great caution (Levene et al. 1990).

• *Glutamate*. Glutamate plays a central role in the pathogenesis of hypoxic–ischaemic injury. Large amounts of glutamate are present in the brain, normally stored in presynaptic terminals and other intracellular locations. During cerebral ischaemia, increased synaptic release and impaired cellular uptake rapidly produce extracellular accumulation of glutamate. Excessive exposure to extracellular glutamate can destroy central neurons. The most important mechanism for glutamate mediated injury is calcium entry through membrane channels that are opened by N-methyl D-aspartate (NMDA) receptors. The mechanism of action of NMDA receptor antagonists is either receptor competition or channel blockade. Several NMDA receptor antagonists have been proved to be effective in experimental brain ischaemia. However, their role in the treatment of human cerebral ischaemia waits clinical testing. The least toxic compound under trial at present is the infusion of magnesium, which is an essential ion in the NMDA receptor. Another readily available NMDA receptor blocker is ketamine; this has also been tried in inborn errors with neurotransmitter effects such as non-ketotic hyperglycinaemia (Ohya et al. 1991).

• *Free radical scavengers*. Free radical scavengers have reduced the severity of hypoxic–ischaemic damage in experimental animals (Wallace and Wraith 1993). Theoretical and experimental studies have tried the use of calcium antagonists, glutamate antagonists, magnesium, free radical scavengers, and stabilization of sulphydryl groups, but none of these methods are at present of proven clinical efficacy in the human. Substances such as MK801 are toxic; calcium antagonists proved dangerous; and at present most interest surrounds the possible use of magnesium infusions and hypothermia. Equally the inhalation of nitric oxide, amyl nitrite, and others is of great interest but not of proven value. Mannitol is a free radical scavenger. Vitamins C and E as antioxidants probably do no harm. The most important clinical dogmas must be to monitor and maintain blood pressure and oxygenation and not to decapitate a compensatory rise or depress respiration by misuse of sedation, and also to treat severe acidosis and maintain supply of glucose substrate.

• *Hyperbaric oxygen*. The advent of hyperbaric chambers in medical centres close to deep sea diving platforms, such as those for North Sea oil, means that the therapy has been tried in many neurological diseases such as multiple sclerosis and cerebral palsy. It is difficult to see the rationale of trying to reverse a gliosed scarred brain by increasing the pO_2. On the other hand, trying to maintain oxygenation and aerobic metabolism in a poorly perfused brain appears superficially to make more sense, as long as we do not produce more toxicity from epoxides or further protective cerebral vasoconstriction. There is no point in increasing the oxygen to ischaemic brain if it has no substrate for oxidative metabolism. Rockswold

337

et al. (2001) claim that hyperbaric oxygenation (HBO) therapy has been shown to reduce mortality of those with severe brain injury by 50% in a prospective randomized trial. One hundred per cent oxygen at 1.5 atmospheres was delivered to 37 patients in a hyperbaric chamber for 60 minutes every 24 hours (maximum of seven treatments per patient). Levels of CSF lactate were consistently decreased 1 hour and 6 hours after treatment. ICP values higher than 15 mmHg before HBO were decreased 1 hour and 6 hours after HBO ($p<0.05$). Increased cerebral metabolic rate of oxygen ($CMRO_2$) and decreased CSF lactate levels after treatment indicate that HBO may improve aerobic metabolism in individuals with severe brain injury.

Maintenance of homeostasis

Homeostatic problems commonly result from the encephalopathy itself, but also increase the risk of permanent damage. Hypothalamic osmoreceptors and glucoreceptors may be dissociated from their effector systems through the brainstem by the compressive effects of shifts and cones. Brainstem distortion will disrupt the connections between the aortic arch receptors, right atrial receptors, chemoreceptors and baroreceptors, and the main centres in the brainstem. All these events will lead to inappropriate homeostatic responses to changes in blood tonicity, sodium concentration, glucose, body temperature, arterial and venous pressure, pCO_2, pO_2, acid base status, and respiratory control.

BIOCHEMICAL HOMEOSTASIS

Hypocalcaemia

Hypocalcaemia is very common in children, particularly in young infants, during the stress of acute illness. One mechanism for hypocalcaemia is failure of normal membrane pumping following hypoxic–ischaemic insult leading to leakage of calcium into the cells or bone. Hypocalcaemic seizures may ensue and be wrongly regarded as being due to brain damage. Correction of hypocalcaemia with a single intravenous bolus of calcium (0.1mmol/kg centrally over 20 minutes) requires ECG to monitor for arrhythmias, and is also short-lived, so administration of calcium in a continuous infusion or in an electrolyte cocktail mixture is most convenient.

Glucose homeostasis

Hyperglycaemia may occur with very high blood glucose levels of over 20mmol/l, simulating diabetes mellitus. There are several reasons: any child under stress develops a hypercatecholin-aemia that will mobilize liver glycogen, and even isolated seizures may be associated with marked hyperglycaemia; high ICP will influence glucose homeostasis giving a diabetic-type glucose tolerance curve (Fig. 10.15) that returns to normal within 24 hours of ICP being relieved; and pontine lesions usually interrupt the sympathetic effector systems from glucoreceptors giving very high blood glucose levels. Children with this type of 'cerebral diabetes' are extremely sensitive to insulin and so insulin should be used cautiously, aiming for normoglycaemia. Two consecutive blood-glucose monitoring (BM) strip tests above 10mmol/l warrant starting insulin infusion at 0.01–0.05 μg/kg/hour.

Hypoglycaemia may cause an encephalopathy or result from brain damage due to dis-

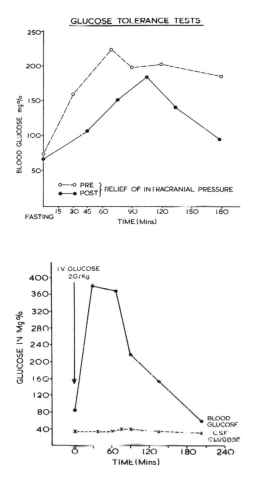

Fig. 10.15. Effect of raised ICP on the glucose tolerance profile.

Fig. 10.16. With loss of cerebrovascular autoregulation there is failure to show an increase in CSF glucose following an intravenous infusion in acute encephalopathy.

sociation of glucoreceptors and hormonal (growth hormone, glucocorticoid and catecholamine) or autonomic adjustment of blood sugar. There may be dissociation between plasma glucose and CSF glucose levels in individuals with lost cerebrovascular autoregulation (Fig. 10.16). Diseases such as Reye syndrome, Leigh's encephalopathy, medium-chain acyl dehydrogenase deficiency (MCADD), multiple acyl-CoA dehydrogenase deficiency (MADD – also known as glutaric aciduria type II) should be remembered in the child presenting with encephalopathy and hypoglycaemia. Hypoglycaemia should be corrected using bolus doses of 10% glucose (5 ml/kg). Five per cent glucose solutions alone should be avoided because of the risk of water intoxication. A plasma glucose measurement must be performed immediately in any patient with acute encephalopathy and then routinely every 4–6 hours.

Hyponatraemia
Hyponatraemia usually associated with hypo-osmolality is common and seen in association with a wide range of acute encephalopathies, especially following asphyxia, meningitis,

head injury, or any cause of raised ICP (Weizman et al. 1982). Fits and impaired consciousness may result if sodium concentration falls below 120 mmol/l.

Hyponatraemia is usually due to water intoxication with haemodilution from inappropriate ADH secretion. Although not suitable for the kidneys it is appropriate for the brain in order to reduce brain and CSF water. It also occurs as a result of distension of the third ventricle, traction on the hypothalamus during coning, or by disruption of the fibres connecting osmoreceptors in the hypothalamus with their effector systems. The child is water intoxicated rather than salt depleted, and there is no fall in weight or dehydration. This is especially likely to occur as a result of intravenous infusions of electrolyte-free solutions. Inappropriate ADH secretion is diagnosed where there are low plasma osmolality and high urine osmolality.

Water intoxication with inappropriate ADH secretion should be anticipated in all acute encephalopathies, and fluid restriction should be started immediately on admission to the hospital. Fluid to maintain circulating volume should be isotonic in order to lessen the risk of a dysequilibrium syndrome and rebound cerebral oedema. Hyponatraemia may result from excessive urinary sodium loss due to mannitol therapy and massive sympathetic discharges. In water overload, the child will be of normal or increased weight (and may show mild pitting oedema), while in sodium depletion they will be dehydrated and weight loss occurs. If fluids are required to replace true sodium loss or expand extracellular volume, normal saline should be used to decrease the risk of cerebral oedema and minimize a dysequilibrium syndrome from sudden changes in osmolality. Routine fluid maintenance should preferably be with glucose in 0.45% saline. Hypertonic saline is administered slowly if serum sodium is less than 120 mmol/l or if there are convulsions when cerebral oedema is likely to occur.

Hypernatraemia

Hypernatraemia used to be an important cause of acute encephalopathy before the modification of infant feeds. Also, there is the condition of central or essential hypernatraemia (Dorn and Rothballer 1973) in which high plasma osmolality and high serum sodium may be seen. However, the possibility of unrecognized diabetes insipidus should be considered because polyuria is associated with severe hypernatraemia.

Acute hypernatraemia is associated with loss of body water, acidosis and a high haematocrit, predisposing to hyperviscosity, thrombosis and massive venous infarction.

If the clinical condition (plasma volume, hydration, and blood pressure) and ICP monitoring are stable, the osmolality should be reduced gradually at a rate not exceeding 1 mOsm per hour, i.e. 24 mOsm per 24-hour maximum. It may take several days to bring the osmolality back to normal without dysequilibrium. There is a 6-hour time gap in equilibration between blood and CSF, so that an osmolar gap exceeding 6 mOsm is likely to be associated with osmotic dysequilibrium and rebound oedema (Habel and Simpson 1976). If fluid is required for tissue dehydration then normal saline should be used to minimize osmolar shifts. Hypovolaemia must always be corrected first with fluid bolus, as renal hypoperfusion will make things worse.

Hyperosmolality may be due to high serum sodium, urea or glucose, but, in addition, in many of these children the osmolality is higher than calculated, thought to be due to so-called idiogenic osmols. It is therefore necessary to measure plasma osmolality and not guess it from urea, sodium and glucose concentrations. The same gradual reduction of osmolality appearing in diabetic ketoacidosis or a fatal cerebral oedema can occur.

Acid base status

Blood gas analysis is mandatory in all cases of acute encephalopathy. Metabolic acidosis is a common complication of many acute encephalopathies such as Reye syndrome, bacterial endotoxaemia, hypernatraemia, uraemia, diabetes, organic acidurias, and aminoacidurias, ketoacidosis from vomiting and starvation, and following hypoxic–ischaemic episodes. Urinary organic acids should be tested in all children with marked metabolic acidosis in order not to miss a treatable inborn error of metabolism. Disorders such as Leigh encephalopathy, MELAS (mitochondrial myopathy, encephalopathy, lactic acidosis and stroke like episodes), maple syrup urine disease, glutaric aciduria, methylmalonic aciduria and biotinidase deficiency may easily be misdiagnosed as acute encephalitis.

The pH of the CSF and that of the blood may show increasing disparity. Carbon dioxide passes freely into and out of CSF, while bicarbonate does not. Acidosis is a potent central stimulator of hyperventilation. With hyperventilation, CO_2 is removed leaving bicarbonate and severe alkalinity will result. The nervous system compensates for this by producing lactic acid, and CSF lactate will rise. Any further sudden rise in pCO_2 in the presence of lactate will result in marked drop in CSF pH. CSF pH below 7.2 will lead to loss of consciousness and a 'Posner encephalopathy' will ensue. Metabolic acidosis should be corrected using bicarbonate, except in diabetic ketoacidosis. However, one should only reduce the pCO_2 by 1.5 kPa (10 mmHg) per hour and avoid sudden rapid changes in ventilator settings to avoid sudden discrepancies between blood and CSF pH.

CARDIOVASCULAR HOMEOSTASIS – CARDIAC RHYTHM ABNORMALITIES

Bradycardia, asystole and ECG changes resembling myocardial infarction may occur secondary to cerebral lesions. There may also be variations in blood pressure unrelated to raised ICP.

Although bradycardia is characteristic of raised ICP, severe tachycardia of up to 200/min may occur in some children, and a marked sinus arrhythmia may be the only abnormality in raised ICP. Adrenaline or atropine may be needed if asystole or severe bradycardia occur that are not immediately abolished by reducing ICP.

ECG abnormalities may occur independent of the rhythm changes, e.g. large Q waves, large T waves, U waves and prolonged QT intervals, have all been reported in subarachnoid haemorrhage or associated with complex partial seizures.

DISORDERS OF RESPIRATORY CONTROL

Respiratory changes, problems with carbon dioxide retention, and its effects on intracranial pressure and CSF acid base status are discussed above. Most children in coma will be ventilated in an intensive care unit. The importance of proper sedation and ventilator technique has already been emphasized. Ventilation is taken over by machine in part because

TABLE 10.4
Respiratory abnormalities in acute encephalopathies

Tachypnoea ≥200/min	Laryngospasm
Bradypnoea <12 per min	Sleep apnoea
Respiratory arrhythmia	Ondine's curse
Gasping	Neurogenic pulmonary oedema
Apnoea	Neurogenic intrapulmonary shunting
Periodic Cheyne Stokes breathing	Neurogenic oesophageal reflux
Central neurogenic hyperventilation	Mendelssohn syndrome
Kussmaul (acidotic) breathing	Diaphragmatic paralysis
Central hypoventilation (respiratory failure)	

of the risk of a respiratory abnormality as a symptom of the encephalopathy and to control CO_2. Respiratory abnormalities are frequent in acute encephalopathies (Table 10.4).

Massive pulmonary oedema may occur in acute encephalopathies due to raised ICP and responds to positive end expiratory pressure ventilation and reduction of ICP. Furosemide should also be given intravenously. Occasionally intrapulmonary shunting causes desaturation and cyanosis which does not respond to raising the inspired oxygen concentration, although nitrous oxide may help.

Central neurogenic hyperventilation with tachypnoea, a very low pCO_2 and alkalosis can be seen without raised ICP in children with subarachnoid haemorrhage, meningitis or hepatic failure.

Gastric abnormalities
Acute gastric erosions, Curling ulcers and hyperchlorhydria are due to autonomic imbalance with marked vagal overactivity. They are commonly associated with coffee-ground aspirate from the nasogastric tube, but a catastrophic haematemesis requiring blood transfusion may occur. Pontine haemorrhages or tumours may be associated with severe haematemesis.

Prophylactic ranitidine is used in all unconscious patients, in patients not established on enteral feeds, and in those with burns or shock when the risk of gastrointestinal bleed is high.

Relaxation of cricopharyngeus with initiation of oesophageal peristalsis and relaxation of the cardia is mediated by the brainstem, so gastro-oesophageal reflux with risk of aspiration of gastric contents is a worry in acute and chronic CNS diseases.

RENAL FUNCTION
Multisystem organ failure occurs in asphyxia, severe shock and meningococcal disease, and requires separate consideration which will not be dealt with here.

Poisoning or renal failure must be corrected by haemofiltration, diuresis or peritoneal dialysis. Occasionally, specific therapy may be needed, e.g. administration of naloxone or chelating agents, or dietary manipulation or plasmaphoresis.

Conclusion
Treatment of acute encephalopathy should begin with a systematic approach with an open

mind regarding the underlying cause. The main principle of treatment is supportive with a 'treat the treatable' approach until the underlying cause is identified. Appropriate recognition and management of infection, raised ICP and seizures, with adequate maintenance of cerebral perfusion, metabolism and oxygenation along with maintenance of homeostasis will minimize morbidity and mortality.

REFERENCES

Aly Hassan A, Lochbuehler H, Frey L, Messmer K (1997) Global tissue oxygenation during normovolaemic haemodilution in young children. *Paediatr Anaesth* 7: 197–204.

Baxter P (1999) Epidemiology of pyridoxine dependent and pyridoxine responsive seizures in the UK. *Arch Dis Child* 81: 431–433.

Bostrom B (1982) Paraldeyhde toxicity during treatment of status epilepticus. *Am J Dis Child* 136: 414–415.

Bruce DA (1984) Effects of hyperventilation on cerebral blood flow and metabolism. *Clin Perinatol* 11: 673–680.

Chambers IR, Jones PA, Lo TY, Forsyth RJ, Fulton B, Andrews PJ, Mendelow AD, Minns RA (2005) Critical thresholds of intracranial pressure and cerebral perfusion pressure related to age in paediatric head injury. *J Neurol Neurosurg Psychiatry* (epub ahead of print).

Clark RS, Carcillo JA, Kochanek PM, Obrist WD, Jackson EK, Mi Z, Wisneiwski SR, Bell MJ, Marion DW (1997) Cerebrospinal fluid adenosine concentration and uncoupling of cerebral blood flow and oxidative metabolism after severe head injury in humans. *Neurosurgery* 41: 1284–1292.

Curless RG, Halzmann BH, Ramsay RE (1983) Paraldehyde therapy in childhood status epilepticus. *Arch Neurol* 40: 477–480.

Dorn JD, Rothballer AB (1973) Essential hypernatraemia. *Arch Neurol* 28: 83–90.

Dutta S, Cloyd JC, Granneman GR, Collins SD (2003) Oral/intravenous maintenance dosing of valproate following intravenous loading. a simulation. *Epilepsy Res* 53: 29–38.

Eden OB, Sills JA, Brown JK (1977) Hypertension in acute neurological diseases of childhood. *Dev Med Child Neurol* 19: 437–445.

Habel AH, Simpson H (1976) Osmolar relation between cerebrospinal fluid and serum in hyperosmolar hypernatraemic dehydration. *Arch Dis Child* 51: 660–666.

Harcourt B, Hopkins D (1971) Ophthalmic manifestations of the battered baby syndrome. *BMJ* 3: 398–401.

Harvey PKP, Higenbotlam TW, Loh L (1975) Chlormethiazole in treatment of status epilepticus. *BMJ* 2: 603–605.

Kimura S, Ohtsuki N, Adachi K, Aihara Y (2000) Efficacy of methylprednisolone pulse and mild hypothermia therapies in patients with acute encephalopathy. *No To Hattatsu* 32: 62–67.

Kochanek PM, Clarke RS, Obrist WD, Carillo JA, Bell MJ, Marim DW (1997) The role of adenosine during the period of delayed cerebral swelling after severe traumatic brain injury in humans. *Acta Neurochir Suppl* 70: 109–111.

Levene ML, Gibson NA, Fenton AC, Papthoma E, Barnett D (1990) The use of a calcium channel blocker, nicardipine, for severely asphyxiated newborn infants. *Dev Med Child Neurol* 32: 567–574.

Lingam S, Bertwistle H, Elliston HM, Wilson J (1980) Problems with intravenous chlormethiazole (Heminevrin) in status epilepticus. *BMJ* 280: 155–156.

Little JR (1978) Modification of acute focal ischaemia by treatment with mannitol. *Stroke* 9: 4–9.

Macdonald JT, Uden DL (1982) Intravenous glycerol and mannitol therapy in children with intracranial hypertension. *Neurol* 32: 437–440.

Mackway-Jones K, Molyneaux E, Phillips B, Wieteska S, eds. (2001) *Advanced Paediatric Life Support – The Practical Approach. 3rd edn.* London: BMJ Books.

Miller JD (1979) The management of cerebral oedema. *BMJ* 21: 152–166.

Minns RA (1977) Clinical application of ventricular pressure monitoring in children. *Zeitschr Kinderchirurg Grenzgebiete* 224: 430–443.

Minns RA (1991) Infectious and parainfectious encephalopathies. In: Minns RA, ed. *Problems of Intracranial Pressure in Childhood. Clinics in Developmental Medicine No. 113/114.* London: Mac Keith Press, pp. 170–282.

Moncada S, Vane JIR (1978) Unstable metabolites of arachidonic acid and their role in haemostasis and thrombosis. *Br Med Bull* 34: 129–135.

343

Morawski K, Telischi FF, Merchant F, Abiy LW, Lisowska G, Mamyslowski G (2003) Role of mannitol in reducing post ischaemic changes in distorsion – product otoacoustic emissions (DPOAEs): a rabbit model. *Laryngoscope* **113**: 1615–1622.

Mori K, Maeda M, Miyazaki M, Iwase H (1999) Misery perfusion caused by cerebral hypothermia improved by vasopressor administration. *Neurol Res* **21**: 585–592.

Munakata M, Kato R, Yokohama H, Haginoya K, Tanaka Y, Kayaba J, Kato T, Takayangi R, Endo H, Hasegawa R, Ejima Y, Hoshi K, Iinuma K (2000) Combined therapy with hypothermia and anticytokine agents in influenza A encephalopathy. *Brain Dev* **22**: 373–377.

Munar F, Ferrer AM, de Nadal M, Poca MA, Pedraza S, Sahuquillo J, Garnacho A (2000) Cerebral hemodynamic effects of 7.2% hypertonic saline in patients with head injury and raised intracranial pressure. *J Neurotrauma* **17**: 41–51.

Myburgh JA, Upton RN, Grant C, Martinez A (1998) A comparison of the effects of norepinephrine, epinephrine, and dopamine on cerebral blood flow and oxygen utilisation. *Acta Neurochir Suppl* **71**: 19–21.

Newberg LA, Steen PA, Milde JH, Michenfelder JD (1984) Failure of flunarizine to improve cerebral blood flow or neurologic recovery in a canine model of complete cerebral ischaemia. *Stroke* **15**: 666–671.

Ohmura A, Nakajima W, Ishida A, Yasuoka N, Kawamura M, Miura S, Takada G (2005) Prolonged hypothermia protects neonatal rat brain against hypoxic–ischaemia by reducing both apoptosis and necrosis. *Brain Dev* (in press).

O'Regan ME, Brown JK, Clarke M (1996) Nasal rather than rectal benzodiazepines in the management of acute childhood seizures? *Dev Med Child Neurol* **38**: 1037–1045.

Ohtsuki N, Kimura S, Nezu A, Aihara Y (2000) Effects of mild hypothermia and steroid pulse combination therapy on acute encephalopathy associated with influenza virus infection: report of two cases. *No To Hattatsu* **32**: 318–322.

Ohya Y, Ochi N, Mizutoni N, Hayakawa C, Watanabe K (1991) Nonketotic hyperglycinaemia: Treatment with NMDA antagonist and consideration of neuropathogenesis. *Pediatr Neurol* **7**: 65–68.

Pierce EG, Lambersten CL, Deutsh S (1962) Cerebral circulation and metabolism during thiopental anaesthesia and hyperventilation in man. *J Clin Invest* **41**: 1664–1671.

Posner JB, Plum F (1967) Spinal fluid pH and neurologic symptoms in systemic acidosis. *N Engl J Med* **277**: 605–613.

Rockswold SB, Rockswold GL, Vargo JM, Erickson CA, Sutton RL, Bergman TA, Biros MH (2001) Effects of hyperbaric oxygenation therapy on cerebral metabolism and intracranial pressure in severely brain injured patients. *J Neurosurg* **94**: 403–411.

Ruf B, Heckmann M, Schroth I, Hugens-Penze M, Reiss I, Borkhardt A, Gortner L, Jodicke A (2003) Early decompressive craniectomy and durapalsty for refractory intracranial hypertension in children: results of a pilot study. *Crit Care* **7**: 133–138.

Scott R C, Neville BGR (1999) Pharmacological management of convulsive status epilepticus in children. *Dev Med Child Neurol* **41**: 207–210.

Shields WD (1989) Status epilepticus. *Pediatr Clin North Am* **36**: 383–393.

Siesjo BK (1981) Cell damage in the brain: a speculative synthesis. *J Cereb Blood Flow Metab* **1**: 155–167.

Sopala M, Danysz W, Quack G (2002) Neuroprotective effects of NS-7, voltage gated Na+/Ca2+ channel blocker in a rodent model of transient focal ischaemia. *Neurotox Res* **4**: 655–661.

Status Epilepticus Working Party (2000) The treatment of convulsive status. *Arch Dis Child* **83**: 415–419.

Wallace G, Wraith JE (1993) Acute encphalopathies in infancy. *Recent Advances in Paediatrics* **11**: 117–131.

Weizman Z, Goitein K, Amit Y, Wald U, Landau H (1982) Combined treatment of severe hyponatraemia due to inappropriate antidiuuretic hormone secretion. *Pediatrics* **69**: 610–612.

Wiles CM (1982) Steroids in neurology. *B J Hosp Med* **28**: 308–322.

Yang YX, Lewis JD (2003) Prevention and treatment of stress ulcers in critically ill patients. *Semin Gastrointest Dis* **14**: 11–19.

11
THE NEUROPATHOLOGY OF NON-ACCIDENTAL HEAD INJURY

Jeanne E Bell

Non-accidental injury (NAI) is a leading cause of death and disability in children, particularly if cerebral injury is part of the spectrum of damage (American Academy of Pediatrics Committee on Child Abuse and Neglect 1993, Jayawant et al. 1998, Conway 1998). Young infants are particularly vulnerable to a form of NAI known as the shaken baby syndrome. The concept of the shaken baby syndrome began to emerge in the 1940s after Sherwood (1930) had described nine infants with subdural haemorrhage (SDH) in whom he considered that trauma was the undisclosed cause. Caffey (1972, 1974) had been aware of the association between SDH and skeletal fractures since the 1940s and he drew attention to the likely severe long term consequences that may result from shaking an infant. He also drew interesting parallels between the effects of non-accidental head injury (NAHI) in surviving infants and the cognitive decline and pathological findings found in boxers who sustain repeated head trauma. Kempe et al. (1962) and Russell (1965) also drew attention to the association between SDH and NAHI. It is noteworthy that the recognition of this syndrome pre-dated modern neuroimaging techniques, which have revolutionized the investigation of previously occult intracranial haemorrhage.

Shaking injuries are potentially life threatening for infants, possibly because of the rapid to and fro movement of the heavy infant head in relation to the adult grasp around the thorax or elsewhere (Brown and Minns 1993). The infant's weak neck muscles fail to protect the head from the full range of imposed movements. The small overall size of an infant relative to the perpetrator also ensures that this is a form of injury virtually confined to the very young. In addition to SDH, which may appear quite trivial in its extent at autopsy, the brain is nearly always acutely swollen and may show parenchymal damage in the form of contusional haemorrhages and axonal injury. These features are further described in this chapter together with recent studies that challenge the view that the axonal injury is traumatic in origin. However, the exact mechanical stresses producing the injury remain unclear (Geddes et al. 2001a,b). Although shaking injury may be sufficient on its own to produce severe clinical sequelae and neuropathological changes, some experts believe that contact injury may also be involved (Duhaime et al. 1987). This additional injury occurs when the infant head impacts on a soft or hard surface during the shaking, with the consequent risk of skull fracture. The infant may also be thrown or dropped after shaking. Brown and Minns (1993) and Krous and Byard (1999) have pointed out that it is irrelevant from the medico-legal point of view whether or not a contact injury occurs in addition to shaking since both are inflicted injuries. Hadley et al. (1989) drew attention to damage in the upper cervical cord in association with NAHI and the importance of this phenomenon is increasingly recognized.

The incidence of NAI in children is not known for certain (Carty and Ratcliffe 1995, Kinney and Armstrong 2002). The difficulty of ascertainment results not just from the duplicity of the perpetrators but also from the failure of healthcare staff to recognize that NAI might have occurred (Lloyd 1998). It is widely acknowledged that infants under 1 year of age are particularly at risk of NAHI, although cases also occur in older children up to 3 years (Caffey 1972, 1974; Hadley et al. 1989; Duhaime et al. 1992). The peculiarly high prevalence of SDH in infants subjected to NAI was recognized early by Kempe et al. (1962), Russell (1965), Guthkelch (1971) and Caffey (1972, 1974). Recent retrospective studies of SDH in children under 2 years of age have established an incidence of between 13 and 21 per 100,000 children per year in the UK (Jayawant et al. 1998), but a prospective study in Scotland revealed a higher incidence of NAHI in infants with an annual incidence of 24.6 cases per 100,000 children under 1 year of age (Barlow and Minns 2000). Estimates in the USA of 1100 fatal cases, and 15,000 seriously injured survivors of NAI, were made in the 1990s (Spear et al. 1992).

NAI should be suspected where there is a clear discrepancy between the history provided and the injuries incurred (Kempe et al. 1962, Billmire and Myers 1985). More recent studies have confirmed that subdural haematoma in an infant is most often due to NAHI and is likely to have a serious outcome (Brown and Minns 1993, Jayawant et al. 1998). The clinical presentation, and the investigations that should be instituted in such cases, are explored elsewhere in other chapters of this text and are well summarized in recent publications (American Academy of Pediatrics Committee on Child Abuse and Neglect 1993, Jayawant et al. 1998). However, it is worth reiterating briefly the main presenting signs and symptoms in the present context since they point to the underlying pathology. A presentation of drowsiness, lethargy or coma may reflect the cerebral oedema and rising intracranial pressure associated with SDH. These signs may also result from the worsening clinical condition of an infant who has not been brought to medical attention immediately after the injury. Uncontrolled convulsions may follow a neglected injury, possibly causing additional hypoxic injury within the brain. The cardinal features of NAHI in infants include SDH in virtually all cases, and retinal haemorrhages are estimated to be present in up to 90% of such infants. Evidence of skeletal trauma is present in up to 70% of cases (Kleinman et al 1995, Geddes et al. 2001a). Recent careful surveys suggest that the vast majority of SDHs occurring in infants are the result of NAI (Jayawant et al. 1998). However, this view is being challenged in some quarters (Geddes et al. 2003, Geddes and Plunkett 2004).

Many studies have emphasized the poor outcome following SDH in infants. At worst the outcome may be fatal, either immediately or shortly after the injury, or the child may survive in a vegetative state. In the study by Jayawant et al. (1998), 27% of infants with SDH had an early fatal outcome, 45% went on to profound disability or later death, and only 27% developed normally. Serious complications in longer-term survivors include epilepsy, mental retardation, spastic quadriplegia and motor dysfunction.

This chapter is concerned with the pathology that underlies these clinical outcomes of NAI. The pathological changes will be described, followed by an account of the dilemmas

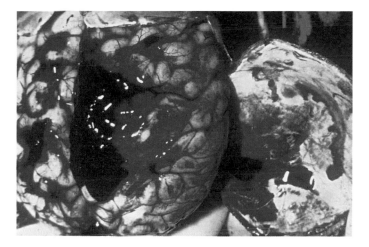

Fig. 11.1. Appearance of the brain at autopsy in a 10-week-old infant dying of NAHI. Reflection of the skull and dura (to the right of the figure) reveals the presence of fresh blood clot overlying the right parieto-occipital region and in continuity with interhemispheric haemorrhage.

and discussion surrounding the pathogenesis of these events. Consideration is given to the differential diagnosis of the pathological findings, and illustrative case histories are provided in addition to guidelines for the neuropathological investigation of NAI.

Pathology of non-accidental injury of the head and of the spinal cord

The pathology of NAI both in the brain and in the spinal cord may be considered as that which occurs quite rapidly after injury, and the delayed complications and sequelae.

EARLY PATHOLOGICAL FEATURES

The neuropathological features seen classically in the early period after injury include SDH, haemorrhage in the globes and/or optic nerves, and cerebral swelling. Skull fractures with possible epidural haemorrhage, subarachnoid haemorrhage, cerebral contusions and haema-tomas are also seen in some cases. In NAHI the acute SDH may be unilateral but is more frequently bilateral (Russell 1965; Guthkelch 1971; Alexander et al. 1990a,b). SDH is usually sited at the parieto-occipital convexity (Fig. 11.1) or in the posterior interhemispheric tissure (Duhaime et al. 1998). The source of the SDH is likely to be torn bridging veins (Fig. 11.2) that are disrupted at or close to their entry point to the superior sagittal sinus (Guthkelch 1971, Caffey 1974, American Academy of Pediatrics Committee on Child Abuse and Neglect 1993). The dura is densely adherent to the inner surface of the infant skull, which predisposes to venous disruption in the context of sudden head movements (Kinney and Armstrong 2002). Infants may display both fresh and older SDH (Figs. 11.1, 11.3), suggestive of repeat episodes of NAHI, and positivity for haemosiderin at histological examination confirms a maturing or old haemorrhage (Duhaime et al. 1998). However, it should be noted that small old haemorrhages, particularly in relation to the tentorium, may

347

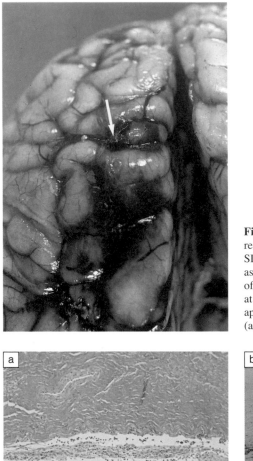

Fig. 11.2. Anterior view of a formalin fixed brain removed from a 10-week-old male infant in which SDH was found at autopsy. The brain is swollen as shown by flattening of the gyri and effacement of the sulci. The right cerebral hemisphere displays at the centre of the field a ruptured bridging vein approximately 1cm from the interhemispheric cleft (arrowed).

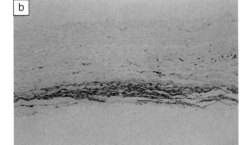

Fig. 11.3. Old SDH was found in the posterior cranial fossa in a child of 12 weeks who had also sustained fresh SDH as a result of NAHI. Both scans show dura mater in the upper half of the field. Deep to the dura (lower half of the field) a layer of pigmented macrophages is present (a) which stained positively for haemosiderin (b). [Haematoxylin–eosin (a) and Perls Prussian blue reaction (b), both ×40.]

be birth related. The presence of a sizeable fresh haematoma may of itself cause raised intracranial pressure, but it is secondarily aggravated by the brain swelling which usually occurs in response to the presence of the haematoma. Cerebral swelling is a very significant early pathological consequence of brain injury, often found with SDH but also occurring as an apparently isolated finding (American Academy of Pediatrics Committee on Child Abuse and Neglect 1993, Kinney and Armstrong 2002). The swollen brain displays flattened gyri and compressed sulci and ventricles (Munger et al. 1993) (Figs. 11.2, 11.4). Very

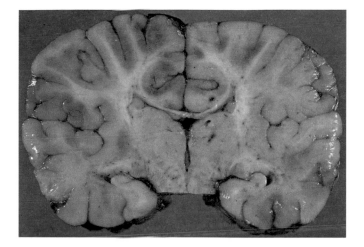

Fig. 11.4. Coronal slice of the cerebrum from a 7-week-old infant with NAHI. The brain is swollen and shows compression of the ventricular system with hypoxia-associated discolouration of brain tissue.

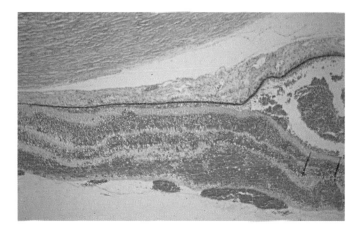

Fig. 11.5. Histological section of the retina confirms fresh haemorrhage in an infant with NAHI. The haemorrhage involves all layers of the retina. [Haematoxylin–eosin ×40.]

severe cerebral oedema may be present by 6 hours after injury (Brown and Minns 1993). There is no evidence to suggest that children with acute brain swelling display a lucent interval (Duhaime et al. 1998). Intraocular haemorrhages may involve the sclera, choroid, vitreous or retina (Fig. 11.5) and there may be evidence of retinal detachment or of previous haemorrhage in the form of haemosiderin laden macrophages (Munger et al. 1993). Subdural and subarachnoid haemorrhage may also be present surrounding the optic nerve.

In a recent paper describing retrospective examination of 37 infants less than 1 year in age who had suffered inflicted head injury, SDH was present in 31, mostly as a thin film,

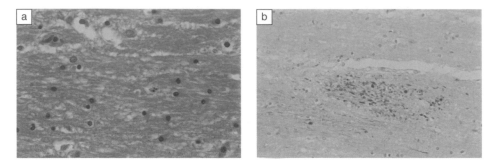

Fig. 11.6. Histological appearance of white matter damage associated with SDH in an infant of 6 weeks. (a) Parenchymal rarefaction with apoptotic glial nuclei (haematoxylin–eosin). (b) Same tissue stained for β-APP confirms the presence of distorted and swollen axons. [Both ×200.]

retinal bleeding in 23, raised intracranial pressure in 30, skull fracture in 16, subscalp bruising in 24, and significant extracranial injury in 15 (Geddes et al. 2001a). In this series, global hypoxia was described in 31 infants and diffuse axonal injury in only two, although focal traumatic axonal injury was present in 31% at the craniocervical junction and in the central white matter in five. Vascular axonal injury was described in 12, characterized by geographic areas of axonal β–amyloid precursor protein (β-APP) staining which lacked axonal balls. This study highlighted some contrasts in cranial pathology between infants who suffered injury before 1 year of age and those who were older. It called into question the nature of the axonal injury, which until this time had been assumed in such cases to be traumatic in origin, and underlined the importance of a comprehensive assessment of all areas of the brain for axonal injury. This study also benefited from the application of immunostains to detect early axonal injury, an analysis that had been lacking from previous studies.

Axonal injury is a highly significant pathological finding in the white matter in head injured infants (Fig. 11.6). The presence of axonal injury is likely to signify serious injury in the brain contributing to the clinical status of coma and leading to a fatal outcome or to a vegetative state. It is important to note, however, that not all cases of NAHI display axonal injury. Axons become irregular in contour and may display so-called retraction balls, which were originally thought to represent physical interruption of axonal continuity, but are now known to reflect disturbance of axonal transport in the context both of trauma and of hypoxic injury. Axonal swellings become visible in routinely stained preparations after 15 hours or so have elapsed (Graham et al. 2002) but may be detected more readily by the use of special stains, particularly immunopositivity for β-APP (Fig. 11.6b), which appears about 2 hours after the injury (Gleckman et al. 1999, Geddes et al. 1997, Graham et al. 2002). Axonal injury may be focal, often underlying an SDH, or widespread in the white matter of the cerebral hemispheres (Shannon et al. 1998). Before the advent of immunocytochemistry it was thought that diffuse axonal injury did not occur in the brainstem of infants (Vowles et al. 1987). However, several recent studies have emphasized the finding of β-APP-positive swollen axons in the medulla and pons of infant brains that were studied

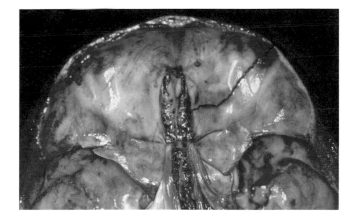

Fig. 11.7. Internal view of the skull displaying a fracture associated with haemorrhage in a 14-month-old child with NAHI.

following trauma-related death, both accidental and non-accidental (Shannon et al. 1998; Oehmichen et al. 1999; Geddes 2001a,b). The study reported by Geddes et al. (2001a,b) is the largest in recent times and concludes that much of the axonal injury is hypoxic rather than traumatic, is focal rather than diffuse (i.e. confined largely to the brainstem), and is significantly different from the pathology of injury both in older children and in adults. However, there was no difference in pathology findings between the group of infants likely to have suffered impact as well as shaking injury and those who had no evidence of impact injury.

The acute phase of traumatic axonal injury is characterized by so-called retraction balls and varicosities. If the patient survives for a number of days or weeks the acute axonal injury is followed by reactive changes including clusters of microglia in the region of damaged axons. β-APP immunoreactivity is down-regulated at this stage. Having faded by eight days post-injury, it is claimed to disappear in axons by 30 days (Geddes et al. 1997). It is important to note, especially for medico-legal purposes, that axonal injury and immunopositivity for β-APP are not specific for trauma-related injury, but also occur following other cerebral insults, notably hypoxia (Shannon et al. 1998, Oehmichen et al. 1999). It is likely that hypoxic injury is a significant contributory factor to the pathology of NAHI (Geddes et al. 2001a,b).

Retinal haemorrhages may be present unilaterally or bilaterally (Fig. 11.5) and occur in up to 95% of cases in NAHI (Kinney and Armstrong 2002), although Geddes et al. (2001a) reported their presence in only 70% of their series. These are usually extensive, multiple, and may involve the periphery of the retina. The optic nerve may also display haemorrhages and/or disruption of tissue.

Fracture of the skull is likely to have resulted from a contact injury, possibly during shaking, and need not involve a very hard surface. The infant skull is rather easily fractured, and such fractures are often bilateral, linear and/or depressed (Fig. 11.7). Skull fracture is

351

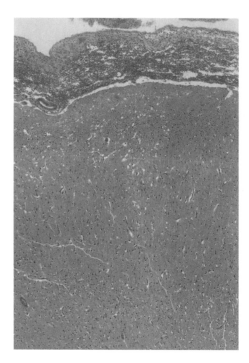

Fig. 11.8. Sections from the cortex of a 7-week-old infant with NAHI and SDH. Subarachnoid haemorrhage is present (seen at the top of the figure). In addition the grey matter is oedematous. [Haematoxylin–eosin ×100.]

present in 25% of cases and may be associated with epidural haemorrhage (Duhaime et al. 1998). Geddes et al. (2001a) found a skull fracture in 36% of their series of NAHI overall and in 16 of 37 affected infants less than 1 year of age. The presence of a contact injury may also be indicated by scalp bruising in the absence of skull fracture, although this finding should be interpreted cautiously (Kinney and Armstrong 2002).

Subarachnoid haemorrhage may be present but is not usually severe unless there are underlying intracerebral haematomas (Fig. 11.8). The presence of subarachnoid haemorrhage may have been revealed during life by examination of the cerebrospinal fluid (CSF). In such cases, the finding of blood in the CSF should not be dismissed as contamination by peripheral blood without further investigation, particularly to establish the presence of xanthochromia (Spear et al. 1992). Xanthochromia is said to be present 1–2 hours after the subarachnoid haemorrhage has occurred (Spear et al. 1992), although a longer interval has been put forward by others (Brown and Minns 1993). Contusional haemorrhages resulting from trauma are more often found in the white matter in the infant compared with the injured adult brain where grey matter contusions occur typically (Graham et al. 2002, Kinney and Armstrong 2002).

Patients in coma as a result of cerebral swelling or severe acute injury may be maintained on a ventilator for some period of hours or days, and in such cases the brain displays the changes of non-perfusion characterized by parenchymal autolysis with no cellular reaction. If some cerebral perfusion is maintained in a comatose patient, early pathological events such as axonal injury become more easily detectable with the passing hours. In particular,

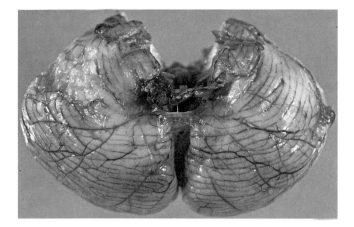

Fig. 11.9. Ventral view of the fixed cerebellum of a child with tonsillar herniation and necrosis. The child had suffered NAHI and had been maintained on ventilation for 36 hours.

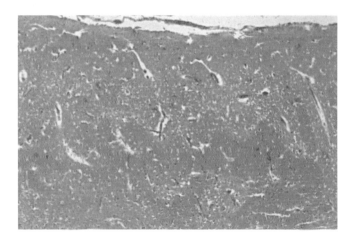

Fig. 11.10. Histological section of the cortex from the brain shown in Fig. 11.9. Variation in staining indicates the presence of recent hypoxic damage and cortical infarction. [Haematoxylin–eosin ×100.]

neurons in the vulnerable regions such as the temporal hippocampus may take on the morphological appearances of acute hypoxia, displaying eosinophilia and shrunken and contracted nuclei (these changes require at least 5 hours after injury to become visible), and β-APP positivity becomes evident in axons by 2 hours after injury and in neuronal cell bodies earlier than that. In particular the brain shows evidence of evolving hypoxic–ischaemic events that may themselves give rise to cerebral oedema (Kinney and Armstrong 2002). Significant cerebral swelling induces herniation of the brain in the supratentorial and infratentorial compartments particularly in the region of the medial temporal lobes and cerebellar tonsils (Fig. 11.9). Widespread cortical infarction may result (Fig. 11.10). Secondary haemorrhages, often small and multiple, may also occur as a result of hypoxia. If the skull has been fractured, brain swelling may lead to spreading fractures of the infant skull, so called because the lines of fracture are increasingly separated. In this context there is a risk of infection, particularly meningitis, if the child survives long enough for this complication to supervene. Delayed presentation of children with NAHI frequently leads to seizures (Hadley et al. 1989), which only increase the risk of hypoxic brain damage. If epilepsy is an early or uncontrolled complication of NAHI, hypoxic damage may occur particularly in the vulnerable neuronal subsets of the temporal hippocampus and brainstem and cerebellum. Such secondary events may be preventable and provide an opportunity for therapeutic intervention in children who survive the immediate injury, although real achievements in this field are still awaited. Delay in seeking medical attention is one factor in this lack of progress, but whether this remains a significant factor at the present time remains unclear.

DELAYED PATHOLOGY CHANGES

The late changes seen in a brain that has been subjected to NAI during infancy depend on the severity of the initial injury and on the degree of the secondary damage. If the infant survives, the residual state of the severely injured brain may be cystic encephalopathy with probable microcephaly and consequent severe cognitive impairment (Kinney and Armstrong 2002). In less comprehensively injured brains, evidence of more focal old infarction and tract degeneration may be present. Hydrocephalus requiring shunting may supervene, particularly in infants who have had subarachnoid haemorrhage. Visual impairment may result from the injury or haemorrhage in the globes or visual tract. Approximately 50% of injured infants develop subsequent epilepsy. The late effects of epilepsy may be present, including hippocampal neuronal loss and gliosis, and these may be bilateral. Some cases display a combination of all of these types of pathology.

If the infant survives, it appears that some smaller subdural haematomas are absorbed. It is unclear how many SDHs persist in infants with NAHI, becoming chronic and evolving to form subdural hygromas. In adults, most SDHs resolve spontaneously (Graham et al. 2002). There is no convincing evidence that significant rebleeding occurs in an SDH in infants in the absence of further significant trauma (Krous and Byard 1999). In particular, there is no firm evidence that rebleeding causes any increase in volume, brain shift or brain oedema as a new event in an older SDH in infants unless a second episode of injury has occurred. However, this remains a matter of controversy.

SPINAL CORD INJURY

SDH in the spinal compartment may accompany NAHI and may be extensive (Fig. 11.11). Although the spinal cord has received much less attention than the brain in the context of shaking injury or other NAI, it is known that trauma to the infant head can cause axonal injury in the brainstem (Shannon et al. 1998) and in the upper cervical cord (Hadley et al. 1989). In the series reported by Geddes et al. (2001a,b), axonal injury was often maximal in the brainstem and was also reported in the cervical spinal roots. In other cases where the cervical cord has been examined specifically, contusions were found at the cervical level in five out of six cases of infant NAI (Hadley et al. 1989). This study also revealed that

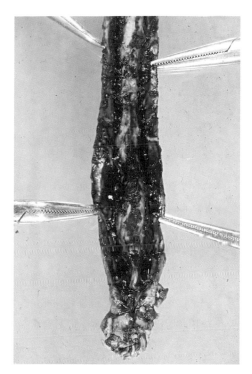

Fig. 11.11. Spinal cord and opened dura mater in a 12-week-old infant with NAI. Extensive SDH and focal subarachnoid haemorrhage is seen in this case. These accompanied bilateral SDH in the cranial compartment.

spinal epidural and subdural haemorrhages were present. In a recent comparative study, β-APP-positive axonal injury was identified in the upper cervical cord in infants with traumatic but not in those with hypoxic brain injury (Shannon et al. 1998). However, it is unlikely that the presence of spinal cord axonal injury would discriminate between accidental and non-accidental injury in an individual case (Kinney and Armstrong 2002). Thus, while β-APP-positive axonal injury is present in the brains of both accidental and non-accidental trauma cases as well as hypoxic–ischaemic cases, present evidence suggests that in the spinal cord, while the first two groups may display positive axons, infants with hypoxic–ischaemic brain injury do not have corresponding positive axonal injury in the cord. Further study of such a potentially discriminatory feature is clearly warranted.

The vertebral column and spinal cord may be the primary site of NAI although less frequently so than the brain (Kleinman and Marks 1992). The results may not be fatal (Swischuk 1969) and may be underreported (Cullen 1975). Fatal cases may show spinal cord hypoxic and focal axonal injury (Fig. 11.12). Bruising in the neck behind or below the ear may be indicative of an injury to the vertebral artery and hence to the cervical cord and medulla. Injury to the vertebral column may be detectable on X-ray, or is revealed at autopsy by the presence of bleeding around the vertebrae. Detection of haemorrhage in this region should prompt more detailed examination of the radiological and pathological appearances. Epidural and subdural congestion and haemorrhage have been reported in sudden unexplained infant death in the past (Swischuk 1969) but it is not clear whether such cases

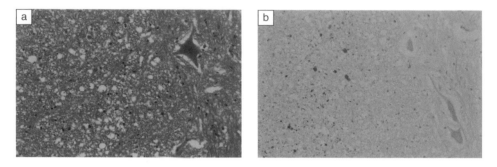

Fig. 11.12. Sections of the thoracic spinal cord from a 2-year-old child with non-accidental spinal injury producing spinal fracture at the level of T12. The child died of associated head injury 24 hours after the assault. (a) The parenchyma shows oedematous changes and recent hypoxic damage to a large spinal neuron (haematoxylin–eosin). (b) Axonal injury is confirmed by positivity for β-APP in axons in the tract to the left of the scan. [Both ×200.]

were the result of NAI. Spinal injury may be associated with concurrent brain haemorrhage or with isolated cerebral swelling. The long term sequelae for infants who survive spinal cord injury may be very profound, and include spastic quadriplegia or paraplegia.

Pathogenesis of non-accidental brain injury

So far as the antecedent circumstances of NAI are concerned, previous debate has centred on whether the changes seen in the infant brain were the result of shaking alone or whether a contact injury was also needed. Proponents of the view that contact is needed to induce the brain injury included Duhaime et al. (1992) and Di Maio (1998), but earlier opinion held that shaking in its own right could produce severe brain injury in an infant (Hadley et al. 1989, Alexander et al. 1990a). In circumstances where impact has been added to shaking injury the further insult of impact is not necessarily predictive of fatal outcome (Alexander et al. 1990b). The mechanistic events underlying NAHI are not well understood and it may be that rotatory movement is more damaging than to-and-fro movement. A view that SDH may be hypoxic in origin has been recently advanced (Geddes et al. 2003), but this has been challenged (Smith et al. 2003).

The primary injury is likely to lead to varying degrees of mechanical distortion of brain tissue and blood vessels within the meninges. Contact injury may result in skull fracture and disruption of meninges, brain tissue and blood vessels. The acceleration/deceleration movements resulting from shaking may induce rotational sheer injury within brain tissue leading to tissue distortion, disruption and contusion (Guthkelch 1971, Hadley et al. 1989, Duhaime et al. 1992, Jayawant et al. 1998, Kinney and Armstrong 2002). The pathogenesis of axonal injury appears to be the result of interrupted axonal transport, which may occur at the moment of injury and is identified by the presence of axonal retraction balls. These were thought initially to be due to physical disruption of axons but are now usually linked to disturbance of normal axonal transport causing localized distensions. Experimental studies show that nodal blebs occur on axons in association with calcium flux and that cytoskeletal abnormalities result in focal accumulation of 68 kD neurofilament protein (reviewed by Graham et al. 2002).

The cause of early diffuse brain swelling is not well understood, but it certainly contributes to raised intracranial pressure with consequent decrease in cerebral perfusion. Factors that have been implicated include immaturity of biomechanical properties, auto-regulation and vasoreactivity as well as poor tolerance of ischaemia/hypoxia and the tendency to post-injury apnoea and hypotension in children (Kinney and Armstrong 2002). Cerebral swelling appears to occur more commonly in children than in adults (Graham et al. 2002) and is associated with early vasodilatation in the brain (Conway 1998). Breakdown of the blood–brain barrier is likely to contribute to cerebral swelling (Brown and Minns 1993). Focal contusions within the white matter are early events and probably result from disruption of tissue in the presence of rotational sheer forces. Lacerations are rare in infantile NAI because of the smooth inner surface of the infant skull (Vowles et al. 1987).

Cerebral hypoxia due to respiratory dysregulation, together with hypotension, may compound the secondary brain insult. Hypoxia is also likely to contribute to damage in vulnerable neuronal subsets but damage may be mediated by excitotoxic transmitters such as glutamate or by the release of free radicals (Conway 1998). Neonatal rats who were subjected to shaking injury displayed pathology similar to that in NAHI in infants and there was evidence of a rise in free radical activity, although treatment with an antioxidant had no apparent neuroprotective effect (Smith et al. 1998). Pro-inflammatory cytokines including tumour necrosis factor α (TNFα) and interleukin 1β (IL1β) are released from activated cells including microglia, and this may be a further complicating factor in the evolving pathology. The cascade of molecular and cellular events that is set in train by traumatic injury, in particular by an episode of shaking, is not fully understood. Investigation of adult human cases, and of mature and immature experimental animals subjected to traumatic insult (re-viewed by Graham et al. 2002) may be informative in this regard about the pathogenesis of NAI in infant brains, despite developmental and interspecies related differences. The infant brain is virtually unmyelinated at birth and the consistency of brain tissue is markedly different from that of the adult (Duhaime et al 1992, Conway 1998). Magnetic resonance spectroscopy has been advocated as an in vivo method of monitoring biochemical cerebral events in shaken infants (Haseler et al. 1997).

In summary, the three most common pathological features found in NAHI are SDH, retinal haemorrhages and diffuse brain swelling. While SDH may be simply the result of disrupted bridging veins, the onset of brain swelling is less easily explicable. To what degree these conditions coexist with axonal injury of hypoxic or traumatic origin is not known. Because SDH is an acute event and is accompanied by cerebral oedema, the classic division of trau-matic lesions into focal and diffuse injury, which is emphasized in mature adult brains, is less relevant to the situation in the infant. The contribution of hypoxic damage to the spec-trum of NAHI has certainly been underestimated in the past.

DIFFERENTIAL DIAGNOSIS OF NAI
Although NAI remains the most likely cause of SDH in the infant, it is important to consider

the range of other possible causes that might lead to SDH, or any of the other pathological findings described above. In times past, SDH was relatively common in the context of birth-related injury and is classically seen following difficult breech or forceps delivery, and associated with tears in the dura mater, but these complications are rare nowadays (Brown and Minns 1993, Conway 1998, Kinney and Armstrong 2002). Retinal haemorrhages are also seen in some newborn infants in the absence of NAI but in these circumstances are not accompanied by SDH (Caffey 1974, Kinney and Armstrong 2002). Retinal haemorrhages are reported to occur rather rarely in accidental falls (Wilkins 1997). In contrast, Plunkett (2001) reported bilateral multilayered retinal haemorrhage in short distance accidental falls whenever it was looked for and always in association with SDH. Other reported causes of retinal haemorrhage include resuscitation, papilloedema, coagulopathy and hypertension (Kinney and Armstrong 2002). However, the prevalence of retinal haemorrhage in conditions other than NAI is not known because the globes are not routinely examined in cases of sudden infant death syndrome (SIDS). The main differential diagnosis for NAI is accidental trauma. The history and pattern of injury are usually helpful in distinguishing between the two. Billmire and Myers (1985) undertook a comparative study of accidental and abusive head injury in infants and showed that the prevalence of skull fracture was higher in the former group than in abuse-related head injury. In contrast, intracranial injury was much higher in NAI than in accidental trauma. As previously stated, Geddes et al. (2001a) reported skull fracture in rather more of the younger children (16/37) with NAHI than in the older children (19%). However, Plunkett (2001), in a retrospective study of observed accidental falls, found skull fracture in only 28% of cases. It is important to distinguish severe accidental trauma such as road traffic accidents from milder accidental trauma. In the context of falls in the home, Billmire and Myers (1985) showed that skull fracture was rare. It is in this context that the Plunkett study (2001) is often quoted, but it is noteworthy that the neuropathology status is not comprehensively reported in this paper, and that the children are often older, making comparison with infant NAHI more problematic. Duhaime et al. (1992) also found that most household falls were neurologically benign and concluded that SDH was much more likely to result from a road traffic accident or inflicted injury. Wilkins (1997) concurred with this view, although Conway (1998) reported that SDH was actually unusual in cerebral injury resulting from vehicle accidents. Haematological disorders, particularly bleeding diatheses, should be excluded as a cause of SDH, which may also arise as a complication of meningitis or of neurosurgical procedures (Jayawant et al. 1998). Axonal injury is known to occur in hypoxic–ischaemic injury of the brain and should not be interpreted as clear-cut evidence of accidental or non-accidental head injury (Geddes et al. 2001a,b; Kinney and Armstrong 2002). The two conditions may not be distinguishable pathologically, and both display β-APP immunoreactivity (Shannon et al. 1998, Gleckman et al. 1999). In a large Australian study of accidental deaths in children, attention was drawn to the rarity of accidents amongst infants of less than 1 year (Byard 2000). This was attributed to their relative immobility.

Intentional infant asphyxia may be difficult to distinguish from SIDS. There may be no distinguishing pathological findings in the brain in these two conditions, or slight swelling and/or gliosis may be present in either. The shaken baby syndrome has been likened in the past to near-miss SIDS, a minority of cases of which reportedly have associated retinal haemorrhages and SDH (Altman et al. 1998), circumstances that surely suggest that concealed NAHI has taken place. Conway (1998) presented a detailed analysis of the differences between SIDS and NAI. Byard (2000) has also highlighted the causes of sudden death in infancy. Geddes et al. (2003) and Geddes and Plunkett (2004) have called into question the whole concept of SDH being indicative of trauma. They have suggested that SDH in infants may rather be secondary to hypoxia, akin to events in SIDS. While Geddes and her colleagues have rightly pressed for better evidence gathering in the context of suspected NAHI, it is noted that recent papers from this group focused on microscopic intradural and subdural haemorrhages in hypoxic infants and inferred that the macroscopic SDHs in allegedly injured infants could also be ascribed to an hypoxic origin. However, it is unlikely that hypoxia could account for associated injuries that could be present, including fractures of the skull, injuries to the neck, and visibly ruptured bridging veins Harding et al. (2004) have again stressed that undue force is required for the triad of subdural and retinal haemorrhages with brain damage to be present in an infant. The diagnosis of NAHI should not rest on the presence of one feature alone. Because of the spectrum of clinical presentation and the uncertainty as to the exact causation of injury, Minns and Busuttil (2004) have recommended that the generic term, NAHI, should be used in preference to SBS.

It is clear from the above discussion that considerable uncertainties still remain regarding the pathogenesis of NAHI and this leads to dilemmas of interpretation. The debate hinges around the following facts. In infants, the SDH is often 'trivial' and certainly not space occupying. The infant may have SDH and severe brain swelling but no evidence of traumatic or even very much hypoxic axonal injury. There may be sufficient injury to the head to cause SDH, putatively caused by disruption of veins, while there is no evidence of traumatic axonal injury. The lack of certainty regarding the time of onset of observed pathological findings only adds to the uncertainties.

One possible chain of events is for the NAI to cause both SDH and diffuse axonal injury, which lead to brain swelling, raised intracranial pressure, cardiorespiratory collapse and rapid death before histological or immunocytological evidence of axonal injury can become evident. A second possibility is that the same injury may cause SDH and localized axonal damage in the brainstem, leading to loss of respiratory drive, generalized hypoxia with evolving evidence of hypoxic brain injury, brain swelling and a fatal outcome. In either case the infant brain may respond to injury more rapidly than a more mature brain. While it might be argued that the apparent absence of diffuse axonal injury implies only a mild injury, the fact that skull fracture is present in at least a proportion of cases confirms that a severe injury has occurred.

CASE STUDY 1

A 3-month-old firstborn infant was left in the care of his father for four hours. When the mother returned the infant was found to be unwell and drowsy and the father declared that the baby had bumped his head on the side of the cot. The infant rapidly became unresponsive and cyanosed, and started to convulse. An ambulance was called and on arrival at hospital the baby was found to have a bulging fontanelle and retinal haemorrhages, and he appeared pale. Imaging showed bilateral SDH and gross brain swelling. Burr holes were performed to decompress the haemorrhages but the baby remained comatose. Brain death tests were performed the next day following which the ventilator was switched off. At autopsy no skull fracture was found but bilateral SDH and brain swelling were confirmed. Subarachnoid haemorrhage was also present. Histological examination of the brain revealed widespread recent cerebral infarction and white matter axonal positivity for β-APP. The father denied that he had shaken the infant but was later convicted on a charge of NAI.

CASE STUDY 2
This 2-month-old female infant was the second child of her mother but the first of her father. The infant was left in the care of her father who made an emergency call to the ambulance service following what was claimed to be a fall from a settee. The infant was unconscious and not breathing, and examination showed bruising of the abdomen and fixed dilated pupils. The baby also had a skull fracture and SDH. Surgery was undertaken to remove the haematoma but to no avail and the infant remained deeply unconscious. Brain death tests were performed 3 days later. At autopsy, the skull fracture and SDH were confirmed. The brain was very swollen, and cerebral contusions were present in the white matter. Histological examination showed focal infarction and diffuse axonal injury. Autolytic changes were present in the cerebellum consistent with lack of perfusion of the brain. The father later admitted that he was responsible for the injuries.

Examination of the child with suspected NAI
In the context of a medico-legal autopsy in an infant where NAHI is suspected, a full clinical history and whole body radiological survey should be obtained. External signs of injury should be looked for, although these may be minimal or absent. The appearances of the scalp, skull, meninges, globes and optic nerves, as well as the external surface of the brain, should be recorded, with photography as necessary. It may be appropriate to retain a specimen of CSF to examine for xanthochromia if this was not available during life. The volume of any haemorrhage, particularly SDH, should be estimated as accurately as possible. Fresh or frozen samples should be retained as necessary for toxicology and microbiology purposes. It is most important to examine the soft tissues of the neck, the cervical spine and epidural region as well as the spinal cord (Kinney and Armstrong 2002).

If the brain is extremely swollen and/or there is suspicion of upper cervical cord injury, the cervical cord should be removed in continuity with the brainstem by exposing the posterior cranial fossa. This approach allows inspection of the cerebellar tonsils in relation to the foramen magnum and reduces any artefactual damage to the upper cervical cord. The brain should be suspended immediately in formalin solution for 2–3 weeks. It is highly desirable if not mandatory to retain the spinal cord, particularly the cervical cord, for later examination. The globes should be retained for later sectioning.

The fixed brain is weighed and photographed. The macroscopic appearances are described including the cranial nerves, particularly the olfactory, optic and oculomotor nerves, and the cranial vessels and leptomeninges. Evidence of shift and herniations as well as gyral injury should be noted. Coronal sectioning of the cerebrum after detachment of the brainstem and cerebellum will reveal the status of the ventricular cavities, together with evidence of contusions or cerebral haemorrhages, particularly in the corpus callosum. Evidence of older damage or malformation should also be sought. The brainstem, cerebellum and spinal cord should be similarly examined. Representative photographs should be taken particularly of any abnormalities. Tissue blocks for histology should include all areas of the cortex, including the temporal hippocampus bilaterally, the basal ganglia and thalami, adequate representation of the central white matter and corpus callosum, and the midbrain, pons, medulla, cerebellum and cord. The importance of comprehensive tissue sampling for accurate detection of axonal injury has been emphasized by Geddes et al. (1997, 2000, 2001a,b). The leptomeninges should be retained in as many blocks as possible in order to detect the presence of meningitis. Any focal lesions or evidence of older brain damage should be sampled, together with areas of possible infarction. Histological examination using routine staining should be supplemented with special stains including luxol fast blue for myelin. Evidence of axonal damage should be sought using antibodies to 68 kD neurofilament protein and β-APP. Assessment for haemosiderin deposition may be required in the meninges Astrogliosis and microgliosis may be visualized using antibodies to glial fibrillary acidic protein and CD68 respectively. Other stains may be appropriate depending on the primary histological findings. All tissues, blocks, slides and photographs should be reliably identified and labelled, and preserved until final decisions about the case have been taken.

Conclusions

The majority of infants and young children in whom subdural and retinal haemorrhages with brain damage are identified are likely to have suffered NAI, and this is an important cause of death and persistent disability. Cerebral damage in the infant is easily induced. Variable degrees of axonal injury, hypoxia and/or contusional injury may be present. In the context of anything other than certain accident, these findings should alert healthcare staff to the suspicion of NAI. However, the attribution of blame can be problematic in cases presenting with atypical pathology, and the lack of basic understanding of infant head injury only compounds this problem. Guidelines exist for the clinical investigation of such cases. The initial pathological events in the brain may be compounded by allegedly secondary events such as hypoxic–ischaemic injury, herniation and further brain swelling. Alternatively these features may be part of the primary response, and they certainly appear very rapidly in many cases. In theory, some of these conditions may be amenable to thera-peutic intervention although this possibility remains limited at present. Delay in seeking medical assistance also reduces the opportunities for preventing secondary damage. The consequences of failing to diagnose episodes of NAI are those of continuing risk for further episodes in the survivors or in their sibs. Serious neurological sequelae in the survivors of infant NAI pose a major burden on society.

> "Guard well your baby's precious head
> shake, jerk and slap it never
> lest you bruise his brain and twist his mind
> or whiplash him dead for ever."
>
> (Caffey 1974)

ACKNOWLEDGEMENTS

Dr Jean Keeling, Dr Ian Rushton, Professor Anthony Busuttil and Dr Colin Smith have provided helpful discussion. Figures 11.1, 11.3, 11.4, 11.5 and 11.7 are photographs kindly provided by Dr Jean Keeling of cases examined jointly with the author. The assistance of Mrs Betty Wyatt in the laboratory investigations, and of Ms Angela Penman in the preparation of the manuscript, is gratefully acknowledged.

REFERENCES

Alexander R, Crabbe L, Sato Y, Smith W, Bennett T (1990a) Serial abuse in children who are shaken. *Am J Dis Child* **144**: 58–60.

Alexander R, Sato Y, Smith, W, Bennett T (1990b) Incidence of impact trauma with cranial injuries ascribed to shaking. *Am J Dis Child* **144**: 724–726.

Altman RL, Kutscher ML, Brand DA (1998) The "shaken baby syndrome". *N Engl J Med* **339**: 1329–1330.

American Academy of Pediatrics Committee on Child Abuse and Neglect (1993) Shaken baby syndrome: inflicted cerebral trauma. *Pediatrics* **92**: 872–875.

Barlow LM, Minns RA (2000) Annual incidence of shaken impact syndrome in young children. *Lancet* **356**: 1571–1572.

Billmire ME, Myers PA (1985) Serious head injury in infants: accident or abuse? *Pediatrics* **75**: 340–342.

Brown JK, Minns RA (1993) Non-accidental head injury with particular reference to whiplash shaking injury and medical–legal aspects. *Dev Med Child Neurol* **35**: 849–869.

Byard RW (2000) Accidental childhood death and the role of the pathologist. *Pediatr Dev Pathol* **3**: 405–418.

Caffey J (1972) On the theory and practice of shaking infants. Its potential residual effects of permanent brain damage and mental retardation. *Am J Dis Child* **124**: 161–169.

Caffey J (1974) The whiplash shaken infant syndrome: manual shaking by the extremities with whiplash-induced intracranial and intraocular bleedings, linked with residual permanent brain damage and mental retardation. *Pediatrics* **54**: 396–403.

Carty H, Ratcliffe J (1995) The shaken infant syndrome. *BMJ* **310**: 344–345.

Conway EE (1998) Nonaccidental head injury in infants: "the shaken baby syndrome revisited". *Pediatr Ann* **27**: 677–690.

Cullen JC (1975) Spinal lesions in battered babies. *J Bone Joint Surg Br* **57**: 364–366.

Di Maio VJ (1998) The "shaken-baby syndrome". *N Engl J Med* **339**: 1329 (letter; author reply 1329–1330).

Duhaime AC, Gennarelli TA, Thilbault LE, Bruce DA, Margulies SS, Wiser R (1987) The shaken baby syndrome. A clinical, pathological and biomechanical study. *J Neurosurg* **66**: 409–415.

Duhaime AC, Alario AJ, Lewander WJ, Schut L, Sutton LN, Seidl TS, Nudelman S, Budenz D, Hertle R, Tsiaras W, Loporchio S (1992) Head injury in very young children: mechanisms, injury types and ophthalmologic findings in 100 hospitalized patients younger than 2 years of age. *Pediatrics* **90**: 179–185.

Duhaime AC, Christian CW, Rorke LB, Zimmerman RA (1998) Nonaccidental head injury in infants the "shaken baby syndrome". *N Engl J Med* **338**: 1822–1829.

Geddes JF, Plunkett J (2004) The evidence base for shaken baby syndrome – we need to question the diagnostic criteria. *BMJ* **328**: 719–720.

Geddes JF, Vowles GH, Beer TW, Ellison DW (1997) The diagnosis of diffuse axonal injury: implications for forensic practice. *Neuropathol Appl Neurobiol* **23**: 339–347.

Geddes JF, Whitwell HL, Graham DI (2000) Traumatic axonal injury: practical issues for diagnosis in medico-legal cases. *Neuropathol Appl Neurobiol* **26**: 105–116.

Geddes JF, Hackshaw AK, Vowles GH, Nickols CD, Whitwell HL (2001a) Neuropathology of inflicted head injury in children. I. Patterns of brain damage. *Brain* **124**: 1290–1298.

Geddes JF, Vowles GH, Hackshaw AK, Nickols CD, Scott IS, Whitwell HL (2001b) Neuropathology of inflicted head injury in children. II. Microscopic brain injury in infants. *Brain* **124**: 1299–1306.

Geddes JF, Tasker RC, Hackshaw AK, Nickols CD, Adams GGW, Whitwell HL, Scheimberg I (2003) Dural haemorrhage in non-traumatic infants: does it explain the bleeding in 'shaken baby syndrome'? *Neuropathol Appl Neurobiol* **29**: 14–22.

Gleckman AM, Bell MD, Evans RJ, Smith TW (1999) Diffuse axonal injury in infants with nonaccidental craniocerebral trauma: enhanced detection by beta-amyloid precursor protein immunohistochemical staining. *Arch Pathol Lab Med* **123**: 146–151.

Graham DI, Gennarelli TA, McIntosh TK (2002) Trauma. In: Graham DI, Lantos PL, editors. *Greenfield's Neuropathology, 7th edn*. London: Arnold, p. 823–898.

Guthkelch AN (1971) Infantile subdural haematoma and its relationship to whiplash injury. *BMJ* **2**: 430–431.

Hadley MN, Sonntag VKH, Rekate HL, Murphy A (1989) The infant whiplash–shake syndrome: a clinical pathological study. *Neurosurgery* **24**: 536–540.

Harding B, Risdon RA, Krous HF (2004) Shaken baby syndrome – pathological diagnosis rests on the combined triad, not on individual injuries. *BMJ* **328**: 720–721.

Haseler LJ, Arcinue E, Danielsen ER, Bluml S, Ross BD (1997) Evidence from proton magnetic resonance spectroscopy for a metabolic cascade of neuronal damage in shaken baby syndrome. *Pediatrics* **99**: 4–14.

Jayawant S, Rawlinson A, Gibbon F, Price J, Schulte J, Sharples P, Sibert JR, Kemp AM (1998) Subdural haemorrhages in infants: population based study. *BMJ* **317**: 1558–1561.

Kempe CH, Silverman FN, Steele BF, Droegemueller W, Silver HK (1962) The battered-child syndrome. *JAMA* **181**: 17–24.

Kinney HC, Armstrong DD (2002) Perinatal neuropathology. In: Graham DI, Lantos PL, editors. *Greenfield's Neuropathology, 7th edn*. London: Arnold, p. 519–609.

Kleinman PK, Marks SC (1992) Vertebral body fractures in child abuse. Radiologic–histopathologic correlates. *Invest Radiol* **27**: 715–722.

Kleinman PK, Marks SC, Richmond JM, Blackbourne BD (1995) Inflicted skeletal injury: a postmortem radiologic–histopathologic study in 31 infants. *AJR* **165**: 647–650.

Krous HF, Byard RW (1999) Shaken infant syndrome: selected controversies *Pediatr Dev Pathol* **2**: 497–498.

Lloyd B (1998) Subdural haemorrhages in infants. *BMJ* **317**, 1538–1539.

Minns RA, Busuttil A (2004) Patterns of presentation of the shaken baby syndrome. *BMJ* **328**: 766.

Munger CE, Peiffer RL, Bouldin TW, Kylstra JA, Thompson RL (1993) Ocular and associated neuropathologic observations in suspected whiplash shaken infant syndrome. A retrospective study of 12 cases. *Am J Forensic Med Pathol* **14**: 193–200.

Oehmichen M, Meibner C, Schmidt V, Pedal I, Konig HG (1999) Pontine axonal injury after brain trauma and nontraumatic hypoxic–ischaemic brain damage. *Int J Legal Med* **112**: 261–267.

Plunkett J (2001) Fatal paediatric head injuries caused by short-distance falls. *Am J Forensic Med Pathol* **22**: 1–12.

Russell PA (1965) Subdural haematoma in infancy. *BMJ* **2**: 446–448.

Shannon P, Smit CR, Deck J, Ang LC, Ho M, Becker L (1998) Axonal injury and the neuropathology of shaken baby syndrome. *Acta Neuropathol* **95**: 625–631.

Sherwood D (1930) Chronic subdural haematoma in infants. *Am J Dis Child* **39**: 980–1021.

Smith C, Bell JE, Keeling JW, Risden RA (2003) Dural haemorrhage in non-traumatic infant deaths: does it explain the bleeding in 'shaken baby syndrome'? Geddes JE et al. A response. *Neuropathol Appl Neurobiol* **29**: 411–413.

Smith SL, Andrus PK, Gleason DD, Hall ED (1998) Infant rat model of the shaken baby syndrome: preliminary characterization and evidence for the role of free radicals in cortical haemorrhaging and progressive neuronal degeneration. *J Neurotrauma* **15**: 693–705.

Spear RM, Chadwick D, Peterson BM (1992) Fatalities associated with misinterpretation of blood cerebrospinal fluid in the "shaken baby syndrome". *Am J Dis Child* **146**: 1415–1417.

Swischuk LE (1969) Spine and spinal cord trauma in the battered child syndrome. *Radiology* **92**: 733.

Towbin H (1967) Sudden infant death related to spinal injury. *Lancet* **ii**: 940.

Vowles GH, Scholtz CL, Cameron JM (1987) Diffuse axonal injury in early infancy. *J Clin Pathol* **40**: 185–190.

Wilkins B (1997) Head injury—abuse or accident? *Arch Dis Child* **76**. 393–396; discussion 396–397.

12

OUTCOME AND PROGNOSIS OF NON-ACCIDENTAL HEAD INJURY IN INFANTS

Robert A Minns, Patricia A Jones, Karen M Barlow

Although extreme shaking may damage the adult brain (Pounder 1997, Carrigan et al. 2000), the young infant brain is particularly vulnerable to shaking injury because the head size is relatively large and heavy in comparison with body size, head control is not yet established and the neck muscles are weak and hypotonic, there is normally a relatively wide extracerebral space in young infants, and there is physiological laxity of the meninges at this age. However, shaking is not the only mechanism of inducing a brain injury in infants; others include shaking with impact, isolated impact injury (acceleration/deceleration) and compression injury. The primary brain injuries will result from 'impact forces' that cause injuries to the scalp, skull and brain in the form of bruising, lacerations, subgaleal haemorrhage, skull fractures, extradural haemorrhages brain contusions and focal subdural haemorrhages, and 'inertial forces' which are consequent on movement of the brain within the cranium with rotational and deceleration forces resulting in concussion, bilateral subdural and subarachnoid haemorrhages, subcortical tears, diffuse axonal injury and intraparenchymal haemorrhage, and injury to the brainstem, cervico-medullary junction and spinal cord. The secondary brain injuries are both hypoxic and ischaemic in origin (central apnoea, hypoxaemia, hypotension, anaemia, hyponatraemia, raised intracranial pressure, low cerebral perfusion pressure, ischaemia, vasospasm, seizures, infection, excito-toxic stress, etc.) and result in diffuse cerebral hypodensities, border zone infarctions and cerebral oedema.

Outcome studies

Studies reporting the outcome and prognosis of non-accidental head injury (NAHI) to infants quote marginally different rates for mortality and neurological and developmental sequelae, although the results are universally poor (Tables 12.1–12.3). In attempting to appraise the literature and deduce an accurate picture of the consequences of NAHI it must be appreciated that there are a number of factors that limit comparability:

(1) While most series are similar in their definition of abusive head injury to infants, the precise definitions may differ slightly. Some studies do not specify how strict the diagnostic criteria were for entry to the study, or whether they were acknowledged/confessed or convicted cases, or whether they remain 'suspected NAHI'. However, the diagnoses in most series have been based on an anomalous history in which the story is incompatible with the mechanism offered, is not unexplained at all, or is inconsistent, together with the

364

recognition of a clinical syndrome consisting of clinical, radiological and ophthalmological features that are all individually consistent with (and sometimes characteristic of) a non-accidental origin. This leads to a presumptive clinical diagnosis of 'suspected' NAHI, inflicted traumatic brain injury or shaken baby (or impact) syndrome. In most series the diagnosis has satisfied 'child case conferences' or child protection proceedings.

(2) Many studies comprise highly selected hospital cases and the outcome may not reflect the broad picture of all NAHIs.

(3) Outcome studies are often different in their design and lack procedural uniformity; most were retrospective and only a few had prospective follow-up; and some lacked a comparison group of accidental head injury in infants, which makes regression analysis for risk factors problematic.

(4) The duration of follow-up was variable and usually short. The mean follow-up interval (from 13 studies) was 15 months ± 13.6 months (Makaroff and Putnam 2003). Only Bonnier et al. (1995) and Barlow et al. (2003) report follow-up through later childhood. The follow-up usually began immediately following the injury or after discharge from hospital, but others define the start point as from the resolution of post-traumatic amnesia, which for 2-year-olds was defined as a return to play activities (Ewing-Cobbs et al. 1998).

(5) The injury severity will undoubtedly influence outcome. A number of studies have nominated a low Glasgow Coma Score to indicate injury severity, but other indices such as 'duration of unconsciousness' or cerebral oedema have additionally been factored in as a measure of cerebral injury severity.

(6) The outcome scales employed to measure global outcome have generally been modifications (e.g. Adelson et al. 1997) of the Glasgow Outcome Scale (Jennett and Bond 1975), which instead of being compared to the pre-injury functional level, is compared to age-appropriate activities in normal children. Global outcome in future studies may be more appropriately assessed by means of the KOSCHI score (Crouchman et al. 2001).

Follow-up of children who have been abused is a difficult research exercise. Investigators eventually make contact with the child and family in only 23% of those originally identified in hospital (Duhaime et al. 1996). The reasons for this are the reluctance of caregivers to revisit painful thoughts and feelings about the original injury; defaulting from long-term follow-up by a very mobile population who are casual about health issues; and changes in the family structure. The children's medical supervisors may be reluctant to recommend them for further medical examinations, and there may be strict legal constraints on locating the child and their new family.

While there is a vast literature on the effects of child abuse, child abuse is a very hetero-geneous diagnosis and much of the literature comprises follow-up studies after emotional, sexual or other types of abuse or neglect, and head injury is often excluded from these studies (Applebaum 1977, Green et al. 1981, Okun et al. 1994). Abuse that has not involved head injury may still be associated with later cognitive, motor or language delay. Dissociating the effects of the brain injury from the effects of other maltreatment or poor social conditions is a challenge and will be more relevant in children who were older at the time of inflicted head injury and those whose head injury was at the mild to moderate end of the severity spectrum.

TABLE 12.1
Prospective studies of outcome following non-accidental head injury

Category	Reference	N	Age at injury	Time to outcome	Series (type of injuries and study)	Outcome measures
Child abuse/ accident/ comparisons with impact	Elmer (1977)	17 matched pairs plus non-trauma matched group	≤12mo	Approx. 8yr	Child abuse, with evidence of impact. Matched for age, sex, race and socio-economic status. Also matched for infantile hospitalization. Identified, prospectively studied 8 years later	Anthropometric measures; language development; self-concept; intellectual functioning; impulsivity; aggression; interim school achievement ratings
NAHI	Ewing-Cobbs et al. (1998)	20	0–6yr (mean 10.6mo)	Mean 1.3mo post-injury	Inflicted TBI (vs 20 non-inflicted). All survivors. Prospective study	Modified Glasgow Outcome Scores; cognitive development; motor functioning; Children's Orientation and Amnesia Test for 3- to 6-yr-olds; "return to play activities" for 0- to 2-yr-olds; Bayley Scales of Infant Development, 2nd edn (Mental and Motor scales); Stanford–Binet Intelligence Scale, 4th edn; McCarthy Scales of Children Abilities
Inflicted TBI	Ewing-Cobbs et al. (1999)	28 survivors	2–42mo (mean 9.28mo)	1–3mo post-injury	Moderate to severe TBI, suspicious for inflicted injury. Algorithm uses: injuries incompatible with stated mechanism, unexplained injuries and old skeletal fractures, delay in seeking treatment, changing history. Comparison group n=28, uninjured, <42mo, same inclusion criteria (except no HI, or no known premorbid neurologic/metabolic disorder, and no prior history of TBI, gestational age ≥32wk, and CT on first day. Prospective study	Bayley Scales of Infant Development–II, Bayley Behaviour Rating Scale, Modified Glasgow Outcome Scale (5 = dead, 1 = good)

Outcome and comments	Dead	Coma/ veg state	Severe disability	Moderate disability	Good recovery
3 groups: abused, accidents, comparison group. No differences in any except anthropometric measures where abused were significantly heavier than others. All 3 groups scored poorly in all aspects, with many developmental problems. Socio-economic status may be as potent a factor as abuse in development of a child. Language difficulties common in all 3 groups					
9/20 with ITBI achieved good recovery and 13/20 had moderate disability, vs 11/20 and 7/20 respectively in non-ITBI group. 9/20 with ITBI scored in "mentally deficient" range vs 1/20 in non-ITBI group, p <0.005. Motor scores similar in both groups, with 5/20 of each group in deficit range. Seizures in 13/20 with ITBI. Hemiparesis in 6/20 with ITBI. Cranial nerve deficits in 4/20 with ITBI. Distribution in non-inflicted group: 11 good recovery, 5 moderate disability, 4 severe disability. Significantly different to NAI group	n/a	0	3	13	4
1 At baseline, and at 3mo FU, the ITBI group scored significantly lower than comparison group on both mental and physical developmental indices, and the distribution of scores differed across the groups at both baseline and FU. 2. At baseline, and at 3mo FU, the ITBI group had less favorable Behaviour Rating Scale than comparison group, and at baseline more with ITBI had scores in non-optimal range. 3. ITBI group had higher rate of impairment in motor quality, orientation/engagement and non-optimal emotional regulation. GOS scores stable from discharge to 3mo FU. At 3 mo FU, Bayley Behaviour Rating Scale results showed: impaired emotional regulation in 12/26, orientation/engagement in 7/25; and impaired motor quality in 12/28. Those with ITBI without oedema/infarct had scores in low-average range at both baseline and FU Children with oedema/infarcts obtained significantly lower mental and motor scores than others with ITBI. Those with oedema/infarct had scores in delayed/ "deficient" range (65–/4)	n/a	0	4	17	7

Continues ➔

TABLE 12.1
(continued)

Category	Reference	N	Age at injury	Time to outcome	Series (type of injuries and study)	Outcome measures
NAHI	Barlow et al. (1999, 2004)	55 met criteria; 25 consented to be included in study	Mean 5.3mo Median 2.36mo	Planned FUs fre-quently delayed because of medico-legal and social circum-stances Mean length of FU was 59mo (median 40mo, range 11–252mo)	NAHI, satisfying a predetermined algorithm that NAHI is the most likely mechanism of injury, and consent of physician and legal guardian. Algorithm: an encephalopathy plus at least two of the following: intracranial haemorrhage, including SDH, RH, rib fractures, skeletal injuries, malicious injuries, and history inconsistent with observed injuries and/or changing histories with time. Cross-sectional and prospective study	Physical examination at least 3mo after hospital discharge, and every 6–12mo thereafter. Assessment based on (i) recorded neurological deficits, and (ii) a calculated developmental quotient (DQ) in gross motor, fine motor and hand function, communication and language abilities: DQ ≤25 = profound impairment, DQ >25–50 = severe impairment, DQ >50–70 = mild impairment, DQ >70–<80 = mild impairment. Modified Glasgow Outcome Score (1 = dead, 5 = good). Seshia's Outcome (1 = normal, 6 = dead). Neuropsychological testing in all cases at least once, included: Bayley Scales of Infant Development (2nd edn) 0–2.5yr; Mental Developmental Index (score of 100 is mean); Psychomotor Developmental Index (score of 100 is mean); Behaviour Rating Scale: total score categorized as Within Normal Limits, Questionable, or Non-optimal; Vineland Adaptive Behaviour Scales; Reynell–Zinkin score used for children with severe visual impairment

Abbreviations:
Coma/veg state = coma/vegetative state
FU = follow-up
GOS = Glasgow Outcome Scores
ITBI = inflicted traumatic brain injury
NAHI = non-accidental head injury
n/a = not applicable
NAI = non-accidental injury
RH = retinal haemorrhage
SDH = subdural haemorrhage
TBI = traumatic brain injury.

Numbers underlined have been used in summations.

Outcome and comments	Dead	Coma/ veg state	Severe disability	Moderate disability	Good recovery
Mortality, total group = 6/55 (10.9%). Outcome in study group: Acquired microcephaly 7/25. Neuromotor assessments: normal neuromotor patterns 10/25, hemiparesis 4/25, ataxia 8/25, tetraplegia 2/25, mixed motor conditions 4/25. Visual function abnormalities (including cortical blindness, visual agnosia, field and acuity defects) 12/25. Epilepsy 5/25. Gross motor function: 11/25 normal, 14/25 with difficulties. Normal functional mobility in 15/25. Fine motor function in upper limb normal 11/25. Speech and language normal 9/25. Abnormal behaviour 13/25. Global Outcome, Seshia Score: 7/25 normal, 5/25 mild difficulties, 6/25 moderate difficulties, 7/25 severe difficulties	1	0	9	5	10

TABLE 12.2
Retrospective outcome studies with outcome categorized by modified GOS score, or similar

Category	Reference	N	Age at injury	Time to outcome	Series (type of injuries and study)	Outcome measures
Child abuse and neglect	Morse et al. (1970)	25	Range: 3mo – 5yr 11mo Mean 24.4mo	2yr – 4yr 5mo post-injury Median = 2yr 11mo Ages at FU: 2yr 9mo – 9yr 10mo Median = 5yr 3mo	Abuse = "any wilful or grossly careless act on the part of caregiver which resulted in overt physical injury". Gross neglect = "omission of caregiver to take minimal precautions for the proper supervision of child's health and/or welfare." Series included survivors of suspected abuse or neglect. Suggested abuse diagnosed only when no other explanation seemed plausible, or on admission of abuse	21/25 families available for interview for FU. All notes reviewed, and all agencies involved contacted, including courts, police, child protection, family service agencies, hospitals, institutions for mentally ill and "mentally retarded", and teachers, etc. 16 children ≤24mo
Acute head injury from abuse	Sinal and Ball (1987)	24 23/24	1–20mo <1yr	Clinical exams at periodic intervals (range 5d – 7yr post-injury)	All with acute head trauma (on CT) after abuse, with following criteria: (i) an admission of abuse; (ii) multiple injuries unexplained by medical history or evaluation, or by social service evaluation; (iii) confirmation of abuse by Dept of Social Services and/or the Court system. 6 cases excluded because CT not performed Whiplash shaken infant syndrome (WSIS) identified if there was a history of being shaken or thrown into the air, without a history of battering of the head. If no history, then Caffey's (1974) guidelines for diagnosis were followed. WSIS n=17 (all <9mo, 14/17 <6mo)	Neurological exam and repeated FU

Outcome and comments	Died	Coma/ veg	Sev dis	Mod dis	Minor dis	Good recov	N/K	Total
4/25 lost to FU								
6/21 normal (15/21 remaining with difficulties); 9/21 mentally retarded; 6/21 emotionally disturbed.	Excl	0	? 5	? 6	? 4	6	—	21
Of 16 children ≤4mo at time of injury, 4 lost to FU, 3 normal.	Excl	0	3	4	2	3	4	16
In no case were any formal charges made on behalf of authorities or convictions obtained								
Died 3/24	3	—	7	5	5	3	1	24
Spastic quadriplegia 4/24								
Spastic diplegia 2/24								
Hemiparesis 1/24								
Blindness 2/24								
Severe mental retardation 6/24								
Moderate/mild mental retardation 4/24								
Developmental delay 6/24								
Mild cerebral palsy 3/24								
Seizures 7/24								
Severe behavioural problems/ADD 2/24								
Normal 3/24								

Continues ➔

TABLE 12.2
(continued)

Category	Reference	N	Age at injury	Time to outcome	Series (type of injuries and study)	Outcome measures
NAHI vs TBI	Goldstein et al. (1993)	40	All <18yr	"At hospital discharge"	All diagnosed with head injury by history, physical exam, evidence of trauma on skull X-ray/CT [NAHI diagnosis given only after review of all medical, social, criminal or family court decisions]	GOS at discharge from hospital
		14 NAHI	1.6yr ± 2.0yr SE			
		26 TBI	7.3yr ± 5.4yr SE			
Whiplash SBS	Fischer and Allasio (1994)	10 survivors	1–12mo (median 3mo)	8–15yr post-injury	Whiplash SBS (intracranial and retinal haemorrhages in the absence of signs of head trauma or skull fracture). From original 25, 4 died, 4 re-injured and excluded. From remaining 17, 10 survivors traced	Review of medical records; telephone interview with parent/grandparents; standardized questions and collection forms
NAI with CNS injury	Johnson et al. (1995)	75 suffered child abuse, 28 with CNS injury:		Extracted from case notes retro-spectively. No indi-cation of FU period given	Admitted as NAI, confirmed child abuse with CNS injury	Apnoea (description of breathing prior to admission, first recorded systolic BP <80, arterial pH at first encounter). Diffuse brain swelling
		15	Mean = 6mo		SIS (physical signs of impact and/or skull fracture)	
		13	Mean = 4mo		SBS (without evidence of direct trauma, i.e. craniofacial bruising or swelling)	
Whiplash SIS	Bonnier et al. (1995)	13	3wk – 21mo	4–14yr post-injury	Whiplash shaken impact syndrome	General exam, neurological exam, psychological evaluation, social evaluation, developmental tests (Gesell, WISC, Ajuriaguerraand Marcelli, Terman)
		12	3wk – 6mo (mean 5.5mo)			
		1	21mo			

Outcome and comments	Died	Coma/ veg	Sev dis	Mod dis	Minor dis	Good recov	N/K	Total
Median GOS in NAHI group = 3 (cf median GOS in accidental TBI group = 4; p=0.004). 8 with neurological complications in NAHI group (vs 10 in accidental TBI): Blindness/visual impairment 3 (vs 0 in accidental TBI) Focal neurological deficit 2 (vs 0 in accidental TBI) Hemiparesis 1 (vs 0 in accidental TBI) Seizures 7 (vs 6 in accidental TBI) Orthopaedic complications 1 (vs 6 in accidental TBI)	5	1		7		1	—	14
At discharge: 3 "normal"; 3 with epilepsy; 1 VP shunt; 2 with cerebral palsy; 1 "vegetative". At long-term FU: 1 "normal" 3 spastic hemiparesis 2 spastic quadriparesis 1 blind; 2 poor vision 1 severe mental retardation 2 behavioural problems 2 motor deficits 4 moderate cognitive deficits 1 no speech	Excl	—	7	2	—	1	—	10
Apnoea common as part of "admitting history" (23/28 required intubation on admission). 21/28 had seizures. 21/28 had diffuse brain swelling. 25/28 were <6mo, 3 were >1yr. None with diffuse cerebral swelling had a good outcome. None with admission GCS ≤8 had a good outcome. Trauma-induced apnoea causes cerebral hypoxia and/or ischaemia, which is more fundamental to outcome than the mechanism of injury.								
All CNS injury:	4	1	7	7	—	9	—	28
SIS (+ impact):	4	1	—	6	—	4	—	15
SBS (– impact):	0	7	—	1	—	5	—	13
1 died (with no sign-free interval) 6/12 severely disabled (with no sign-free interval) 5/12 moderate–severe disability, all requiring special education – developed signs after a sign-free interval 1/12 normal – remained sign free at 3 yr post-injury 2/12 blind; 2/12 visual impairment 3/12 tetraplegia/hemiplegia; 2/12 hemiparesis 4/12 microcephaly 4/12 epilepsy 9/12 psychomotor retardation 6/12 psychiatric problems 11/12 mental retardation	1	0	6	5	—	1	—	13

Continues ➔

TABLE 12.2
(continued)

Category	Reference	N	Age at injury	Time to outcome	Series (type of injuries and study)	Outcome measures
NAHI (SIS)	Duhaime et al. (1996)	84 (total group) 14 FU	<2yr Mean = 6.4mo	 5.3–15.3yr (average 9yr) post-injury (age 5.5–15.5yr)	NAHI (SIS)	Telephone interview. Modified GOS
NAI	Haviland and Russell (1997)	15	1–30mo (mean 3mo)	3mo–3yr post-injury	NAI (severe injuries inconsistent with history; clinical, radiological and/or ophthalmic evidence suggesting NAI; and sufficient clinical confidence in diagnosis to involve police and social services)	Description of disability: Severe = physical, "mental disability", totally dependent; Mod = severe hemiparesis, blindness, developmental delay; Mild = hemiparesis and seizures
NAHI	Gilles and Nelson (1998)	14	53d – (mean 12mo 6d)	4–34mo post-injury (mean 17mo 12d post-injury)	Confirmed NAHI, "witnessed, confession, conviction, or physical evidence of injury without trauma history", grouped into diffuse hypoattenuation (mean age 5mo) or focal cerebral hypoattenuation (mean age 16mo)	Children's Outcome Score (COS), Denver II developmental testing
NAHI	Barlow and Minns (1999)	17	1–20mo (mean 5.1mo)	3–122mo (mean age 33mo)	Combination of using ICD codes, examining intensive care and neurology ward admission details, and hospital social work department case files. All cases defined as acute encephalopathy plus at least 2 of the following: RH, skeletal fractures, inconsistent history, SDH, other malicious injury	Sheisa outcome scale (1 = normal to 6 = dead) (includes neurological deficits,seizures and seizure control, and functional outcome, based on developmental quotient. Intracranial pressure/MAP/CPP

374

Outcome and comments	Died	Coma/ veg	Sev dis	Mod dis	Minor dis	Good recov	N/K	Total
22 died; 62 survived, of whom 14 could be traced: 3 blind, nonverbal and wheelchair-dependent 1 blind, mental retardation and seizures 2 hemiparetic, severe learning disabilities and behavioural problems 2 moderate disabilities, perceptual impairments, memory and attention deficits (special schools) 1 hemiparetic 1 vegetative, died 5 yr post-injury 5 good outcome, functioning in normal school, but 3 repeated grades/have special tutors; 2 behavioural problems	1	—	6	2		5	—	14
At discharge: 2 died 9 severely disabled 3 moderately disabled 1 normal, and still normal at 3 months FU (no further FU recorded in this patient) At FU:	2	—	7	4	1	1	—	15
Poor in both groups (focal vs diffuse/hypoattenuation), mean COS III/IV. 3 died, 6 severe/very severe developmental delay; 3 moderate delay; 3 mild delay. Motor deficit 9/14: hemiparesis 4, quadriparesis 5. Visual loss 10/14. Epilepsy 3/14. Microcephaly 8/14. Cerebral infarction developed in all survivors (most common was hemispheric necrosis after swelling, ipsilateral to ASDH). A range of infarctions (PCA 4/14; CM branch of ACA 4/14; and border zone 4/14). No lucid interval (9/9) found in these children, typical of severe concussive syndrome. 11/14 EPTS, with progression of symptoms in 9	3	3	6	2	0	0	—	14
No differences between those with impact ⊥ shaking, and those with pure whiplash SBS. Lowest CPP significantly related to outcome, p≤0.005. Lowest MAP significantly related to outcome, p=0.039. Mean maximum ICP did not correlate significantly with outcome, p=0.251	2	0	3	3	2	7	—	17

Continues ➔

TABLE 12.2
(continued)

Category	Reference	N	Age at injury	Time to outcome	Series (type of injuries and study)	Outcome measures
Hypoxic–ischaemic encephalopathy, excluding accidental trauma	Rao et al. (1999)	73: 47 NAI, 26 medical conditions	1d – 15yr. Boys, mean = 12mo. Girls, mean = 18mo	Not stated ("long term")	26 with "medical conditions" (11 with sepsis, 3 SIDS/near-miss cot death, 1 smoke inhalation, 2 seizures, 9 cardiac arrest). None had skull fracture, RH, bruising, soft tissue injury or scalp injury. 47 no identifiable medical reason for admission, but NAHI features (16 had skull fracture, 14 rib(s) fracture, 19 long bone fractures, 21 RHs, 15 skin bruising, 6 petechial rash, 1 necklace calcification, 8 scalp haematoma,18 tense fontanelle). Dx of NAHI made based on a combination of clinical and radiological findings, and the exclusion of identifiable cause for hypoxic–ischaemic injury or bleeding	Reversal sign (in hypoxic–ischaemic cerebral injury) on CT (described as diffusely decreased density of the cerebral cortical grey and white matter with a decreased or lost grey–white interface or reversal of the grey–white matter densities and relative increased density of the thalami, brainstem and cerebellum)
NAHI	Barlow et al. (2000)	44	1–34mo (mean 5.9mo) length of FU in survivors = 3yr)	3mo – 18yr (median	All cases defined as acute encephalopathy plus at least 2 of the following: RH, skeletal fractures, inconsistent history, SDH, other malicious injury	Identification of early post-traumatic seizures: number, length and duration of seizures; status epilepticus classified as (1) responsive to medication with episodes of status epilepticus; or (2) unresponsive to medication ± status epilepticus. Time from 1st hospital admission to 1st seizure. Seisha's 6 point outcome (includes both neurological and developmental outcome)
SBS	Kivlin et al. (2000)	Total 123:		1mo – 5yr post-injury (mean 26mo)	Shaken baby syndrome, characterized by SDH, bone injuries and inconsistent history	Neurological assessment. Visual assessment in 87 survivors (done 1mo – 7yr post-injury, mean 21mo)
		99	0–12mo			
		24	13–36mo			

Outcome and comments	Died	Coma/ veg	Sev dis	Mod dis	Minor dis	Good recov	N/K	Total
NAHI group: 13/47 died, 34/47 survived. 7 mild/moderate impairment (developmental delay, swallowing difficulties, visual problems). 25 severe impairment (severe mental retardation and/or physical disability with reduced quality of life). 2 lost to FU. Reversal sign carried a poor prognosis with irreversible brain damage, and was highly associated with child abuse. Cerebral atrophy in 15/47 NAHI group, and 4/26 Medical group. Medical group: 13/26 died, 13/26 survived (4 mild impairment, 9 severe impairment)	13	—	25	7	—	—	2	47
	13	—	9	4	—	—	—	—
Seizure (EPTS) activity in 14/44 (10 with multifocal and 4 with focal seizure activity). Subclinical seizures noted in 4 children. Presence of seizures and whether those seizures were intractable was significantly related to outcome: n=42, p = 0.017 Most of those with intractable seizures had a poor outcome, and only 1 with intractable seizures had a normal outcome. At FU, 8 children had epilepsy (5 intractable epilepsy defined as at least 1 seizure/day despite medical treatment). Severity of EPTS was not related to development of post-traumatic epilepsy. At FU those with epilepsy had significantly greater disabilities than epilepsy-free group (p<0.0001)	6	0	8	8	6	14	2	44
Global outcome: 49/87 (56%) good vision 17/87 (20%) poor vision 2/87 (2%) poor in one eye 12/87 (14%) good at discharge, no FU 7/87 (8%) no information 26/87 severely disabled with hemiparesis, ataxia and severe developmental delay 8/87 attention deficit disorder, or mild speech delay Mortality 29.3%	36		26	8	—	22	31	123

Continues →

377

TABLE 12.2
(continued)

Category	Reference	N	Age at injury	Time to outcome	Series (type of injuries and study)	Outcome measures
TBI	Kieslich et al. (2001)	318 Abuse: 21 (6.6%)	64 were <2yr. Not specified, but inferred <2yr	Mean FU 8.9yr post-injury (range ?-25 yr)	TBI ("physical abuse")	GOS score. Post-traumatic epilepsy (PTE). Frankfurt Mental Outcome Scale
SBS	King et al. (2003)	364	<5yr (median 4.6mo, range 7d – 58mo)	At discharge from hospital	SBS ICD codes: (1988 – Mar 1996): 995.5, E967.0, E967.1, E967.9 (Apr 1996 –1998): 995.55, 995.54, E967.0, E967.9	Paediatric Cerebral Performance Category (PCPC), where 1 = normal and 6 = brain death. (PCPC is associated with functional outcome at 6mo FU)

Abbreviations:
ACA = anterior cerebral artery
ADD = attention deficit disorder
ASDH = acute subdural haematoma
CM = callosomarginal branch of ACA
Coma/veg state = coma/vegetative state
EPTS = early post-traumatic seizures
Excl = excluded
FU = follow-up
Good recov = good recovery
GOS = Glasgow Outcome Scores
ITBI = inflicted traumatic brain injury
Minor dis = minor or mild disability
Mod dis = moderate disability
NAHI = non-accidental head injury
NAI = non-accidental injury
N/K = not known
PCA = posterior cerebral artery
RH = retinal haemorrhage
SBS = shaken baby syndrome
SDH = subdural haemorrhage
Sev dis = severe disability
SIS = shaken impact syndrome
TBI = traumatic brain injury.

Numbers underlined have been used in summations.

Outcome and comments	Died	Coma/ veg	Sev dis	Mod dis	Minor dis	Good recov	N/K	Total
Outcome by cause not given. PTE in 43.8% <2-yr-olds (vs 20.5% in 2- to 6-yr-olds, and 13.3% in >6-yr-olds)								
All TBI (<2 yr):	Excl.	4	17	8	11	24	—	64
Abuse	Excl.	3	9	3	4	2	–	21
Mortality 69/364 (19%). 295 survived, of whom 65 "well", 162 with neurological deficit, and 192 with visual impairment. 251/295 (85%) required ongoing care. On PCPC scale, 21/295 survivors (7%) rated as "normal"	69	34	143	—	97	21	—	364

TABLE 12.3
Retrospective outcome studies with outcome descriptors other than GOS

Category	Reference	N	Age at injury	Time to outcome	Series (type of injuries and study)
Child abuse	Martin (1972)	42 survivors	Not specified	Evaluations at 4–6mo after treatment started and subsequently every 6–12mo thereafter, for up to 3yr	"Child abuse" defined as significant physical trauma unexplained by history or admitted by parents; repeated unexplained physical trauma; neglected children who are seriously suspected of being abused and who have siblings with documented abuse. Excluded if a single diagnosis of neglect, failure to thrive, or affective deprivation.
NAI	Hensey et al. (1983)	50	1mo – 13yr (mean 3.1yr)	At least 4yr post-injury	NAI/abuse. SDH in 1/50
CP population and ITBI	Diamond and Jaudes (1983)	Total 86. Postnatal onset of CP 18/86. With history of child abuse 8/18 All alive	<11 mo	Up to 17yr post-diagnosis of CP	From a total of 86 CP children, 18/86 had postnatal onset of CP. 8/18 ascertained as having histories of child abuse as the cause of disability. 7/8 had normal prenatal, perinatal, postnatal and developmental histories before incident
SBS without evidence of impact or other injuries	Ludwig and Warman (1984)	20 cases (out of 1250 records reviewed)	1–15mo (mean 5.8mo, median 3mo)	Not given. Assumed to be short – perhaps hospital discharge	Cases selected if admission of injury by solely shaking, or suspicion by staff when history and evaluation could not account for the child's injuries. Cases excluded if other evidence of abuse (external head trauma, skull fracture, multiple skeletal fractures, burns, patterned or severe bruising)
NAI (incl. NAHI)	Oates et al. (1984)	39, all survivors. 8 NAHI	11 <1yr, 8 1–2yr, 19 "just over" 2yr	Mean 5.5yr post-injury. Mean age at re-assessment was 8.9yr (4.6–14.4yr)	"Child abuse" (group matched for age/sex/social class). Injuries included bruising, fractures, skull fractures, head injury with skull fracture, malicious injury and near-drowning; 8/39 head injuries
NAI (incl. NAHI)	Oates (1984)	39, all survivors	Same as above	Same as above	Same group as above (1 too disabled to answer questions)

380

Outcome measures	Outcome and comments
Revised Yale Developmental Schedules (including Gesell Developmental Schedules, Stanford–Binet Form L-M, and Merrill–Palmer Scale of Mental Tests)	Retarded function 14/42 (defined as IQ or DQ<80). Mean IQ or DQ of retarded function group = 69 (range 19–79). Language delay in 4/14 (and also in 12/28 who were considered not retarded). Neurological sequelae in 18/42 (including hemiparesis, focal signs, optic atrophy), of whom 11 also had retardation. Experience shows it is very difficult to follow abusive families, as they tend to be very mobile and unreceptive to repeated evaluation from the institution that first involved them with legal/family/personal interventions. Many tests difficult to perform routinely because of child's behaviour or medical problems
Unsatisfactory outcome. Poor physical development. Emotional disturbance. Poor educational progress	Unsatisfactory outcome 26/50 (52%). Poor physical development 7/50 (14%). Emotional disturbance 18/50 (36%). Poor educational progress 11/50 (22%). Epilepsy 1/50 (2%)
Neurological	In 8 HBI children: 4/8 spastic quadriplegia; 1/8 spastic triplegia; 1/8 hemiplegia; 2/8 hemiparesis. 1/8 seizures; 1/8 severe mental retardation; 3/8 moderate mental retardation; 4/8 mild mental retardation. Researchers also found a group of 8/18 CP children who were abused after the carer became aware of the CP: here a different type of abuse was described, occurring later, at ages up to 9yr
Neurological examination	Mortality 3/20. Morbidity 10/20. Blindness 4/20. Visual loss 3/20. Motor deficit 5/20. Seizures 7/20. Developmental delay 6/20. No apparent deficit 7/20. Researchers noted that even those who apparently escaped without sequelae may manifest some abnormality if followed up for a long period, suggesting that these cases had a relatively short FU period
WISC-R; Mecham Verbal Language; Schonell and Schonell Reading Test; Children's Personality Questionnaire; Rutter Behavioural Questionnaire, completed by school teacher	Mean Wechsler score = 95. Mean performance score = 95. Full Scale Intelligence Quotient (n=38): mean = 95 (range 65–127) vs 106 in comparison group. Full Scale Intelligence Quotient, head injured (n=8): mean = 90 vs 107. Verbal Language (Vineland Social Maturity Scale): mean = 92 vs 106. Reading test, on average 14.3mo behind their chronological reading age (range 12 – >36 months), vs 4.8mo delay in comparison group. Teachers questionnaire, abnormal behaviour in 21/38 (antisocial 13/38, neurotic 6/38, undifferentiated 2/38, vs 5/38, 1/38 and 1/38 respectively in comparison group)
Piers–Harris self-concept scale. Children's Personality Questionnaire. Vineland Social Maturity Scale	Mean score 51.4, vs 60.9 in comparison group. Mean 3.5, vs 5.2 in comparison group. No differences. Behavioural questionnaire as above

Continues ➜

TABLE 12.3
(continued)

Category	Reference	N	Age at injury	Time to outcome	Series (type of injuries and study)
NAHI (incl whiplash SBS and "head squeezing"	Frank et al. (1985)	4 survivors:			Admitted shaking or squeezing child
		Case 1	3mo	1yr	"Violently shaken"
		Case 2	5wk	? (at subsequent readmission)	"Admitted shaking child"
		Case 3	6wk	5mo	Head squeezed
		Case 4	4mo	10mo (at readmission with further injuries)	"Admitted shaking child"
					None had skull fracture; only one had SDH; all had RH, and all showed CT abnormalities on day 1 of admission
Whiplash-SBS	Hadley et al. (1989)	13	Range 1.5–14mo Median 3mo	Autopsy/"review"	Presumed isolated whiplash–shake injury, determined by clinical history of shake without direct cranial trauma (ascertained by multiple interviews, notes cross-referenced by all individuals investigating each case). They also had no physical evidence of external craniofacial trauma, or skull/facial fractures. Criteria: (1) documented history of infant shaking as admitted by carer/perpetrator, and (2) no historical, clinical, radiographic evidence of direct impact trauma to craniofacial region
SBS	Wilkinson et al. (1989)	14	2–28mo (mean 10.5mo)	>12mo post-injury in survivors	SBS, defined as findings of intraocular haemorrhage plus intracranial injury in the absence of external signs of head trauma
NAI and accidental injury	DiScala et al. (2000)	1997 NAI vs 16,831 accidental injuries. Child abuse = 15 cases Child abuse = 1238 cases	Newborn – 4yr <1mo 1–12mo	Hospital discharge	All cases reported were either *established* child abuse, or established as accidental injury. "Suspected child abuse" cases were excluded

Outcome measures	Outcome and comments
	All 4 severely disabled
Neurological exam	Mental retardation, quadriparesis, blindness
Neurological exam	Quadriparesis, blindness
Neurological exam	Bilateral upper motor neurone abnormalities, blindness, poor head control
Neurological exam	Partial blindness, spasticity
Complete autopsies on 6/8 who died	Mortality 8/13.
All had cranial SDH, cerebral contusions, and marked swelling with herniation.	5 survivors, all with clinical pattern of profound encephalopathy
One had evidence of extracalvarial contusion, in fascia.	
None had skull fracture.	
5/6 had epidural and/or SDH of the spinal cord at the cervicomedullary junction.	
4/6 had evidence of ventral spinal contusions at high cervical levels	
Intraocular haemorrhages classified by type and extent.	11/14 children were <12mo old.
Type (mutually exclusive):	2/14 died.
mild: intraretinal haemorrhages only = 1;	Mean age of children with severe-type retinopathy was 6.4mo (SD 3.7mo), vs 14.6mo (SD 9.8mo) in children without severe-type RH.
moderate: subhyaloid haemorrhage, all lesions <2 disc areas in size = 2; severe: subhyaloid haemorrhage, any lesion >2 disc areas in size, or vitreous haemorrhage = 3.	3/14 had unilateral RH; 11/14 had bilateral RH.
	Mean retinopathy score 4.4 points, median 4 (5 cases had highest score of 6, 5 had scores 2–3, 4 had scores 4–5).
Extent (sum of categories):	At FU (n=8), all continued to exhibit retinal abnormalities: retinopathy
Any haemorrhage in the following areas: macula (>1 disc diameter [DD] from disc, within 2 DD of fovea) = 1; peripapillary (within 2 DD of disc margin, excluding macula) = 1, periphery (outside macula or peripapillary regions) = 1	scores 2–3 in 3 cases; scores 4–5 in 3 cases, and 2 remained severely affected with score of 6.
	4 lost to FU.
	Children with bilateral RH tended to have more severe acute neurological injury
Functional status at time of discharge, including vision, hearing, speech, self-feeding, bathing, dressing, walking, bladder and bowel control, cognition and behaviour.	1239/1997 cases were found to have head injuries.
	843/1239 had intracranial injury (68%).
	Mortality of all child abuse cases 253/1997 (12.7%).
	Survived child abuse 1744/1997 (87.3%).
Each function rated as either: age appropriate, impaired, or unable.	8.7% of child abuse cases had 4 or more functional limitations (i.e. were more severely disabled) than the accidentally injured group, where only 2.7% were in the poorest function group.
Number of functions deficient calculated	14.8% of abuse group required ICP monitoring, vs 2.3% of accidentally injured group

Continues ➔

383

TABLE 12.3
(continued)

Category	Reference	N	Age at injury	Time to outcome	Series (type of injuries and study)
NSBS, with photographed RH	McCabe and Donahue (2000)	30	1–39mo (mean 9.3mo)	1st FU at approx. 2mo post-injury and continued for at least 6mo. Overall FU at 1–36mo (mean 8.2mo)	Confirmed cases of SBS, all with RHs that had been photographed. Diagnosis of SBS given when bilateral RHs were observed in a situation where the injury was not consistent with the history, when present, or if there had been a history of a previous suspicious episode in a lethargic infant. Perpetrator identified in all 30 cases, and majority prosecuted successfully
NAHI	Nassogne and Bonnier (2001)	37	1–15mo	Deficits detected at different times	NAHI
Suspected ITBI	Lo et al. (2003)	16	2wk 3d – 28wk 6d (median 7wk)	OFC measures: 24–92wk post-injury (median 67.9wk). MRI performed at 1wk 1d – 134wk 5d (median FU period 19.86 weeks)	Survivors of NAHI

Abbreviations:
FU = follow-up
ICP = intracranial pressure
ITBI = intentional traumatic brain injury
NAHI = non-accidental head injury
NAI = non-accidental injury
OFC = occipitofrontal circumference
RH = retinal haemorrhage
SBS = shaken baby syndrome
SDH = subdural haemorrhage.

Outcome measures	Outcome and comments
Ophthalmological exam at FU clinic for 20/22 of the survivors. 2/22 by telephone interview. Repeated clinic visits for survivors until findings stabilized, including examination of vision, ocular motility, presence of amblyopia, and resolution of intraocular haemorrhages	8 died – all had unreactive pupils on admission. 22 survived (all had reactive pupils). 23/30 had no midline shift of the brain at presentation (21 of these survived, the other 2 had unreactive pupils). 7 had brain midline shift, and 6/7 died, including 2 with brainstem midline shift and uncal herniation. Resolution of RHs: by 1mo in 7 cases, by 2mo in 5, by 3mo in 4, and by 4mo in 2. Remaining 2 resolved by 9mo and 11mo respectively. 6/22 had poor vision in at least one eye after resolution of RH (due to optic atrophy, retinal fibrosis, traumatic cataract and retinal scarring). All 8 who died were visually unresponsive at presentation: therefore visual responsiveness is highly suggestive of survival. 12 initially had fix-and-follow vision (all lived, but 2 subsequently lost this in at least one eye), 18 presented without fix-and-follow in at least one eye: of these 8 died, 3 never regained fix and-follow and showed no other improvement, and 7 eventually regained fix-and-follow
Neurological	Mortality 3/37 Blind 3/37 Severe visual deficit 5/37 Hemiplegia/tetraplegia (detected within 1mo) 9/37 Increased OFC (detected after 4mo) 12/37 Hemiparesis (at 1 year) 6/37 Psychomotor delay (at 1yr) 28/37 Epilepsy (detected within 2yr) 12/37 Behavioural disturbances (detected within 4yr) 19/37 Mental retardation (detected within 5yr) 34/37 Learning deficits (detected within 6yr) 34/37
Sequential MRI (median 3 per patient, range 2–4 scans). Cerebral atrophy (measurement of ventriculo/cortical ratio on coronal images). Microcephaly (serial OFC measures)	8/15 with microcephaly showed progressive increase in bifrontal ventricular diameter, and ventriculo/cortical ratio, indicating cerebral atrophy was the cause of the microcephaly. Acquired microcephaly found in 15/16 over a mean FU of 67.9wk. The serial OFC measurements dipped to more than 2SD below the mean, indicating failure to maintain a normal head growth pattern. Severe disability 1 Severe developmental delay 2 Moderate developmental delay 6 Mild developmental delay 4 Alive with age appropriate development 3

TABLE12.4
Summary of outcome data from Tables 12.1–12.3

Outcome measure	Cumulated	Ludwig and Warman (1984)	Sinal and Ball (1987)	Hadley et al. (1989)	Wilkinson et al. (1989)	Goldstein et al. (1993)	Bonnier et al. (1995)	Johnson et al. (1995)	Duhaime et al. (1996)	Haviland and Russell (1997)	Gilles and Nelson (1998)	Barlow and Minns (1999)	Barlow et al. (1999)	Rao et al. (1999)	Barlow et al. (2000)	Kivlin et al. (2000)	McCabe and Donahue (2000)	Nassogne and Bonnier (2001)	King et al. (2003)
Mortality (n)	(20.6%) 197	3	3	8	2	5	1	4	22	2	3	2	6	13	6	36	8	3	69
Population (N)	956	20	24	13	14	14	13	28	84	15	14	17	55	47	44	123	30	37	364

Modified GOS scores	Morse et al. (1970)	Sinal and Ball (1987)	Goldstein et al. (1993)	Fischer and Allasio (1994)	Bonnier et al. (1995)	Johnson et al. (1995)	Duhaime et al. (1996)	Haviland and Russell (1997)	Gilles and Nelson (1998)	Barlow and Minns (1999)	Ewing-Cobbs et al. (1998)	Barlow et al. (1999)	Ewing-Cobbs et al. (1999)	Rao et al. (1999)	Barlow et al. (2000)	Kivlin et al. (2000)	Kieslich et al. (2001)	King et al. (2003)	Total	%
1 = Dead	n/a	3	5	n/a	1	4	1	2	3	2	n/a	1	n/a	13	6	36	n/a	69	146	19.7
2 = Vegetative state	0	0	1	0	0	1	0	0	3	0	0	0	0	25	0	0	3	34	42	5.0
3 = Severely disabled	3	7	7	7	6	7	6	7	6	5	3	9	4	7	8	26	9	143	286	34.2
4 = Moderately disabled	6	10	0	2	5	7	2	4	2	7	13	5	17	2	14	8	2	97	211	25.2
5 = Good outcome	3	3	1	1	1	9	5	1	0	0	4	10	7	0	14	22	2	21	113	13.5
Lost to follow-up	4	1	0	0	0	0	0	1	0	0	0	0	0	0	2	31	0	39	78	9.3
Total	16	24	14	10	13	28	14	15	14	17	20	25	28	47	44	123	21	364	837	

Seizures (n)	Population (N)	
12	37	Nassogne and Bonnier (2001)
8	36	Barlow et al. (2000)
5	25	Barlow et al. (1999)
3	14	Gilles and Nelson (1998)
13	20	Ewing-Cobbs et al. (1998)
3	14	Duhaime et al. (1996)
20	28	Johnson et al. (1995)
4	12	Bonnier et al. (1995)
3	10	Fischer and Allasio (1994)
7	14	Goldstein et al. (1993)
7	24	Sinal and Ball (1987)
7	20	Ludwig and Warman (1984)
1	50	Henscy et al. (1983)
1	8	Diamond and Jaudes (1983)
(30.2%) 94	312	

Blindness (n)	Population (N)	
3	37	Nassogne and Bonnier (2001)
4	14	Duhaime et al. (1996)
2	12	Bonnier et al. (1995)
1	10	Fischer and Allasio (1994)
3	14	Goldstein et al. (1993)
2	24	Sinal and Ball (1987)
1	4	Frank et al. (1985)
4	20	Ludwig and Warman (1984)
(14.8%) 21	135	

Continues →

387

TABLE12.4
(continued)

Outcome measure	Cumulated	Ludwig and Warman (1984)	Frank et al. (1985)	Wilkinson et al. (1989)	Fischer and Allasio (1994)	Bonnier et al. (1995)	Gilles and Nelson (1998)	Barlow et al. (1999)	Rao et al. (1999)	Kivlin et al. (2000)	McCabe and Donahue (2000)	Nassogne and Bonnier (2001)	King et al. (2003)
Visual impairment (n)	(45.3%) 263	3	1	5	2	2	10	12	7	19	6	4	192
Population (N)	581	20	4	8	10	12	14	25	47	87	22	37	295

Outcome measure	Cumulated	Bonnier et al. (1995)	Gilles and Nelson (1998)	Barlow et al. (1999)	Lo et al. (2003)
Microcephaly (n)	(50.7%) 34	4	8	7	15
Population (N)	67	12	14	25	16

388

Continues →

	Macrocephaly (n)	Population (N)
Barlow et al. (1999)	4	25

Intellectual/cognitive deficits (n)	Population (N)	Profound	Severe	Moderate	Mild
Martin (1972)	14	42				
Elmer (1977)	9	17				
Diamond and Jaudes (1983)	8	8		1	3	4
Hensey et al. (1983)	11	50				
Sinal and Ball (1987)	10	24		5		4
Fischer and Allasio (1994)	5	10		1		4
Bonnier et al. (1995)	11	12				
Duhaime et al. (1996)	9	14				
Ewing-Cobbs et al. (1998)	9	20				
Barlow et al. (1999)	16	25	4	3	2	7
Nassogne and Bonnier (2001)	34	37				
Lo et al. (2003)	12	15	2	6		4
	(53.7%) 148	275				

389

TABLE12.4
(continued)

Outcome measure	Cumulated	Studies (n / N)
Behavioural/emotional (n) problems / Population (N)	(38.4%) 80 / 208	Hensey et al. (1983) 18/50; Oates et al. (1984) 4/8; Sinal and Ball (1987) 2/24; Fischer and Allasio (1994) 2/10; Bonnier et al. (1995) 6/12; Duhaime et al. (1996) 3/14; Barlow et al. (1999) 13/25; Ewing-Cobbs et al. (1999) 13/28; Nassogne and Bonnier (2001) 19/37
Any motor deficit (n) / Population (N)	(38.1%) 150 / 395	Martin (1972) 18/42; Diamond and Jaudes (1983) 8/8; Hensey et al. (1983) 7/50; Ludwig and Warman (1984) 5/20; Frank et al. (1985) 4/4; Sinal and Ball (1987) 10/24; Fischer and Allasio (1994) 7/10; Bonnier et al. (1995) 5/12; Duhaime et al. (1996) 8/14; Ewing-Cobbs et al. (1998) 5/20; Gilles and Nelson (1998) 9/14; Barlow et al. (1999) 14/25; Ewing-Cobbs et al. (1999) 15/28; Kivlin et al. (2000) 26/87; Nassogne and Bonnier (2001) 9/37

Cranial nerve deficits (n) / Population (N)

Study	Cranial nerve deficits (n)	Population (N)
Barlow et al. (1999)	5	25
Ewing-Cobbs et al. (1998)	4	20
	9	45

Hemiparesis (n) / Population (N)

Study	Hemiparesis (n)	Population (N)
Nassogne and Bonnier (2001)	6	37
Barlow et al. (1999)	4	25
Gilles and Nelson (1998)	4	14
Ewing-Cobbs et al. (1998)	6	20
Duhaime et al. (1996)	3	14
Bonnier et al. (1995)	2	12
Fischer and Allasio (1994)	3	10
Goldstein et al. (1993)	1	14
Sinal and Ball (1987)	1	24
Diamond and Jaudes (1983)	3	8
	(18.7%) 33	178

Continues ➔

TABLE 12.4
(continued)

Outcome measure	Cumulated		
Quadriparesis (n)	17	5 — Gilles and Nelson (1998)	
Population (N)	48	14	
		3 — Bonnier et al. (1995)	2 — Fisher et al. (1994)
		12	10
		3 — Frank et al. (1985)	4 — Diamond and Jaudes (1983)
		4	8

Quadriparesis (n): 17 / Population (N): 48

- Gilles and Nelson (1998): 5 / 14
- Bonnier et al. (1995): 3 / 12
- Fisher et al. (1994): 2 / 10
- Frank et al. (1985): 3 / 4
- Diamond and Jaudes (1983): 4 / 8

Normal (n): (10.9%) 47 / Population (N): 431

- King et al. (2003): 21 / 295
- Barlow et al. (1999): 8 / 25
- Haviland and Russell (1997): 1 / 15
- Duhaime et al. (1996): 0 / 14
- Bonnier et al. (1995): 1 / 12
- Fischer and Allasio (1994): 3 / 10
- Sinal and Ball (1987): 3 / 24
- Ludwig and Warman (1984): 7 / 20
- Morse et al. (1970): 3 / 16

TABLE 12.5
Traumatic brain injury (non-inflicted): mortality

	Cumulative total	Calculated %	References
Infants and children <3yr	10/456	2.19%	Musemeche et al. (1991) Duhaime et al. (1992) Michaud et al. (1992) Berney et al. (1994) Chiaviello (1994a,b) Jones et al. (2003a,b)
Older children	63/1618	3.89%	Musemeche et al. (1991) Michaud et al. (1992) Berney et al. (1994) Chiaviello (1994a) Jones et al. (2003a,b)

Mortality

Fatalities occur from forms of child abuse that do not involve head injury (Kempe et al. 1962, Elmer and Gregg 1967, Lynch and Roberts 1982, Hensey et al. 1983). The average mortality rate reported in these studies is 7%. The average mortality rate for NAHI in children under 2 years of age, was calculated, from relevant studies listed in Table 12.4, to be around 20%. This may be an underestimate because it is likely that some infant fatalities are non-accidentally caused but unrecognized from the antecedent clinical or imaging features or because of an incomplete autopsy that did not include examination of the spinal cord or the eye. Extended autopsies have shown otherwise unrecognized evidence of injury at the cervico-medullary junction, atlanto-occipital ligament, spinal cord contusions and subdural haemorrhage, and occipital periosteal haematomas. Hadley et al. (1989) reported a series of 13 children who died without any physical examination evidence of trauma although all perpetrators had confessed to shaking them. Five of the six who had autopsies had evidence of spinal epidural or subdural blood at the cervico-medullary junction and four had ventral upper cervical cord contusions.

Fatalities due to accidental head injuries in infants are rare. The literature estimates mortality rates of 2% for infants and children under 3 years and 4% for older children (Table 12.5). This exaggerated mortality in inflicted brain injury may be due to the mechanism of infliction, as well as the anatomic vulnerability of the infant brain and immaturity of neuroprotective mechanisms.

Morbidity

DEVELOPMENTAL AND GLOBAL OUTCOME

All investigators agree that there is a high incidence of severely disabled children with gross developmental delay in infant survivors of NAHI (Tables 12.1 and 12.4). The high morbidity appears at variance with what might be predicted from the sometimes relative mildness of the presenting symptoms, imaging findings or conscious state. Severely disabled children are frequently blind, nonverbal and cognitively impaired, have epilepsy and behavioural

393

problems, are wheelchair dependent, and rely on adults for their daily care throughout their life. Averaging estimates or quoted values from the relevant literature shows an incidence of severe disability of 34%. Moderate disability includes perceptual and cognitive (memory and attention) difficulties, hemiplegia, and a requirement for special education and rehabilitation therapy. This occurs in 25% of survivors. Children with good outcome or mild impairment frequently function in the normal education stream but may require remedial help and may display behavioural problems.

In prospective studies comparing accidental and non-accidental injuries the global outcome following inflicted traumatic brain injury (TBI) was worse than that after accidental TBI. Only 20% in the inflicted group were found to have a good outcome compared to 55% following accidental TBI (Bruce and Zimmerman 1989, Ewing-Cobbs et al. 1998).

A 'good' or normal neurodevelopmental outcome following NAHI can be expected in approximately 11% of cases (Table 12.4).

ABSENCE OF 'CATCH UP' AND A 'SIGN FREE INTERVAL'
Older children who suffer traumatic brain injury characteristically show an improvement in their motor, cognitive and social function scores, particularly in the first six months following injury (Dumas et al. 2001, Fragala et al. 2002, Tomlin et al. 2002): further improvement by 5 years compared to the first assessment at 12 months post-injury was noted in 12 of 40 survivors of severe TBI (Carter et al. 1999), although plateauing in neuropsychological function after the first year may occur (Yeates et al. 2002).

The recovery curves over three months, for children surviving NAHI were flat and failed to show the expected catch-up (Haviland and Russell 1997, Ewing-Cobbs et al. 1999).

In a seminal work, Bonnier et al. (1995) were the first to present their findings on the long-term follow-up of 'whiplash shaking injury syndrome'. Approximately half of their cohort displayed a sign free interval, apparently recovering completely after the shaking, as evidenced by no detectable deficits in neurological, psychomotor and general examinations in the interim. All but one of these children became disabled after an interval of between 6 months and 5 years. Interruption of brain growth took 4 months to appear; long-track signs took 6–12 months to emerge; epilepsy appeared after 2 years and behavioural and neuropsychological signs (severe anxiety, pervasive developmental disorder, hyperkinetic behaviour) became evident after 3–6 years.

'Delayed behavioural deficits' following brain injury in early life may be related to the degree of functional maturity of the brain region–behaviour relationship; in much the same way as the evolution of an infantile hemiplegia, the behavioural deficit becomes manifest at a time remote from the primary injury

NEUROLOGICAL ABNORMALITIES
Motor deficits in the form of hemiplegia, tetraplegia, and diplegia are seen in 38% of cases. Quadriplegia (35%) and hemiplegia (18%) were the commonest acquired motor disorders (Table 12.4).

The contralateral hemiplegia may be due to: (i) a cortical lesion from cortical laminar necrosis and infarction or contusion, with accompanying epileptic seizures, homonymous hemianopia and aphasia; (ii) white matter oedema and subsequent ischaemia at the centrum semiovale; (iii) tears at the grey–white matter junction with axonal fractures from the cortex sliding over the underlying white matter; (iv) diffuse axonal injury; (v) cerebral peduncle injury (occasionally with accompanying IIIrd cranial nerve lesion) (Weber) where the hemispheres rotate on the brainstem; (vi) pontine injury (with an accompanying VIth and VIIth cranial nerve lesion—Millard Gubler) and (vii) medullary injury, where the brainstem and upper cervical cord form the pivot of the 'lash of the whip'; (viii) lateral column contusion of the cervical cord, which may occasionally be responsible for homolateral hemiplegia (but usually tetraplegia); or (ix) direct carotid trauma with subsequent ischaemia.

Since most babies have a left occipito-anterior presentation at birth, the subsequent position of comfort is normally with the head to the right. Shaking will therefore be slightly away from the midline and asymmetrical, with a likelihood of cortical or other injury to the right hemisphere, making a left hemiplegia theoretically more likely. Barlow et al. (2003) found a 3:1 predominance of left over right hemiplegia in survivors of NAHI, in contrast to hemiplegic cerebral palsy where a 2:1 predominance of right over left hemiplegia is normally found.

Cranial nerve deficits
Cranial nerve defects have been reported in 20% of cases at follow-up in two studies (Ewing-Cobbs et al. 1998, Barlow et al. 2003). These took the form of individual or multiple deficits involving the IIIrd, IVth, Vth, VIth, VIIth, VIIIth, and bulbar (IXth to XIIth) cranial nerves.

EPILEPTIC SEIZURES
Early post-traumatic seizures are common (Barlow et al. 2000). They have been found with a frequency of 32–79% in children presenting with NAHI (Bonnier et al. 1995, Johnson et al. 1995, Haviland and Russell 1997, Ewing-Cobbs et al. 1998, Gilles and Nelson 1998, Barlow et al. 2000, Nassogne and Bonnier 2001, King et al. 2003). They may be the commonest presenting clinical feature (Haviland and Russell 1997).

The incidence of epilepsy in survivors of NAHI is 30% (Table 12.4). O the 36 survivors in our own series, 8 developed post-traumatic epilepsy, and in 5 cases this was classified as 'intractable' or 'refractory' (one or more seizures per day despite anticonvulsant treatment) (Barlow et al. 2000). Post-traumatic epilepsy following accidental head injury occurs less frequently, between 5% and 15% (Annegers et al. 1980, Ewing-Cobbs et al. 1998).

The origin of early post-traumatic seizures is multifactorial and includes (i) cerebral hypoxia (increased synaptic excitatory amino acids and receptor density), (ii) laminar grey matter shearing that isolates the cortex from reticular control and results in intractable seizures, and (iii) pressure-induced seizures. Intractable seizures are a common feature of other laminar dissociations such as laminar necrosis and laminar dysplasia. GABAergic inhibition is particularly affected since anticonvulsant drugs such as benzodiazepines are ineffective. The seizures generally cease within 5 days. Epilepsy at follow-up is a consequence of the widespread brain damage, which involves the cortex and highly epileptogenic regions of the child's brain such as the frontal lobe and hippocampus.

PATTERNS OF BRAIN DAMAGE

Resolution of the acute brain injury is followed by evolution of the long term brain damage patterns that are recognized from follow-up imaging studies. These include the following.

Chronic subdural haematoma

An acute subdural haemorrhage implies haemorrhage within 3 days; subacute, from 3 days to 3 weeks; and a chronic subdural haematoma, more than 3 weeks (Choux et al. 1986, Brown and Minns 1993).

Subdural hygroma

In the absence of a recent infection or new trauma to the arachnoid membrane, the subdural hygroma evolves from degradation of a previous subdural haematoma.

Ventricular abnormalities

Ventricular abnormalities (exvacuo hydrocephalus) are noted in approximately 50% of NAHI cases at follow-up. Post-traumatic hydrocephalus, particularly following brain contusion or acute SDH, occurs in less than 3% of cases following accidental head injury. An early onset (weeks later) is due to haemorrhage in the subarachnoid space or ventricles, while a later onset (over months) is due to post-haemorrhagic fibrosis in the subarachnoid space. (Meyers et al. 1983, Oi and Matsumoto 1987).

Cerebral infarction patterns

Border zone infarction occurs between the anterior and middle cerebral artery, with brain atrophy, in some 80% of survivors of diffuse brain swelling and coma. Similarly, focal brain swelling at presentation with focal neurological deficits is followed by hemispheric or uni-lateral frontal infarction patterns in the distribution of the callosal marginal branch of the anterior cerebral artery, as a result of subfalcine herniation (Zimmerman et al. 1979, Cohen et al. 1986, Gilles and Nelson 1998). Arterial territory ischaemic strokes following trauma are most frequent in the posterior circulation. The commonest patterns after NAHI were superior cerebellar, internal carotid, and in the terminal branches of the middle cerebral artery.

Hemispheric oedema and infarction should be considered secondary to strangulation only when there is clinical or other evidence such as absent venous pulsation in the ipsilateral retina, absence of carotid pulsation and contralateral hemiparesis, and Doppler confirmation or imaging, or autopsy evidence of ischaemia in the internal carotid territory.

Cerebral atrophy and microcephaly

Cerebral atrophy is well recognized after various brain insults by the widening of the extra-axial space with increased prominence of the sulci, widening of the subarachnoid space and dilated ventricles. It is seen after perinatal hypoxic–ischaemic encephalopathy, intra-cranial haemorrhage or meningitis in 91% of those who develop microcephaly. Cerebral atrophy ensues in adults after severe brain trauma in 28% of cases, but the incidence increases to 83% in those who have suffered an acute SDH, and can first be recognized two weeks after the head injury (Tomita et al. 1990).

Lo et al. (2003) determined the frequency of cerebral atrophy and microcephaly in a group of children surviving a non-accidental head injury. These children had semi-quantitative measurements made on sequential MRI, along with serial head circumference measurements over a median follow-up period of 20 weeks. Microcephaly was detected in 94% of cases over a median follow-up of 16 months. There was a significant reduction in the head circumference compared to presentation (p<0.001). It is accepted that the head circumference is abnormally increased at the time of presentation as a result of acute raised intracranial pressure. Cerebral atrophy was the cause for the microcephaly in 53% of cases, evident from as early as 9 days after presentation, and all cases started less than 4 months after the shaking injury. Onuma et al. (1995) reported five children with severe cerebral atrophy on CT after accidental head injury, and all were associated with a poor outcome and first detected two weeks after the injury. Cerebellar atrophy has also been a late MRI finding in a high percentage (46%) of infants who suffered severe head trauma (Soto-Ares et al. 2001).

Proposed pathophysiological mechanisms for the cerebral atrophy include (i) diffuse necrosis resulting from cerebral oedema and traumatic vascular accidents, (ii) excitotoxic neuronal necrosis following the injury (Lipton and Rosenberg 1994), and (iii) interference with neurodevelopmental processes of infancy (dedrogenesis, axogenesis, synaptogenesis, synaptic stabilization, glygenesis and myelation) (Yakovlev and Lecours 1967, Evrard 1992, Bonnier et al. 1995).

Global slowing of brain growth
A global brain insult will result in a global slowing of brain growth and microcephaly, with a proportional loss of cortex and white matter, so that the ventricular–cortical ratios remain constant. This may be the origin of the microcephaly in those cases not associated with obvious cerebral atrophy on brain scan.

Malacia and cystic encephalomalacia
This is a distinctive brain pattern that evolves into the more gross atrophic image seen later. Malacic changes consequent on hypoxic–ischaemia (which on MRI are hyperintense on T_2 and hypointense on T_1 and FLAIR) give rise to cystic and multicystic encephalomalacia. Localized damage results in focal porencephaly which may become confluent with the lateral ventricle (McPhillips 2002).

Secondary subdural haemorrhage
Where the acute injury has caused bilateral SDHs (plus or minus diffuse CT hypodensity), the resultant severe atrophy (independent of whether or not subduro-peritoneal shunting was performed), may result in later subdural bleeding because of a marked craniocerebral disproportion (Fig. 12.1). Further subdural peritoneal shunting of this collection would induce yet further bleeding in the subdural space.

VISUAL IMPAIRMENT
Blindness occurs in 15% of survivors after NAHI and there is some visual impairment in

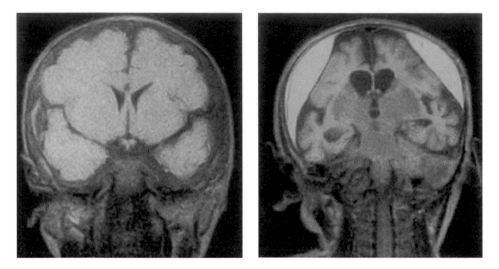

Fig. 12.1. An 8-week-old girl presented with a short history of vomiting, irritability, lethargy, epileptic seizures, bilateral retinal haemorrhage, two bruises on the left side of the face and a bruise behind one ear. Examination showed a bulging fontanelle.

(a) CT revealed bilateral subdural haemorrhage and reduced T_1 signal intensity in the frontal and occipital white matter. No focal intra-cerebral haemorrhage was identified.

(b) Extensive brain shrinkage occurred over the next 3 months. On follow-up CT at 6 months post-injury, large secondary bilateral subdural haemorrhages are seen, with extensive brain atrophy.

45% (Table 12.4). Resolution of the retinal haemorrhages is variable and depends on the multiplicity of regions and layers involved. We have seen some cases where 90% of the haemorrhage has resolved within a week and others where they are substantially present 6 weeks after admission; however, retinal haemorrhages have resolved in nearly all cases by 4 months. Of those patients having reactive pupils at initial presentation, 27% still have poor vision in at least one eye after nearly 7 months and the remainder have at least 'fix and follow vision' (McCabe and Donahue 2000).

The causes of visual impairment after NAHI are related to both anterior and posterior visual pathway damage. Visual impairment results most commonly from brain injury in the form of cortical blindness (the retention of pupillary light reflexes in the absence of vision) and is due to bilateral brain injury posterior to the optic chiasm. Given the significantly high intracranial pressure, the mechanism is raised pressure compressing the posterior cerebral artery at the edge of the tentorium with consequent ischaemia to the optic radiations and calcarine cortex with later occipital lobe atrophy. Unilateral encephalomalacic changes correspond to homonymous hemianopia. Other causes of visual impairment following NAHI include optic atrophy, retinal fibrosis, traumatic cataract and retinal scarring, and macular folds.

COGNITIVE FUNCTION

Caffey (1972) postulated that many cases of mental retardation might be due to unrecognized abusive head injury in infancy. The incidence of global learning difficulties following NAHI is 54% (Table 12.4). The incidence in a matched accidental head injury group of patients was 5% (Ewing-Cobbs et al. 1998).

Cognitive outcome following NAHI may be estimated from the language domains of developmental assessments in young infants and children and more formally assessed with psychometric testing in older children. Following developmental testing at 1 and 3 months, 45% of children scored in the "deficient" range at initial cognitive assessment and in a low-average range on repeat testing, with persistent deficits in attention/arousal, emotional regulation and motor coordination, and all tested significantly below the comparison group (p<0.0001) (Ewing-Cobbs et al. 1998, 1999). A fall in IQ (to below 80) between the ages of 3 and 6 years has been noted in the group with a 'sign-free' interval at follow-up (Oliver 1975, Bonnier et al. 1995).

The causes for the severe cognitive deficit are multifactorial but result from multiple severe cortical brain lesions together with interruption of associative white matter pathways.

BEHAVIOURAL AND EMOTIONAL SEQUELAE

There are numerous studies reporting behaviour and emotional sequelae of child abuse generally but fewer that concentrate specifically on NAHI. Abused children generally have a higher frequency of anxiety and depression, fewer friends, lower ambition and lower self-esteem; they are shy, serious and subdued, perform lower on intelligence testing, are delayed in language and reading ability and show abnormal behavioural profiles (Martin and Beezley 1977, Hensey et al. 1983, Goldson 1991). One third of abused children were antisocial, one sixth were neurotic and barely half were normal, all significantly different from a comparison group (Oates 1984, Oates et al. 1984).

The incidence of emotional and behavioural sequelae following NAHI is at least 38% (Table 12.4). The Behavioural Rating Score was less favourable in an inflicted group by comparison with an accidental group immediately after injury (p<0.0001), and again at 3 months follow-up (p<0.005). There was limited recovery in the NAHI group in terms of energy interests and toy exploration at baseline, with increasing deficits in affect, frustration, tolerance and adaptation to change at follow-up (Ewing-Cobbs et al. 1999). The emotional abuse may antedate the injury and be compounded later by inadequate psychosocial environment as well as prolonged hospitalization and sometimes multiple fostering placements. These emotional problems may also contribute to poor educational attainment. Given the young age of infants abused by shaking it is unlikely that pre-injury psychological trauma would contribute to later behavioural problems in the way it does to older children. Head injury in young adults is known to be associated with a lifetime risk of depression (Holsinger et al. 2002).

Outcome of legal proceedings

There is a surprising lack of prosecutions for NAHI (successful or otherwise) and one can only theorize about the reasons for this, but undoubtedly a major reason is the lack of certainty of the medical diagnosis and postulated mechanism of injury, in a condition where the injury is not witnessed, and in the absence of a single pathognomonic denominator of abuse it is perhaps not surprising that prosecutors are less inclined to pursue criminal charges because conflicting medical opinion confuses juries. In a large collaborative Canadian study, two thirds of 364 cases were the subject of an ongoing police investigation. Criminal charges were laid in 26% of cases and 7% resulted in conviction for assault (King et al. 2003). Haviland and Russell (1997) studied the current care conditions and prosecutions for NAHI and reported prosecutions in 20% of cases (with one still outstanding). Fewer than half of the children were still under the protection of a care order, and 69% of survivors had been returned to their previous homes with no successful prosecutions being made. In Scotland to date, of the 49 cases where legal proceedings were known to have been brought, 25 resulted in convictions of the perpetrator.

Prognostic risk factors
PREMORBID FACTORS
Some of the risk factors for the acute injury will have an additional influence on the outcome following the injury. In Liverpool, predisposing risk factors for non-accidental injury generally included male gender, an unmarried mother, low birthweight, previous injury to children, low maternal age, and the presence of environmental stress factors in the family (Sills et al. 1977).

Pre-injury factors that may influence outcome after NAHI are: (i) antecedent injury (both overt and covert), (ii) ongoing postnatal environmental factors, and (iii) pre-existing medical and developmental abnormalities.

Alexander et al. (1990a,b) noted that inflicted injuries in young children were frequently preceded by other forms of maltreatment, and emphasized the repetitive nature of child maltreatment and the tendency for perpetrators to engage in increasingly more violent assaults. A previous medical encounter within the 6 weeks prior to the admission with brain injury was noted in 28% of cases, of which one third occurred because the earlier abuse was not recognized (Kivlin et al. 2000). Jayawant et al. (1998) found that 12% of cases had a previous history of abuse and all died at the subsequent admission.

During the acute admission with NAHI brain imaging may show evidence of a pre-existing injury in the form of cerebral atrophy, subdural hygroma and ex vacuo ventriculomegaly in 45% of cases despite the absence of a history of earlier brain injury (Ewing-Cobbs et al. 1998).

Environmental factors such as family instability and disadvantaged socio-economic conditions result in several crucial prognostic factors that have a bearing on the outcome after acute traumatic brain injury such as the quality of parenting, the emotional environment and affective relationship between the mother and child.

Preterm birth and low birthweight will influence outcome because of the injury severity to a relatively immature nervous system as well as being a risk factor for the head injury to occur in the first place. The antecedent quality of child care is seen when the average weight of such children at birth is on the 30th centile, and at admission on the 10th centile (Bonnier et al. 1995).

The acute brain injury may add to preexisting neurodevelopmental problems, with correspondingly poorer outcomes. Twenty per cent of 86 children with cerebral palsy were

TABLE 12.6
Acute clinical and physiological factors influencing outcome after inflicted/accidental head injury

Feature	Outcome	Reference
Following NAHI		
GCS <8	None with 'good' outcome	Johnson et al. (1995)
Cerebral hypoxic–ischaemic injury (apnoea, BP<80 mmHg, ETT, EPTS, blood transfusion, diffuse brain swelling)	None with 'good' outcome (major determinant)	Johnson et al. (1995)
Coma, apnoea, diffuse brain swelling, or hypoxia–ischaemia	Predictive of poor outcome	Kemp et al. (2003)
Lowest CPP Lowest MAP	Poor outcome	Barlow and Minns (1999)
Diminished level of consciousness Require intubation Seizures (acute) Apnoea	Poor outcome	Duhaime et al. (1996)
Non-reactive pupils (on presentation) (Conversely reactive)	Died (p<0.001) (Conversely lived)	McCabe and Donahue (2000)
Require IPPV	Poor vision (p<0.041)	McCabe and Donahue (2000)
Initial visual perception good	See well at follow-up (p<0.0041)	Kivlin et al. (2000)
Injury severity	Poorer outcome	Ewing-Cobbs et al. (1999)
Longer period unconscious	Poorer outcome	Ewing-Cobbs et al. (1999)
Specific retinal findings	Poor final vision	Mills (1998)
Lack of visual response (on presentation)	Mortality	Mills (1998)
Diffuse retinal haemorrhages	Poor neurological outcome	Mathews and Das (1996)
Extensive preretinal/macular haemorrhages	Poor or profound visual loss	Wilkinson et al. (1989)
Cerebral injury	Visual loss	Han and Wilkinson (1990)
Deceleration of head growth	Long-term neurological sequelae	Bonnier et al. (1995)
Following severe accidental traumatic brain injury		
Duration (as percentage of total monitoring time) of age-specific derangement of CPP	Survival (p=0.003) and poor outcome (p=0.004) after accidental TBI	Jones et al. (2003b)
Primary areflexia and secondary brain swelling/oedema, indicated by low GCS score	Adverse outcome	Feickert et al. (1999)
Somatosensory evoked potentials	Long-term (poor) outcome (using GOS and Health Utilities Index) at 1 and 5yr after brain injury	Carter et al. (1999)
Minimum CPP of 43–45 mmHg and maximum ICP of 35 mmHg	Poor short-term outcome (dead, vegetative or severe disability,) after TBI	Chambers et al. (2001)
Primary disturbance of consciousness >24hr, GCS <7, increased ICP with CPP <50 mmHg, age at accident <2yr, physical abuse, and development of post-traumatic epilepsy	Unfavourable long-term outcome (mean 8.75yr)	Kieslich et al. (2001)

TABLE 12.6
(cont'd)

Feature	Outcome	Reference
Abbreviated Injury Scale score, Injury Severity Score, GCS (measured at the scene, and at 6, 24 and 72hr), length of coma, and initial discharge site	Outcome at discharge (<17yr old)	Massagli et al. (1996b)
AIS, ISS, GCS, pupils, and discharge GOS	Outcome at 5–7 years later	Massagli et al. (1996a)
Cumulative risk factors: (i) GCS at 24hr following injury; (ii) presence of hypoxia on admission; (iii) CT findings of subarachnoid haemorrhage, diffuse axonal injury and brain swelling	Poor outcome (6mo post-injury) after TBI in children aged <15yr	Ong et al. (1996)
GCS, duration of impaired consciousness, number of intracranial lesions seen on CT/MRI	Children <6yr Related to outcome at baseline, 3 and 12mo post-injury	Prasad et al. (2002)
Inflicted brain injury	Poorer GOS and cognitive outcome	
Pupillary abnormalities	Poorer motor outcome	
Age and ISS alone	Not associated with outcome	
Injury severity (lower GCS scores at admission and 24hr post-injury)	Poorer performance in physical and cognitive domains at 6mo post-injury in 2- to 12-yr-olds	Anderson et al. (2001)
Pre-injury behavioural and family functioning measures	Related closely to psychosocial outcome	
The younger the age, lower GCS, higher PRISM score at admission	Mortality and dependent functions more likely	Thakker et al. (1997)
	Children aged 2–16yr, with severe head injury:	Sharples et al. (1995)
(i) Lower mean cerebral blood flow and lower mean CMRO$_2$ in first 24hr post-injury	(i) Poorer outcome	
(ii) After 24hr, mean CBF and mean CMRO$_2$	(ii) No difference between good and poor outcome	
Injury severity (lower GCS scores at admission and 24hr post-injury)	Poorer performance in physical and cognitive domains at 6mo	Anderson et al. (2001)
	Post-injury in 2- to 12-yr-olds	
Pre-injury behavioural and family functioning measures	Related closely to psychosocial outcome	
Pre-injury factors, TBI severity, measures of the post-injury family environment	Predict outcome at 6 and 12mo post-injury	Taylor et al. (1999)
S100β protein serum levels	Poor outcome (hospital discharge and 6mo outcome) after accidental TBI	Spinella et al. (2003)

TABLE 12.7
Imaging findings influencing outcome after NAHI

Diffuse brain swelling	Poor morbidity	Gilles and Nelson (1998)
Midline shift	89% died	Gilles and Nelson (1998)
Infarct/oedema on acute CT	Lower mental and motor scores	Ewing-Cobbs et al. (1998)
Bilateral diffuse hypodensity ('big black brain')	Most important predictor of outcome	Duhaime et al. (1993)
DAI (signature)	Not solely related to outcome	Johnson et al. (1995)
'Reversal sign' (Han et al. 1989 definition)	Poor prognosis and irreversible brain damage	Rao et al. (1999)
Polar atrophy at 20 days	Abnormal outcome	Sinal and Ball (1987)
Diffuse cerebral swelling	No 'good' outcome	Sinal and Ball (1987)

TABLE 12.8
Treatment influences on outcome after NAHI

Aggressive management	No influence on outcome	Duhaime et al. (1996, 1998)
CPP/MAP	Related to outcome	Barlow and Minns (1999)

found to be the subject of abuse. In these cases the cerebral palsy was due to the abuse in 50% and a cause for the abuse in a similar percentage. Rarely the same child has cerebral palsy resulting from abuse and is additionally later abused (Diamond and Jaudes 1983). Both head trauma and the broader spectrum of injury have been reported in the cerebral palsy population (Mac Keith 1974, Solomons 1979).

ACUTE BRAIN INJURY FACTORS (PRIMARY AND SECONDARY BRAIN INJURY)
Clinical, imaging and treatment factors that have a bearing on the outcome after NAHI are tabulated in Tables 12.6, 12.7 and 12.8.

Age or maturational level at the time of any global brain injury is thought to have a significant influence on outcome (Johnson and Almli 1978). In one study, the age at which young children suffered NAHI was estimated at 6.2 months ± 2.7 months, and the age at injury of those who died from their injury was 7.7 ± 7.2 months (Makaroff and Putnam 2003). Table 12.9 summarizes the existing literature that relates age at time of injury to outcome.

POST-INJURY FACTORS
Additional brain injuries or abnormal influences on neurodevelopment may contribute to the final outcome, such as persistent adverse environmental influences; different forms of abuse such as emotional abuse or neglect, which may have serious cognitive consequences; and additional brain injury from periods of status epilepticus or prolonged seizures, decompensated raised intracranial pressure from ventriculoperitoneal shunt blockage or infection, or where there has been inadequate or absent treatment for the neurological problems. While not minimizing their potential adverse effect in all children, these post-

TABLE 12.9
Influence of age on outcome

Younger age taken into care/adoption	Favourable outcome	Hensey et al. (1983), Howe (1998)
TBI <2yr	Worse outcome compared to those who were >2yr at time of TBI	Kretschmer (1983)
Infant brain	More susceptible to insults than adult brain	Brazier (1975), Dennis (2000)
Injury at critical developmental periods	Worse outcome	Levin et al. (1982)
Young children with diffuse brain injury	Worse memory and cognition than in older children	Ruijs et al. (1994)
Young brain	Late post-traumatic epilepsy	Jennett (1973, 1974), Kretschmer (1983), Gjerris (1986), Kieslich and Jacobi (1995), Kieslich et al. (2001)
Infants and preschool children with severe TBI	High mortality and adverse neurobehavioural outcome	Ewing-Cobbs et al. (1995), reviewing the majority of relevant studies
Younger child with TBI (inflicted and non-inflicted)	Reduced scores on development and outcome scales	Goldstein et al. (1993), Duhaime et al. (1996), Adelson et al. (1997)
Injury <6mo	6/7 severe disability	Duhaime et al. (1996)
Injury >6mo	3/5 good outcome	Duhaime et al. (1996)
Injury <6mo	Poor prognosis	Wilkinson et al (1989), Duhaime et al. (1996)
Age at injury	Predicts attentional-inhibitory control and cognitive outcome (younger do worse)	Dennis et al. (2001)
Diffuse brain injury in the young brain	Associated with a transient arrest of experience-dependent plasticity	Fineman et al. (2000)
Young children with brain injuries	Requirement for more social/family support than adolescents (rated by educational psychologists)	Brooks et al. (2003)
Mean age at injury 5.2 ± 3.2mo Mean age at injury 6.5 ± 2.8mo Mean age at injury 5.9 ± 8.0mo Age not significantly different between these groups	No impairment Mild impairment Moderate impairment	Makaroff and Putnam (2003), review of literature

injury factors will be most evident in children with milder deficits following the acute injury. The most important factor in this period is the possibility of re-injury.

A summary of the important associations between pre-injury, injury and post-injury factors and outcome is shown in Figure 12.2.

Re-injury rate

It is not unusual for re-injury to be a feature of accidental events in primary school-age children,

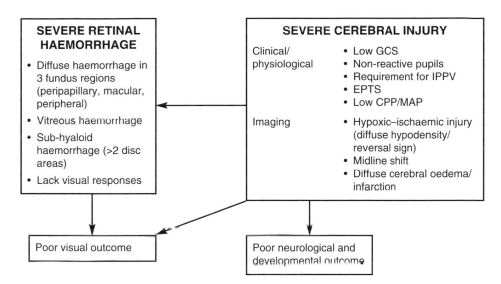

SEVERE RETINAL HAEMORRHAGE	SEVERE CEREBRAL INJURY	
• Diffuse haemorrhage in 3 fundus regions (peripapillary, macular, peripheral)	Clinical/ physiological	• Low GCS • Non-reactive pupils • Requirement for IPPV • EPTS • Low CPP/MAP
• Vitreous haemorrhage • Sub-hyaloid haemorrhage (>2 disc areas) • Lack visual responses	Imaging	• Hypoxic–ischaemic injury (diffuse hypodensity/ reversal sign) • Midline shift • Diffuse cerebral oedema/ infarction

Poor visual outcome

Poor neurological and developmental outcome

Fig. 12.2. Schematic presentations of the associations between severe retinal haemorrhage, severe cerebral injury, and visual, neurological and developmental outcome. (*Abbreviations:* IPPV = intermittent positive pressure ventilation, CPP = cerebral perfusion pressure; MAP = mean arterial pressure; EPTS = early post-traumatic seizures.)

and between 15% and 44% of such children had multiple occurrences of head trauma with loss of consciousness (Klonoff et al. 1993, Michaud et al. 1993).

Three years after hospitalization following general child abuse or neglect, one third of the children are again suspected victims of further physical abuse or neglect (Morse et al. 1970). Other investigators have found a re-injury rate for child abuse generally (not specifically head injury) of between 10% and 30% (Cohn 1980, Lynch and Roberts 1982, Hensey et al. 1983). Such a high percentage suggests either that the decision to return the child to the home where they were injured was wrong, or that there was inadequate supervision. A study by Murphy et al. (1992) similarly found that 31% of cases that had initially been brought before a court on Care and Protection Petitions were dismissed, but that 29% of these dismissed cases had substantiated reports of further mistreatment, and 16% were eventually returned to the courts. This was more likely where the parent was diagnosed as psychotic or with other personality disorders. Authorities would obviously be more alert to the possibility of a second injury particularly if the child is returning to the original home, but the subsequent injury may be subtle and as difficult to diagnose as sometimes is the initial injury.

The re-injury may not be the second injury, but the third, fourth or later. Some 27% of children admitted with NAHI in one series had earlier been seen in a casualty department and sent home before a final admission with fractures and other injuries that led to the diagnosis of abuse. This is explicable given the many different ways in which child abuse may present; for example, a child may present with hypoxic–ischaemic encephalopathy as the sole manifestation of non-accidental injury without any external markers of injury (Rao et al. 1999).

When children are returned to their home there is a very real risk of a further NAHI and as many as two thirds in one study of survivors of shaken baby syndrome who were returned to their home were re-injured (Fischer and Allasio 1994).

Given the importance of a past history of social work intervention as a predictor for acute NAHI, this re-injury rate emphasizes the importance of addressing outstanding social issues if the child is to be returned to the abusive household.

Progressive brain damage

Some patients appear to deteriorate after severe head injury, and it may be difficult to distinguish true dementia from severe multiple cognitive deficits, and for infants and young children this may simply be a result of a reduction in plasticity potential that far outlasts the acute effects of the injury. Brain damage can be followed by events such as reactive synaptogenesis, re-routing of axons to unusual locations and altered axon-retraction processes. The neuronal circuitry changes are considered to be developmental growth processes triggered in response to neuronal loss rather than as a specific healing process (Finger and Almli 1985).

In a long term follow-up study of children (median age 4.4 years), three of the 40 whose status changed deteriorated, and two of these had suffered accidental head injury (Carter et al. 1999). From our own database of 150 surviving children after either severe or moderate accidental TBI (GCS ≤12), or minor TBI with an ISS score of ≥16, who were followed up for a maximum of 24 months, 7% showed a deterioration in global outcome (GOS score) between two successive assessments. With more sophisticated outcome measuring tools we suspect that the number deteriorating is likely to be considerably more.

Sequential MRI in children suffering NAHI shows increasing abnormality suggestive of ongoing brain injury (Fig. 12.3). A possible explanation for this relates to the ApoE genotype: the presence of an ApoE e4 allele has been found to hasten the onset of dementia (Graham 1999, Nemetz 1999). Alternatively, recent pathological studies have suggested persistence of destructive cytokines (IL-1) in the brain white matter for prolonged periods after the injury (C Smith, personal communication 2003).

Summary

An overview of the outcome after shaken baby syndrome and other forms of NAHI is seen in Table 12.10, where 20% of cases have suffered a fatal outcome and 59% are left with severe or moderate disability (Fig. 12.4). There are frequent motor deficits, epilepsy, microcephaly, visual impairment, severe learning disability, and behavioural and emotional sequelae, and the children may still remain at risk of a further injury.

The reasons for the devastating mortality and morbidity figures following shaken baby syndrome and other NAHIs have been postulated under each of the specific deficits outlined above, but in general are likely to be due to:

(i) the fact that this is a very severe brain injury and more severe than was originally appreciated or than is recognized at the time of the child's presentation. Autopsy evidence

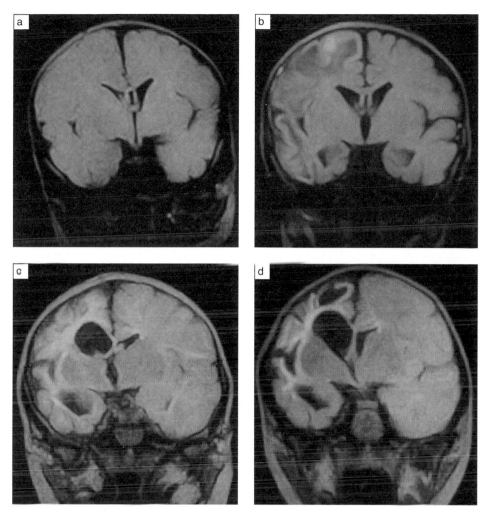

Fig. 12.3. A 5-week-old boy who presented with acute encephalopathy, multiple rib fractures, bilateral retinal haemorrhages and bilateral subdural haematomas with resultant raised intracranial pressure requiring neurointensive care: sequential MRI at (a) 1 day, (b) 11 days, (c) 9 months and (d) 2.3 years after presentation. The scans show the development of asymmetrical cerebral atrophy continuing after 9 months and up to 2.3 years.

has shown additional tears, contusions in cerebrum, brainstem and spinal cord unrecognized by conventional imaging to date. The very severe secondary neuronal injury is evidence of severe TBI, and child abuse in the very young is associated with extremely high CSF glutamate concentrations (Ruppel et al. 2001);

(ii) the early hypoxic–ischaemic injury resulting from the apnoea and hypoxia, hypotension and low cerebral perfusion pressure is likely to be a major contributor (similar to perinatal hypoxic–ischaemic injury) to the poor outcome;

407

TABLE 12.10

Overview of outcome features after NAHI, from cumulated literature sources

Feature	%
Mortality	20.6
Vegetative state	5.0
Severe disability	34.2
Moderate disability	25.2
Any motor deficit	38.2
Quadriparesis	35.4
Hemiparesis	18.7
Cranial nerve deficits	20.0
Seizures	30.2
Microcephaly	50.7
Macrocephaly	16.0
Blindness	14.8
Visual impairment	45.3
Intellectual/cognitive deficits	53.7
Behavioural/emotional problems	38.4
At risk of further injury	≤40.0
Normal	10.9

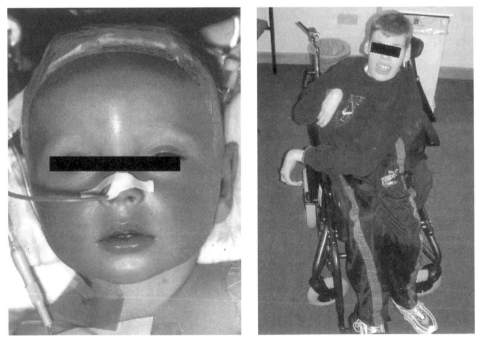

Fig. 12.4. (a) Infant photographed during acute admission with an encephalopathy, bilateral subdural haematoma, retinal haemorrhages and bruising due to a non-accidental head injury. (b) Nearly 20 years later he remains confined to a wheelchair with a mixed spastic and dyskinetic tetraparesis, learning and visual impairments, and scoliosis, and he is dependent for all activities of daily living.

(iii) a cascade of neurotrophic factors may continue to cause neuronal loss after the trauma has ceased;

(iv) the very young age of these infants. MNDA receptor-bearing neurones are highly sensitive to both excitotoxic stimulation (Ikonomidou et al 1989) and transient global blockade of MNDA receptors (Ikonomidou et al. 1999) during the first two weeks of life but not after 21 days of age in experimental animals, i.e. excessive and inadequate stimulation during this 'critical period', results in demise of a large percentage of neurones. It is now accepted that head injury in young children has a substantially worse outcome than that in the later years because of the interference with the normal neurodevelopmental growth processes.

Apart from the primary and secondary injuries detailed at the beginning of this chapter, there are also tertiary brain injuries (chronic subdural haematoma, post-traumatic hydrocephalus, growing skull fracture, cerebral atrophy and microcephaly) and quaternary injuries that take the form of secondary positional deformity, scoliosis and wind-sweeping, contractures, persistent vegetative state and the altered family dynamics.

It is clear from the above that many aspects of the lives of these children who have been abused require some ongoing medical care, but nursing, therapy, social work and sometimes protracted legal involvement dominates their future lives in the long term. Further research, particularly in areas such as the motor disorder, and cognitive and functional (ADL) sequelae, is necessary in an attempt to modify the serious disabilities these children have unwittingly suffered.

REFERENCES

Adelson PD, Clyde B, Kochanek PM, Wisniewski SR, Marion DW, Yonas H (1997) 'Cerebrovascular response in infants and young children following severe traumatic brain injury: a preliminary report.' *Pediatr Neurosurg* **26**: 200–207

Alexander R, Sato Y, Smith W, Bennett T (1990) 'Incidence of impact trauma with cranial injuries ascribed to shaking.' *Am J Dis Child* **144**: 724–726.

Alexander R, Crabbe L, Sato Y, Smith W, Bennett T (1990) 'Serial abuse in children who are shaken.' *Am J Dis Child* **144**: 58–60.

Anderson VA, Catroppa C, Haritou F, Morse S, Pentland L, Rosenfeld J, Stargatt R (2001) 'Predictors of acute child and family outcome following traumatic brain injury in children.' *Pediatr Neurosurg* **34**: 138–148.

Annegers JF, Grabow JD, Groover RV, Laws ER, Elveback LR, Kurland LT (1980) 'Seizures after head trauma: a population study.' *Neurology* **30**: 683–689.

Appelbaum AS (1977) 'Developmental retardation in infants as a concomitant of physical child abuse.' *J Abnorm Child Psychol* **5**: 417–423.

Barlow KM, Minns RA (1999) 'The relationship between intracranial pressure and outcome in non-accidental head injury.' *Dev Med Child Neurol* **41**: 220–225.

Barlow KM, Thompson E, Minns RA (1999) 'Neurological outcome of non-accidental head injury.' *Eur J Paediatr Neurol* **3**: 139–140.

Barlow KM, Spowart JJ, Minns RA (2000) 'Early posttraumatic seizures in non-accidental head injury: relation to outcome.' *Dev Med Child Neurol* **42**: 591–594.

Barlow KM, Thompson E, Johnson D, Minns RA (2004) 'The neurological outcome of non-accidental head injury.' *Pediatr Rehabil* **7**: 195–203.

Berney J, Favier J, Froidevaux AC (1994) 'Paediatric head trauma: influence of age and sex. I. Epidemiology.' *Child's Nerv Syst* **10**: 509–516.

Bonnier C, Nassogne M-C, Evrard P (1995) 'Outcome and prognosis of whiplash shaken infant syndrome: late consequences after a symptom-free interval.' *Dev Med Child Neurol* **37**: 943–956.

Brazier MAB (1975) *Growth and Development of the Brain. Nutritional, Genetic, and Environmental Factors. International Brain Research Organization Monograph Series, Vol. 1.* New York: Raven Press.

Brooks BM, Rose FD, Johnson DA, Andrews TK, Gulamali R (2003) 'Support for children following traumatic brain injury: the views of educational psychologists.' *Disabil Rehabil* **25**: 51–56.

Brown JK, Minns RA (1993) 'Non-accidental head injury, with particular reference to whiplash shaking injury and medico-legal aspects.' *Dev Med Child Neurol* **35**: 849–869.

Bruce DA, Zimmerman RA (1989) 'Shaken impact syndrome.' *Pediatr Ann* **18**: 482–484.

Caffey J (1972) 'On the theory and practice of shaking infants. Its potential residual effects of permanent brain damage and mental retardation.' *Am J Dis Child* **124**: 161–169.

Carrigan TD, Walker E, Barnes S (2000) 'Domestic violence: the shaken adult syndrome.' *J Accid Emerg Med* **17**: 138–139.

Carter BG, Taylor A, Butt W (1999) 'Severe brain injury in children: long-term outcome and its prediction using somatosensory evoked potentials (SEPs).' *Intensive Care Med* **25**: 722–728.

Chambers IR, Treadwell L, Mendelow AD (2001) 'Determination of threshold levels of cerebral perfusion pressure and intracranial pressure in severe head injury by using receiver-operating characteristic curves: an observational study in 291 patients.' *J Neurosurg* **94**: 412–416.

Chiaviello CT, Christoph RA, Bond GR (1994a) 'Infant walker-related injuries: a prospective study of severity and incidence.' *Pediatrics* **93**: 974–976.

Chiaviello CT, Christoph RA, Bond GR (1994b) 'Stairway-related injuries in children.' *Pediatrics* **94**: 679–681.

Choux M, Lena G, Genitori L (1986) 'Intracranial haematomas.' In: Raimondi AJ, Choux M, di Rocco C, editors. *Head Injuries in the Newborn and Infant.* Heidelberg: Springer Verlag, p 203–216.

Cohen RA, Kaufman RA, Myers PA, Towbin RB (1986) 'Cranial computed tomography in the abused child with head injury.' *AJR* **146**: 97–102.

Cohn AH (1980) 'The pediatrician's role in the treatment of child abuse: implications from a national evaluation study.' *Pediatrics* **65**: 358–361.

Crouchman M, Rossiter L, Colaco T, Forsyth RA (2001) 'Practical outcome scale for paediatric head injury.' *Arch Dis Child* **84**: 120–124.

Dennis M (2000) 'Childhood medical disorders and cognitive impairment: biological risk, time, development, and reserve.' In: Yeates KO, Ris MD, Taylor HG, editors. *Pediatric Neuropsychology, Research, Theory and Practice.* London: Guilford Press, p 3–22.

Dennis M, Guger S, Roncadin C, Barnes M, Schachar R (2001) 'Attentional–inhibitory control and social–behavioral regulation after childhood closed head injury: do biological, developmental, and recovery variables predict outcome?' *J Int Neuropsychol Soc* **7**: 683–692.

Diamond LJ, Jaudes PK (1983) 'Child abuse in a cerebral-palsied population.' *Dev Med Child Neurol* **25**: 169–174.

DiScala C, Sege R, Li G, Reece RM (2000) 'Child abuse and unintentional injuries: a 10-year retrospective.' *Arch Pediatr Adolesc Med* **154**: 16–22.

Duhaime AC, Alario AJ, Lewander WJ, Schut L, Sutton LN, Seidl TS, Nudelman S, Budenz D, Hertle R, Tsiaras W (1992) 'Head injury in very young children: mechanisms, injury types, and ophthalmologic findings in 100 hospitalized patients younger than 2 years of age.' *Pediatrics* **90**: 179–185.

Duhaime A-C, Bilaniuk LT, Zimmerman R (1993) 'The "big black brain": radiographic changes after severe inflicted head injury in infancy.' *J Neurotrauma* **10** Suppl. 1: S59 (abstract).

Duhaime AC, Christian C, Moss E, Seidl T (1996) 'Long-term outcome in infants with the shaking-impact syndrome.' *Pediatr Neurosurg* **24**: 292–298.

Duhaime AC, Christian CW, Rorke LB, Zimmerman RA (1998) 'Nonaccidental head injury in infants—the "shaken-baby syndrome".' *N Engl J Med* **338**: 1822–1829.

Dumas HM, Haley SM, Rabin JP (2001) 'Short-term durability and improvement of function in traumatic brain injury: a pilot study using the Paediatric Evaluation of Disability Inventory (PEDI) classification levels.' *Brain Inj* **15**: 891–902.

Elmer E (1977) 'A follow-up study of traumatized children.' *Pediatrics* **59**: 273–279.

Elmer E, Gregg GS (1967) 'Developmental characteristics of abused children.' *Pediatrics* **40**: 596–602.

Evrard P, Miladi N, Bonnier C, Gressens P (1992) 'Normal and abnormal development of the brain.' In Rapin I, Segalowitz SJ, editors. *Child Neuropsychology.* Amsterdam: Elsevier Science, p 11–44.

Ewing-Cobbs L, Duhaime A-C, Fletcher JM (1995) 'Inflicted and noninflicted traumatic brain injury in infants and preschoolers.' *J Head Trauma Rehabil* **10**: 13–24.

Ewing-Cobbs L, Fletcher JM, Levin HS, Francis DJ, Davidson K, Miner ME (1997) 'Longitudinal neuropsychological outcome in infants and preschoolers with traumatic brain injury.' *J Int Neuropsychol Soc* **3**: 581–591.

Ewing-Cobbs L, Kramer L, Prasad M, Canales DN, Louis PT, Fletcher JM, Vollero H, Landry SH, Cheung K (1998) 'Neuroimaging, physical, and developmental findings after inflicted and noninflicted traumatic brain injury in young children.' *Pediatrics* **102**: 300–307.

Ewing-Cobbs L, Prasad M, Kramer L, Landry S (1999) 'Inflicted traumatic brain injury: relationship of developmental outcome to severity of injury.' *Pediatr Neurosurg* **31**: 251–258.

Feickert H-J, Drommer S, Heyer R (1999) 'Severe head injury in children: impact of risk factors on outcome.' *J Trauma Inj Infect Crit Care* **47**: 33–38.

Fineman I, Giza CC, Nahed BV, Lee SM, Hovda DA (2000) 'Inhibition of neocortical plasticity during development by a moderate concussive brain injury.' *J Neurotrauma* **17**: 739–749.

Finger S, Almli CR (1985) 'Brain damage and neuroplasticity: mechanisms of recovery or development?' *Brain Res* **357**: 177–186.

Fischer H, Allasio D (1994) 'Permanently damaged: long-term follow-up of shaken babies.' *Clin Pediatr* **33**: 696–698.

Fragala MA, Haley SM, Dumas HM, Rabin JP (2002) 'Classifying mobility recovery in children and youth with brain injury during hospital-based rehabilitation.' *Brain Inj* **16**: 149–160.

Frank Y, Zimmerman R, Leeds NM (1985) 'Neurological manifestations in abused children who have been shaken.' *Dev Med Child Neurol* **27**: 312–316.

Gilles EE, Nelson MD (1998) 'Cerebral complications of nonaccidental head injury in childhood.' *Pediatr Neurol* **19**: 119–128.

Gjerris F (1986) 'Head injuries in children—special features.' *Acta Neurochir Suppl* **36**: 155–158.

Goldson E (1991) 'The affective and cognitive sequelae of child maltreatment.' *Pediatr Clin N Am* **38**: 1481–1496.

Goldstein B, Kelly MM, Bruton D, Cox C (1993) 'Inflicted versus accidental head injury in critically injured children.' *Crit Care Med* **21**: 1328–1332.

Graham DI, Horsburgh K, Nicoll JA, Teasdale GM (1999) 'Apolipoprotein E and the response of the brain to injury.' *Acta Neurochir Suppl* **73**: 89–92.

Green AH, Voeller K, Gaines R, Kubie J (1981) 'Neurological impairment in maltreated children.' *Child Abuse Negl* **5**: 129–134.

Hadley MN, Sonntag VK, Rekate HL, Murphy A (1989) 'The infant whiplash–shake injury syndrome: a clinical and pathological study.' *Neurosurgery* **24**: 536–540.

Han DP, Wilkinson WS (1990) 'Late ophthalmic manifestations of the shaken baby syndrome.' *J Pediatr Ophthalmol Strabismus* **27**: 299–303.

Han KB, Towbin RB, De Courten-Myers G, McLaurin RL, Ball WF (1989) Reversal sign on CT: effect of anoxic/ischemic injury in children. *AJNR* **10**: 1191–1198.

Haviland J, Russell RIR (1997) 'Outcome after severe non-accidental head injury.' *Arch Dis Child* **77**: 504–507.

Hensey OJ, Williams JK, Rosenbloom L (1983) 'Intervention in child abuse: experience in Liverpool.' *Dev Med Child Neurol* **25**: 606–611.

Holsinger T, Steffens DC, Phillips C, Helms MJ, Havlik RJ, Breitner JC, Guralnik JM, Plassman BL (2002) 'Head injury in early adulthood and the lifetime risk of depression.' *Arch Gen Psychiatry* **59**: 17–22.

Howe D (1998) *Patterns of Adoption: Nature, Nurture and Psychosocial Development.* Oxford: Blackwell Scientific.

Ikonomidou C, Mosinger JL, Salles KS, Labruyere J, Olney JW (1989) 'Sensitivity of the developing rat brain to hypobaric/ischemic damage parallels sensitivity to N-methyl-aspartate neurotoxicity.' *J Neurosci* **9**: 2809–2818.

Ikonomidou C, Bosch F, Miksa M, Bittigau P, Vockler J, Dikranian K, Tenkova TI, Stefovska V, Turski L, Olney JW (1999) 'Blockade of NMDA receptors and apoptotic neurodegeneration in the developing brain.' *Science* **283**: 70–74.

Jayawant S, Rawlinson A, Gibbon F, Price J, Schulte J, Sharples P, Sibert JR, Kemp AM (1998) 'Subdural haemorrhages in infants: population based study.' *BMJ* **317**: 1558–1561.

Jennett B (1973) 'Trauma as a cause of epilepsy in childhood.' *Dev Med Child Neurol* **15**: 56–62.

Jennett B (1974) 'Early traumatic epilepsy. Incidence and significance after nonmissile injuries.' *Arch Neurol* **30**: 394–398.

Jennett B, Bond M (1975) 'Assessment of outcome after severe brain damage. A practical scale.' *Lancet* **1**: 480–484.

411

Johnson D, Almli CR (1978) 'Age, brain damage, and performance.' In: Finger S, editor. *Recovery from Brain Damage: Research and Theory*. New York: Plenum Press, p 115–132.

Johnson DL, Boal D, Baule R (1995) 'Role of apnea in nonaccidental head injury.' *Pediatr Neurosurg* **23**: 305–310.

Jones PA, Andrews PJD, Easton VJ, Minns RA (2003a) 'Traumatic brain injury in childhood: intensive care time series data and outcome.' *Br J Neurosurg* **17**: 29–39.

Jones PA, Minns RA, Lo TYM, Andrews PJD, Taylor GS, Ali S (2003b) 'Graphical display of variability and inter-relationships of pressure signals in children with traumatic brain injury.' *Physiol Meas* **24**: 201–211.

Kemp AM, Stoodley N, Cobley C, Coles L, Kemp KW (2003) 'Apnoea and brain swelling in non-accidental head injury.' *Arch Dis Child* **88**: 472–476.

Kempe CH (1971) 'Paediatric implications of the battered baby syndrome.' *Arch Dis Child* **46**: 28–37.

Kempe CH, Silverman FN, Steele BF, Droegemueller W, Silver HK (1962) 'The battered-child syndrome.' *JAMA* **181**: 17–24.

Kieslich M, Jacobi G (1995) 'Incidence and risk factors of post-traumatic epilepsy in childhood.' *Lancet* **345**: 187.

Kieslich M, Marquardt G, Galow G, Lorenz R, Jacobi G (2001) 'Neurological and mental outcome after severe head injury in childhood: a long-term follow-up of 318 children.' *Disabil Rehabil* **23**: 665–669.

King WJ, MacKay M, Sirnick A; Canadian Shaken Baby Study Group (2003) 'Shaken baby syndrome in Canada: clinical characteristics and outcomes of hospital cases.' *CMAJ* **168**: 155–159.

Kivlin JD, Simons KB, Lazoritz S, Ruttum MS (2000) 'Shaken baby syndrome.' *Ophthalmology* **107**: 1246–1254.

Klonoff H, Clark C, Klonoff PS (1993) 'Long-term outcome of head injuries: a 23 year follow up study of children with head injuries.' *J Neurol Neurosurg Psychiatry* **56**: 410–415.

Kretschmer H (1983) 'Prognosis of severe head injuries in childhood and adolescence.' *Neuropediatrics* **14**: 176–181.

Levin HS, Eisenberg HM, Wigg NR, Kobayashi K (1982) 'Memory and intellectual ability after head injury in children and adolescents.' *Neurosurgery* **11**: 668–673.

Lipton SA, Rosenberg PA (1994) 'Mecahnisms of disease: axcitatory amino acids as a final common pathway for neurologic disorders.' *N Engl J Med* **330**: 613–622.

Lo TYM, McPhillips M, Minns RA, Gibson RJ (2003) 'Cerebral atrophy following shaken impact syndrome and other non-accidental head injury (NAHI).' *Pediatr Rehabil* **6**: 47–55.

Ludwig S, Warman M (1984) 'Shaken baby syndrome: a review of 20 cases.' *Ann Emerg Med* **13**: 104–107.

Lynch MA, Roberts J (1982) *Consequences of Child Abuse*. London: Academic Press.

Mac Keith R (1974) 'Speculations of non-accidental injury as a cause of chronic brain disorder.' *Dev Med Child Neurol* **16**: 216–218.

Makaroff KL, Putnam FW (2003) 'Outcomes of infants and children with inflicted traumatic brain injury.' *Dev Med Child Neurol* **45**: 497–502.

Martin H (1972) 'The child and his development.' In: Kempe CH, Helfer RE, editors. *Helping the Battered Child and His Family*. Philadelphia: Lippincott, p 93–114.

Martin HP, Beezley P (1977) 'Behavioral observations of abused children.' *Dev Med Child Neurol* **19**: 373–387.

Massagli TL, Jaffe KM, Fay GC, Polissar NL, Liao S, Rivara JB (1996a) 'Neurobehavioral sequelae of severe pediatric traumatic brain injury: a cohort study.' *Arch Phys Med Rehabil* **77**: 223–231.

Massagli TL, Michaud LJ, Rivara FP (1996b) 'Association between injury indices and outcome after severe traumatic brain injury in children.' *Arch Phys Med Rehabil* **77**: 125–132.

Matthews GP, Das A (1996) 'Dense vitreous hemorrhages predict poor visual and neurological prognosis in infants with shaken baby syndrome.' *J Pediatr Ophthalmol Strabismus* **33**: 260–265.

McCabe CF, Donahue SP (2000) 'Prognostic indicators for vision and mortality in shaken baby syndrome.' *Arch Ophthalmol* **118**: 373–377.

McPhillips M (2002) 'Non-accidental head injury in young infants.' In: Rutherford M, editor. *MRI of the Neonatal Brain*. Edinburgh: WB Saunders, p 261–269.

Meyers CA, Levin HS, Eisenberg HM, Guinto FC (1983) 'Early versus late lateral ventricular enlargement following closed head injury.' *J Neurol Neurosurg Psychiatry* **46**: 1092–1097.

Michaud LJ, Rivara FP, Grady MS, Reay DT (1992) 'Predictors of survival and severity of disability after severe brain injury in children.' *Neurosurgery* **31**: 254–264.

Michaud LJ, Rivara FP, Jaffe KM, Fay G, Dailey JL (1993) 'Traumatic brain injury as a risk factor for behavioral disorders in children.' *Arch Phys Med Rehabil* **74**: 368–375.

Mills M (1998) 'Funduscopic lesions associated with mortality in shaken baby syndrome.' *J AAPOS* **2**: 67–71.

412

Morse CW, Sahler OJ, Friedman SB (1970) 'A three-year follow-up study of abused and neglected children.' *Am J Dis Child* **120**: 439–446.

Murphy JM, Bishop SJ, Jellinek MS, Quinn D, Poitrast JF (1992) 'What happens after the care and protection petition? Reabuse in a court sample.' *Child Abuse Negl* **16**: 485–493.

Musemeche CA, Barthel M, Cosentino C, Reynolds M (1991) 'Pediatric falls from heights.' *J Trauma Inj Infec Crit Care* **31**: 1347–1349.

Nassogne MC, Bonnier C (2001) 'Diagnosis and long-term outcome of shaken infants.' *J Pediatr Puericult* **14**: 235–239.

Nemetz PN, Leibson C, Naessens JM, Beard M, Kokmen E, Annegers JF, Kurland LT (1999) 'Traumatic brain injury and time to onset of Alzheimer's disease: a population-based study.' *Am J Epidemiol* **149**: 32–40.

Oates RK (1984) 'Personality development after physical abuse.' *Arch Dis Child* **59**: 147–150.

Oates RK, Peacock A, Forrest D (1984) 'The development of abused children.' *Dev Med Child Neurol* **26**: 649 656.

Oi S, Matsumoto S (1987) 'Post-traumatic hydrocephalus in children. Pathophysiology and classification.' *J Pediatr Neurosci* **3**: 133–147.

Okun A, Parker J, Levendosdy A (1994) 'Distinct and interactive contributions of physical abuse, socioeconomic disadvantage, and negative life events to children's social, cognitive, and affective adjustment.' *Dev Psychopathol* **6**. 77–98.

Oliver JE (1975) 'Microcephaly following baby battering and shaking.' *BMJ* **2**: 262–264.

Ong LC, Selladurai BM, Dhillon MK, Atan M, Lye MS (1996) 'The prognostic value of the Glasgow Coma Scale, hypoxia and computerized tomography in outcome prediction of pediatric head injury.' *Pediatr Neurosurg* **24**: 285–291.

Onuma T, Shimosegawa Y, Kameyama M, Arai H, Ishii K (1995) 'Clinicopathological investigation of gyral high density on computerized tomography following severe head injury in children.' *J Neurosurg* **82**: 995–1001.

Pounder DJ (1997) 'Shaken adult syndrome.' *Am J Forensic Med Pathol* **18**: 321 324.

Prasad MR, Ewing-Cobbs L, Swank PR, Kramer L (2002) 'Predictors of outcome following traumatic brain injury in young children.' *Pediatr Neurosurg* **36**: 64–74.

Rao P, Carty H, Pierce A (1999) 'The acute reversal sign: comparison of medical and non-accidental injury patients.' *Clin Radiol* **54**: 495–501.

Ruijs MBM, Keyser, A, Gabreels FJM (1994) 'Clinical neurological trauma parameters as predictors for neuropsychological recovery and long-term outcome in paediatric closed head injury: a review of the literature.' *Clin Neurol Neurosurg* **96**: 273–283.

Ruppel RA, Kochanek PM, Adelson PD, Rose ME, Wisniewski SR, Bell MJ, Clark RS, Marion DW, Graham SH (2001) 'Excitatory amino acid concentrations in ventricular cerebrospinal fluid after severe traumatic brain injury in infants and children: the role of child abuse.' *J Pediatr* **138**: 18–25.

Sharples PM, Stuart AG, Matthews DS, Aynsley-Green A, Eyre JA (1995) 'Cerebral blood flow and metabolism in children with severe head injury. Part 1: Relation to age, Glasgow Coma Score, outcome, intracranial pressure, and time after injury.' *J Neurol Neurosurg Psychiatry* **58**: 145–152.

Sills JA, Thomas LJ, Rosenbloom L (1977) 'Non-accidental injury: a two-year study in central Liverpool.' *Dev Med Child Neurol* **19**: 26–33.

Sinal SH, Ball MR (1987) 'Head trauma due to child abuse: serial computerized tomography in diagnosis and management.' *South Med J* **80**. 1505–1512.

Solomons G (1979) 'Child abuse and developmental disabilities.' *Dev Med Child Neurol* **21**: 101–105.

Soto-Ares G, Vinchon M, Delmaire C, Abecidan E, Dhellemes P, Pruvo JP (2001) 'Cerebellar atrophy after severe traumatic head injury in children.' *Child's Nerv Syst* **17**: 263–269.

Spinella PC, Dominguez T, Drott HR, Huh J, McCormick L, Rajendra A, Argon J, McIntosh T, Helfaer M (2003) 'S-100beta protein-serum levels in healthy children and its association with outcome in pediatric traumatic brain injury.' *Crit Care Med* **31**: 939–945.

Taylor HG, Yeates KO, Wade SL, Drotar D, Klein SK, Stancin T (1999) 'Influences on first-year recovery from traumatic brain injury in children.' *Neuropsychology* **13**: 76–89.

Thakker JC, Splaingard M, Zhu J, Babel K, Bresnahan J, Havens PL (1997) 'Survival and functional outcome of children requiring endotracheal intubation during therapy for severe traumatic brain injury.' *Crit Care Med* **25**: 1396–1401.

Tomita H, Ito U, Saito J, Maehara T (1990) 'Cerebral atrophy after severe head injury.' *Adv Neurol* **52**: 553.

413

Tomlin P, Clarke M, Robinson G, Roach J (2002) 'Rehabilitation in severe head injury in children: outcome and provision of care.' *Dev Med Child Neurol* **44**: 828–837.

Wilkinson WS, Han DP, Rappley MD, Owings CL (1989) 'Retinal hemorrhage predicts neurologic injury in the shaken baby syndrome.' *Arch Ophthalmol* **107**: 1472–1474.

Yakovlev P, Lecours A (1967) 'The myelogenetic cycles of regional maturation of the brain.' In: Minkowski A, editor. *Regional Development of the Brain in Early Life*. Oxford: Blackwell, p 3–70.

Yeates KO, Taylor HG, Wade SL, Drotar D, Stancin T, Minich N (2002) 'A prospective study of short- and long-term neuropsychological outcomes after traumatic brain injury in children.' *Neuropsychology* **16**: 514–523.

Zimmerman RA, Bilaniuk LT, Bruce D, Schut L, Uzzell B, Goldberg HI (1979) 'Computed tomography of craniocerebral injury in the abused child.' *Radiology* **130**: 687–690.

13
CHILD PROTECTION AND THE PREVENTION OF ABUSE

Jacqueline YQ Mok

Head injury is the most common cause of morbidity and mortality in physically abused children. In a retrospective epidemiological study in Scotland a mortality rate of 2% was reported (Barlow et al. 1998). The most frequently encountered form of inflicted head injury in infants is the shaken baby syndrome (SBS), characterized by subdural haemorrhage (SDH), diffuse parenchymal brain injury and retinal haemorrhages. There may or may not be accompanying skeletal or soft tissue injuries to other parts of the body. The clinical presentation is usually nonspecific, the infant could be acutely ill or asymptomatic, and non-accidental injury may not be suspected. Even after a diagnosis is made, difficulties remain with the management of the infant and family, because of the conflicting interests between the clinical needs of the child, and the ensuing child protection investigations. Child abuse is also costly both in human terms and in its financial consequences. This chapter will address the child protection issues as well as the prevention of non-accidental head injury (NAHI).

Difficulties with diagnosis
The average incidence of NAHI was calculated over a 15-year period in Scotland as 0.04 cases per year per 1000 children under the age of 5 years, with 55% of all cases occurring in children less than 1 year of age (Barlow et al. 1998). This is likely to be an underestimate, due to the retrospective nature of the study. A population-based study in south Wales and south-west England found a higher incidence of 12.8 per 100,000 children per year, rising to 21 per 100,000 children per year in children under 1 year of age (Jayawant et al. 1998). This study also showed the clear relation between SDH and fractures, other traumatic injury, retinal haemorrhages, and a previous history of child abuse in the family. Despite this, a significant number of these cases were not fully investigated in an appropriate way.

The full clinical spectrum is not always present. In its most subtle form, the diagnosis is frequently overlooked, but its more serious expression can also be missed. At one extreme is a well infant with an increasing head circumference, in whom there is no suggestion of any form of maltreatment. At the other, the infant may present acutely collapsed, with or without seizures, when there is a need to exclude infectious and metabolic causes. Where there is no evidence of trauma to the head, the diagnosis is often delayed. The baby's carers may misrepresent or have no knowledge of the cause of the brain injury. In milder cases

TABLE 13.1
Predictors of correct diagnosis of abusive head trauma*

Variable	Odds ratio	(95% confidence interval)
Abnormal respiratory status	7.23	(2.4–21.3)
Seizures	6.67	(2.5–17.3)
Facial/scalp injuries	4.81	(2.1–11.0)
Parents not living together	2.49	(1.1–5.7)

*Jenny et al. (1999).

of shaking, the infant may have a history of poor feeding, vomiting, lethargy or irritability occurring intermittently for days or weeks prior to the initial presentation. These symptoms are often attributed to mild viral illnesses, feeding difficulties or infantile colic.

Underdiagnosis of shaking injuries

Jenny et al. (1999) examined 173 children under 3 years old with NAHIs over a 5-year period. The diagnosis of abusive head injury was made when there was a confession of intentional injury by an adult caregiver, an inconsistent or inadequate history given by the caregiver, associated unexplained injuries, or a delay in seeking care. Fifty-four (31.2%) of the abused children had been seen by physicians at initial presentation, when the diagnosis was not recognized. The average time to correct diagnosis among these children was 7 days (range 0–189 days). Nine variables were found to be significantly associated with missing the diagnosis of abusive head trauma by univariate analysis. These were: (1) age younger than 6 months; (2) not from minority race; (3) parents living together; (4) no facial and/or scalp injury; (5) absence of seizures; (6) normal mental status; (7) normal respiratory status; (8) vomiting at first visit; (9) irritability at first visit. Of these, four independent variables predicted the correct diagnosis at the first visit (Table 13.1). Applying a logistic regression model constructed from the data, it was found that if none of the four factors were present, the probability that abusive head trauma would be recognized was less than 20%.

Reluctance on the part of clinicians to entertain a diagnosis of non-accidental injury often leads to delay. Lack of corroboration from the history makes it difficult to time the injury. The medico-legal issues are usually protracted and stressful for clinicians, who feel that they need to prove the case 'beyond reasonable doubt'. Other reasons that lead to an underdiagnosis of non-accidental injuries include a fear of 'confronting parents', a loss of doctor–patient relationship, a mistrust of other professionals, and an ignorance of child protection procedures. As a result other diagnoses are entertained: the SDH could have arisen around the time of birth, it could have been caused by minor trauma, or it could be 'idiopathic'. There is minimal scientific evidence on which to base clinical opinions on causation of SDH around the time of birth and early infancy (Salman and Crouchman 1997). There is even less evidence on which to base a diagnosis of 'idiopathic SDH' because the diagnostic criteria and incidence of idiopathic SDH are unknown, its predisposing factors are ill-defined, and its natural history remains a mystery.

TABLE 13.2

Features associated with inflicted vs accidental head injury*

- Delay in seeking medical help
- Vague or absent history/no eye witnesses
- History inconsistent with physical examination
- Younger age (<1 year)
- Previous involvement with social services
- Associated retinal haemorrhages/long bone or rib fractures
- Admission to intensive care

*DiScala et al. (2000).

Abuse or accident?

Recent media coverage of court cases with widely divergent medical opinions illustrates the dilemma of distinguishing between inflicted and accidental causes of head injury. Much of our understanding of brain injury in child abuse has come from extrapolations from research into road traffic accidents. In a study of 40 consecutive cases of severe head injury admitted to a paediatric intensive care unit, 14 were due to inflicted head trauma. In the accidental cases of head injury, the most common mechanism of injury was road traffic accidents involving passengers (6/24), cyclists (6/24), or pedestrians (4/24). Features that were associated with inflicted head injury included a history inconsistent with the physical examination, parental risk factors such as alcohol or drug abuse, previous social service intervention, and a past history of child abuse or neglect (Goldstein et al. 1993). Experience recorded over 10 years in Western Australia also confirmed the high incidence of non-accidental injury in a cohort of children less than 2 years of age presenting with subdural haematomas (Tzioumi and Oates 1998). These authors found that the commonest cause was non-accidental injury, found in 55% of cases. Important clinical features were significantly higher incidence of retinal haemorrhages with associated long bone and rib fractures in the abused children, and delay in presentation for medical attention. Another comparative analysis of 1997 children injured by abuse versus those injured accidentally (n = 16831) was reported recently from the USA. The study population included newborn infants to children of 4 years. During the 10-year study period, child abuse accounted for 10.6% of all blunt trauma to patients younger than 5 years. When compared to accidental injuries, children who were injured non-accidentally were significantly younger (12.8 vs 25.5 months) and were more likely to have a pre-injury medical history (53% vs 14.1%) and retinal haemorrhages (27.8% vs 0.06%). Non-accidental injuries included physical abuse (53%) and shaking (10.3%), while accidentally injured children were hurt mainly by falls (58.4%) and by motor vehicle accidents (37.1%). Abused children were also more likely to sustain intracranial, thoracic and abdominal injuries, and to require admission to the Intensive Care Unit (DiScala et al. 2000). Features associated with inflicted head trauma are summarized in Table 13.2. A systematic interpretation process must be applied to help in the decision whether non-accidental injury has occurred; and Kemp (2002) has proposed a series of essential baseline radiological, ophthalmological, haematological, biochemical and post-mortem investigations.

417

TABLE 13.3
Risk factors for child abuse and neglect

Child	Preterm birth/low birthweight
	Difficult temperament
	Evidence of prior abuse or neglect
	Delayed cognitive/motor development scores
Mother	Young age at birth of child
	Short birth intervals
	Lack of prenatal care
	History of previous abortion/stillbirth/child death
	Low educational attainment
	More children <6 years
	Alcohol and drug abuse
	Depression
	Lack of preparation for parenting
	Social isolation
	Separation from own mother at age 14
	Victim of physical abuse/domestic violence
	Financial/social/emotional stresses
Other	Male unemployment
	Housing difficulties

Risk factors and early indicators

For all forms of child maltreatment, various factors have been identified that are associated with an increased risk of maltreatment. Published studies have focused on the identification of children who are at high risk for abuse. It is assumed that by identifying high-risk populations the efficiency of child abuse prevention programmes will be increased. Leventhal et al. (1989) concluded that as early as the postpartum period, clinicians could identify some families who were at high risk of maltreatment and other major adverse outcomes resulting from poor parenting. Review of the children's medical records from birth until the fourth birthday showed that child abuse or neglect, non-organic failure to thrive, and changes in the child's caregiver occurred more frequently in those infants identified by clinicians at birth to be of high risk, compared to the control group. Some of the recognized risk factors are outlined in Table 13.3. Factors may relate to the child themselves, their parents' background, the home and family environment, or the wider social and cultural context.

However, most of the research strategies used to identify children at high risk for abuse have been fraught with difficulties. Risk factors are not specific for abuse, although knowledge of risk factors is important for primary prevention. The outcome is difficult to define because of the wide spectrum of child abuse and neglect. There are also problems with choice of a specific control group, clear definitions of the risk factors, and lack of information on the temporal sequence between risk factor and abuse. Detection bias can also arise because of unequal follow-up and review of the abused and non-abused children (Leventhal 1982).

Attempts have been made to predict the occurrence of abuse from identified risk factors, but such checklists lack specificity, are inaccurate, and can be potentially dangerous.

Researchers have therefore sought indicators that might enable an earlier diagnosis of maltreatment. Powell (2003) used the Delphi technique to identify physical, behavioural and developmental indicators in the child, parental factors, and a 'clustering of signs' that were thought to be early indicators of abuse and neglect. Early indicators are signs and symptoms that should alert practitioners at an early stage that the child has been subjected to maltreatment. Practitioners still require clinical acumen, experience and skills to move from a possible indication to a firm diagnosis of abuse.

In performing a thorough assessment, it is important to obtain detailed medical, social and family histories from records kept by medical and nursing staff in primary care and the community as well as in hospital. Failure to review all available information on the family may result in the diagnosis being missed or delayed, thus exposing the child and siblings to repeated abuse. Shaking of children is not usually an isolated event, and serial abuse has been reported (Alexander et al. 1990). Consideration must be given to the nature of the harm caused, the likely or possible causes, and the circumstances in which the harm occurred. The framework suggested by the Department of Health (2000) centres on an assessment triangle with three interrelated domains – the child's developmental needs, parenting capacity, and family and environmental factors. The interaction or influence of these dimensions on each other should be explored, and the results used to guide intervention and prevention strategies. At all times the welfare of the child is of paramount importance, and the assessment should concentrate on the harm that has occurred as a result of the mal-treatment. The assessment of the carers should be about the carers, with the carers, rather than against the carers. There are problems surrounding the risk assessment, however. Most risk assessment is focused on the mother, whereas men are responsible for more homicides in young children, as well as physical and sexual abuse. It is worth remembering that many single parent families are not single adult households, and risk can therefore fluctuate over time. In addition, stressful life events may increase or decrease the risk of reports of child abuse, depending on the presence of social support.

Management

When NAHI is suspected, it is best to separate the clinical care of the infant from the child protection investigation. Where the child presents acutely ill, the urgent medical needs take precedence over the child protection enquiry. However, there must not be undue delay in involving the child protection team, as siblings may be put at risk of continued abuse.

In their population-based study, Jayawant et al. (1998) found that only 22 of 33 children identified with SDH had the basic investigations of a full blood count, coagulation screen, computed tomography or magnetic resonance imaging, skeletal survey or bone scan, and ophthalmological examination (Table 13.4). Clear guidelines are now available for the clinical, laboratory and radiological management of babies in whom a diagnosis of NAHI is suspected (Kemp 2002, Jaspan et al. 2003).

A full multidisciplinary assessment should be part of the child protection enquiry, and involve joint discussions with colleagues in social work and the police. At the earliest stages of any suspicion of a shaking injury, this formal interagency discussion enables sharing of information on the child and family, as well as planning of the investigative process

TABLE 13.4
Mandatory investigations in cases of subdural haemorrhage in infants*

- Full multidisciplinary assessment of child and family
- Full paediatric case history with documentation of all possible explanations for injury
- Social background and police information
- Thorough clinical examination with documentation and clinical photographs of all injuries
- Ophthalmological examination of both eyes through dilated pupils, by ophthalmologist
- Radiological assessment by CT or MRI of head, repeat at 7–14 days
- Full blood count, repeat over first 24–48 hours
- Coagulation screen
- Biochemistry – urea and electrolytes, liver function tests
- Infection screen
- Skeletal survey supplemented with a bone scan, or repeat skeletal survey at 10–14 days

---

*Kemp (2002).

(Scottish Executive 1998, Department of Health 2003). The initial referral discussion/strategy meeting must take place as soon as there is a suspicion of maltreatment being the cause of the SDH. This is important so that a thorough investigation can be conducted before the issues become clouded by time and comparison of explanations by caregivers. Prompt notification also allows the police to explore the probable scene of the injury and elicit information from the caregiver before any defensive reactions have developed. A risk assessment must be done on the siblings or other children within the household, to ensure their current and future safety (Department of Health 2000).

The clinical team should include a paediatrician who can resuscitate and stabilize the baby while investigations and diagnostic radiological studies are being done. Specialists in paediatric radiology, neurology, neurosurgery and ophthalmology as well as the lead clinician in child abuse should form the diagnostic team. The paediatrician who works with the child protection team is responsible for taking a broad but detailed history from the caregivers. Information regarding symptom onset, as well as the chain of caregivers, needs to be quickly passed on to the police. The principal aims of a full clinical assessment are to: (1) establish the need for immediate treatment; (2) provide a comprehensive assessment of the injuries; (3) provide information that might support the suspicion as well as, in due course, sustain criminal proceedings and care plans; (4) plan any ongoing health care.

In keeping with the recommendations from the Cleveland Inquiry in the UK (Butler-Sloss 1988), a list of approved doctors who have experience and knowledge in the needs of children who might have been abused should be drawn up in each area. Each health authority should commission a comprehensive child protection service where a lead clinician is identified to ensure that there are appropriate guidelines and procedures in place, and that all staff are aware of and adhere to these (Scottish Executive Health Department 2000, Department of Health 2003).

The joint paediatric–forensic examination is intended to encompass within a single examination the child's need for medical care and the need to obtain and document fully any forensic evidence (Mok et al. 1998). The lead paediatrician in child protection, together with the forensic medical examiner (police surgeon) should undertake the joint paediatric–

forensic examination, drawing on the paediatrician's expertise in the assessment of the child's development and his/her general physical health, while the police surgeon assists with the description and interpretation of any injuries found in terms of their possible causation and whether the cause was likely to be accidental or non-accidental. The police surgeon would also collect appropriately any samples that might be useful for forensic laboratory analysis. As far as possible the police should take any photographs of physical injuries, with both doctors present. The paediatrician and police surgeon should document and describe any injuries seen, and postulate a cause as to how they might have happened with rough estimates of when the injuries might have occurred. The expert opinion of experienced paediatric radiologists is always essential when dating the ages of bony injuries or SDHs (Jaspan et al. 2003). While it may be feasible to postulate likely risk factors that might have predisposed to the injury, doctors should never attempt to identify the culpable person. This is best left to police investigations and for the jury to decide.

Social work investigations will be helped by participants at an interagency meeting (case conference), which should be attended by senior clinicians directly involved with the child and family. One of the functions of the case conference is to decide whether to place the child's name on the Child Protection Register, and whether it is in the child's best interest to return him/her to the carers. Discharge from hospital should be carefully planned and coordinated, again with the medical needs separate from the child protection issues. There may or may not be criminal proceedings arising from the police investigations, but civil proceedings should always follow, looking at the welfare of the child. Figure 13.1 outlines the child protection investigations in cases of NAHI.

Costs of child abuse
Apart from the morbidity and mortality caused by NAHIs, child abuse is costly in its effects on the family and its financial consequences. In the United Kingdom, the estimated direct cost was £735 million per annum, incurred by personal social services for the children and families involved, Home Office services (courts, probation, police and prisons), and health services. Indirect costs are more difficult to estimate, and range from delinquency to mental health services and marriage guidance counselling. Impossible to measure are costs incurred by dysfunctional adults damaged by abuse in childhood, and the cost to individuals and society brought about by people unable to function to their full potential in the education system, at work or in their personal relationships, including their relationships with their own children (National Commission of Inquiry into the Prevention of Child Abuse 1996).

Prevention
Child abuse is one of the most complex areas of paediatrics and child health, and a major public health problem. Most efforts, both at a local and a national level, tend to focus on responding to the abuse once it has occurred, rather than preventing it happening. The National Commission of Enquiry into the Prevention of Child Abuse (1996) recognized that most forms of child abuse are preventable, and the responsibility for this has to be accepted by all sectors of society, from the national government to individuals. The Commission acknowledged that narrow technical definitions of child abuse did not provide an adequate

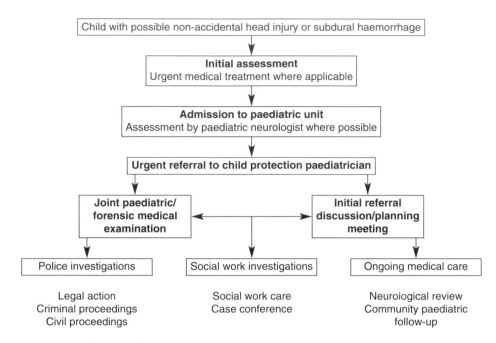

Fig. 13.1. Child protection investigations in non-accidental head injury.

framework within which to develop effective prevention strategies. Therefore a broader definition was adopted, where child abuse was defined as "anything which individuals, institutions, or processes do or fail to do which directly or indirectly harms children or damages their prospects of safe and healthy development into adulthood."

PRIMARY PREVENTION

The most effective primary prevention is the active promotion of the well-being of all children, coupled with a refusal by society as a whole to tolerate conditions and systems known to harm them. The Scottish Child Protection Audit and Review (Scottish Executive 2002) found that many children experience serious levels of hurt and harm. They live in conditions and under threats that should not be tolerated in a civilized society. Many adults and children have little confidence in the child protection system and are reluctant to report concerns about child abuse and neglect. Among its recommendations was the promotion of positive childhood initiatives that focus on every child's right to life, health, decency, and development. Strategies should include discouraging corporal punishment of children as well as other forms of violence, making health care more accessible to all children, and education of young people for parenthood. Parenting skills can be taught in local community centres or clinics, or in schools as part of the Personal and Social Development programme, and should include an overview of normal developmental expectations of children, positive parenting techniques, acquisition of social skills and problem solving, as well as management of anger and conflict.

422

Dukewich et al. (1996) examined maternal and child factors that placed young mothers at risk of abusing their children. The strongest direct predictor of abuse potential in the young mothers was lack of preparation for parenting, which included knowledge and attitudes about children's development. However, its effects could be partially mediated by the mother's psychological predisposition for coping under stress.

SECONDARY PREVENTION

Secondary prevention strategies aim to identify early indicators for child abuse, so that appropriate interventions can be offered. Community nursing services such as health visiting could be used to prevent child abuse at both a primary and secondary level. However, the success reported by these programmes is variable. Browne (1995) reviewed the role of health visitors in the prevention of child abuse and neglect, and concluded that accurate prediction of high-risk families required more than one screening procedure, to reduce the number of false positives. Few health visitor interventions were deemed to be successful, indicating that greater support and training was required for community nurses if they were to be used to prevent child abuse and neglect. More recently, a systematic review and meta-analysis was performed to evaluate the effectiveness of home visiting programmes on parenting and quality of the home environment. Relevant outcomes were reported in 34 studies, with 17 using the Home Observation or Measurement of the Environment (HOME) scores, 27 reporting other measures of parenting, and 10 reporting both types of outcomes. Twelve studies were entered into the meta-analysis, which showed a significant effect of home visiting programmes on the quality of the home environment as measured by the HOME score. Other positive parenting outcomes reported were better interaction between mother and child; lower rates of reported difficulties in the mother–infant relationship; greater positive feedback and more praise of the child; improved parental handling of aggressive behaviour in their child; and appropriate parental developmental expectations of the child (Kendrick et al. 2000).

The majority of studies used professional home visitors, mainly community nurses, but teachers, social workers and lay workers could also be used. However, the follow-up periods in the studies varied, with shorter studies (follow up periods of less than 2 years) showing a greater treatment effect compared to those with follow-up periods of greater than 2 years. It is therefore likely that the effect of home visiting on the quality of the home environment reduces over time.

INCREASING PUBLIC AWARENESS

Interventions aimed at improving parenting can only be part of a wider preventive child health strategy. Other recommendations highlighted in the National Commission of Inquiry into the Prevention of Child Abuse (1996) included the need to improve statistical information on the state of Britain's children. It also stressed changes in legislation, so that children should receive the same protection as adults, which would mean removing from the statute book the defence of 'reasonable chastisement'. In the United Kingdom, heated debate continues as to whether shaking children, blows to the head, and the physical punishment of very young children should be made unlawful. Children should not be seen as possessions, but as individuals with rights and developing responsibilities. It must therefore be recognized that child protection is everyone's responsibility, and that greater public awareness and involvement are essential.

At local, national and international levels, public awareness has been raised by campaigns that underline the dangers of shaking a baby. Previous studies show that between 25% and 50% of adults and adolescents do not recognize the dangers of shaking a baby. A 'Don't Shake the Baby' project was conducted in one county of Ohio, USA, targeting 15,708 parents of newborn babies (Showers 1992). The primary goal was to inform parents about the dangers of shaking, with the secondary objective of providing positive ways of coping with the crying infant. Twenty-one percent of the parents returned a response postcard in the educational package, with three-quarters stating that they found the information useful. Approximately half indicated that subsequent to reading the material, they were less likely to shake their babies. In the London Borough of Newham, the Area Child Protection Committee carried out research to provide information for their 'Don't Shake the Baby' publicity campaign. The aims of the research were to ascertain the levels of awareness of the dangers of shaking babies, and to investigate the extent to which parents and carers had felt like shaking or had shaken their babies. The participants who were interviewed included 83 mothers, 56 fathers, and 152 secondary school students. Of the mothers interviewed, half were not fully aware of the dangers of shaking, 10% admitted to shaking their babies, and 25% had felt like shaking their baby. The researchers found great difficulties in getting men to complete the questionnaire. Forty-six of 50 fathers were aware of the dangers of shaking babies, while 17 of 31 had felt like shaking the baby and one admitted to having done so. Of the school students surveyed, 67% of girls and 39% of boys were fully aware of the dangers of shaking. Of the respondents who had felt like shaking or who had actually shaken their baby, the majority identified crying to be a particular problem (Sampson and Shepherd 1996).

Given the relationship between a lack of awareness of the dangers of shaking and actually shaking a baby, an important part of a prevention strategy would be a publicity campaign, targeting women, men and young people of all social and ethnic groups. Public ignorance about the dangers of shaking a baby might have been added to by outdated professional advice to 'shake' babies who were found apparently apnoeic. There may also be a belief that, when punishing children, 'a shake is better than a smack'. Particular efforts are needed to target fathers who generally do not attend baby clinics or parent and toddler groups. It is not known which medium (leaflets, posters, videos, or television campaigns) is most effective at public education, but all should list local and national help lines and community organizations that can provide support for parents. Literature should also be available in ethnic minority languages, and for those with poor literacy skills.

Conclusion

The major trigger factor for shaking is incessant crying. Therefore clinicians should try to identify and treat the cause of the baby's persistent crying. Professionals dealing with children, such as those in health, education and early years' services, often miss or respond inadequately to signs of abuse. Among health professionals, there must be a greater awareness of the varied presentations of a shaking injury, and less reluctance to make a diagnosis, followed by prompt referral to the multi-agency team for a child protection investigation.

Current interagency arrangements for protecting children depend on good working relationships between key agencies in health, the police and social services. Critical to the success of child protection are strong leadership and effective management structures to improve supervision, coordination and accountability. Unfortunately, deficiencies exist in the system, as highlighted in the Scottish Child Protection Audit and Review (Scottish Executive 2002). This multi-agency audit found that despite state intervention, about two-thirds of children were either not protected or only partially protected, or their needs were not fully met. Children and their families did not always get the help they needed when they needed it. There was duplication of effort by the agencies, and energies were directed at meeting system requirements rather than the needs of the child. In his inquiry into the death of Victoria Climbié, Lord Laming (2003) also emphasized the importance of better education, training, and quality monitoring of front-line staff who do this work.

At a primary prevention level, the long-term strategy should be improved education of all young people on the vulnerability of babies, normal developmental expectations, and parenting skills, before they embark on parenthood. Support groups for parents of children who have survived shaking injuries have been active in promoting prevention programmes. At a public and professional level, conferences on shaken baby syndrome help to raise awareness of the problem; to develop multidisciplinary strategies and guidelines on working together; and perhaps, by raising political awareness, foster the development of a national strategy to prevent shaking injuries to infants. Although there is an increasing awareness of the dangers of shaking babies, there remains a need to develop the most effective medium for public education and preventive work. More work is also needed to identify the gaps in service provision and the needs of vulnerable young parents. Further research must be done to define the clinical presentations, diagnostic criteria, incidence and natural history of 'idiopathic subdural haemorrhages', especially in infants who present clinically well with increasing head circumference.

REFERENCES

Alexander R, Crabbe L, Sato Y, Smith W, Bennett T (1990) Serial abuse in children who are shaken. *Am J Dis Child* **144**: 58–60.

Barlow KM, Milne S, Aitken K, Minns RA (1998) A retrospective epidemiological analysis of non-accidental head injury in children in Scotland over a 15 year period. *Scott Med J* **43**: 112–114.

Browne K (1995) Preventing child maltreatment through community nursing. *J Adv Nurs* **21**: 57–63.

Butler-Sloss E (1988) *Report of the Inquiry into Child Abuse in Cleveland 1987*. London: HMSO.

Department of Health (2000) *Framework for the Assessment of Children in Need and their Families*. London: Department of Health.

Department of Health (2003) *What to Do if You're Worried a Child Is Being Abused – full report*. London: Department of Health.

DiScala C, Sege R, Guohua L, Reece RM (2000) Child abuse and unintentional injuries. A 10 year retrospective. *Arch Pediatr Adolesc Med* **154**: 16–22.

Dukewich TL, Borkowski JG, Whitman TL (1996) Adolescent mothers and child abuse potential; an evaluation of risk factors. *Child Abuse Negl* **20**: 1031–1047.

Goldstein B, Kelly MM, Bruton D, Cox C (1993) Inflicted versus accidental head injury in critically injured children. *Crit Care Med* **21**: 1328–1332.

Jaspan T, Griffiths PD, McConachie NS, Punt JAG (2003) Neuroimaging for non-accidental head injury in childhood: a proposed protocol. *Clin Radiol* **58**: 44–53.

Jayawant S, Rawlinson A, Gibbon F, Price J, Schulte J, Sharples P, Sibert JR, Kemp AM (1998) Subdural haemorrhages in infants: population based study. *BMJ* **317**: 1558–1561.

Jenny C, Hymel Lt Col KP, Ritzen A, Reinert SE, Hay TC (1999) Analysis of missed cases of abusive head trauma. *JAMA* **281**: 621–626.

Kemp AM (2002) Investigating subdural haemorrhage in infants. *Arch Dis Child* **86**: 98–102.

Kendrick D, Elkan R, Hewitt M, Dewey M, Blair M, Robinson J, Williams D, Brummell K (2000) Does home visiting improve parenting and the quality of the home environment? A systematic review and meta-analysis. *Arch Dis Child* **82**: 443–451.

Lord Laming (2003) *Inquiry into the Death of Victoria Climbié*. London: HMSO (online: www.victoria-climbie-inquiry.org.uk).

Leventhal JM (1982) Research strategies and methodologic standards in studies risk factors for child abuse. *Child Abuse Negl* **6**: 113–123.

Leventhal JM, Garber RB, Brady CA (1989) Identification during the postpartum period of infants who are at high risk of child maltreatment. *J Pediatr* **114**: 481–487.

Mok JYQ, Busuttil A, Hammond HF (1998) The joint paediatric–forensic examination in child abuse. *Child Abuse Rev* **7**: 194–203.

National Commission of Inquiry into the Prevention of Child Abuse (1996) *Childhood Matters*. London: HMSO.

Powell C (2003) Early indicators of child abuse and neglect: a multi-professional Delphi study. *Child Abuse Rev* **12**: 25–40.

Salman M, Crouchman M (1997) What can cause subdural haemorrhage in a term neonate? *Paediatrics Today* **5**: 42–45.

Sampson A, Shepherd J (1996) *Newham ACPC Don't Shake the Baby Campaign. A Report and Recommendations for the London Borough of Newham. Commentary Series No. 53*. London: University of East London Centre for Institutional Studies.

Scottish Executive (1998) *Protecting Children – A Shared Responsibility: Guidance on Inter-Agency Cooperation*. Edinburgh: HMSO.

Scottish Executive (2002) *It's Everyone's Job to Make Sure I'm Alright. Report of the Child Protection Audit and Review*. Edinburgh: HMSO.

Scottish Executive Health Department (2000) *Protecting Children – A Shared Responsibility: Guidance for Health Professionals in Scotland*. Edinburgh: HMSO.

Showers J (1992) 'Don't Shake the Baby': the effectiveness of a prevention campaign. *Child Abuse Negl* **16**: 11–18.

Tzioumi D, Oates RK (1998) Subdural hematomas in children under 2 years. Accidental or inflicted? A 10 year experience. *Child Abuse Negl* **22**: 1105–1112.

14
SHAKEN BABY SYNDROME AND POLICE PROCEDURE

Philip Wheeler

This chapter is based on my experiences in recent years of dealing with cases of shaken baby syndrome (SBS) and advising police officers on how to investigate them. I have not attempted to universalize the language or the procedures of the UK police forces. However, I am very aware of many cases of child abuse reported from countries other than the UK. In spite of some procedural differences, the sort of information a police officer needs to collect is essentially the same wherever the case may have taken place. I have also included some health and medical information, so that the reader may understand the extent to which they can expect a police officer to be aware of medical issues. As a result of the training of police officers, the Home Office Report on SBS (Wheeler 2002), and other articles and training events, police officers in the UK are much more aware now of the medical issues involved in these investigations.

There are few police forces in Great Britain that have not had to deal with cases of SBS resulting in the death or serious injury to a child in the last 10 years. Indeed, some forces have dealt with many cases. Until recently though, there was no real collective wisdom among the police services of this country as to how these cases should be managed and investigated.

Assessing numbers of cases

It is difficult to give accurate figures for the number of cases investigated by police in the United Kingdom. Between 2000 and 2003, advice was given to officers in the UK and abroad on 100 cases to as many as six forces in one week, as a result of the National Crime Faculty referral system.

Police forces in the UK record these cases in differing ways. Some show them as grievous bodily harm, assault to the head, infanticide, murder, or manslaughter. This makes a detailed knowledge of numbers of cases involving shaking very difficult to assess.

One police force in the south of England collated their figures for crimes of this type in late 2002. Their survey showed that between September 1999 and October 2002 there were 21 reported crimes where a baby had been shaken, causing serious injury. Of these, three were classed as murder, a further seven were being dealt with as serious assaults where the baby survived, and another was classified as manslaughter. Other cases were ongoing at the time with no investigative result.

The lack of knowledge of numbers of cases in the field of medicine is no different. There are no records available that a researcher could access in order to tell them the number of cases being dealt with in any one year by hospitals in the UK. A similar story pertains in the coroners' courts. Accurate recording of figures by all agencies was in fact one of the recommendations in the Home Office Report in 2002.

The best projection of numbers of SBS cases within the population comes from studies in the late 1990s in Scotland and Wales and from the UK study carried out by Hobbs (2003). The Barlow and Minns study in Scotland in 2000 showed that the incidence of SBS cases was 24.6 per 100,000 children under 1 year of age (Barlow and Minns 2000). The incidence of subdural haematoma in children under 2 years in Wales during 1993–1995 was 10.13 per 100,000 children, but by 1997 had risen to 12.45 per 100,000 (Kemp and Price 1998).

In a UK and Republic of Ireland study in 1998 to 1999, the annual incidence of subdural haematoma in babies was 12.54 per 100,000 infants aged between 0 and 2 years of age. For infants between 0 and 1 year of age the incidence was found to be 24.1 per 100,000 births (Hobbs 2003). For such large studies these are remarkably similar findings.

The recording of numbers of cases of SBS, shaken impact syndrome, abusive head trauma, non-accidental head injury or whatever nomenclature is chosen, needs to be addressed by all agencies in the future.

What happens in SBS
The reason that police forces become involved in SBS investigations is that shaking a baby or infant until serious injury or death results is a serious form of child abuse. SBS is therefore a medical diagnosis but also a criminal act worthy of police investigation. The most frequent triggering event for babies to be shaken is accepted to be the inconsolable crying of an infant. However, there have been other triggers, e.g. food refusal or the inability of a carer to get on with a task because of a crying baby, and even the act of a baby spitting out a dummy have been triggers to severe and violent assaults on babies in the past, both here and in other parts of the world.

The child is sometimes gripped under the armpits in the classic shaken baby grip as the baby's head flails backwards and forwards, the chin often hitting the baby's chest. The head not only flails from front to back but also from side to side as the child is violently shaken. Often, the baby is gripped by a limb and there are cases where the child has been swung around the head of the abuser by a leg. The result of this violent shaking makes the baby's head move forcibly backwards and forwards. This in turn causes shearing of the blood vessels within the brain itself. The shearing of the vessels causes subdural or subarachnoid bleeding, which is the collection of blood visible when the skull is opened at post-mortem examination.

The constellation of injuries occurring is very stereotyped and is now universally recognized by physicians (Wheeler 2001). They are: (1) retinal haemorrhages (bleeding in the layer at the back of the eye); (2) subdural and/or subarachnoid haemorrhages (bleeding in the membranes that cover the brain); and (3) cerebral oedema (or swelling of the brain).

Other signs associated with shaken baby injuries are:
- skull fractures, often resulting from the impact when a child is thrown or hit against a hard surface
- fractures of the posterior arches of the ribs near the spine due to the manner in which the abuser grips the baby

- fractures of the clavicles (the collarbones)
- fractures of the long bones due to gripping or twisting actions
- bruising to the skin, head, face and body.

It is extremely important that the investigator becomes familiar with the medical issues in shaken baby cases. Although medical language is complex and unfamiliar to police officers, it must be a prerequisite to working on a case that investigating officers make themselves acquainted with the injuries involved in shaking a baby to death or injury. This applies equally to magistrates, legal counsel and the judiciary. Without such knowledge it is difficult for the investigating officer to know where to find and make the best use of expert opinion on the medical aspects of the case.

A member of the Attorney General's staff in Utah, USA sums this up: "Successful prosecution of a shaken baby case demands that the prosecutor learn the medical dynamics of the syndrome and understands the significance of the collection of injuries most often associated with shaking cases" (Parrish 2001).

Police officers charged with investigating these cases should be in no doubt about the violent nature of the injuries that the child has endured. The American Academy of Paediatrics (2001) states: "The act of shaking, leading to shaken baby syndrome is so violent that individuals observing it would recognize it as dangerous and likely to kill the child. Shaken baby syndrome injuries are the result of violent trauma. The constellation of these injuries does not occur with short falls, seizures or as a consequence of vaccination. Shaking by itself may cause fatal or serious injuries."

Definition and terminology

In the 19th century, a French pathologist named Tardieu was writing about his findings of cases of babies where blood was found on the surface of the brain at autopsy. These were possibly the first recorded findings of subdural haematoma in infants (Tardieu 1860).

In the USA in the 1940s, Caffey noticed babies being brought to his radiology department with chips from the bones associated with subdural haematomas. He coined the term 'whiplash shaken baby syndrome' in two fascinating articles in the early 1970s (Caffey 1972, 1974).

At the same time in England, Dr Norman Guthkelch wrote in the *British Medical Journal* about cases of shaken baby injuries at Hull Royal Infirmary (Guthkelch 1971).

More recently, Reece and Kirschner from Massachusetts and Chicago University Hospitals expanded the definition of SBS. They stated, "The terms 'shaken baby syndrome (SBS)' or 'shaken impact syndrome (SIS)' refer to the signs and symptoms, as well as the clinical, radiographic, and sometimes autopsy findings resulting from violent shaking of an infant or young child. SBS /SIS are often used interchangeably and are synonymous with other descriptive items used in the earlier scientific literature, such as 'whiplash shaken baby syndrome' and 'shake/slam syndrome'" (Reece and Kirschner 1998).

Current research is centred around (1) whether impact (including soft impact) is necessary (Duhaime 1987); (2) correlation of the pathology seen at autopsy in a minority of cases with the clinical and imaging studies of the majority; and (3) studies on the long-term follow-up.

The complex medical terminology used by doctors is a problem for both police and jurors alike. The investigating officer can improve this situation a little by ensuring that officers taking statements have a glossary of medical terms. This can also be produced for the jury to help them to follow the evidence given.

Assessing the evidence
The central aim of any investigation is to establish whether the child has been injured or died as a result of shaken baby injuries and not other causes.

Survey after survey in the USA and latterly in Great Britain have pointed to the male caregiver as being the main perpetrator of this crime. It might be easy to take the view that male figures in the baby's life should be the foremost suspects in a case of SBS. However, that would lead us to miss the detailed investigation needed to assess significant others in the baby's life, such as female babysitters, carers and other relatives. The watchword for the investigators is to be open-minded in establishing the suspect. Equally, it needs to be assessed whether there was one perpetrator or more than one, though the latter scenario is indeed rare.

The investigator must also be aware of the temptation to assume that this incident is an isolated moment of madness on the part of whoever has injured the child. This may or may not be so. If not, this leaves the child (or siblings) vulnerable to future injury. There is a natural tendency for the team, in their efforts to be empathetic and sympathetic to the bereaved parent, to believe the initial story given.

If one adds to this the many other problems of taking an SBS case through to court (see Chapter 15), then it can be seen that only the most detailed of investigations will suffice.

The most difficult issue to deal with for the investigator is probably that of timing the injuries. It would be extremely easy were police officers able to ask a doctor to give the exact time that the baby was injured. Sadly, this is not yet possible in medical science.

What doctors can say is the condition the child was in after receiving the injuries. This in itself may help the case but only as part of a full and thorough investigation citing all the other circumstances and timings around the injury.

Starling et al. (1995) showed that 36 of 37 perpetrators who later confessed to shaking their children were the same persons who identified the initial symptoms. Video reconstruction of the circumstances leading up to the injury is extremely useful. The investigator should be prepared to be innovative and ask the suspect to take part in a video reconstruction.

The failure to collaborate between disciplines is a major problem in shaken baby investigations. When child protection teams undertake the investigation the procedure is clearly laid down. A referral is made, often from the hospital social services team, and a strategy meeting is held. This will involve the professionals who have dealt with the case thus far, including health visitors, doctors, casualty doctors, police and social services.

All of these have an important role to play in getting any investigation off to a good start. Unfortunately many investigations into SBS cases are not done by child protection detectives brought up in this discipline. There have been many examples within the UK in recent years where the investigation has started without a strategy meeting taking place.

It is also clear that the lack of training in investigating these cases has been a problem for police in the past. The lack of Crown Prosecution Service (CPS) specialist lawyers to agree to take these difficult cases forward has been another factor in cases being dropped before court. The dearth of relevant experts in the field is one more problem for the police investigator to overcome.

EARLY INVESTIGATION

The investigating officer needs to be aware of the *Investigator's Guide to Shaken Baby Syndrome* (Wheeler 2002). They should ensure that the lessons learned by other police forces are used to good effect in their case. The investigator should also realize that this case is not unique and they can obtain advice from other experts and comparative cases.

In this regard the investigators will have to be aware that there are others investigating similar cases across the country, or who have expertise in doing so recently. There is also a register of 'experts' for investigators to call upon kept at the National Crime and Operations Faculty, based at the Police Staff College in Bramshill, Hampshire, England. All of this is standard and well-known procedure for the trained police investigator. These days it goes by the grandiose title of 'comparative case analysis'.

One of the keys to a successful investigation of this kind is to realize from the start that it is going to be multidisciplinary in nature. Police officers cannot hope to investigate the case without the cooperation of their colleagues in other agencies. They should also understand that by using the skills and knowledge of the professional childcare network they will save themselves an inordinate amount of time. Professionals working in hospitals will know where to locate files, who to speak with about medical investigations and how to help with other enquiries. The support of people working in these areas is invaluable.

COLLABORATING WITH MEDICAL PROFESSIONALS

By using the hospital social services as a conduit to doctors and nurses much time can be saved in locating health staff and arranging statement times. The same can be said of locating records and other hospital-based evidence. Police access to records is straightforward in cases where the child has died but can be more complex when the child has survived. The social services team is a key player in the initial investigation as a whole, and in terms of getting access to medical records. It often happens that cases are transferred from one hospital to another because of bed space or better equipment and expertise. In this case it is important to use the social workers from both hospitals as a conduit for information.

It is essential to realize from the outset that the case will revolve to a great extent around medical professionals, their actions and observations, and their expert testimony. There are rarely witnesses to a shaking event. It is also important to acknowledge that although it was a few seconds of injury to a child, it will necessitate taking statements from many people. In the 'Australian nanny' case in 1999, no less than 236 statements were taken and eventually over 100 witnesses were prepared to give evidence had the case gone to full trial. A total of 56 of these were medical professionals. The case went to the Old Bailey after nanny Louise Sullivan shook a baby in her care to death. She pleaded guilty to involuntary manslaughter.

The importance of knowing the medical issues behind the birth of a child as well as its early developmental stages is illustrated by questions regarding birth trauma or complications. It is recognized that some children can have retinal haemorrhages as a result of birth trauma. However, these haemorrhages will disappear within a short time after the birth. As retinal haemorrhages are an important diagnostic pointer in SBS, it is important to establish whether or not they were caused by birth trauma. This is another reason for investigators to be aware and up to date with new medical research into such issues.

The younger the child, for example up to 5 or 6 weeks of age, the more important it is for the consultant ophthalmologist to tell the investigator whether any haemorrhages were the result of birth trauma or not. After this period any retinal haemorrhages are probably not the result of birth trauma but should still be covered in statements in case it is put forward by the defence at a later stage. The investigator should be using information from medical professionals that relates to the period from the baby's birth to the time of the shaking incident to investigate the full circumstances behind the incident.

At this early stage the birth records of the child have to be obtained, along with any health visitor records kept by the local clinic. The birth records will help to show whether the baby was injected with a vitamin K supplement at birth (given to prevent failure of clotting of the blood). Failure to administer this is a frequent defence and it should be established whether the midwife did actually administer the medication at birth. As the child is likely to be very young, it should not be difficult to trace the midwife who was present at the birth.

The issue of children being injured by vaccinations they receive is a common defence put forward by lawyers on behalf of their clients. There are many professionals giving evidence, rightly or wrongly, about vaccination damage to children in courts in the USA at present.

LOOKING FOR MOTIVE

The investigator should look for motives at the earliest opportunity. There are many potential motives for abuse in the shaken baby case. It is extremely important that the investigator should be aware of these in their investigative strategies. Uncontrollable crying is the single most common reason for babies being shaken.

The shaking is often carried out because it thwarts the perpetrators' activities. There are several examples of cases where inability of the carer to watch television or play computer games because of a crying baby have been the trigger for the abuse. Figure 14.1 is a somewhat simplified model of 'causality' in SBS cases but it is a useful one for the investigator to bear in mind.

There are many motives for the abuse to consider, including:
• the medical or physical condition of the child may cause frustration for the caregiver

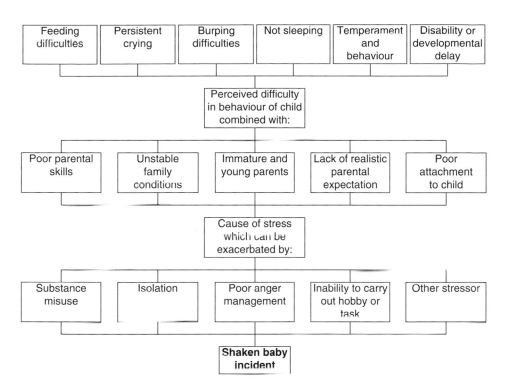

Fig. 14.1. Possible risk and motive factors in the shaken baby syndrome case.

- childcare responsibilities interfering with the caregiver's work or recreation (TV programme, video game, favourite video). All have featured in SBS cases as motives for the abuse
- a triggering event provoking anger and frustration, e.g. soiling nappies, crying, inability to feed, vomiting
- alcohol or drug misuse by the parent(s)
- lack of parental experience (child's first weekend away with an estranged father)
- problems with the domestic relationship, e.g. an unwanted pregnancy
- lack of attachment to the child on the part of one or both of the parents
- financial difficulties and other causes of stress such as problems at work or lack of sleep
- the offender deliberately tortures or abuses the child as part of their antisocial and sadistic nature. Although applicable to a minority of SBS cases, it has been true in some. The possibility of a final SBS incident being part of a pattern of abuse should not be ruled out and should be investigated accordingly.

Some of these factors may well come as a surprise to experienced detectives, but the investigating team must be aware of them. This is especially so of any detective sent to examine the scene. If an examiner is not aware that they should look for evidence of motive, it will often not be considered. Motive must be analysed when examining the scene of an alleged shaken baby case.

SCENE EXAMINATION

One of the most common mistakes made by investigators in shaken baby cases is to assume that because it is a shaken baby case there is no scene to examine. This is very far from the truth. In fact there will be several scenes to consider, all of which will require as meticulous an examination as other scenes of serious crimes.

The following are the main points to consider in examining the SBS scene. Several are common to the usual crime scene but some may not be apparent to the individual investigator working alone. Some of the actions may well be overlooked because investigators do not see the relevance or need to carry out the procedure.

An example of this is the telephone records of the house or the mobile phone records of the suspect where the child has become symptomatic. The seizing of these records is routine in major investigations. However, it would be interesting to discover how many times phone records are currently examined in SBS cases.

The records will tell you many things and deserve careful analysis. For example, this type of evidence was given at the Louise Woodward trial (*Commonwealth* v *Woodward* 1998) in which a young British woman was convicted of the involuntary manslaughter of the child for whom she was caring. Evidence was given of a friend phoning her during the day and being able to hear the baby, Matthew, gurgling and playing away happily in the background, thus indicating that the child was well until a particular point in the day at least.

In one case in London in 2002, the grandmother of the child routinely phoned at lunchtime to say hello and coo down the phone at her new grandchild and did so on the day that the child was injured. This helped to show that the child was reacting in a normal way up to that time. The father of the baby was convicted of grievous bodily harm. In another London case the perpetrator telephoned several people after the shaking to explain what had happened. When collated, there were several similar but different explanations given by phone to friends and relatives, all of whom were seen by the investigators. In this last case (*R* v *Dafonte* 2001) the father was initially tried for grievous bodily harm and then for murder as the child died some few months later. Investigators should be aware that they must look at these cases with an eye to the fact that the baby could well die some weeks or months down the line.

Telephone evidence may be useful in refuting stories put forward to explain injuries.

Key steps in an SBS investigation

Many of the suggestions below are routine and normal parts of any murder enquiry. However, because the relevance of the action is often not seen by investigators in the SBS case they are not carried out. Due to the fact that the case is often run by a single detective sergeant with a detective constable there are often not enough personnel to do many of the things suggested here and some get forgotten, at the expense of the case. This is to be regretted and surely points to the need to have a full team working on the case at the outset. This can be scaled down when much of the early work is completed. The following represents a 'checklist' of investigative tasks.

• In many cases of SBS the initial referral will come from the hospital. Therefore speedy access may be needed to several scenes to prevent tampering or reconstruction. The main scene will be the one where the child becomes symptomatic. Remember that this can be confused in childminder cases where a childminder was caring for the child and the parents have taken the child home, unaware of any previous injuries due to the child supposedly being 'asleep' when collected.

- The baby will require thorough examination and for the results of that examination to be documented.
- Examine original clothing, look in the laundry basket or other areas for washing storage to find vomit or blood-stained clothing that may have been taken off. There have been several examples of carers changing the baby's clothes prior to hospital attendance because of dirty clothing caused by the incident.
- Be aware of discarded nappies and any blood in the stools. This may indicate internal injury. Has the nappy been changed regularly during the day, indicating that the child has been well tended by the carer?
- The child should be photographed as soon as possible and then other photographs taken a few days later. Consultation with the ophthalmic pathologist will be useful in cases where the child dies so that they can achieve the best photographic evidence.
- All bruises, marks, etc. should be body charted prior to the post-mortem examination.
- The hospital should be asked to ensure that the child is scanned using magnetic resonance imaging and computed tomography unless doctors advise against moving the child. A full skeletal survey should also be obtained.
- Where the hospital has a 'retcam' (a machine to examine and photograph children's retinas), ensure that the photographs are made available. Also ensure that all notes and diagrams made by doctors are obtained. These can often be overlooked. Doctors may sometimes have taken their own photographs for their notes or for later presentation in training or for other reasons. Always be sure to ask if this is the case.
- At the domestic scene look for motive evidence, i.e. what the carer would have been doing at the time, whether there are soiled and discarded nappies, whether there are half-full feeding bottles or spills of milk or vomit on or near where the child is normally fed or in the cot. Look for any items indicating special medical needs for the baby.
- Look for evidence of a normal routine being carried on in that particular day. At one scene the pillows had been moved to safeguard the child from falling from the bed. In the morning the caregiver would take the baby back to bed with her after the parents had left. This indicated that the baby was well after the parents had left for work. At another scene milk was found on worktops indicating that a feed had been attempted by the carer, thus indicating wellness at that time and a possible motive for the shaking incident. Feeding problems can lead to frustration with a baby and have also been the motive for shaking incidents to occur.
- There may be medication at the scene that the child or the carer is taking. This should be removed and analysed as in any other routine investigation.
- Always assess the house for evidence of child safety and any neglect issues. This is particularly important if there is another child in the house. The well-being of the other children of the family will be another consideration for the strategy meeting, and a

decision would have to be taken as to whether to remove the other child or children from possible harm.

- Searches should include rooms and any vehicles (e.g. cars, prams) where the baby is kept.
- Photographs of all scenes should be taken in the normal way. Video footage should also be taken of the house and the baby's equipment, such as the cot, high chair, changing table or other place used to change the baby's nappy. Any bathing equipment, including the bath, should also be imaged. A common story given by carers to explain away injuries is that the child slipped in the bath while being washed.
- Diagrams should be made of positions of baby equipment such as cots, changing tables and any other paraphernalia. Measurements of the heights of chairs, couches, beds and other furniture should be taken. One of the most common stories given for injuries is that the child had rolled from a bed or a couch. This needs to be tested by reference to medical experts who will be able to give their opinions on whether this could have caused the injuries. (The consensus among experts is that short falls do not cause the type and severity of injuries seen in the shaken baby episode).
- Examine, photograph and take samples of floor coverings, especially around areas such as the cot or changing table. It may be that a week into the case one or other of the carers will 'remember' that 2 weeks ago there was a fall incident from the changing table and use that as an excuse for the injuries.
- Look for trace evidence near where the child might routinely be laid. If there is a shake and a slam on to a hard surface then the baby will be slammed near to where they are usually placed. A carer who does not have a very strong bond with a child is unlikely to keep the child with him or her all the time. Find out where they routinely put the child while they carry on with their daily life and carry out a forensic examination of the area around for traces of blood and hair from the baby's head. If there is an explanation for injuries by a fall and clash against a hard surface then examine the area where it supposedly happened for trace evidence or DNA evidence.
- Look for any evidence of induced illness such as salt, insulin, or medication such as methadone.
- Examine calendars, diaries and bills for evidence of any recent stressor in the lives of the parents that may be a secondary trigger to the shaking event.
- Look at photograph albums of the family to see that appropriate handling is being carried out. Are there any home videos that show inappropriate handling on the part of one or both parents or others?
- Seize any records available to show the health record of the child or any developmental charts, usually issued by the local health visiting service.
- Examine letters and any evidence of records of childcare kept for the local authority. Are they up to date, forged or altered in any way?
- Ensure that house-to-house questioning is done in the area around the premises. Were there crying incidents? Did anyone hear the parent or carer becoming exasperated with the child? Was there a time when the child cried and suddenly stopped? Was there a thud or other noise at that time? Many SBS enquiries are carried out without any questions being asked of neighbours who will often have much information to give.

- Ensure that anyone called to the house, such as the ambulance personnel or a neighbour who may arrive before police, are shown the photographs of the subsequent scene to see if it reflects the scene as they found it.
- Ensure that the emergency services' telephone tape is seized as in all other major enquiries and record what the initial story is to the ambulance personnel. Does that fit with the story given to any absent carer or the hospital staff? What is happening in the background? In one case the telephone operator asked whether the baby was choking on food, and the parent replied no, thus ruling this out as a possible defence later.
- Examine, document, and test and recreate any pattern of events that the suspect may try to say happened to explain away the injuries, e.g. "I was asleep and the block fire alarm went off, the baby fell off my chest on to the pipes." Ensure that this scenario is recreated and tested. Think laterally in light of the scene as to how a suspect might later explain the injuries to the child.

RECONSTRUCTION

In many cases the explanation given by the cargiver will be that the child was being fed or washed or having some interaction with the carer and the child 'just went limp'. In other cases the explanation will be that the caregiver was carrying the child and the baby fell from their arms. Sometimes the explanation will simply be that the baby fell from a couch or bed. All of these are common stories given in these cases.

Seasoned investigators of proven cases of SBS will be well aware of many of these excuses and explanations. They should be aware that many of them will explain the circumstances but in reverse, i.e. they will give symptoms resulting from the injury as the cause of the injury. For example, the baby may well have stopped breathing, after being shaken. The baby may well have had a seizure, after being shaken.

"One of the most common insufficient explanations of a baby suffering from severe inflicted head trauma is that the baby fell from a couch. In fact, this explanation has been heard so much in Shaken Baby Syndrome cases that legal and other professionals jokingly refer to it as the 'killer couch'" (Parrish 2001).

One of the ways to test these types of stories is to use video reconstruction. In many cases the suspect will be so convinced of the strength of their story that they will agree to the request to recreate the last moments before illness of their baby. This device is an extremely useful investigative tool and fairly simple to arrange.

A uniformed inspector or chief inspector independent of the Investigation can be used to facilitate the reconstruction, which is filmed throughout, with the suspect giving a commentary as to what they say actually happened. The suspect will quite often inadvertently give the investigator the evidence they need to take the case forward. The reconstruction will also serve to show that the suspect admits that they were alone with the child when the baby's collapse happened. Such reconstructions can be powerful for a jury, especially after medical evidence that catastrophic collapses in babies are extremely rare and attributable to traceable symptoms.

It should be stressed that the local CPS should be consulted in the event of a reconstruction in order to give advice. The maxim, as with any investigation under Police and Criminal

Evidence Act rules, should be fairness. Therefore the suspect should be allowed free rein to express what happened and simply go through the actions as requested by the independent Chief Inspector. This will help to place the suspect at the scene alone when the catastrophic collapse happened. It will also show the investigator much of what happened in the lead-up to the incident. In cases where the suspect is guilty this will often be truthfully reconstructed but with the shaking left out. It will certainly be useful to identify trigger points for the assault.

When measuring equipment and furniture the investigator should be aware that a defence lawyer may well use a biomechanical defence strategy to prove that a child could have secured injuries from falling from a couch or low height. Investigators should be aware of the complicated calculations used by experts in biomechanics. These often serve to confuse the jury still further than the medical evidence.

THE POST-MORTEM EXAMINATION

One of the most important points to note about the post-mortem examination in a case of SBS is that the result will not be declared from the outset. An experienced pathologist may give their opinion but further tests will be needed to confirm the cause of death.

The child's brain will be removed and fixed in formalin solution for a period. This can take from 4 weeks to some months. The full pathology report may therefore not be available at the time a decision is made to take the case to court. It may be that the suspect has already been charged with an offence prior to the child dying. The local authority solicitors will also want to be made aware of the progress of the case if there are other children in the family. Care proceedings on their behalf will be taken to ensure that they are safe.

Once again this emphasizes the multi-agency nature of these cases. Investigators who are not well versed in child protection procedures should ensure close liaison with the child protection team who can attend strategy meetings and advise on civil proceedings.

In the case of a suspicious death, the system is well established that a Home Office appointed pathologist will carry out the examination. What is not so well established in child death cases is that a paediatric pathologist should accompany that examination to give advice on their area of expertise. The difficulty at the present time is the distinct lack of paediatric pathologists in the whole of the United Kingdom.

The CPS should be made aware that these experts need to be consulted independently and that there will be an obvious cost implication in doing so.

A full skeletal survey and examination of the eyes for retinopathy are crucial parts of the post-mortem examination in SBS (for more details on these injuries see Chapters 5 and 8). The investigator should consult with the ophthalmic pathologist who will be examining the eyes to ascertain what photographs will be most useful and should be taken at the subsequent post-mortem examination. This consultation rarely happens and it means that the resulting photographs are not always the most appropriate ones for gathering evidence.

The pathologist should shave the head of the baby to look for evidence of bruising or impact injuries, although some do not. The pathologist should also remove the eyes of the child for independent examination by an ophthalmic pathologist. Some remove the back third of the eyes only and some refuse to remove the eyes for humanitarian reasons, thinking of the parents.

A recent case points to the benefits of removing the eyes from the baby at autopsy. At first the pathologist was reluctant to remove the eyes and then upon seeking the normal National Crime Faculty advice the police asked him to do so. Upon examination by the ophthalmic pathologist the eyes were found to have not only retinal haemorrhages but also evidence of blunt force trauma, thus strengthening the case of abuse against the suspect. The case resulted in life imprisonment for the defendant. The moral is, be aware of what samples are needed from the autopsy and do not be afraid to say to the pathologist what you want and why you want them.

The back of the child should be dissected and the spine and muscles photographed. The spinal cord should be photographed in situ and then taken out for examination. The pathologist will be looking for evidence of lack of oxygen due to squeezing and shaking, cracked or broken ribs due to the forceful holding around the ribs, and the effects of the shaking on the lungs, heart and colon. The pathologist should be asked to take a blood sample from the haematoma itself in case this issue becomes a defence ploy at a later stage in the proceedings.

Retinal haemorrhages are extremely important to the diagnosis of SBS. There have been many studies around retinal haemorrhages and child abuse. Most studies agree that these haemorrhages occur in at least 80% of shaken baby cases and they can be either bilateral (in both eyes) or unilateral (occurring in just one eye). It has already been noted that some retinal haemorrhages are missed in casualty wards due to lack of qualified doctors to do the examination or because the right examination is not done.

INTERVIEWING THE SUSPECT

Unfortunately the literature on SBS offers little information dealing with interviewing the suspect.

By the time a suspect has emerged in shaken baby cases the person responsible for the injuries may have given details of their version of events many times. They may be asked by the ambulance service for details; they may have to relate the circumstances to a general practitioner; they will certainly have to give a version of events to a partner or to an employer in child minder cases; at the hospital they will be 'interviewed' by a triage nurse regarding the circumstances and eventually by an emergency doctor. Potentially then, a suspect will have had to explain their side of events to people five or six times before the police begin their interviewing. Unfortunately police will not be able to intervene in these 'interviews' as most take place prior to their involvement. In some cases a mistake is made by those asking questions by enquiring whether the baby has been shaken, thus alerting the perpetrator to think of alibis. In other cases doctors, in their efforts to save the child, interview parents together, thus allowing stories to be concocted or subliminally suggested to the non-abusing partner.

It is extremely important that police obtain and record all of the accounts given to the various health professionals at the different stages of the process. These can be analysed for discrepancies and used when interviewing any suspects to detect any stories they have fabricated.

The first police interview with parents or other carers in these cases is likely to be in

439

the hospital after the report by the social services to police. All the normal rules of separate interviewing will apply in this case, but as mentioned above police should be aware that of necessity, doctors will have asked many of the same questions prior to their arrival.

Once again it goes without saying that the watchwords for investigators in these circumstances are open mindedness and compassion. The interviewer at the hospital should take time to explain why and how police are involved and that they are merely trying to ascertain why the baby is in ill health at the present time. It can be pointed out to the parents that detailed knowledge of how the baby became ill can help the doctors to save the baby's life.

There may be several statements taken from the parent or carer at this time. The parents will obviously be traumatized and may want to have breaks prior to completing their version of events. The point of these initial statements, from either parent or caregiver, is to obtain an explanation from the suspect for the baby's injuries that can be assessed by the medical experts and later used in an interview.

A suspect may give several different explanations to various doctors and family members for the child's injuries. It may be useful for an analyst to chart these differing explanations prior to the interview of the suspect. Police analysts, drawing timelines and reconstructing events, are commonplace in serious cases. They should be used in SBS cases also.

When a formal interview of the suspect takes place the normal rules of interview strategy and consultation with police force expert interviewers apply. The suspect should be allowed to give a free narrative account of what has happened in the life of the child and his/her carers in the last 48 hours.

The interview should then detail the injuries that the child has sustained and the suspect told about what the doctors have said about those injuries. The interview should concentrate then upon the onset of symptoms and who would have been present at that crucial time.

In this part of the interview it is important that the interviewer has some idea of what the symptoms of SBS are and what the medical findings are in this particular case. Therefore, the interviewer should be well briefed in what the circumstances of the case and the injuries are. It is preferable that the interviewers will have had some training at least in what SBS is and the common responses of suspects.

This is so that the interviewer is in a position to say to the suspect why their explanations of the child's injuries are not possible, due to the nature and severity of injuries and the opinions of the medical experts in the case.

At this stage it may be useful to introduce the video reconstruction of the time when the suspect says that the child became symptomatic. Here the time line of events prepared by the analyst will be very useful. There will be a sequence of events chart requested by the investigator to place everyone's movements over the previous 24 hours. There will also be the analysis of the various statements made by the suspect when explaining the circumstances of the injury. Both of these should be used to put discrepant stories to the suspect. The interview should be videotaped, either taking place in a specially equipped video suite or, where none exists, a video should be set up in the room. This will allow the medical experts in the case to review the explanations given by the suspect and to say whether those explanations are medically possible.

Another option in the interview is to use a doll of the same weight as the child. This prop can easily be obtained from a local toy shop and weighted with shot or sand to make it heavier. The suspect should be asked to go through the various routines that the child had, such as feeding, burping and changing, and how the suspect would have dealt with each eventuality and procedure. Where there are witnesses available to any of these procedures or witnesses of previous poor handling by the parent then they should be interviewed using the doll as a prop also. The witness interview could easily take place in the child protection video suite. Of course the doll should be listed as an exhibit in the case.

Although some experienced detectives may not wish to use this technique initially they should be encouraged to do so. There are now several examples of good video interviews with excellent evidence to show for their efforts from several murder enquiries around the country.

After the suspect has been allowed to give their version of events and it has been explained that this could not be so the interview may develop into a more confrontational style, using the doll as a prop once more. Again, the footage should be made available to the medical expert in the case to give their opinion on the veracity of the statements and explanations.

The suspect may well say that they found the baby lifeless in the cot. The investigators of SBS murders and assault cases must be prepared for an aggressive defence to be mounted by the defendant and their legal team. There are several avenues that defence lawyers will go down. Many of these are repeated time and time again in cases both here and in the USA.

TIMING THE INJURY

One of the most difficult areas for investigators is timing the injury and tying someone down to having caused the injuries at that time. As has been noted already it is extremely difficult for pathologists and doctors to time injuries such as this in as precise a way as the police would like. Doctors and pathologists can only use their expertise and knowledge of the condition and symptoms the child had at the time they became symptomatic.

The other main player in timing the injuries and tying down the suspect is of course the analyst. The latter is crucial in establishing the timeline of events in the case. In cases where murder squad detectives are running the case the analyst is automatic. Unfortunately, many of these cases are investigated by one officer on a small team with few resources and limited access to analysts. Consequently they are presented to the CPS as difficult cases in the first instance and thus never progress to court.

This was the case in the past and the reason why several cases were never taken to court. A study at Cardiff University has recently helped to point out how these cases were dealt with in the last decade by social services and police agencies (Cobley et al. 2002). The conclusions were that they were dealt with very poorly. In more than 60 cases examined by the study the highest number of statements taken by police to investigate the case was just 10! These included several murders.

EXAMINING DEFENCE STRATEGIES

It will sometimes be argued that other illnesses such as osteogenesis imperfecta or glutaric acidura type 1 are responsible for the injuries to the child. These need to be ruled out from

441

the start, even if at first there is no suggestion that these are an issue. Many children are mistakenly treated for meningitis at entry to the hospital casualty department. This in itself provides a difficulty for the investigator who will have to engage experts in meningitis to rebut any suggestion that the child died in this way.

The vaccination damage defence is now a common one in shaken baby cases. However, medical research tells us repeatedly that vaccinations have been found to be safe overall.

If a 'vaccine defence' is being argued then it is very important that the actual vaccine itself is identified. The company producing the vaccine should be contacted and their global safety database examined for any similar claims. The investigator should work closely with the company producing the vaccine to ensure that this defence avenue is blocked if appropriate.

Several cases have reached courts and the defence of finding the baby lifeless and then shaking to revive has been used. The importance of the multidisciplinary team comes to the fore in this instance. They must be given all relevant documents and X-rays, along with circumstances to help them decide whether the child would have been lifeless through some other cause.

When a nanny or other trained carer is alleging this scenario it is important to ascertain what training they have received in this regard. It is very important that the investigator keeps up to date with medical literature that deals with SBS. In all the main medical journals there are frequent articles and letters concerning new research. The investigator should be prepared to source articles from an internet medical database such as PubMed (www.ncbi.nlm.nih.gov/PubMed) and to visit medical libraries. Internet searches should be used to research defence witnesses and their previous papers.

In doing this the researcher will establish from articles exactly who the main experts are in each particular field. In a world made smaller by the internet, we should be prepared to speak with such experts and use them in our cases if necessary to disprove defence claims that babies died from falls from couches.

Defence strategies used in both the Woodward case in Boston and the Sullivan case in London included alleged blood disorders in the infant. In the Woodward case it was alleged that baby Matthew had a bleeding disorder, which caused bleeding in the brain some days before the death. In this way the defence hoped to widen the time line to bring in more people who might have been responsible for the death – in this case his parents.

In the Sullivan case the strategy employed was to allege that the baby had a bleeding disorder from birth, genetically inherited from parents. In this latter case it may be that the parents have to undergo blood tests to refute the claim.

In both of these cases the investigator should be employing the services of a good haematologist. The help desk at the National Crime Faculty is a point of reference in this instance and will provide details of the relevant experts.

In some cases there will be an absence of retinal haemorrhages in the eyes of the child and this will be used to show the jury that the baby has not been shaken. This is where knowledge of the nature of SBS is important. Not all shaken baby cases have retinal haemorrhages associated with them. In other cases the retinal haemorrhages that do exist can be a result of birth trauma.

In some SBS cases complicated biomechanical defences have been put forward to explain head injuries babies have experienced. This is where the importance of video reconstruction with a doll, using the same hold and for the same period becomes useful. This again can be shown to the medical experts for comment as to whether such handling could cause the injuries sustained. The interviewer should remember, however, that the suspect would minimize the shaking event and rarely show the amount of force they have used.

The investigator has to use all the strategies at their disposal to challenge defence arguments. Childminders will often have been on a childcare course where they have learned first aid. Any training like this that the carer has received should be fully researched and documented in order to establish if a carer has specifically been trained not to pick up a lifeless child and shake them as a resuscitation attempt.

IN COURT

When the case is eventually in court the prosecution should have ensured that the expert witnesses have met to discuss their common points of evidence. It may well be a good idea to begin the case with an objective explanation from an independent doctor as to what SBS is. Graphics packages written by Dr Jim Lauridsen at Alabama University are available to help this. These can be found on the website of the National Center on Shaken Baby Syndrome (www.dontshake.com).

This type of presentation will help the jury to understand what injuries are being looked for and how the injuries occur. In short, it will help to explain a very complicated injury to a member of the public who is sitting on a jury.

The prosecution should prepare a good 'jury bundle'. This should contain a glossary of terms and drawings of the brain and eye. These should be labelled with the terminology that they will hear throughout the trial from doctors. These drawings can be found at most teaching hospitals or on the many internet web sites.

KEEPING UP WITH RESEARCH

The investigator must be aware of any developments in the medical controversy surrounding SBS injuries. An article by Geddes et al. (2001) was hyped by the media and headlines read that even a gentle shake could cause SBS. Of course this was seized upon by defence solicitors and careful perusal of the article is needed to rebut any defence claims.

The Geddes et al. article has been reviewed and studied by many doctors. One of these is an eminent American doctor from Louisville, Kentucky, Dr Betty Spivack. In her review of the article she states: "In contrast to some of the media hoopla about the article there is nothing to support 'gentle shaking' as the cause of the observed pathology. While the authors do comment on the features of the infant neck which predispose to the craniocervical injuries which they observed, these are factors which have been described for 30 years. They provide no mechanism whereby 'gentle shaking' might cause subdural haematomas, retinal haemorrhages or cerebral traumatic axonal injury of any grade" (Spivack 2003). The investigator must be aware of such developments in any medical controversies surrounding SBS injuries.

The key issue for any investigator in a suspected SBS case is to remember that thorough and extensive research is the way to ensure that every possible angle is covered. In order for this research to be as thorough as possible, investigators must be acquainted with a knowledge of the basic medical issues surrounding shaken baby cases. Liaison with other agencies is of course also essential to solving these cases, which keep on occurring, and will continue to do so until prevention strategies help to bring down the incidence of deaths from SBS.

REFERENCES

American Academy of Pediatrics (2001) Statement on shaken baby syndrome. *J Am Acad Pediatr* **107**: 206–210.
Barlow K, Minns RA (2000) Annual incidence of shaken impact syndrome in young children. *Lancet* **356**: 1571–1572.
Caffey J (1972) On the theory and practice of shaking infants. *Am J Dis Child* **124**: 161–169.
Caffey J (1974) The whiplash shaken infant syndrome: manual shaking of the extremities with whiplash induced intracranial and intraocular bleedings, linked with residual permanent damage and mental retardation. *Pediatrics* **54**: 396–403.
Hobbs C (2003) The National Subdural Haematoma in Infancy Study. Paper presented to the European Conference on Shaken Baby Syndrome, Edinburgh, May 2003.
Cobley C, Sanders T (2003) Shaken baby syndrome – child protection issues when children sustain a subdural heamotoma. *J Soc Welfare Fam Law* **25**: 101–119.
Commonwealth v Woodward (1998) Supreme Judicial Court for Suffolk County, Middlesex Superior Court. Case number 97-433.
Duhaime AC, Generelli T, Thibault J (1987) The shaken baby syndrome: A clinical, pathological and biomechanical study. *J Neurosurg* **66**: 409–414.
Geddes JF, Hackshaw AK, Vowles GH, Nichols CD, Whitwell H (2001) Neuropathology of inflicted head injury in children, patterns of brain damage. *Brain* **124**: 1290–1298.
Guthkelsch AN (1971) Infantile subdural haematoma and its relationship to whiplash injuries. *BMJ* **2**: 430–431.
Kemp A, Price J (1998) Subdural haemorrhages in children, a population based study. *BMJ* **317**: 1538–1561.
Parrish R (2001) The unique challenge of investigating shaken baby syndrome cases. Lecture notes from the National Crime Faculty Special Interest Seminar on Shaken Baby Syndrome Deaths, Kenilworth, England, June 2001.
Reece R, Kirschner R (1998) A medical explanation of the causes of shaken baby syndrome. *Natl Cent Shaken Baby Syndr Q* Summer: 4–5.
Spivack B (2003) Review of Geddes article. *Q Child Abuse Med Update* **10**: 15.
Starling S, Holden J, Jenny C (1995) Abusive head trauma: the relationship of perpetrators to their victims. *Pediatrics* **5**: 259–262.
Tardieu A (1860) Services et mauvais traitments. *Ann Hyg Publique Medecin Legale* **13**: 361–398.
Wheeler P (2002) *A Report into the Police Investigation of Shaken Baby Syndrome Murders and Assaults in the United Kingdom*. London: Home Office Police Research Award Scheme.
Wheeler P (2003) Shaken baby syndrome – an introduction to the literature. *Child Abuse Rev* **12**: 401–415.

15
LEGAL ASPECTS OF SHAKEN BABY SYNDROME

Cathy Cobley

Over the last few years the phrase 'shaken baby syndrome' (SBS) has become part of everyday vocabulary in the developed world. Although recognized as a form of severe child abuse as far back as 1860 (Tardieu 1860), the impetus for the recent growth in awareness came initially from the USA, beginning with the work of American paediatric radiologist Dr John Caffey who in 1972 called for a nationwide programme to educate the public about the dangers of shaking babies (Caffey 1972). Public and professional awareness of the phenomenon increased in the USA during the 1980s and 1990s, and following several high-profile cases during the 1990s, there was a similar increase in awareness in the UK. As awareness increased, there was a corresponding growth of research into SBS, although very little UK based research existed until the late 1990s. The majority of research that was conducted in the USA initially focused on the medical aspects of the problem – SBS was seen primarily as a medical problem with comparatively little research being conducted on socio-legal aspects (e.g. Aoki and Masuzawa 1984, Duhaime et al. 1987, Fischer 1994, Duhaime 1996, Lancon 1998). However, in recent years it has come to be accepted that the effective management of cases of SBS involves consideration, not only of the medical aspects of an individual case, but also of the social and legal aspects. As a result, research is now expanding beyond the medical issues involved and is focusing on the social and legal consequences of a child being shaken. This chapter is based on the results of a research project undertaken in Wales and south-west England into the legal and social consequences when a child sustains a subdural haemorrhage (SDH) and discusses the legal issues that may arise when a child is shaken, in relation to both child protection proceedings and criminal investigations and prosecutions.

Research

SDH is often the first clinical noted on computed tomography/magnetic resonance imaging or at post-mortem examination that alerts a paediatrician to a likely diagnosis of SBS. The first population-based case series study of infants who had experienced SDH was published in the UK in 1998 (Jayawant *et al.* 1998). This study revealed important details on the epidemiology, associated features, and investigation of SDH, and suggested that, in the absence of alternative explanations, many clinicians were not eliminating the possibility of child abuse in their diagnostic work-up in all cases. However, although the study indicated that there were shortcomings in the evidence available on which to base subsequent decisions, it provided no detail on the social and legal decision-making process and outcomes. It was therefore decided to undertake further research to investigate the quantity and quality of evidence recorded when SDH is detected and during subsequent investigations, and to evaluate the use made of such evidence in the decision-making processes that determine the social and legal consequences for the victims of SBS and their families.

The research was funded by the Nuffield Foundation and was undertaken by a multi-disciplinary team from the Cardiff Family Studies Research Centre in Wales, which was established to promote research collaboration between Cardiff University and the University of Wales College of Medicine. The research was undertaken on a cohort of 68 children under the age of 2 years who had sustained SDH between 1992 and 1998 in Wales and south-west England. Medical records were accessed in each of the 68 cases. In cases where a child protection referral was made, access was negotiated to social service records and, where relevant, to the records of the family courts (Cobley and Sanders 2003). A child protection referral had been made in 54 of the cases and the records of the police and social services were accessed in each of these cases. An application for a care or supervision order had been made in 16 cases, and the relevant court records were accessed in 9 of these cases. The records of the Crown Court were also accessed in the 13 cases which resulted in a trial on indictment. Access to the records of the Crown Prosecution Service (CPS) and magistrates' courts was agreed at the outset of the research. However, it subsequently became apparent that these records are routinely destroyed 3 years after a case has been concluded and so, because of the retrospective nature of the research, these records could not be accessed. As a result we 'lost track' of 7 cases in the cohort after the police had charged a suspect. Key data from the records were identified, extracted, and entered onto data collection schedules designed for the study. Each case was given a unique identifier so that personal details could not be identified. To maintain complete confidentiality, all the data were coded numerically using a closed format system where textual information could not be entered, making case identification impossible. Data were subsequently analysed using the Statistical Package for Social Science (SPSS).

Results

THE CHILDREN

The 54 cases where non-accidental head injury (NAHI) was suspected consisted of 38 boys and 16 girls. The age of the children ranged between 0.5 and 23 months, with a mean age of 5.4 months. Fourteen of the children died immediately or shortly following their injury, giving a fatality rate of approximately 25%. The 54 children lived predominantly in two-parent families. The mothers and their partners tended to be much younger than the national mean age of parents of newly born babies, although the fathers' age reflected the national average. The occupational class of the caregivers (which provides a broad measure of social standing) was strongly skewed towards the lower end of the scale, and a large number of the victims lived in households where unemployment and material deprivation were common.

CLINICAL INTERVENTION AND THE DECISION TO REFER

The child was found to have coexisting injuries, most of which were considered to be non-

446

accidental, in 44 of the 54 referred cases. The injuries included fractures and/or bruises. Retinal haemorrhages were present in 36 cases. Information on medical opinion was drawn from reports written by clinicians who either had direct contact with the child during admission to hospital, or were invited to provide an expert opinion to support child protection and legal procedures. Up to five medical opinions were offered in any one case. The opinions were scaled according to the degree to which the clinicians believed that the SDH was as a result of NAHI, from 1 (definite NAHI) to 7 (definitely not NAHI). The mean opinion in each case ranged from 1.5 to 2.49, where 1 represents definite, 2 is probable and 3 is possible NAHI, showing that clinicians felt that NAHI was definite, probable or possible in most cases. A conflict of medical opinion during the child's admission to hospital as to the cause of the SDH was recorded in 10 of the 54 cases where a child protection referral was made.

THE CHILD PROTECTION PROCESS

In cases where the child was referred to social services, 95% were referred within 6 days of admission, with 20 being referred on the day of admission, nine within 1 day of admission, seven within 2 days, and four within 3 days. A case conference was convened following referral in 47 of the cases. No conference was convened in the remaining seven cases because in six of these cases the child had died and in the remaining case the agencies discounted the possibility of NAHI at a very early stage in their investigations. The child was placed on the child protection register following the first case conference in 38 cases. Five of the children had died by the time the conference was convened, NAHI was discounted in one further case, and in three cases it was decided at the conference that there was no risk to the child as the perpetrator was no longer living with the family.

The decision was taken to work with the family on a voluntary basis in 19 of the cases where the child was registered and proceedings were initiated in the family courts in the remaining 16 cases. A care order was applied for and granted in 13 cases and two supervision orders were applied for and granted. A care order application was unsuccessful in only one case, where, although the threshold criteria in section 31 of the Children Act 1989 had been satisfied, by the time of the final hearing the order was not deemed to be necessary in the best interests of the child. Court records could be traced in only nine of the 16 cases. Two of these cases were concluded in the family proceedings court, four were transferred to care centres in the county court, and three were transferred to the High Court due to the complexity of the case. No interim orders were deemed necessary in two of the cases where the child was being accommodated by the local authority. In the remaining seven cases between three and 11 interim care orders were made before the case was concluded.

EXPERT MEDICAL OPINIONS IN THE CHILD PROTECTION PROCESS

In total 40 medical witnesses provided expert evidence relating to the cause of the SBS in the nine cases reviewed. These were predominantly paediatricians (19), radiologists (9), and paediatric neurologists (3). (Seven other clinicians gave evidence which was not specific to the cause of the injuries.) There was a greater degree of consensus among the experts in the civil courts than there had been during the child's admission to hospital (see above). Only one expert was uncertain as to the cause of the injury, one thought it was probably not NAHI and one thought is was definitely not NAHI (the latter two experts had both been instructed by the parents). The remaining 37 experts thought the injury was definitely (12), probably (23), or possibly (2) NAHI.

CRIMINAL INVESTIGATIONS

A referral was made to the police on the day of admission to hospital in 14 cases, with a further 16 cases being referred within 1 day of admission and another 6 cases within 2 days of admission. The general pattern of referral times is very similar to the pattern of referrals to social services. The overall mean time between admission to hospital and referral to police was 2.55 days, which is slightly longer than the equivalent mean referral time to social services (1.98 days), suggesting that the initial referral was usually made to a social worker. In all cases the police investigation was started on the day of referral.

One or more suspects were arrested in 34 of the cases. The victim's parents were most likely to be suspected of having harmed the child. The arrested suspects included 25 fathers, 20 mothers, five partners of the mother, and one childminder. One or more charges were made in 25 cases. Twenty-one males and eight females were charged, with joint charges being brought in four cases. In total three suspects were charged with murder, three were charged with manslaughter, 11 were charged with causing grievous bodily harm (GBH) with intent, eight were charged with inflicting GBH, two were charged with assault occasioning actual bodily harm (ABH), and two were charged with assault. In five cases a charge of neglect (on the basis of failing to seek appropriate medical assistance for the child) under section 1 of the Children and Young Persons Act 1933 was brought in addition to the specific offences relating to the SDH.

Due to the destruction of records it was not possible to trace seven of the cases after charge, and therefore it was only possible to view files in 13 cases that resulted in a trial on indictment. In five of these cases the defendant was the victim's mother, in seven cases the defendant was the victim's father, and in one case the defendant was the partner of the victim's mother. Seven of the 13 defendants entered a guilty plea at arraignment to one or more of the offences charged. In one case the defendant pleaded guilty to manslaughter, in five cases the defendant pleaded guilty to one or more charge of inflicting GBH on the victim, and in one case the defendant pleaded guilty to a charge of wilfully ill-treating the child under section 1 of the Children and Young Persons Act 1933.

The defendant denied that they were criminally liable for the injuries to the child in six cases. In three of these cases the victim had died – one defendant pleaded not guilty to murder and two defendants pleaded not guilty to manslaughter. In two of the cases where the child had survived the defendant pleaded not guilty to offences involving GBH. In the final case the defendant pleaded not guilty to assault occasioning ABH and the CPS offered no evidence. Therefore a contested trial took place in five cases. One defendant was convicted of manslaughter following a contested trial and three defendants were acquitted of all charges. In the one remaining case the defendant was acquitted of causing the SDH, but was convicted of neglect by failing to seek medical assistance for the child.

In total nine defendants were sentenced, eight having been found to have caused the SDH and one having been found guilty of neglect. Of these, seven were sentenced to an immediate custodial sentence (two fathers following convictions for manslaughter, three fathers and one mother following one or more convictions for inflicting GBH, and one father following a conviction for assault). One mother convicted of inflicting GBH was placed on probation for 3 years and the mother convicted of neglect was given a suspended custodial sentence.

Entering the child protection and criminal justice systems – the clinicians' decision to refer

The clinician's decision to refer a case as possible NAHI is crucial to the success of the overall management of a case. In the absence of a referral, no action will be taken to protect the child, no criminal investigation will be instigated, no one will be punished for abusing the child, and the child may be returned to a potentially abusive home. The increase in awareness of SBS in recent years is now resulting in more detailed guidance for clinicians on the investigation of children with SDH (Kemp 2002), but the research did find that there were socioeconomic differences between the cases which were referred as possible NAHI and those which were not. The mean age of the group of 14 children who were not referred was 8.9 months, significantly higher than the mean age of the 54 referred children. The non-referred children were more likely to be living with married parents, and the occupational status of the caregivers of these children was significantly higher than the caregivers of the referred children. While the non-referred group of cases included recognized medical causes of SDH and witnessed major accidental injury, this was not so in all of the cases in the group and the research does signal a need to investigate further the extent to which the age of the child and social background of the caregivers might influence clinical suspicion of NAHI (Sanders et al. 2003)

Proving abuse in legal proceedings – when is a suspicion of NAHI substantiated?

Once a suspicion of NAHI has been raised and a referral made, cases enter the child protection and criminal justice systems where the police and social services work with the clinicians to determine whether the suspicions of NAHI can be substantiated. As the cases proceed through the system(s), a process of evidence building takes place. The cases have to pass through a succession of evidential 'gateways' before proceeding, with each gateway requiring a higher threshold of evidence than the one before. The question at what stage during this process a suspicion is substantiated or proved depends on the criterion adopted for substantiation. Arguably a suspicion can only be proved with absolute certainty when a perpetrator admits the abuse, and maintains that admission over time. The research found that this happens in only a small number of cases involving suspected SBS (see below). In several of the cases in the research cohort, an admission was made during the police investigations, only to be retracted at a later date. However, there are degrees of proof that fall short of absolute certainty, and one approach would be to say that a suspicion of NAHI may be said to be substantiated by a finding of fact by a court of law. This may be a finding in a criminal court that an individual has committed a criminal offence that resulted in the injury to the child, or it may be a finding in the civil courts that the state intervention (in

449

the form of a care or supervision order in relation to the child) is justified. In England and Wales this means that the court is satisfied that the threshold criteria contained in section 31(2) of the Children Act 1989 are satisfied – i.e. that the child concerned is suffering, or is likely to suffer, significant harm, and that the harm, or likelihood of harm, is attributable to the care given to the child, or likely to be given to them if the order were not made, not being what it would be reasonable to expect a parent to give to them. However, even this criterion for substantiation is not without difficulty. Before such a finding can be made in the criminal courts, the court must be satisfied of the defendant's guilt beyond all reasonable doubt. A lower standard of proof is required in civil courts in that the court need only be satisfied on the balance of probabilities, although the House of Lords has indicated that, in cases of child abuse, the more serious the allegation, the greater the weight of evidence required to establish the allegation on the balance of probability (*Re H* 1996). Thus a finding of abuse may be made in the civil courts in a particular case but, on the same evidence, a criminal prosecution may result in the defendant's acquittal. The research found that, of the 54 cases referred as possible NAHI, only three resulted in both a criminal conviction and a finding of abuse in the civil courts. A finding of abuse in the civil courts was made in a further 13 cases, and a criminal conviction based on causing SDH resulted in a further five cases, bringing the total number of cases where a finding of abuse was made by a court to 21 – a substantiation rate of less than 40%.

However, it is clear from the research that cases may not result in a finding of abuse by a court for a variety of reasons, and it would be unjustifiable to classify those cases that did not proceed to court as 'unsubstantiated' suspicions. While it is true that, in the criminal justice system, the cases usually did not proceed to trial because they failed to meet the evidential criteria required to proceed – e.g. there was insufficient evidence to arrest, charge, or convict a suspect – in many of these cases the lack of evidence centred on who caused the SDH rather then how it was caused (see below). Furthermore, in the child protection system cases that may well have met the threshold criteria did not proceed because it was not thought to be necessary in the interests of the child – e.g. the local authority had sufficient evidence to meet the threshold criteria but decided to work with the family on a voluntary basis without the need to resort to court orders. Although many of these cases were not proved in the strict legal sense, those responsible for the investigations and those working with the family clearly felt that the initial suspicion had, for practical purposes, been substantiated.

Who shook the baby (and does it matter)?

Although clinical investigations may define whether any injuries sustained by a child are recent, old, or of varying ages, they are seldom more specific, and establishing the timing of an injury with any precision is notoriously difficult. This is a particular problem in cases of SBS, where SDH may not be detected for some time after it has been caused. The research found that the child had been admitted to hospital on at least one previous occasion in 50% of the cases referred as possible NAHI, with one child having been admitted on four previous occasions before SDH was detected. In many cases of child abuse, the child will have been in the care of two or more caregivers during the 'window of opportunity' when the injury could have been inflicted, which often makes identification of the person responsible for causing the injuries impossible. Problems of identification are exacerbated by the reluctance of caregivers to admit to having shaken the child. The research found that 60% of caregivers offered no explanation when asked about the cause of the injury and 28% alleged that the cause was accidental. Other explanations included blaming a partner or a sibling, or birth complications. Only four caregivers had made an admission of shaking by the time of the first case conference and a further six subsequently admitted during police investigations that they had shaken the child. However, although all those who admitted shaking were charged with a criminal offence, the admission did not necessarily guarantee a guilty plea or a conviction. Two of the 10 suspects were acquitted at trial – one where the admission was excluded as being unreliable and one where the jury appeared to decide that the defendant did not have the necessary *mens rea* for manslaughter as the act of shaking was not 'dangerous' in the sense required (see below).

The fact that a single perpetrator cannot be identified is not necessarily fatal to child protection proceedings. If the injuries must have been caused by one of two caregivers with whom the child is living, the courts have little difficulty in finding that the threshold criteria in section 31 of the 1989 Act have been satisfied. Cases where the care of the child is shared between a number of caregivers are more problematic. In *Lancashire County Council v B* (2002), a 7-month-old child was found to have sustained serious head injuries, comprising SDHs, retinal haemorrhages and cerebral atrophy. The child had been admitted to hospital on three occasions over a period of 6 weeks prior to the diagnosis of the injuries. During this period the child had been living with her mother and father, but was cared for on weekdays by a childminder, who had a child of her own of a similar age. On the day of each admission to hospital, the injured child had been in the care of the childminder during the day. The local authority applied for a care order in relation to the injured child and also applied for a care order in relation to the childminder's child on the basis that, if the child-minder had been responsible for the injuries, she presented a risk to her own child. It was found as a matter of fact that in the 6 weeks prior to the diagnosis of the injuries, the injured child had experienced at least two episodes of violent shaking which resulted in the injuries, and that the injuries had been caused either by the child's mother or father, or by the childminder. All three possible perpetrators were said to make less than satisfactory witnesses, and the court found that it was not possible to identify who had actually inflicted the injuries. The House of Lords decided that, in cases where the care of a child is shared, as long as the injuries must have been caused by one of the primary caregivers (which may include a childminder), the threshold criteria are capable of being satisfied in relation to the injured child. However, where the local authority is applying for a care order on the basis of possible future harm, the criteria could be satisfied only on proven facts. Therefore, as it had not been established that the childminder was responsible for causing the injuries, the threshold criteria could not be satisfied in relation to her own, uninjured, child.

Although child protection proceedings may be successful even if the perpetrator cannot be identified, this will usually be an insurmountable hurdle in criminal investigations. Even if a court is satisfied that the injuries must have been caused by one of two caregivers, although care proceedings may be successful, unless it can be proved that one caregiver failed to

451

intervene to prevent the other causing the harm (and would thus be liable for aiding and abetting the assault), a conviction based on causing the injuries is not possible (Lane and Lane 1985), even though caregivers may be convicted of an offence of neglect under section 1 of the Children and Young Persons Act 1933 on the basis that they did not seek medical attention for the child as soon as reasonably practicable. The research found that, in comparison with the limited conflict between medical opinion as to the causation of the injury (see above), the majority of the cases that did not proceed to trial, or did not result in a conviction, failed because the prosecution could not establish who had inflicted the injury on the child. Although both caregivers were arrested in 17 cases, joint charges were brought in only four of these cases. Two of the cases where there were joint charges were discontinued by the CPS after charge on the grounds that there was insufficient evidence to secure a conviction as the perpetrator could not be identified. Only one of the remaining two cases proceeded to trial on indictment, where the father was convicted of manslaughter and the mother was convicted of an offence of neglect. Furthermore, of the four defendants who were acquitted of causing the injury following a contested trial, three were acquitted because the prosecution failed to establish that they were responsible for the assault on the child. Thus the crucial issue in criminal investigations in cases of SBS appears to be who rather than how. This problem is not, of course, unique to cases of SBS. The National Society for the Prevention of Cruelty to Children (NSPCC) established a working group to consider the problems encountered in prosecuting parents, and the issue has also been considered by the Law Commission (2003), whose recommendations resulted in the enactment of a new offence of causing or allowing the death of a child under section 5 of the Domestic Violence, Crime and Victims Act 2004.

Keeping the family together: parental cooperation and child protection proceedings
One of the key principles underlying the Children Act 1989 is that children are best cared for by both parents wherever possible and that the state and courts should intervene only where it will make improvements for the child. Social workers are encouraged to work in partnership with the parents in the best interests of the child and, by virtue of Part III of the 1989 Act, every local authority has a general duty to safeguard and promote the welfare of children in their area who are in need and, insofar as is consistent with that duty, to promote the upbringing of such children by their families by providing a range and level of services appropriate to those children's needs. Furthermore, a court may make an order with respect to a child under the Act only if it considers that doing so would be better for the child than making no order as all. These principles are clearly reflected in practice in the cases in the research cohort. Although the child was placed on the child protection register in 38 cases, in 19 of these cases no further proceedings were taken and the local authority worked with the family on a voluntary basis to ensure the child's safety. Following a risk assessment, the victims were most likely to be returned to both parents or placed in temporary foster care with a view to their being returned to their families in due course. Only a small minority of the children were placed with relatives or adopted. The research therefore supports the hypothesis that the main objective was for the rehabilitation of children with their families whenever possible. However, this is a potentially problematic area as it was not clear how

the risks of future abuse were assessed. It is possible that victims were rehabilitated with their families because it was believed that the risk of a further SDH diminished as the child grew older.

Three children died of their injuries after being placed on the register, and a court order was sought in the remaining 16 cases. Although few caregivers were prepared to admit to having shaken the child, this did not necessarily prevent them from cooperating with the child protection investigations. In each case a subjective assessment of the level of cooperation of the caregivers was made, based on information contained in the records. A measure of association was performed (Cramer's V) which showed a significant inverse association between the level of cooperation of both the mother ($p<0.005$) and the father ($p<0.003$) and the subsequent decision to apply for a care order. Thus caregivers who cooperated with the child protection investigations enhanced the likelihood of working with the local authority on a voluntary basis and accordingly reduced the risk of a care order application being made.

Court files were accessed in nine of the cases where an application was made for a care or supervision order. The care plan proposed by the local authority involved the long-term placement of the child with both parents in seven cases, placement of the child in foster care in one case, and adoption of the child in one case, reflecting the position following the risk assessment in those cases that did not proceed to the family courts. Previous research has also found that returning the child to parental care (reflecting the Children Act emphasis on this principle) is the most common plan following care proceedings (Hunt and Macleod 1999). This research found that by the final hearing in care proceedings, firm plans had been made for 120 of the 131 children in the original study, and that parental care was the most common plan (47% of children). However, although the number of cases analysed in this part of the study is very small, the percentage of care plans involving return to parental care is noticeably higher in cases of SBS than in previous, more general, research studies and may reflect professional perceptions of the risk of further abuse. Furthermore, although eight of the nine children had elder siblings, only one sibling was made the subject of a care order, which suggests that elder children are not thought to be at risk.

Criminal offences, convictions and culpability – perceptions of SBS
CRIMINAL OFFENCES
In England and Wales, the majority of criminal offences consist of two essential elements, technically referred to as the '*actus reus*' and the '*mens rea*', which must exist contemporaneously before criminal liability will arise. The *actus reus* consists of the external elements of the offence, which will usually include acts or, exceptionally, omissions in specified circumstances, and may also include prohibited consequences (such as harm or death). In cases where a child has experienced harm through shaking, providing that causation can be established (i.e. that the injuries were caused by the shaking) the actus reus of a criminal offence will be satisfied. The actual offence will depend on the seriousness of the harm caused – whether actual or grievous bodily harm, or death. The *mens rea* consists of the fault element required for the offence, which may be satisfied by intention, recklessness, or in some cases negligence. The perceived gravity of a criminal offence, which is reflected

in the sentence imposed, is influenced by the consequences of the defendant's actions and the culpability of the defendant. Intention is the most culpable state of mind. Thus where a child has died as a result of being shaken, if the jury is satisfied that the defendant either intended the child's death, or intended to cause the child GBH, a conviction for murder will result and the defendant will receive a mandatory sentence of life imprisonment. However, if the necessary intention cannot be proved, the defendant will be convicted of manslaughter if the jury is satisfied that he or she has committed an unlawful dangerous act. Manslaughter attracts a maximum sentence of life imprisonment, although the usual sentence for manslaughter arising from a single incident of abuse is between 2 and 4 years. If the child survives, but is seriously injured, the defendant may be convicted of an offence involving GBH. If it is found that he intended the GBH, he will be convicted of an offence under section 18 of the Offences Against the Person Act 1861 and be subject to a maximum sentence of life imprisonment. However, if the defendant is found to have been only reckless, in that he foresaw only that some harm may be inflicted, he will be convicted of an offence under section 20 of the 1861 Act, which is subject to a maximum sentence of 5 years imprisonment. If the child experiences less serious harm, the defendant may be convicted of an offence of assault occasioning ABH under section 47 of the 1861 Act, subject to a maximum sentence of 5 years imprisonment, or alternatively an offence of wilfully assaulting, ill-treating or neglecting the child under section 1 of the Children and Young Persons Act 1933, subject to a maximum sentence of 10 years imprisonment. Murder and offences under section 18 of the 1861 Act are therefore the two most serious offences that may be charged when a child has been shaken. Both offences require finding of intention and are referred to as offences of specific intent.

Is Shaking Perceived as an 'Intentional' Act?

Intention is a subjective state of mind, and in the absence of an admission from the defendant that he or she intended the harmful consequences of their actions, proving intention to the criminal standard of proof can be difficult. In cases where there is a direct attack on the victim, a jury may have little difficulty in deciding that the defendant intended the harmful consequences. But cases such as shaking a child can be more problematic. Following the case of *R* v *Woollin* (1999), if a jury is satisfied that a particular incident of shaking is virtually certain to result in the prohibited consequences to the child (either death or GBH), and that the defendant was aware of this, the jury may find that s/he intended the harm. However, it appears that in cases of SBS, juries are rarely given the opportunity to find intention in this way, and even if they are, they decline to make the finding. The research found that, of the 13 defendants who were tried in indictment, 11 were initially charged with offences of specific intent (three with murder and eight with section 18 offences). By the time the cases came to trial, the charges had been reduced to ones requiring only recklessness in seven of these cases, and so only four defendants continued to face a charge of an offence of specific intent – two were indicted for murder and two for section 18 offences. At trial, one defendant was acquitted of murder and the other defendant charged with murder pleaded guilty to manslaughter, which was accepted by the prosecution. Likewise, one defendant was acquitted of a section 18 offence and the other defendant charged with section 18 pleaded guilty to an offence under section 20 of the 1861 Act, which was accepted by the prosecution. Therefore, no convictions were obtained for offences of specific intent.

The circumstances in which SBS occurs can vary considerably, and thus the perceived culpability of perpetrators will also vary. At one end of the spectrum, an otherwise loving and responsible caregiver under extreme pressure may have lost control on an isolated occasion and shaken a child. If the caregiver immediately seeks assistance for the child, cooperates with any investigation, and works with professionals to ensure that the event is not repeated, the perceived culpability of that caregiver will usually be limited. However, at the other end of the spectrum a child may be subjected to continued and sustained physical abuse over a significant period of time and a shaking incident or incidents may be part of a pattern of prolonged abuse. The perceived culpability of the perpetrator of such abuse will inevitably be significantly higher and, arguably, should be reflected in any resulting conviction and sentence. The extent of coexisting injuries detected in the study cohort, a significant number of which had been caused on separate occasions, combined with the fact that in 50% of cases the child had at least one previous admission to hospital prior to the detection of SDH, suggests that at least some of the cases in the study cohort arguably fell within the upper range of the spectrum of culpability. If so, the absence of convictions for offences of specific intent is, prima facie, surprising but perhaps reflects a wider, general perception of SBS as involving less culpable actions than other forms of abuse.

Is Shaking Perceived as a 'Dangerous' Act?
The perceived culpability of the perpetrator in cases of SBS can also impact on decision-making in cases involving offences not requiring specific intent. In cases where the child has died, even if the perpetrator can be identified and it can be established that their actions caused the child's death, a conviction for manslaughter is not inevitable. The defendant may be convicted if the jury is satisfied that s/he has committed an unlawful dangerous act. For the act to be dangerous, it must be one that all sober and reasonable people would inevitably recognize must subject the other person to, at least, the risk of some harm resulting therefrom, albeit not necessarily serious harm (*R* v *Church* 1966). Therefore if the jury do not perceive shaking a child to be dangerous in this sense, an acquittal will result. One case in the research cohort provides a striking example of this. A father was charged with murdering his 5-month-old daughter. He admitted during the police investigations that he had shaken the child and it was not disputed that the shaking had caused the injuries which resulted in the child's death. When he was committed for trial, the charge was reduced to manslaughter. At his trial he pleaded not guilty. Although he did not retract the admission of shaking, he maintained that it was not a dangerous act in the sense required. After 5 hours' deliberation, the jury agreed and acquitted him of manslaughter. This decision may seem bizarre to those who are all too familiar with potential consequences of shaking a young child, but it does serve to highlight the need to educate parents and caregivers on the dangers of shaking.

Sentencing in cases of SBS
Sentencing in any case of child abuse has the potential to raise emotive issues. The Court

of Appeal has considered the basis on which sentences should be generally determined in such cases: "It is perhaps worthwhile to pause for a moment to consider the basis upon which the Court must try to arrive at the proper sentence in cases such as these, which are amongst the most difficult which a judge has to deal with so far as sentencing is concerned. First of all it is necessary of course to punish someone who has committed this sort of offence. Secondly it is necessary to provide some sort of expiation of the offence for the defendant. Thirdly, it is necessary to satisfy the public conscience. Fourthly, there is the necessity to deter others from committing this sort of offence, by making it clear that that this sort of behaviour will result in condign punishment" (*Durkin* 1989).

In cases where an intention to cause GBH is proved, the Court of Appeal has made it clear that the finding of intention must be reflected in the sentence. In the *Attorney General's Reference* (2001), a father was convicted of causing GBH with intent by shaking his 5-month-old daughter, causing SDH and severe brain damage. He was initially sentenced to 2½ years imprisonment, but the Court of Appeal expressed the view that following a not guilty plea, the appropriate sentence for an isolated incident involving a baby giving rise to a section 18 offence by an offender of previous good character, would be of the order of 4 or 5 years imprisonment and increased the sentence in the case to one of 3 years imprisonment. However, as previously noted, proving intention in cases of SBS is frequently an insurmountable hurdle, or at least one which the prosecution tend to avoid facing.

Even if intention is not present, or cannot be proved, the Court of Appeal has made it clear that "offences of physical violence to a child, particularly one's own child, must of necessity attract punishment and punishment of a quite severe kind" (*R v Scott* 1995). Sentences for offences which can be committed recklessly or negligently inevitably vary considerably, according to the facts of each individual case. Furthermore, in these cases perceptions of an offender's culpability may potentially have a considerable impact on the sentencing decision. A review of sentencing practice in cases of SBS in England and Wales suggests that the members of the judiciary responsible for sentencing offenders tend to share the perception previously identified that shaking is distinct from other forms of abuse, such as striking a child.

A review of sentencing in cases of child abuse in general indicates that in manslaughter cases arising from a single incident of abuse, the usual sentence is between 2 and 4 years (*Bashford* 1988, *Hall* 1997), although this may rise to 6 years if the violence involved is severe (Horscroft 1985). Sentences for a section 20 offence against a child typically range between 12 months and 2 years imprisonment (*Cavanagh* 1994). As far as sentences in cases of SBS are concerned, anecdotal evidence from police officers suggests that there is no consistency in sentencing practice and that sentences are often regarded as being too lenient (Wheeler and McDonagh 2002). The two defendants in the research cohort who were convicted of manslaughter received sentences of 3 and 4 years imprisonment – clearly within the usual range for offences of child abuse in general. However, of the six defendants who were sentenced for a section 20 offence, although one received a sentence of 18 months imprisonment, two received sentences of 12 months imprisonment (one of which was reduced to 6 months on appeal), two received sentences of only 9 months imprisonment (one of which was suspended for 2 years on appeal), and one was placed on probation for

3 years. Thus two-thirds of those sentenced for section 20 offences received sentences below the usual range for cases of child abuse in general, a fact which may be indicative of judicial perceptions of shaking. However, given the small number of cases in the study cohort that resulted in a criminal conviction, further research on sentencing practice in cases of SBS is needed before any firm conclusions can be drawn.

Despite a lack of empirical evidence as to sentencing practice, comments made by the Court of Appeal give a clear indication of judicial perceptions of shaking. In *R* v *Scott* (1995), Kay J said: "It is necessary to . . . look at the particular acts that resulted in the injuries that this poor child suffered. They were not blows. They were not offences of throwing a child to the floor, or against some object as this Court sometimes has to consider. They were simply shaking a child and shaking a child in circumstances where the appellant, an otherwise loving father, was finding it difficult to cope with a very young baby. It is unfortunate that the appellant aggravated what he had done by failing to report the matter immediately to hospital staff. However it may be that the precise mechanism of the injury was something outside the experience of the appellant, and there was a degree of failure on his part to relate the one to the other."

In *R* v *Terence Hulbert*, Alliot J accepted the defence submission that shaking could be distinguished from a blow or blows, stating "[shaking] is, as it were, an involuntary expression of the exasperation that no parent has not at some stage or another felt when a child reacts, as this child did, on this occasion."

Similar comments have been made in the Court of Appeal on other occasions (e.g. *R* v *Robert Graham* 1997), suggesting that shaking a child is not perceived in the same light as other forms of physical child abuse, despite the fact that the consequences of shaking for the child can be significantly more severe than striking a child.

Legal aspects of SBS in other jurisdictions – are there lessons to be learnt?

The research undertaken in England and Wales provides an important insight into the legal and social consequences for victims of SBS in the jurisdiction and also highlights some of the hurdles faced as cases progress through the child protection and criminal justice systems. The research confirms several of the findings of research projects undertaken elsewhere (Wheeler and McDonagh 2002). As far as the incidence of SBS is concerned, the study which preceded the research in England and Wales reported an annual incidence of SDH in children under 1 year of 21 per 100,000 children, and it was estimated that NAHI accounted for 82% of these cases (Jayawant *et al* 1998). In Scotland, Barlow and Minns (2000) have reported an annual incidence of 24.6 per 100,000 children under 1 year. In relation to the victims and fatality rates, the research findings confirm studies carried out in the USA in the 1990s which found that boys were almost twice as likely to be victims of SBS as girls, with the majority of victims being under 6 months of age and 23–50% of the victims dying as a result of the injuries sustained.

In the past only limited research has been published in the UK, and any research published in other jurisdictions has tended to focus on medical issues, with comparatively little emphasis being placed on socio-legal aspects of the problem. In this respect the research in England and Wales, with its emphasis on the social and legal consequences for

457

the child, is thought to be unique to the jurisdiction, and increasing attention is now being focused on legal aspects of the problem. A similar trend can be seen in other jurisdictions, as more research is being undertaken on socio-legal aspects of SBS. This provides the potential to draw on research findings from other jurisdictions with a view to improving the overall management of cases. However, although there are undoubtedly lessons to be learnt, research findings from one jurisdiction may not necessary be directly applicable to another jurisdiction as any cultural or legal differences between the jurisdictions must be taken into account.

ENCOURAGING GOOD PRACTICE IN CASES OF SBS OR IMPOSING LEGAL OBLIGATIONS? A TALE OF TWO JURISDICTIONS

The starting point for effective management of cases of SBS must be increased awareness of the condition. The need to educate members of the public and professionals about the causes of SBS and the potential consequences for the young children must be treated as a priority. Clinicians in all jurisdictions are now being encouraged to adopt a high index of suspicion when SDH is detected in a young child, but, as previously noted, unless a child protection referral is made or the police are informed of the suspicion, no legal consequences, whether in the form of child protection or criminal prosecution, will follow. Whereas in England and Wales, systems are in place to facilitate the reporting of suspected abuse, and detailed guidance is available to all professionals as to the steps that should be taken, both within their own profession and on an interagency basis (e.g. *Working Together to Safeguard Children*, Department of Health 1999), there exists no mandatory duty to report. In contrast, in the USA, between 1963 and 1966 all states passed some type of statute requiring, inter alia, health care professionals to report suspected child abuse and neglect, and imposed sanctions for failing to report. Although the American experience of mandatory reporting has not been without its problems, it has undoubtedly succeeded in bringing more cases of child abuse to the attention of the authorities (Small 1992). However, although the possibility of a mandatory duty to report was considered by an interdepartmental working group established as part of a review of child care law in 1985 (DHSS 1985), the law in England and Wales imposes no such obligation. It seems that in England and Wales, professionals are expected to work together bound by mutual trust and professional guidance rather than by a legal duty, and there seems little possibility of a mandatory duty to report being imposed in the foreseeable future.

A further example of the willingness of the USA to impose legal obligations on professionals, as opposed to encouraging good practice, is the provision of educational material to parents of young children. Prevention efforts can be targeted at the parents and caregivers of young children through a variety of sources. In the UK, the NSPCC has launched campaigns aimed at warning people about the dangers of shaking babies (NSPCC 1998), and copies of prevention posters have been sent to every Area Child Protection Committee in England and Wales (Wheeler and McDonagh 2002). However, no formal mechanism exists to ensure that all parents of newborn children are provided with information about the dangers of shaking. Experience in the USA suggests that one of the most effective prevention strategies is to provide information on the potentially fatal consequences of shaking to parents of newborn children in a hospital setting. A programme initially developed at the Children's Hospital of Buffalo, New York, presents education to new parents about the dangers of SBS through a video, an SBS educational brochure, and a discussion with a member of the nursing staff, following which the parents sign an acknowledgement/evaluation form (Lithgo 2001). Such programmes are run on a voluntary basis by certain hospitals, but some states have gone further and imposed legal obligations on health care providers to ensure that relevant information is given to parents of young children. For example, the Public Health Law in New York requires hospitals to provide a brochure containing health information to prospective parents who are making arrangements for delivering at the hospital. In October 2001, the law was amended so that the information provided must now also include a description of the dangers of shaking infants and young children. The description must include information on the effect of shaking, appropriate ways to manage the causes of shaking, and discussion on how to reduce the risks of shaking.

The effectiveness of imposing a legal obligation to provide educational material requires further research. An evaluation of the voluntary programmes in the USA suggests that they have significantly reduced SBS injuries, but it is argued that, as the programmes are delivered during the post-delivery stay in hospital (a time when parents are thought to be most receptive to the information), they are more effective than merely providing educational material before the child is born, which is all that is required by law. While continuing efforts are being made in the UK to heighten awareness of SBS among parents and caregivers, as with mandatory reporting of suspected abuse by clinicians, there is no prospect of a similar legal obligation being imposed in the foreseeable future.

SHARING RESEARCH FINDINGS: PERCEPTIONS OF SBS AND PUNISHMENT

One of the key findings of the research in England and Wales was that perceptions of SBS appeared to influence decision-making throughout the child protection and criminal justice systems, and this was particularly apparent when cases came before a criminal court (see above). Yet very little is actually known about the attitude of members of the public towards the perpetrators of SBS and about what is perceived to be an appropriate consequence of a prosecution. With increasing numbers of cases being identified and, with improved police investigation, more convictions expected in the future, research into attitudes regarding punishment in cases of SBS would help to inform appropriate decision-making and encourage consistency. Research in this area has already been conducted in the USA and, while legal and cultural differences mean that the findings may not accurately reflect attitudes in England and Wales, drawing on such findings can be a valuable starting point in designing a research project.

The research in the USA (Kussman 1999) investigated the attitudes of young adults regarding the appropriate punishment for perpetrators of SBS, in relation to both criminal sanctions and levels of restriction on contact with children. The study found that those who were aware of SBS adopted a more punitive approach on both scales, indicating the significance of educating the public about the dangers of shaking and suggesting that, as awareness of SBS grows, society's response may become more punitive. Interestingly, as injury history and severity increased, male perpetrators were rated lower on the criminal sanction scale than female perpetrators, suggesting that males were perceived by the public as being less culpable than females in cases of SBS. Yet, in England and Wales, the research found that the sentences imposed on male perpetrators were significantly higher than those imposed on female offenders. Clearly, further research is needed on both public and professional perceptions of SBS and how these perceptions influence decision-making in the management of cases.

Conclusion

The increase in awareness of the incidence of SBS in England and Wales originated within the medical profession and there is now a growing body of literature available on medical aspects of SBS, although there remains a need for further research, particularly on the mechanics and timing of the injury. In comparison, social and legal aspects of SBS remained largely unexplored until recent times. Now, however, a clear picture of the issues to be considered in this context is beginning to emerge, as the results of the research project outlined in this chapter indicate. SBS is now coming to be recognized as a clearly definable medical condition that requires integration of specific clinical investigation, management, and interdisciplinary community intervention. Clinical diagnosis of the injuries remains the starting point, but it is now recognized that appropriate legal intervention, in terms of both child protection and criminal prosecution, play an equally crucial role in the successful management of cases of SBS.

REFERENCES

Attorney General's reference (No 34 of 2000) (2001) 1 Cr App R (S) 359.
Aoki N, Masuzawa H (1984) Infantile acute subdural hematoma: clinical analysis of 26 cases. *J Neurosurg* **61**: 273–280.
Bashford (1988) 10 Cr App R (S) 359.
Barlow K, Minns RA (2000) Annual incidence of shaken impact syndrome in young children. *Lancet* **356**: 1571–1572.
Caffey J (1972) On the theory and practice of shaking infants: its potential residual effects of permanent brain damage and mental retardation. *Am J Dis Child* **124**: 161–169.
Cavanagh (1994) 15 Cr App R(S) 589.
Cobley C, Sanders T (2003) Shaken Baby Syndrome: Child protection issues when children sustain a subdural haemorrhage. *J Soc Welfare Fam Law* **25**: 101–119.
Department of Health (1999) *Working Together to Safeguard Children*. London: DoH.
Department of Health and Social Security (1985) *Review of Child Care Law: Report to Ministers of an Interdepartmental* Working Party. London: HMSO.
Duhaime AC (1996) Long-term outcome in infants with the shaking-impact syndrome. *Pediatr Neurosurg* **24**: 292–298.
Duhaime AC, Gennarelli TA, Thibault LE, Bruce DA, Margulies SS, Wiser R (1987) The shaken baby syndrome: a clinical, pathological and biomechanical study. *J Neurosurg* **66**: 409–415.
Durkin (1989) 11 Cr App R (S) 313.
Fischer H (1994) Permanently damaged: long term follow-up of shaken babies. *Clin Pediatr* **33**: 696–698.
Hall (1997) 1 Cr App R (S) 406.
Horscroft (1985) 7 Cr App R (S) 254.
Hunt J, Macleod A (1999) *The Best-Laid Plans: Outcomes of Judicial Decisions in Child Protection Proceedings*. London: HMSO.
Jayawant S, Rawlinson A, Gibbon F, Price J, Schulte J, Sharples P, Sibert JR, Kemp AM (1998) Subdural haemorrhages in infants: a common and serious problem. *BMJ* **317**: 1558–1561.
JH (2001) 1 Cr App R (S) 551.

Kemp AM (2002) Investigating subdural haemorrhage in infants *Arch Dis Child* **86**: 98–102.

Kussman E (1999) *Attitudes Regarding Punishment of Perpetrators of Shaken Baby Syndrome*. Unpublished thesis, University of Wisconsin.

Lancashire County Council v *B* (2002) 2AC 147.

Lancon A, Haines D, Parent A (1998) Anatomy of the shaken baby syndrome. *New Anatomist* **253**: 13–18.

Lane and Lane (1985) 82 Cr App R 5.

Law Commission (2003) *Children: Their Non-Accidental Death or Serious Injury (Criminal Trials)*. Law Com No. 282. London: The Stationary Office.

Lithgo G (2001) New York passes new SBS law. *SBS Quarterly*, Winter 2001 (online, http://www.dontshake.com).

Mason (1994) 15 CR App R (S) 745.

NSPCC (1998) Handle with Care. London: National Society for the Prevention of Cruelty to Children.

Piggott (1999) 1 Cr App R (S) 392.

Re H (Minors) (1996) Ac 563, HL.

R v *Church* [1966] 1 QB 59.

R v *Scott* (1995) 16 Cr App R (S) 451.

R v *Robert Graham* (1997) 2 Cr App R (S) 264.

R v *Terence Hulbert* (1998) EWCA Crim 2758, Court of Appeal 2 October.

R v *Woollin* [1999] AC 2.

Sanders T, Cobley C, Coles L, Kemp A (2003) Factors affecting clinical referral of young children with a subdural haemorrhage to child protection agencies. *Child Abuse Rev* **12**: 358–373.

Small M (1992) Policy Review of Child Abuse and Neglect Reporting Statutes. *Law Policy* **14**: 29.

Tardieu A (1860) Etude medico-legale sur les services et mauvais traitments exerces sur des enfants. *Ann Hyg Publ Med Leg* **13**: 361–398.

Wheeler P, McDonagh M (2002) *A Report into the Police Investigations of Shaken Baby Murders and Assaults in the UK*. London: Home Office.

16
ASSESSMENT AND DECISION-MAKING IN NON-ACCIDENTAL HEAD INJURY CASES: A SOCIAL WORK PERSPECTIVE

Elaine Ennis

This chapter explores assessment and decision-making for children diagnosed with non-accidental head injuries (NAHIs) from a social work perspective. It complements the chapters by Mok (Chapter 13) and Wheeler (Chapter 14) on prevention, protection and police investigations, and focuses on tertiary prevention, i.e. professional intervention once abuse has been identified, where protection from further harm and the promotion of the child's welfare are the main objectives. There is also discussion of a pilot case study conducted in 2000/2001 based on a small sample drawn from the database of NAHI cases collated over a period of 15 years in Scotland (Barlow et al. 1998; see also Chapter 4). Legislation and policy references in this chapter are mainly to the Scottish legislative framework because the study took place within that jurisdiction.

The context for assessment and decision-making

There is consensus among professionals that cases of NAHIs present complex challenges in terms of diagnosis, treatment and longer-term management. The point has been made throughout this book that head injuries are among the most serious forms of child abuse and result in high mortality and morbidity rates (Barlow et al. 1998). Where children survive the injuries, sequelae diagnosed soon afterwards may have life-long implications for children's development and functioning (Ludwig and Warman 1984, Fischer and Allasio 1994, Haviland and Russell 1997, Andrew et al. 1998; see also Chapter 12). In other cases, surviving children may appear initially to have no ill-effects; however, studies have shown that problems may not manifest themselves until up to 5–6 years after the head injuries (Bonnier et al. 1995, 2003). Some researchers advocate follow-up of surviving children over a 15- to 20-year period (Parrish 2001). Behavioural impairments following injuries may cause greater stress to families than physical disabilities (Andrew et al. 1998). The implications for planning for children who have sustained NAHIs are far-reaching both in terms of protecting those children from further abuse and in promoting their welfare.

In order to intervene effectively for the child, it is necessary for social workers to consider siblings, parents (both non-abusing and the perpetrators of injuries, although it is by no means always possible to identify the abuser) and, indeed, the totality of the child's environment. Workers need to understand the child's system (family, extended family,

community) (Minuchin 1974; Palazzoli et al. 1978; Garbarino 1986, 1987, 1992) and pro
fessional systems (health, civil and criminal processes, housing, education, social security)
– and to work effectively within them.

The role of social work is determined by legislative frameworks [e.g. Children (Scotland)
Act 1995], national and local child protection guidance (e.g. Scottish Office 1998, Scottish
Executive 2000) and the conceptual, theoretical and practice frameworks adopted by the
profession. Enquiry reports also have a significant impact on policy and practice (e.g.
O'Brien 2003). Although social work has a distinctive and pivotal role in child protection
cases it may only be fulfilled through work in partnership with other professionals, and in
doing so all parties' duties and contributions are defined in government policy (e.g. Scottish
Office 1998, Scottish Executive 2000).

There is also the concept of partnership with families, which although not enshrined
in statutes is nevertheless an important theme in official guidance. There are unique
challenges associated with partnership; the realities of deploying the positive resources of
parents and families to protect and promote the welfare of a child while retaining a clear
focus on factors that may endanger a child again and impede development have to be
addressed (Petrie and James 2002). Enquiry reports and research studies testify to the poor
outcomes for children when decision-making processes take insufficient account of these
tensions (Department of Health 1991, Munro 1999, Reder and Duncan 1999). It is also a
matter of debate how far true partnership can be achieved between professionals and parents when all are aware of the imbalance of power in child protection work.

Finally, in cases of NAHIs it is likely that social work intervention will be provided
by professionals based in hospitals, community-based teams (children and families and/or
children with disabilities teams), health centres, and criminal justice services (both community
and prison-based). In addition, oversight, supervision and consultation will involve senior
managers and other local authority specialists such as lawyers.

A specialist knowledge base and integration with a wide perspective on children and families

There is no doubt that cases of NAHI evoke high levels of anxiety among professionals.
Reactions are shaped both by the complexity of the professional task and by publicity given
to high-profile cases where expert evidence may appear to conflict, as noted earlier in this
volume. Wheeler (2002) has highlighted the importance for police officers of an up-to-date,
reliable and specialist knowledge base including an understanding of medical terminology,
the biomechanics of injury, the types of injuries that may be sustained, their progression,
and likely outcomes for the child, risk factors (see also Chapter 13), investigation, current
medical and courtroom controversies, and prevention.

The same specialized knowledge base is necessary for social workers involved in NAHI
cases. To that end, research literature, training courses, conferences, and IT tools such as
websites (e.g. www.dontshake.com) and CD-ROMs (e.g. Wheeler and McDonagh 2001)
are important professional development tools for acquiring and maintaining expertise.
Continuing professional development also requires effective supervision and management
to complement training.

In the social work role, a specialist knowledge base underpins the capability to:

- evaluate family histories and circumstances and also to listen with a critical ear to explanations of injuries in assessment (although it is explicitly a police role to investigate, and challenge as appropriate, those accounts where a crime may have been committed)
- advocate for the child (Hudlett 2001) taking a long-term (potentially life-long if adoption is considered) view of needs as well as protection in the more immediate term using knowledge of possible outcomes (Haviland and Russell 1997; Ludwig and Warman 1984; Bonnier et al. 1995, 2003; Andrew et al. 1998; see also Chapter 12)
- promote understanding of NAHIs among professional colleagues and families (a role combining education and counselling skills)
- challenge erroneous facts and opinions based on unreliable sources when decisions are being made about a child
- promote confidence in discussions with colleagues, e.g. to seek amplification where necessary to understand the implications of a particular condition for the child and to explain social work perspectives
- recognize and work with disbelief that injuries could have been caused by particular caregivers and to acknowledge that professionals may be susceptible to overlooking areas of enquiry, misinterpreting information, or missing diagnoses in their practice (Jenny et al. 1999; Munro 1999, 2002; see also Chapter 13).

However, the literature has highlighted the inadvisability of employing too narrow a research and theoretical base in work with families where concerns about children have been validated (Department of Health 1995, Reder and Duncan 1999). Therefore, in addition to the specialized knowledge base associated with NAHIs, theoretical linkages are necessary with the wider research literature on child protection and on children and families more generally.

In recent years, significant progress has been made in the development of assessment tools such as the Department of Health's *Framework for the Assessment of Children in Need and their Families* (2000), which draws on widely validated theory such as ecological approaches (Garbarino 1992), and research in child development and parenting capacity in addition to more specific child protection research. Developmental work is continuing (Cleaver et al. 2002) and some have proposed 'bespoke' assessment tools to complement the original framework for use in specific practice situations such as serious physical abuse (Dale et al. 2002, Frude 2003).

In Scotland, the Child Protection Audit and Review (Scottish Executive 2002) led to the formation of a Review and Action Team, which is developing an integrated assessment tool specific to the Scottish context and for use by all child protection professionals.

The underpinning principles of assessment tools include:

- The child is best understood and protected, and has his or her welfare best promoted, by taking an holistic view of their context.
- The complex and subtle interrelationships between the characteristics of a child, his/her parents, and their parenting capacity, the close and extended family, and structural issues such as housing, community resources, income, employment and status are key to the

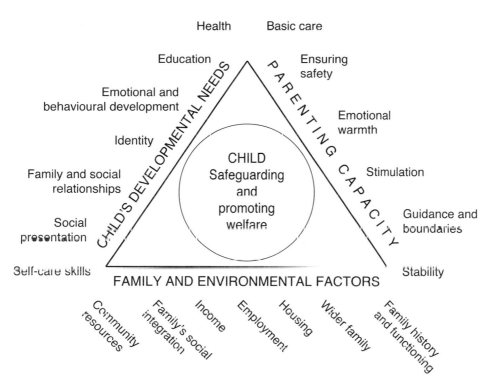

Health   Basic care

Education   Ensuring safety

Emotional and behavioural development

Identity

CHILD Safeguarding and promoting welfare

Family and social relationships

Stimulation

Social presentation

Guidance and boundaries

Self-care skills

Stability

PARENTING CAPACITY

CHILD'S DEVELOPMENTAL NEEDS

FAMILY AND ENVIRONMENTAL FACTORS

Community resources   Family's social integration   Income   Employment   Housing   Wider family   Family history and functioning

Fig. 16.1. The assessment framework (Department of Health 2000).

assessment and intervention processes (Fig. 16.1). Good assessment stems from informed analysis of those interrelationships rather than a mechanistic accumulation of data that are not subjected to interpretation.

- Risk assessment is central to the assessment process and not a separate, unrelated entity. Specificity in risk assessment, e.g. in terms of undesirable behaviours (Moore 1996), is preferable to more generalized, nonspecific statements.
- The ultimate purpose of assessment is both to protect the child (and any other children in the household) and to ensure that his/her needs are met; the two processes are intimately related rather than alternative choices.
- The process of the assessment should identify areas of strength in the child's situation – which may be actual or potential protective factors – as well as areas of vulnerability.
- Areas of vulnerability may be cumulative in such a way that the sum of them (and therefore the significance for the child now and in the future) is greater than individual factors might suggest if viewed in isolation.

Additionally, core values grounded in codes of ethics and discourse in children's rights and human rights drive social work intervention in child protection, as delineated by (McCarrick et al. 2000):

- All children have rights, in particular a basic right to have their needs met.

465

- Assessment must be child centred; its prime focus must be the child. Where there is a conflict of interest between parents and children, the child's interests must have priority.
- Honesty with parents and children is important. Parents and children have the right to respect.
- Assessment should take place with the parents and children, it should not be something that is done to them.
- Assessment should be undertaken in a way that is sensitive to race, culture, class, and disability. However, sensitivity to these issues by the worker must not result in a failure to protect the child.

Finally, an appropriately supportive culture is essential to good practice. The anxiety associated with child protection cases has already been noted, and NAHI cases are particularly distressing in that they challenge cultural beliefs and norms about parenting, the vulnerability of small babies and their rights to protection and nurture. Professionals need explicit permission within organizational cultures to express the emotional impact of a case (Morrison 1997) and to do so in a safe space such as discussion with colleagues, supervision, mentoring or consultation sessions (Munro 2002).

Similarly, exploratory yet purposeful discussions about the dimensions of a case are increasingly viewed as integral to good practice in assessment, planning and decision-making. A "dialectic mindset [which] should pervade the ethos of the workplace" was advocated by Reder and Duncan (1999) in their study of fatal child abuse, and similar points have been made elsewhere (Morrison 1997).

What is known to help us make appropriate decisions for children who have sustained NAHIs?

Within the context just outlined, assessment and decision-making are informed by research studies and insights from professional practice.

RESEARCH LITERATURE

Distinct themes emerge from follow-up studies of children who have sustained NAHIs.

First, the outcomes in medical terms are generally poor with a high proportion acquiring neurological and developmental problems (Ludwig and Warman 1984; Fischer and Allasio 1994; Bonnier et al. 1995, 2003; Haviland and Russell 1997; see also Chapter 12). The outcomes are generally worse than those for children who sustain accidental head injuries (Haviland and Russell 1997). One study focused on social and behavioural effects of traumatic brain injury and found clear evidence of lower levels of self-esteem and adaptive behaviour and higher levels of loneliness, and of maladaptive and aggressive/antisocial behaviours (Andrew et al. 1998).

Second, there are relatively few longer-term studies that trace the social and legal consequences for the child, the child's family and the abuser, if identified, although work by Cobley et al. (2003) is an extensive UK study of decision-making. One English study found a low rate of convictions and the majority of the children returned to their families of origin (Haviland and Russell 1997). In the USA, Fischer and Allasio (1994) studied 21 surviving children, six of whom were returned to homes where the injuries happened, and four of these children were re-injured. In the Scottish pilot study four of five cases resulted in convictions, one child died, three children returned to their families, and one child was placed in out-of-home care, although the small sample size and case study methodology mean findings are 'anecdotal rather than statistical' like those in the Haviland and Russell (1997) study.

However, more studies have retrospectively explored the characteristics and social circumstances of the child and the family before and around the time the head injuries were inflicted. From these we have learned that children are likely to be under 1 year of age and that most cases occur when the children are under 4 months old (Carty and Ratcliffe 1995, Barlow and Minns 2000). Studies generally concur that boys are victims more often than girls and also that their abusers are usually males (birth fathers, stepfathers, and mothers' partners), although female caregivers are also known to be responsible in some cases (Parrish 2001, Wheeler 2002). An important caveat to these studies is that they are based on cases presented for emergency treatment: the true incidence and prevalence of NAHIs – and therefore, the social characteristics of all the families implicated – are not known and are the subject of continuing study.

Mok in this volume has identified child abuse risk factors (Table 13.3, p. 420) and has highlighted earlier involvement with social services and parental behaviours (Table 13.2, p. 419) such as delay in seeking medical treatment for the child and histories that are inconsistent with observed injuries, vague or absent among a range of factors which help clinicians to distinguish inflicted injuries from accidents.

Other studies have highlighted combinations of factors such as inconsistent history with injuries at admission; parental characteristics such as substance misuse, earlier social work intervention, and past history of child abuse or neglect (Goldstein et al. 1993). In another, higher incidence rates of specific types of injuries with delay in seeking treatment (Tzioumi and Oates 1998) were noted.

In a study in Newcastle upon Tyne, England, San Lazaro (2000) noted that 47% of her sample had been taken to accident and emergency departments on at least two occasions before the head injuries were sustained. In that study, 61% of the children were the result of unplanned pregnancies and it was noted that families had undergone fairly significant changes in circumstances prior to injuries.

The Scottish pilot study noted domestic abuse and mental health problems, and to a lesser extent substance misuse and troubled childhoods in the families studied. One child was admitted to hospitals on three occasions before the head injury, while another child had a sibling who was the focus of a child protection investigation at the time of injury. Congenital disability was a factor in one of the cases.

A literature review of abusers in NAHIs concludes that our knowledge of the psychological and biological characteristics of abusers remains imperfect (Hobart Davies and Garwood 2001) and that more work is needed to understand relationships between these, care of a child and other as yet unidentified factors. Nevertheless, the authors noted the predominance of males in the literature; the consensus that in most cases, although not all, abusers sought to control specific behaviours such as crying which were aversive to them; and the lack of evidence thus far on birth order and sex (combinations of child and parent/caregiver) as risk factors.

There is consensus in the wider child protection research literature that mental health problems, substance misuse and domestic abuse may adversely affect parenting capacity in a number of ways such as psychological unavailability, volatility of mood, lack of awareness of physical dangers, diversion of money and material resources from child care, distorted attributions and misperception of normative infant behaviours (Cleaver et al. 1999). Important lessons from these authors' overview study of the literature on parenting capacity are that: (1) children's vulnerability is increased when parental mental health problems or substance misuse coexist with domestic abuse, and (2) as an investigation progresses, the prevalence of these issues will increase incrementally.

Specific studies reviewed by Milner and Dopke (1997) and summarized in Hobart Davies and Garwood (2001) focus more closely on parenting capacity and variables in NAHIs cases. They consider: psychophysiological factors; pyschopathology; isolation and social support; the caregiver–child relationship; child behaviour; infant temperament and caregiver sensitivity; expectations, perceptions, and attributions regarding child behaviour; and situational factors.

The literature on crying is pertinent to several of those variables and suggests that this is often the trigger that precipitates the assault on the child by a caregiver (Carty and Ratcliffe 1995). Hobart Davies and Garwood (2001) tentatively propose an heuristic for use in risk assessments while calling for more research focused on the complex and dynamic interrelationships of variables. Difficult infant behaviour, attribution of infant behaviour, substance misuse, parent physiological reactivity, stress overload, and poor coping impulse control are proximal risk factors that are associated with the shaking incident. Distal factors that may help professionals in identifying high-risk families in secondary prevention strategies include the parents' own development and histories, psychopathology, parent sensitivity/attachment, expectations of infant behaviour, infant temperament, and isolation/ social support.

Finally, the literature on prognosis is particularly relevant in assessment and decision-making in NAHI cases. A review of child maltreatment literature (Jones 1998) identified the following features as significant in predicting the chances of good outcomes for children:
- the absence of residual disability, developmental delay, or special educational needs despite abuse
- less severe forms of abuse or neglect
- non-abusive or corrective relationships with peers, siblings or a supportive adult
- ability in children to develop healthy attributions about the abuse they experienced
- children and families who are both able and willing to cooperate with agencies and who participate in therapeutic work
- good partnerships between professionals and families
- children and families who are able to address psychological aspects of the abuse.

ISSUES ARISING IN PRACTICE
Role and task in the early phases of work with the child's family
Mok (Chapter 13) and Wheeler (Chapter 14) have explored the investigation of NAHIs from a medical and police perspective. From the social work perspective, the main purpose of

investigation is to protect the child from further abuse and to promote their welfare together with that of any siblings in the household. (The initial planning meeting will determine whether emergency legal measures are necessary to protect the injured child and any siblings). The findings of medical and police colleagues are vital to that endeavour.

Similarly, the work carried out by social workers contributes to the work of medical and police colleagues. Hudlett (2001) has noted that social work intervention is guided by the unifying principle of "What is best for the child? . . . Everything the social worker will research, observe, gather and take into account and analyze will culminate in an assessment that will set into motion the plans and processes that will best reintegrate the broken child."

The network created by social workers within hospital, primary health, community, and criminal justice settings is recognized by Wheeler (Chapter 14) as an important conduit for information.

Distinctive features of NAHI cases include:
- The child is unable to give an account of what happened
- Medical colleagues may determine what has happened to a child but will be unable to say who caused the injuries. The time of injuries will also be difficult to establish
- Awareness that deficient assessment may contribute to a child's return to a home where abuse is repeated (Showers and Apolo 1986, Alexander et al. 1990, Fischer and Allasio 1994, Hudlett 2001) or disproportionate intervention which places the family at risk of 'system abuse' (Scottish Executive 2000). Careful planning of the investigation is vital.
- Time factors are important in the planning process: clinical investigations may span a number of days before conclusions can by drawn by medical colleagues; police investigations may result in an abuser being identified and charged within a short space of time or may be inconclusive as a result of insufficient evidence; the injured child may need treatment spanning days or weeks
- The seriousness of the case will be felt acutely: the possibility exists of a child death and a murder enquiry by police colleagues (Wheeler 2002).

The research literature reviewed in this chapter illustrates the many facets to be addressed in assessment and decision-making, with information and observations drawn from a wide range of sources. In addition to the child protection register, hospital (including accident and emergency departments), social work, housing and primary health records, consideration is also given to adult services (e.g. mental health, drug and alcohol and criminal justice) since there is some UK evidence that specialization of services sometimes reinforces the separation between services for adults and for children, with consequences for the sharing of concerns and information (Hetherington 2001, Centre for Research on Families and Relationships 2002). The assessment is also strengthened by eliciting information about the way any services have been used in the past, i.e. whether there was cooperation and good outcomes, since this will indicate how services offered in the future might be perceived. Where there was a poor outcome, further enquiries may reveal reasons, e.g. lack of self-esteem and self-efficacy in one or both parents, and the possible contribution of domestic abuse, mental health problems, or substance misuse.

The emotional atmosphere is likely to be particularly highly charged in the early stages of intervention and will be expressed in a wide range of ways including grief, anger, hostility, sadness, bewilderment and shock. The police investigation may or may not identify the person responsible for the injuries. Whatever the outcome, caution in interpreting expressed emotion prematurely is necessary (Hudlett 2001, Vendola 2002). For non-abusing parents or caregivers and extended family members, there is considerable emotional work necessary to process what has happened to the child, to accept that someone close to them may have inflicted injuries and to begin to appreciate consequences for the child, the relationship, extended family, their community status, and material matters such as income and housing. Carers who have been responsible for the abuse may also express a range of emotions. Contact with family members in the early phase of work allows for observation and interpretation of reactions on a number of occasions.

In interviews with parents and caregivers, clarity of language is important (Hudlett 2001) and attention to commonly used terms may be helpful in understanding the social context and relationship dynamics. Mok (Chapter 13) has discussed 'single parent' which may mean a single parent living alone or may encompass a parent with partner(s) who may or may not live in the household. Other examples are 'father' (birth father or stepfather) and 'shared care'. Assertions that care of the child is shared by both parents may for instance, mask feelings of resentment, emasculation and shame in some men if, for example, other forms of status such as employment and material success are denied them. The use of genograms and ecomaps aids clarity and understanding (Reder and Duncan 1999).

Sustaining intervention following the child's discharge from hospital
Where an abuser is identified and charged with an offence, consequences for other carers, the surviving child, and any siblings may include loss of income, a house move, unwelcome notoriety in a neighbourhood, and partisan behaviours in extended family and friends. These are additional stressors in what is already a complex situation. The provision of practical services and emotional support to adults is likely to be important while the assessment continues. However, professionals are mindful of the necessity to keep the child and siblings at the centre of their attention. Differential time scales within civil and criminal justice systems may also contribute to the complexity of the case especially if incidents occur such as the breach of bail conditions. In all cases, close cooperation between medical personnel, child protection staff, and the judicial system is critically important (Showers and Apolo 1986).

In situations where an abuser is not identified but where NAHIs are confirmed, decision-making for the injured child and siblings is rendered very difficult. Farmer and Owen's (1995) study of child protection plans analysed the level of agreement between professionals and families on commission (who abused or neglected a child), culpability (who was to blame), and risk (how likely was abuse or neglect to recur). Their study showed that social workers were more likely to have to manage situations where there was no agreement at all on these factors or where there was agreement on only two. Agreement on all three was relatively rare (18% of the sample). In NAHI cases where no abuser has been identified, workers may encounter perceptions of the child's situation, which differ markedly from their own and their colleagues'. Additionally, it is not unusual for the lack of criminal proceedings to be viewed as proof that intervention in the family by professionals in matters of child care is unwarranted intrusion. Misunderstanding of civil (child protection) and criminal processes, and the different levels of proof needed in them, underlies this, and explanation of the differences is necessary.

In some cases, minimization of the shaking incident and the outcomes for the child has been noted. Comments from a family member to the effect that, "It was a one-off" or "at least he didn't die" may provide insights into family dynamics, parenting capacity and the implications for the child's future.

Implications of the outcomes of head injuries

The poor outcomes for children with NAHIs in neurological, developmental, social and behavioural terms are highly significant in assessment and decision-making. Children at high risk of NAHIs are vulnerable by virtue of their size, extreme youth, physical immaturity, and family and social circumstances. Their vulnerability is compounded by the consequences of injuries and the turbulence experienced by families in the period following admission to hospital.

Assessment and decision-making are continuous processes, which need to take account of, and react to, changes in circumstances as they occur. This necessitates the best possible engagement with family members and close networking with professionals charged with follow-up assessment, treatment and therapies in order to ascertain the progress made by the child and to continue the assessment of parenting capacity.

The emotional impact of caring for a child who has sustained NAHIs is considerable for parents, siblings and extended family members. The literature emphasizes the importance of adaptation to the realities of the child's condition and needs over a period of time and the implications for professionals in the amount and detail of information provided during this period (Splaingard 2001).

Additionally, the practical aspects of care are likely to be more complex and may necessitate domiciliary support services, financial review, help with transport, housing moves, or adaptations and respite care.

Where the injured child is placed in an out-of-home placement, foster carers will need the same attention to emotional and practical support from their workers.

Practical and emotional support to the family in conjunction with the range of treatment and therapies provided by colleagues in health services contribute to the achievement of a good outcome for the child and any siblings. An example from the Scottish pilot study is help given to the non-abusing carer to prepare a simple account of what happened to her child in readiness for conversations with parents of accidentally injured children in hospitals and clinics.

There remains, however, the necessity to review risk assessments throughout the intervention. Lack of compliance with medical advice, inappropriate use of medication, and missed appointments, particularly when these occur despite advice, support and practical help, are alerting signs as are more general signs of neglect.

Throughout the intervention, awareness of the wider literature on children with disabilities will inform assessment (Westcott and Cross 1996, Kennedy 2002) including vulnerability to rejection, segregation, stigmatization (Wolfensberger 1972) and abuse (Garbarino 1987).

471

Violence and aggression

The investigation and assessment may reveal that the child's injuries took place in a situation where parents or caregivers have histories marked by violence and aggression. Information on earlier crimes of violence may emerge and if so, will be integrated into risk assessments. Clear and regular communication with criminal justice services will benefit assessment and decision-making in relation to the child and the abuser (court reports, aggression risk assessments, parole and after-care).

Domestic abuse may also be identified, and the extensive literature on this topic encompasses frequency and severity of injury to adult victims (Dobash and Dobash 1992, Kelly 1992, Hester and Radford 1995) and the psychological consequences for adult victims who may also be parents, e.g. entrapment, degradation, and loss of self-esteem and self-efficacy (Kirkwood 1993). The difficulties involved in leaving abusive relationships, and the potential for the risk of violence to adults and children to increase when a move is effected, have been documented (Pahl 1985, Kirkwood 1993). In these circumstances, adult victims' reactions to workers from statutory agencies may be clouded by fear of the consequences of their intervention, e.g. children being removed from their care.

The psychological and emotional impact of domestic abuse on children is known to have long-term adverse consequences for their development and functioning (Margolin and Gordis 2000). Work by Zeanah et al. (1999) has shown that children as young as 6 weeks old display signs of disturbance in reaction to domestic abuse incidents.

An understanding of domestic abuse issues may illuminate understanding of circumstances prior to the NAHIs including the fact that the child may have been adversely affected prior to the physical assault. In the period following discharge from hospital, case management will need to address additional complex factors in keeping the child, siblings and victimized parents safe. The physical, emotional and psychological effects of domestic abuse on a parent coupled with care for a child who has sustained serious abuse, carry significant implications for assessment, decision-making and the provision of services.

The Scottish pilot study, for example, revealed how intimidation of a victim may continue through telephone calls and mail despite the abuser's separation from the family. The benefits of longer-term social work intervention for mothers – and their children – as they emerged from abusive relationships were also evident. The ability to return to an agency for help when it was needed was both desired and welcomed.

Longer-term considerations

The practical issues raised here are a small selection of those likely to be encountered in NAHI cases.

Two final points should be made. Differential time scales are recognized to be features in work with families where adult problems coexist with child care concerns, i.e. an adult's recovery or ability to change circumstances may take more time to achieve than is reasonable for a child to wait given their more immediate developmental needs.

The importance of time scales was a theme in the Scottish pilot study. The criminal justice system, when invoked, moved at a slower pace than the civil child protection system and child care decisions had to be made while awaiting the outcome of a criminal trial.

There is also a tension between the processes of deregistration, the revocation of statutory orders, the longer-term needs of children and families, and resources. Where risk to a child is reduced and good outcomes are achieved, deregistration and the revocation of orders are clearly appropriate. However, the literature shows we are only just beginning to understand the longer-term implications for children with NAHIs and to appreciate the types of support and intervention that will be most beneficial in later years. The study by Andrew et al. (1998), for example, suggests that the social and behavioural problems identified have considerable implications for the child's well-being, family stress, school, leisure and community activities. More work in follow-up studies should illuminate our understanding of the challenges faced by children who have been injured and their families, and the implications for professional intervention and resources over a number of years. Findings are likely to provide additional evidence for the support of primary and secondary prevention strategies.

The pilot study and the database of Scottish cases of NAHI

The Royal Hospital for Sick Children in Edinburgh is a centre for research into NAHI. The NAHI multidisciplinary interest group meets to share findings and agreed that not enough was known about the management of NAHI cases in civil and criminal justice processes. Permission and access to records were granted by health and social work agencies so that a small scale, cross-case analysis study could be carried out during 2000/2001. A sample of five cases was selected from the database by Minns and coworkers. It was acknowledged at the outset that sample size and methodology would preclude generalization across similar NAHI cases and would be more akin to a 'snapshot' at a particular point in time. Nevertheless, it was anticipated that the study would highlight issues in decision-making, which would provide useful pointers for practice in shaken baby syndrome cases and a foundation for a funding bid for a larger study based on the database.

The pilot study used four sources of data: (1) the research database (see Chapter 4); (2) medical records; (3) social work records in the hospital and the community; (4) discussions with medical staff and social workers in the hospital and the community.

Its aims were to examine a small sample of cases where NAHIs had occurred and to explore both the ways in which decision-making and available information were used in civil and criminal processes, and the relation between decision-making and the outcomes for the children involved, i.e. protection from significant harm and responses to children in need.

FINDINGS: THE CHILDREN'S CIRCUMSTANCES PRIOR TO AND AT THE POINT OF ADMISSION TO HOSPITAL

Participating children

There were three boys and two girls in the sample group. The children were between 5 weeks and 31 weeks old when the injuries occurred, with four of them no older than 12 weeks when admitted to hospital. One child died soon after admission and the other four children survived.

Of the five children, three were first-born children while the other two were the second child in their families. Two appeared to have had uncomplicated births and good health in the early weeks, one had a slightly more complicated birth and good health subsequently, and information was not available on one child. One child was born preterm, had a low birthweight and was diagnosed with a craniosyntosis syndrome.

Parents: relationships, rights and responsibilities
One child was born to parents who were married to one another and both had parental rights and responsibilities.

Three children were born to birth parents who lived in the same household, and one child was born into a family where the birth mother was living with her partner (the child's stepfather). Information was not available on whether the four men had acquired parental rights and responsibilities.

Contact with universal services and any early concerns about the children
All five children were in families in contact with their GPs and health visitors although contact was limited in one case. The child with the disability was causing concern to the health visitor because of poor weight gain and concerns around handling in the home. A child protection investigation had begun when the injuries occurred. A child protection investigation was underway in another family in relation to a sibling when the child in the study sustained NAHIs. Three families were not involved with social work services prior to the children's admissions to hospital with NAHI.

There were no records of any deaths of children in the families at an earlier time. Of the children who had older siblings, one sibling had received Accident and Emergency department treatment and was the focus of a child protection investigation when the child in the sample group was injured. Of the children in the study, one child had been seen in an Accident and Emergency department or admitted to hospital on three known occasions prior to the admission with NAHI. The child protection investigation had been underway when the head injuries occurred.

Parents' histories and circumstances
The mothers in the sample group were aged between 18 and 22 years while the fathers/step-father were aged between 19 and 25 years.

There was more detail on the mothers' circumstances than the fathers' in the records studied, and issues such as presence or absence of mental health problems, substance misuse, domestic abuse, and childhoods marked by traumatic loss and change were not recorded in all cases. Nevertheless, records noted that one family had all four of these factors, one family had three of these factors, two families had two factors, and records were unavailable for the remaining family. Domestic abuse and mental health problems were noted in particular.

Employment details were not available in two cases. Two families had neither parent in employment, and in one family both parents were employed, the mother having returned to employment soon after the birth.

Three of the families in the pilot study were recorded in hospital records as belonging to Social Class 5 (Office for National Statistics), while no category was recorded for the remaining two families. Perhaps not surprisingly, more information about the adults' own histories, including employment, was recorded for the families deemed to belong to Social Class 5 than for those who were not ascribed a Social Class category.

Treatment of the injuries, explanations of injuries, and acceptance of responsibility
All the children were diagnosed with serious NAHIs. One child died shortly after admission, and the treatment of the other children ranged from 10 days to almost 7 weeks.

Explanations were provided for the head injuries in four cases. In the fifth case an explanation was offered for an earlier injury but not for the head injuries. Explanations changed over time; two different accounts were given in three cases, and three accounts in one case (the final accounts being the ones where responsibility was admitted for injuries or where an individual was charged with an offence). Earlier explanations included a third party's handling of the child, accidents caused by siblings, and children slipping from a parent's arms.

In four of the five cases, the birth father admitted responsibility for the injuries or was charged with causing them. The child's crying was mentioned frequently as a trigger incident.

FINDINGS; THE OUTCOMES OF DECISIONS TAKEN WITHIN CIVIL AND CRIMINAL JUSTICE PROCESSES
Action taken to protect the child
All five children were admitted to hospital. A child protection order was taken in one case. The other three surviving children were not subject to emergency legal protection measures.

Case conferences were held about all the surviving children and siblings between 7 and 18 days after admission. The conference about the child who died took place after the trial of the person accused of inflicting the fatal injuries.

All the surviving children were registered under the category of certain physical abuse and siblings were also registered on the child protection register.

All the surviving children were referred to the Reporter to the Children's Hearing System (Grounds section 52 [2] [d] of the Children [Scotland] Act 1995 and section 52 [2] [e] where applicable to siblings). In three cases, supervision requirements were imposed on the children in the sample group and any siblings. In two of these cases, the family home was specified, and in the third case, an out-of-home placement was initially made. Where a supervision requirement was not imposed, work was carried out under section 56 (4) (b).

Criminal justice system
No charges were preferred in the case where no one admitted responsibility for the injuries. The father of the child who died was charged with murder and remanded in custody. The charges against the other three fathers were under section 12 of the Children and Young Persons Act (1937) in one case and section 14 of the Criminal Procedures (Scotland) Act 1995 in the other two. The three men were bailed, with varying conditions ranging from no access to any children, to supervised access to the child in the study. Bail conditions were breached frequently in two of the cases.

475

Convictions and disposals

One father was convicted of murder and sentenced to life imprisonment. Two fathers were convicted of causing severe injury and endangerment to health with a custodial sentence in one case and a community-based sentence in the other. The outcome of one trial was not known. Interim and then full exclusion orders were necessary in one case to protect the children.

The children in the sample group at the point of data analysis

The surviving children were between 23 months and almost 3½ years old when the data were analysed. All were registered as having special needs, and sequelae included seizures, delay in some or all areas of development, poor head growth, weakness on one side of the body, and divergent squints. One child appeared to be meeting developmental milestones, although this was relatively early in the follow-up period.

All the children had had their names removed from the child protection register at the point of data analysis. None of the children had been subjected to further abuse at the point when data were analysed.

The supervision requirement had been discharged in one case, had been varied in another to give greater protection to the child, and one child had been freed for adoption. In the fifth case, work had taken place under section 56 (4) (b) of the Children (Scotland) Act 1995.

At the point of data analysis, the children in the sample group were in noticeably different family structures from those at the time of their injuries with new stepfathers and siblings in some of the families.

Conclusion

This chapter has explored aspects of assessment and decision-making from a social work perspective. It has explored the way in which social workers are required to respond in enquiry and investigation work, the principles of sound risk and welfare assessment and some of the implications for longer-term involvement with children and their families. The pilot study provided valuable insights into the management of NAHI cases in civil and criminal processes in Scotland. A larger scale study is planned which will draw on the extensive research database and a wider range of agency sources.

ACKNOWLEDGEMENTS

Grateful thanks are extended to all the professionals at the Royal Hospital for Sick Children in Edinburgh and to the local authority for participating in the pilot study.

REFERENCES

Alexander R, Crabbe L, Sato Y, Smith W, Bennett T (1990) Serial abuse in children who are shaken. *Am J Dis Child* **144**: 58–60.

Andrew TK, Rose FD, Johnson DA (1998) Social and behavioural effects of traumatic brain injury in children. *Brain Injury* **12**: 133–138

Barlow KM, Minns RA (2000) Annual incidence of shaken impact syndrome in young children. *Lancet* **356**: 1571–1572.

Barlow KM, Milne S, Aitken K, Minns RA (1998) A retrospective epidemiological analysis of non-accidental head injury in children in Scotland over a 15 year period. *Scot Med J* **43**: 112–114.

Bonnier C, Nassogne MC, Evrard P (1995) Outcome and prognosis of whiplash shaken infant syndrome: Late consequences after a symptom-free interval. *Dev Med Child Neurol* **37**: 943–956.

Bonnier C, Nassogne MC, St Martin C, Mesplies B, Kadhim H, Sebire G (2003) Neuroimaging of intra-parenchymal lesions predicts outcomes in shaken baby syndrome. *Pediatrics* **112**: 808–814.

Carty H, Ratcliffe J (1995) The shaken infant syndrome: Parents and other carers need to know of its dangers. *BMJ* **310**: 344–345.

Centre for Research on Families and Relationships (2002) Family policy in Scotland. Research briefing. *Child Fam Social Work* **2**: 109–120.

Children (Scotland) Act 1995. Edinburgh: HMSO.

Cleaver H, Unell I, Aldgate J (1999) *Children's Needs – Parenting Capacity. The Impact of Parental Mental Illness, Problem Alcohol and Drug Use, and Domestic Abuse on Children's Development*. London: HMSO.

Cleaver H, Walker S, Meadow P (2002) *Assessing Children's Needs and Circumstances; the Impact of the Assessment Framework. Summary and Recommendations*. London: Department of Health.

Cobley C, Sanders T, Wheeler P (2003) Prosecuting cases of suspected shaken baby syndrome – a review of current issues. *Crim Law Rev* **Feb**: 93–106.

Dale P, Green R, Fellows R (2002) Babies in danger. *Commun Care* **7–13 March**: 34–35.

Department of Health (1991) *Child Abuse: A Study of Inquiry Reports 1980-1989*. London: HMSO.

Department of Health (1995) *Child Protection: Messages from Research*. London: HMSO.

Department of Health (2000) *Framework for the Assessment of Children in Need and their Families*. London: HMSO.

Dobash RE, Dobash RP (1992) The nature and antecedents of violent events. *Br J Criminol* **24**: 269–288.

Farmer E, Owen M (1995) *Child Protection Practice: Private Risks and Public Remedies*. London: HMSO.

Fischer H, Allasio D (1994) Permanently damaged; long-term follow-up of shaken babies. *Clin Pediatr* **33**: 696–698.

Frude N (2003) A framework for assessing the physical abuse of children. In: Calder MC, Hackett S, eds. *Assessment in Child Care: Using and Developing Frameworks for Practice*. Lyme Regis, Dorset: Russell House Publishing, pp. 193–213.

Garbarino J (1986) Where does social support fit into optimising human development and preventing dysfunction? *Br J Social Work* **16** (Suppl): 23–37.

Garbarino J (1987) *Special Children-Special Risks: The Maltreatment of Children with Disabilities*. New York: De Gruyter.

Garbarino J (1992) *Children and Families in the Social Environment*. New York: De Gruyter.

Goldstein B, Kelly MM, Bruton D, Cox C (1993) Inflicted versus accidental head injury in critically injured children. *Crit Care Med* **21**: 1328–1332.

Haviland J, Russell RIR (1997) Outcome after severe non-accidental head injury. *Arch Dis Child* **77**: 504–507.

Hester M, Radford L (1995) Safety matters! Domestic violence and child contact, towards an inter-disciplinary response. *Represent Child* **8**: 49–60.

Hetherington R (2001) How the law and welfare combine for children and families where is parental mental illness: inter-country comparisons of professional practice. *Soc Work Eur* **8**: 29–36.

Hobart Davies W, Garwood MM. (2001) Who are the perpetrators and why do they do it? In: Lazoritz S, Palusci VJ, eds. *The Shaken Baby Syndrome: A Multidisciplinary Approach*. New York: Haworth Maltreatment & Trauma Press, pp. 41–54.

Hudlett J. (2001) The medical social worker, child advocacy and the shaken baby. In: Lazoritz S, Palusci VJ, eds. *The Shaken Baby Syndrome: A Multidisciplinary Approach*. New York: Haworth Maltreatment & Trauma Press, pp. 225–236.

Jenny C, Hymel Lt Col KP, Ritzen A, Reinert SE, Hay TC (1999) Analysis of missed cases of abusive head trauma. *JAMA* **281**: 621–626.

Jones DPH (1998) The effectiveness of intervention. In: Adcock M, White R, eds. *Significant Harm: its Management and Outcome*. Croydon, Surrey: Significant Publications.

Kelly L (1992) The connection between disability and child abuse: a review of the research evidence. *Child Abuse Rev* **1**, 157–167.

Kennedy M (1997) Disability and child abuse. In: Wilson K, James A, eds. *The Child Protection Handbook, 2nd edn*. London: Bailliere Tindall, pp. 147–171.

477

Kirkwood C (1993) *Leaving Abusive Partners: From the Scars of Survival to the Wisdom for Change*. London: Sage.

Ludwig S, Warman M (1984) Shaken baby syndrome: A review of 20 cases. *Ann Emerg Med* **13**: 104–107.

Margolin G, Gordis EB (2000) The effects of family and community violence on children. *Ann Rev Psychiatr* **51**: 445–479.

McCarrick C, Over A, Wood P (2000) A framework for assessment in child protection. In: Baldwin N, ed. *Protecting Children, Promoting Their Rights*. London: Whiting & Birch, pp. 186–221.

Minuchin S (1974) *Families and Family Therapy*. London: Tavistock.

Moore B (1996) *Risk Assessment: A Practitioner's Guide to Predicting Harmful Behaviour*. London: Whiting & Birch.

Morrison T (1997) Emotional competence in child protection organizations: Fallacy, fiction or necessity. In: Bates J, Pugh R, Thompson N, eds. *Protecting Children: Challenges and Change*. Aldershot, Hampshire: Ashgate Publishing, pp. 193–211.

Munro E (1999) Common errors of reasoning in child protection work. *Child Abuse Negl* **23**: 745–758.

Munro E (2002) *Effective Child Protection*. London: Sage Publications.

O'Brien S (2003) *Report of the Caleb Ness Inquiry*. Edinburgh: Edinburgh & the Lothians Child Protection Committee.

Pahl J (1985) *Private Violence and Public Policy*. London: Routledge &d Kegan Paul.

Petrie S, James AL (2002) Partnership with parents. In: Wilson K, James AL, editors. *The Child Protection Handbook, 2nd edn*. London: Bailliere Tindall, pp. 387–402.

Palazzoli M, Bossolo L, Cecchin E, Prata G (1978) *Paradox and Counter Paradox*. New York: Jason Aronson.

Parrish R (2001) *Executive Summary April 2001 of the Third National Conference on Shaken Baby Syndrome*. Ogden, UT: National Center on Shaken Baby Syndrome.

Reder P, Duncan S (1999) *Lost Innocents: A Follow Up Study of Fatal Child Abuse*. London: Routledge.

San Lazaro C (2000) Injuries from bouncy chairs. Paper presented at the BASPCAN Study Day on Subdural Bleeds, Leeds, 19 May 2000.

Scottish Executive (2000) *Protecting Children: A Shared Responsibility, Guidance for Health Professionals in Scotland*. Edinburgh: Scottish Executive Health Department.

Scottish Executive (2002) *It's Everyone's Job to Make Sure I'm Alright. Report of the Child Protection Audit and Review*. Edinburgh: HMSO.

Scottish Office (1998) *Protecting Children: A Shared Responsibility. Guidance on Inter-Agency Co-operation*. Edinburgh: HMSO.

Showers J, Apolo J (1986) Criminal disposition of persons involved in 72 cases of fatal child abuse. *Med Sci Law* **26**: 243–247.

Splaingard M (2001) Brain injury rehabilitation in children with non-accidental trauma. In: Lazoritz S, Palusci VJ, eds. *The Shaken Baby Syndrome: A Multidisciplinary Approach*. New York: Haworth Maltreatment & Trauma Press, pp. 225–236.

Tzioumi D, Oates RK (1998) Subdural haematomas in children under 2 years. Accidental of inflicted? A 10 year experience. *Child Abuse Negl* **22**: 1105–1112.

Vendola MJ (2002) Dynamics of the non-offending mother. SBS Quarterly **Spring**: 1–3, 6–7.

Westcott H, Cross M (1996) *This Far and No Further: Towards Ending the Abuse of Disabled Children*. Birmingham: Venture Press.

Wheeler P (2002) *A Report into the Police Investigation of Shaken Baby Murders and Assaults in the United Kingdom*. London: The Home Office.

Wheeler P, McDonagh M (2001) *Shaken Baby Syndrome*. CD-ROM. London: Home Office Police Research Award Scheme.

Wolfensberger W (1972) *The Principle of Normalization in Human Services*. Toronto: National Institute on Mental Retardation.

Zeanah C, Boris N, Heller S, Hinshaw-Fuselier S, Larrieu J, Lewis J, Palomino R, Roviaris M, Valliere J (1997) Relationshp assessment in infant mental health. *Inf Ment Health J* **18**: 182–197.

Zeanah C, Danis B, Hirshberg L, Benoit D, Miller D, Heller S (1999) Disorganized attachment associated with partner violence: a research note. *Inf Ment Health J* **20**: 77–86.

GLOSSARY OF TERMS

Nina Punt

acute – of rapid onset; in some contexts, implies of recent onset

aetiology – the cause of a disease

afebrile – without fever, normal body temperature

agonist – a substance that acts on cells to produce an effect similar to one of the body's normal chemical messengers; cf. antagonist

albumin – blood protein sometimes given intravenously to treat shock

alopecia – absence of hair from places where it would normally grow

amblyopia – poor sight not due to any detectable disease

amniocentesis – withdrawal of a sample of fluid from around a baby in the uterus in order to test for abnormalities such as Down syndrome or spina bifida

anaemia – reduction of the oxygen-carrying pigment, haemoglobin, in the blood

angiogram – imaging of the blood vessels produced either by X-rays (conventional invasive angiography) after injection of radio-opaque material, or by special magnetic resonance imaging (MR angiography, q.v.)

anorexia – loss of appetite

anoxia – a lack of oxygen in the tissues

antagonist – a substance that produces an opposite effect to one of the body's normal chemical messengers, or to another drug, which it inhibits; cf. agonist

anterior – towards the front

anterior fontanelle – the more frontal of the openings in the skull of a baby where the coronal, frontal, and sagittal sutures have not yet closed together; the 'soft spot'

antero-posterior – from the front to the back, i.e. a face-on view

antibiotics – substances used to treat infections caused by certain organisms, usually bacteria

anticonvulsant – a drug that reduces the frequency or severity of epileptic seizures

Apgar score – a method of rapidly assessing the general state (breathing, heart rate, colour, muscle tone, and response to stimuli) of a baby immediately after birth; an infant scoring 10 points at five minutes after birth would be in optimum condition

aphasia – a language disorder affecting the content and generation of speech

apnoea – stopping of breathing from any cause

apoptosis – genetically-programmed cell death with no inflammatory reaction; cf. necrosis

APTT – one of the clotting factors in the blood

arachnoid – the middle of the three membranes covering the brain and spinal cord

arrhythmia – any deviation from the normal rhythm of the heart

artefact – something made by man, or a computer, that makes a disease or abnormality appear to be present, e.g. faulty staining of a microscope slide

arteriovenous malformation – a cluster of abnormal blood vessels on or in the brain or spinal cord, which may burst and/or cause epilepsy

artificial respiration or ventilation – a procedure for maintaining the flow of air into and out of a patient's lungs by way of mouth-to-mouth respiration or, in hospital, a mechanical respirator or ventilator

aspiration – the withdrawal of fluid from the body by means of suction, usually through a syringe

astrocyte – a type of cell found throughout the central nervous system

asystole – a condition in which the heart no longer beats

ataxia – shaky limb movements and/or unsteady gait caused by the brain being unable to coordinate limb movements properly

atrophy – the wasting away of a normally developed organ or tissue due to degeneration of cells; occurs through under-nourishment, disuse or ageing, or following damage

attenuation – the extent to which beams of X-rays are reduced by passing through body tissues

autonomic – refers to bodily functions that are not under conscious control, such as heartbeat, salivation, etc.

autopsy, *see* post-mortem examination

avulsion – forcible separation, e.g. the scalp being torn away from the skull bone

axial – through the body, as to divide it into upper and lower parts

axon – a nerve fibre

axoplasm – the semifluid material within an axon

basal cisterns – the cerebrospinal fluid spaces around the base of the brain

basal ganglia – large masses of grey matter buried within the white matter of the cerebrum. These are involved with voluntary movements at a subconscious level

benign communicating hydrocephalus – a condition seen in the first 18 months of life in which there is abnormally rapid head growth and some enlargement of the cerebral ventricles; it is called benign because it is self-limiting, only very rarely requires treatment, and is not associated with any complications

bilateral – relating to both sides of the body or of an organ, or both of a pair of organs, e.g. the eyes; cf. unilateral

bilirubin – the breakdown products of haemoglobin; *see* jaundice

biopsy – the removal of a small piece of tissue for microscopic examination

blood culture – checking a blood sample for infection by micro-organisms

blood pressure – the pressure of blood against the walls of the main arteries

blood sugar (blood glucose) level – the concentration of glucose in the blood

bolus – a soft mass of chewed food, a liquid, or a pharmaceutical preparation that is ready to be swallowed

bone window views – electronic manipulation of CT scans to examine bones, e.g. the skull; performed at the same time as CT to examine the soft tissues, e.g. the brain, during a head scan

bradycardia – slowing of the heart rate to less than 50 beats per minute

brainstem – the enlarged extension upwards within the skull of the spinal cord

brainstem death – the permanent functional death of the centres in the brainstem that control breathing, circulation, pupillary and other vital reflexes

brittle bone disease – *see* osteogenesis imperfecta

burr hole – a circular hole drilled through the skull for the release of intracranial tension or to facilitate procedures such as biopsy or pressure measurement

callus formation – the mass, containing bone-forming cells, that forms around bone ends following a fracture

calvarium – the vault, or top part, of the skull

canthus – the angle at which the upper and lower eyelids meet

capillary refill time – the time it takes for the small blood vessels (the capillaries) to refill with blood after pressure has been exerted; a slow capillary refill time would indicate a state of shock

cardiopulmonary resuscitation (CPR) – attempts to restart the beating of the heart and restart spontaneous breathing

cardiorespiratory arrest – when the heart stops beating and breathing ceases

cardiotochography – the electrical monitoring of the fetal heart rate and rhythm, plus measurement of the strength and frequency of the maternal uterine contractions

carotid arteries – two main arteries, situated in the neck, that supply blood to the head, neck and brain

cartilage – connective tissue on the surface of a bone within a joint

catheter – a flexible tube for insertion into a narrow opening for the introduction or removal of fluids

CAT scan – computerized (axial) tomography, q.v.

cavernous sinuses – two cavities at the base of the skull, behind the eye sockets, into which blood drains from the upper part of the head, including the brain

centile - a line on a chart or graph to measure average height, weight, etc.; for example, the 10th centile means 10% of the population will be smaller, and 90% will be bigger, at that age

central nervous system (CNS) the brain and spinal cord

centrifuge – a machine for separating components of different densities in a liquid

cephalohaematoma – a swelling on the head, usually of a newborn, caused by a collection of fluid between one of the skull bones and its covering membrane

cerebellar peduncle – the brain tissue connecting the pons and cerebellum

cerebral – referring to the cerebrum

cerebral cortex – the outer layer of the cerebrum responsible for memory, intellect, initiating voluntary activity, etc.

cerebral hemisphere – one of the two halves of the cerebrum

cerebral irritation – inflammation of, or the disturbance of the normal functioning of, the cerebrum

cerebral perfusion pressure (CPP) – the difference between blood pressure and intracranial pressure. If the cerebral perfusion pressure falls below a critical limit, brain damage will occur

cerebrospinal fluid (CSF) – the clear fluid that surrounds the brain and spinal cord and

481

fills the cerebral ventricles

cerebrum – the largest part of the brain, composed of the two cerebral hemispheres. Responsible for all voluntary activity in the body and all intelligent behaviour

cervical – relating to the neck or, alternatively, relating to the neck of an organ

cervico-medullary – describes the region at the junction of the brainstem and the cervical spinal cord

choroid – the layer of the eyeball between the retina and the sclera

choroid plexus – the areas that produce cerebrospinal fluid within the ventricles of the brain

chronic – a disease of long duration involving slow changes; in some contexts, implies the delayed effects of an event occurring some time previously

cistern – spaces outside the brain containing cerebrospinal fluid

clinical – the study of patients and their diseases, as opposed to the study of diseases in laboratory settings

clonic – rhythmical limb movements in convulsive epilepsy

CNS – central nervous system, q.v.

coagulation (blood) – the process whereby blood changes from a liquid to a solid state, i.e. clotting

coagulation screen (or coagulation profile) – a series of laboratory tests to check the ability of the blood to clot

coagulopathy – disorder of blood clotting

colic – severe abdominal pain; often, in babies, caused by wind in the intestine

comminuted fracture – a fracture where a bone is broken in more than one place

computed (computerized) tomography (CT) – the production of cross sectional 'slices' of different parts or organs the body with an X-ray scanner, using a powerful computer

concussion – a period of unconsciousness due to an injury to the brain

condyle – the rounded protuberance at the end of some bones

congenital abnormalities – abnormalities present from before birth

coning – prolapse of the brainstem through the foramen magnum as a result of raised intracranial pressure, often with damaging or fatal consequences

conjunctiva – the membrane that covers the front of the eye and lines the inside of the eyelids

contralateral – affecting the opposite side of the body, cf. ipsilateral

contrecoup – injury on the opposite side to the actual site of impact; for example, a blow to the back of the head could cause the brain to be pushed against the inside of the skull at the front; cf. coup

contusion – bruise

convexity subarachnoid space – the space between the arachnoid and the pia, over the upper surface of the brain

convulsion – an involuntary contraction of the muscles producing contortion of the body and limbs

coronal – a section through the body that would divide it into back and front parts

coronal suture – the join between the frontal and parietal bones of the skull

corpus callosum – the band of nerve tissue that connects the two cerebral hemispheres

cortical visual impairment – impairment of vision caused by damage to the brain, as

482

opposed to damage to the eyes or the nerves that run between the eyes and the brain

costo-chondral junction – the junction of rib and cartilage

coup – injury at the actual site of impact; cf. contrecoup

CPR – cardiopulmonary resuscitation, q.v.

cranial fossa (*plural* fossae) – a compartment within the skull

cranial sutures – the joins between the bones of the skull

craniectomy – an operation to open the skull, in which some of the bone is removed

cranio-cervical junction – where the skull joins on to the spine

craniotabes – small dents on the inside of the skull giving a copper-beaten effect

craniotomy – an operation to open the skull, in which a trapdoor is made in the bone

crenated – describes the crinkling of the walls of red blood cells seen in some blood
disorders or when a specimen of blood has been stored for a prolonged time

cribiform plate – the perforated bone that forms the roof of the nasal cavity, separating it
from the cranial cavity

CSF – cerebrospinal fluid, q.v.

CT – computerized tomography, q.v.

cutaneous – relating to the skin

cyanosis – bluish discoloration of the skin caused by an inadequate amount of oxygen in
the blood

cyst – an abnormal sac or cavity filled with liquid or semi-solid matter

cytotoxic – refers to a drug that damages or destroys cells by inhibiting cell division; used
to treat various types of cancer

decerebrate attacks – episodes of intermittent abnormal posturing indicative of a severe
and acute insult to the brain

defibrination – the removal of fibrin from a sample of blood

dementia – a chronic disorder of mental processing caused by organic brain disease

dendrite – the part of a neurone (nerve cell) that makes contact with other neurones and
receives nerve impulses

diabetes insipidus – a disorder of metabolism that is due to a deficiency of the pituitary
hormone vasopressin

diabetes mellitus – a disorder of metabolism that is due to a lack of the pancreatic hormone
insulin

diaphysis – the central part, or shaft, of a long bone; cf. epiphysis

diastasis – separation; *see* sutural diastasis

diastolic – referring to the measurement of blood pressure; diastolic pressure is the lower
of the two measurements, when the ventricles are relaxing; cf. systolic

diathesis – a tendency to develop certain diseases

diencephalic – refers to the midbrain (diencephalon), the highest part of the brainstem

diffuse axonal injury – widespread traumatic axonal damage in the brain

dilatation – the enlargement or expansion of a cavity or hollow organ

dilated – made larger, by instruments, drugs, or muscle action

diplopia – double vision. An awareness of two images of a single object

distal – away from the point of attachment or middle of the body, e.g. a nerve fibre that is far from the central nervous system, or the part of a limb furthest from the body

diuresis – increased output of urine by the kidneys

diuretic – a drug used to increase the volume of urine produced by the kidneys

Doppler technique – a technique that uses ultrasound waves to demonstrate the structure of tissues;it is used in the diagnosis of tumours and other soft tissue lesions, and also for investigating the functioning of the heart and arteries

dura mater (dura) – the thickest and outermost of the three coverings of the brain and spinal cord

dysphasia – a disorder of language affecting the generation and content of speech and its understanding, caused by disease of the dominant hemisphere, usually the left

dystonia – a disorder of posture caused by disease of the basal ganglia

echogenic – of an ultrasound scan, having a bright appearance due to absorption and reflection of ultrasound waves by a body tissue

EEG – electroencephalogram, q.v.

effusion – the presence of excess blood or tissue fluid in an organ, body cavity, or tissue

electroencephalogram (EEG) – the trace of a recording of electrical activity in different parts of the brain

emphysema – air in the tissues

encephalomalacia – an area of brain tissue that has wasted away as a result of disease or injury; cf. leukomalacia

encephalopathy – any of various diseases that affect the functioning of the brain

endothelium – the layer of cells that lines the heart and blood vessels, as well as the lymphatic vessels; cf. epithelium

endotracheal tube – a tube that has been introduced into the trachea, or windpipe, to aid breathing

ependyma – the membrane that lines the ventricles of the brain

epilepsy – a group of disorders of brain function characterized by recurrent attacks that have sudden onset, e.g. major (tonic/clonic or grand mal) seizures, and absences (petit mal seizures); caused by uncoordinated electrical brain activity

epileptogenic – having the capacity to provoke epileptic seizures

epiphenomenon – a symptom or event that occurs at the same time as a disease or injury, but is not the cause of the disease or injury

epiphysis – the end of a long bone; cf. diaphysis

epithelium – the tissue that covers the external surface of the body and lines hollow structures such as the stomach and bowel; cf. endothelium

erythrocyte – a red blood cell, the function of which is to transport oxygen from the lungs to the rest of the body within the arteries

ethmoid bone – one of the bones in the floor of the front part of the skull

excoriation – the destruction and removal of the surface of the skin by scraping, chemical, or other means

extensor – a muscle that causes the straightening of a limb or other part

external auditory meatus – the passage leading from the pinna (the exterior part of the ear) to the eardrum

external ventricular drain – apparatus used to drain excess cerebrospinal fluid from the cerebral ventricles to the outside, as opposed to ventricular shunting, which drains the fluid into a body cavity

extracerebral – outside the brain

extracranial – outside the skull

extradural haematoma – an accumulation of blood between the dura and the skull

exudate – the liquid that escapes through the walls of blood vessels, usually as a result of inflammation

falx cerebelli – the fold of the dura which dips inwards between the posterior parts of the cerebellar hemispheres

falx cerebri – the fold of the dura which dips inwards between the cerebral hemispheres

febrile – feverish, having a high temperature

fibrin – the final product of the process of blood clotting

fibrinogen – a coagulation factor in the blood that aids the final stage of clotting

fibrinolysis – the process by which blood clots are removed from the circulation; in health, there is a balance between coagulation and fibrinolysis in the body, and an increase of fibrinolysis leads to excessive bleeding

fibroblast – a type of cell found in connective tissue (the tissue that supports, binds or separates other tissues and organs) and also in scar tissue, but not in the brain and spinal cord; cf. glial cell

flexor – a muscle that causes bending of a limb or part of the body

focal – referring to the principal site, or a localised area, of infection or other disease

fontanelle – a skin covered opening in the skull of an infant due to the sutures having not yet closed

foramen (*plural* foramina) – an opening or hole in a bone

foramen magnum – the hole in the occipital bone, at the base of the skull, through which the spinal cord passes

formalin – a solution of formaldehyde and water used as a sterilizing agent or fixative

fossa – a depression or hollow

fovea – a small area of the retina at the back of the eye

fracture margins – the edges of bone on either side of a fracture site

frenulum – any of the folds of mucus membrane under the tongue or between the lips and the gums

frontal lobe – the anterior (front) part of each cerebral hemisphere, concerned with voluntary movement, behaviour, learning, and personality

fronto-parietal – towards the front, top and sides of the head

full blood picture – examination of the blood for any abnormalities

fundoscopy – examination of the fundus of the eye using a fundoscope

fundus (*plural* fundi) – the back of the eyeball that can be viewed through the pupil using an instrument (fundoscope)

galactosaemia – an inability to utilize the sugar galactose, which is present in milk; affected children fail to develop normally unless galactose is eliminated from their diet

gastroenteritis – inflammation of the stomach and intestines causing vomiting and diarrhoea

gastro-oesophageal reflux – a condition in which the stomach contents come up into the oesophagus because the normal mechanisms of keeping the stomach contents down are impaired in some way

gestation – the period during which a fertilized egg develops into a baby

Glasgow coma score – a system used to determine a patient's level of consciousness after a head injury: 15 is fully conscious, whereas 7 would indicate a coma

glial cells – connective tissue cells within the nervous system; cf. fibroblast

gliosis – scarring of nerve tissue in the brain or spinal cord

glutaric aciduria – a very rare inherited metabolic disorder

glycogen – carbohydrate stored in the liver and muscles

Gram stain – a method of staining bacteria cells that highlights the differences in the structure of the cell walls

grand mal seizures – *see* epilepsy

granulocyte – a type of white blood cell

greenstick fracture – an incomplete fracture of a long bone in children, their bones being more flexible and less likely to snap completely in two

grey matter – the darker coloured tissue of the central nervous system containing the cell bodies of neurones; cf. white matter

grey/white matter differentiation – the difference in appearance on scanning of the grey matter compared with the white matter of the brain

gyrus (*plural* gyri) – a raised part of the cerebral cortex between two sulci (clefts)

haematocrit – the volume of red blood cells in the blood, expressed as a fraction of the total volume of blood

haematology – the study of blood and associated disorders

haematoma – an accumulation of blood within the tissues that clots to form a solid swelling

haemoglobin – the substance in the red blood cells that transports oxygen around the body

haemorrhage – the escape of blood from a ruptured blood vessel

haemorrhagic contusions – bruises

haemorrhagic disease of the newborn – a temporary disturbance of blood clotting affecting infants on the second to fourth day of life and caused by vitamin K deficiency

haemosiderin – an insoluble substance containing iron salts present inside certain cells

heart rate – the number of times per minute that the heart pumps

hemianopia – blindness in one half of the visual field; can be unilateral, affecting only one eye

herniation – the protrusion of an organ or tissue out of its normal place in the body

heterogeneous – showing variability or difference between populations

high dependency unit – a unit for patients who do not need the very high levels of care and supervision given in the intensive treatment unit (ITU), but do require a greater level than can usually be provided on a normal hospital ward

hippocampus – a prominence in part of the temporal horn of each lateral ventricle of the brain

histology – the study of the structure of tissues using staining techniques and microscopy

homeostasis – the physiological process whereby the internal systems, such as blood pressure and temperature, are kept stable despite external conditions

homonymous hemianopia – loss of the corresponding half of the normal visual field in both eyes

hydrocephalus – an abnormal increase in the amount of cerebrospinal fluid in the ventricles of the brain; it may be caused either by an obstruction to the outflow of the fluid, or by failure of re-absorption of the fluid into the cerebral venous sinuses

hygroma – a type of fluid collection over the surface of the brain; it may develop from the liquefied remains of a subdural haematoma

hyperacute – of very rapid onset, usually in the context of radiological appearances

hyperaemia – abnormally increased blood supply to a part of the body

hypercapnia – synonym hypercarbia; excess carbon dioxide in the blood; cf. hypocapnia

hyperdensity – excessive or abnormally increased density of a tissue or fluid on CT, usually assessed with respect to brain tissue

hypernatraemia – the presence of an abnormally high concentration of sodium in the blood; cf. hyponatraemia

hypertension – elevation of the arterial blood pressure to above the normal range

hypertonia – an abnormal increase in the state of slight contraction of healthy muscles

hyperventilation – rapid breathing

hyphaema – a collection of blood in the eye in front of the iris

hypocapnia – low concentration of carbon dioxide in the blood; cf. hypercapnia

hypodensity – reduced density

hypoglycaemic – a deficiency of glucose in the bloodstream

hyponatraemia – the presence of an abnormally low concentration of sodium in the blood; occurs, for example, in dehydration

hypoplasia – underdevelopment of an organ or tissue

hypotension – reduction of the arterial blood pressure to below the normal range

hypothalamus – a region in the floor of the third ventricle where important centres for the control of body temperature, thirst, hunger, sexual function, emotions and sleep are located

hypothermia – reduction of body temperature below the normal range

hypotonia – an abnormal decrease in the state of slight contraction of healthy muscles

hypovolaemia – decrease in the volume of blood circulating the body

hypoxia – a deficiency of oxygen in the tissues

hypoxic–ischaemic brain injury – injury caused by an inadequate flow of oxygen-containing blood to the brain or part of the brain, leading to a deficiency of oxygen in the tissues

iatrogenic – a condition brought about by medical treatment

idiopathic – describing a condition or disease the cause of which is not known

immunohistochemistry – a technique used to detect microscopic amounts of chemicals within cells

infarction – the death of the whole or part of an organ occurring when the blood supply to the tissue is obstructed (e.g. by a blood clot), or diminished for long enough to cause irreversible damage

infection screen – various tests carried out to check for infection in any part of the body, e.g. urine, blood, wound swabs, etc.

infratentorial – below the tentorium

INR – a measurement of blood clotting

intensive treatment (care) unit (ITU or ICU) – a unit designed to give intensive care to a selected group of very seriously ill patients

interhemispheric – between the two cerebral hemispheres

interictal – between two epileptic seizures

intracerebral – within the cerebrum

intracranial – within the skull

intracranial pressure (ICP) – the pressure inside the skull

intraparenchymal – within the parenchyma or substance of an organ

intraretinal haemorrhage – bleeding within the retina at the back of the eye

intrathecal – within the coverings (meninges) of the brain and/or spinal cord

intravenous (i.v.) – into or within a vein

intravenous contrast enhancement – the infusion into a vein of a substance that will make certain structures and certain abnormalities of brain tissue more apparent on imaging

intraventricular haemorrhage – bleeding within the ventricles of the brain

intubation – the introduction of a tube into part of the body

ipsilateral – affecting the same side of the body; cf. contralateral

ischaemia – an inadequate flow of blood to a part of the body, caused by constriction or blockage of the blood vessels supplying it

isotonic – describing solutions that are of the same concentration

jaundice – yellowing of the skin and/or whites of the eyes caused by an excess of bilirubin in the bloodstream

laceration – a tear in tissue

lambdoid suture – the joint between the parietal and occipital bones of the skull

lamina – a thin membrane or layer of tissue

lateral – situated at, or relating to, the side of an organ or organism

lateral scout radiograph – a view taken before making a CT scan to show the plane and thickness of the slices and the extent of the area of the head that is going to be scanned

leptomeningeal cyst – a collection of fluid contained within the arachnoid membrane

lesion – an area of tissue with impaired function as a result of damage, disease, or wounding

lethargic – sluggish, inactive and/or unresponsive

leukomalacia – an area of cerebral white matter that has wasted away as a result of disease or injury; cf. encephalomalacia

leukocyte – *see* white blood cell

lumbar puncture – a procedure to take cerebrospinal fluid for examination from the dural lined sac or cavity that surrounds the spinal cord and nerve roots via a hollow needle inserted into the spinal canal through the skin; *see also* traumatic lumbar puncture

lymphocyte – a type of white blood cell that usually fights infections

lysosome – an enzyme containing structure within a cell

macrocephaly – abnormally large head; cf. microcephaly

macrophage – a scavenger cell, the purpose of which is to remove foreign material, bacteria, or dead cells; cf. microglia

macroscopic – visible to the naked eye

macula – a spot on the retina at the back of the eye

macular haemorrhage – a flat area of altered skin colour caused by bleeding under the skin

magnetic resonance angiography (MRA) – examination of the blood vessels by MRI; *see also* angiogram

magnetic resonance imaging (MRI) – a technique based on the absorption and transmission of radio waves by hydrogen protons (usually in water molecules) in tissues placed in a strong magnetic field; computers are then used to map out any variations in tissue signals, thereby producing images of the tissues

malacia – wasting away of an organ or tissue

mandible – the lower jawbone

mass effect – the displacement of brain structures by, for example, a tumour, haemorrhage or hydrocephalus

mastoid – part of the temporal bone containing the middle and inner ear

medulla oblongata – the lowest part of the brainstem

medulloblastoma – a type of brain tumour that develops most frequently in childhood

meninges – the three membranes that cover the brain and spinal cord, consisting of the dura mater (the outermost layer), the arachnoid mater, and the pia mater (the innermost layer)

meningitis – inflammation of the meninges due to infection by bacteria, viruses or chemicals; causes headache, fever, loss of appetite, dislike of light and noise, and stiff neck; unless treated promptly, can lead to seizures, damage, or even death

metabolic screen – tests to check that the metabolism is functioning correctly

metabolism – the chemical and physical changes in the body that enable it to grow and function; includes the building of tissues and organs and the release of energy

metaphysis – the growing portion of the long bones; this lies between the end of the bone and the shaft

metopic suture – the continuation of the sagittal suture, joining the frontal bones in the forehead region

microbiology – the isolation and identification of micro-organisms that cause disease

microcephaly – abnormally small head; cf. macrocephaly

microglia – scavenger cells in the central nervous system (the brain and spinal cord); cf. macrophage

microscopic – too small to be seen with the naked eye.

midline structures – structures such as the pituitary gland, hypothalamus, and corpus callosum, which are situated between the two cerebral hemispheres

mitochondria – structures concerned with energy production within cells

morbidity – refers to having an illness or disease, or a complication of treatment

MR – magnetic resonance

MRA – magnetic resonance angiography, q.v.

MRI – magnetic resonance imaging, q.v.

mucosa – the moist membrane lining tubes and cavities of the body, e.g. the nasal sinuses, the respiratory tract, the gastrointestinal tract, etc.

myelin – the sheath around the axons of certain neurones

myelomeningocele – a developmental defect whereby the backbone has not formed properly, and therefore part of the spinal cord and its coverings are exposed; often referred to as 'spina bifida'

myocardium – the specialized muscle forming the walls of the heart

nasogastric feeding – food and liquid being given to a patient via a tube that passes through the nose and into the stomach

nasotracheal tube – a tube that passes through the nose and into the trachea to aid breathing when attached to a ventilator

necrosis – cell death with marked inflammatory response; cf. apoptosis

neonatal – the time from birth up to 6 weeks old

neurodevelopment – the relationship between the nervous system and development

neurologist – a doctor who specializes in the functioning and diseases of the nervous system, including the brain, spinal cord, and peripheral nerves

neurone (nerve cell) – a specialized cell that transmits electrical nerve impulses

neuropsychological – the relationship between the nervous system and behaviour

neuroradiologist – a doctor who specializes in the interpretation of imaging (ultrasound, X-ray, CT and MRI) of the brain and spinal cord in order to diagnose disorders of the central nervous system

neurosurgeon – a surgeon who specializes in the treatment of diseases of the brain and spinal cord, such as head injuries, hydrocephalus, tumours, intracranial haemorrhage, etc.

neurotransmitter – a chemical messenger released by a nerve ending to be picked up by an adjacent nerve or muscle or gland

neurotrophic – relating to the growth of neural tissue

neutrophil – a type of white blood cell that usually fights bacterial infection

normotensive – blood pressure within the normal range

obstetric – describing the care given to women during pregnancy, birth, and up to about six weeks after the birth

occipital bone – the bone which forms the back and part of the base of the skull

occipital lobe – the part of the brain lying at the back of the head that is concerned with vision

occipitofrontal circumference – the measurement around the head at its widest point, around the forehead and the occiput

occiput – the back of the head

ocular fundus (*plural* fundi) – the back of the inside of the eye that can be seen through the pupil using an instrument

oedema – excess build-up of fluid in body tissues, often causing swelling

ophthalmologist – a doctor who studies and treats diseases of the eyes

ophthalmoscope – an instrument for examining the inside of the eye using a beam of light

opisthotonic – the arching backwards of the head, neck, and spine

optic disc – the first part of the optic nerve, at the back of the eye

optic nerve – the nerve leading from the back of the eye to the visual cortex of the brain

oral – taken by mouth, or relating to the mouth

orbit – the cavity in the skull that contains the eye

organic acids – chemicals found naturally in the body tissues and body fluids, abnormal quantities of which may be a marker of certain disorders of body chemistry or metabolism

orthoptist – a specialist in the detection, measurement and non-surgical treatment of abnormalities of vision and eye movements

osmosis – the passage of water through a membrane from a solution of lower concentration to one of higher concentration, thereby equalizing the concentration

ossified – converted into bone

osteogenesis imperfecta – synonym brittle bone disease; a group of congenital conditions in which the bones are abnormally brittle

osteomyelitis – inflammation of the bone marrow

osteopaenia of prematurity – poor mineralization of bones in babies born preterm

oximeter – an instrument for measuring the amount of oxygen being carried in the blood

oxygen saturation – the amount of oxygen in the bloodstream

palsy – paralysis

papilloedema – swelling of the first part of the optic nerve (the optic disc)

parafalcine – alongside the falx, between the cerebral hemispheres

parenchyma – the working part of an organ, as opposed to the supporting tissues

parenchymal haemorrhage – bleeding within the brain substance

parenteral – given any way other than through the mouth, e.g. fluids given by intravenous infusion

parietal – towards the top and sides of the head

parietal lobe – the part of the brain lying beneath the crown (top) of the skull and the ears, between the frontal and occipital lobes

parieto-occipital – towards the top and back of the head

parkinsonism – a clinical picture of tremor, rigidity and lack of spontaneous movements, with an expressionless face and shuffling gait; can be caused naturally by Parkinson's disease, or by certain drugs

partial thromboplastin time (PTT) – one of the measures of blood clotting

pathogen – an organism, such as a bacterium, that produces disease

pathognomonic – describes a sign or symptom that is characteristic of, or unique to, a particular disease

pathologist – a doctor who specializes in the study of disease processes using bodily fluids and tissue samples taken from living patients or at autopsy

pathophysiology – the study of disturbed function of the body and its organs

perfusion – the passage of fluid through tissues, e.g. the passage of blood through lung tissue to enable oxygen to be absorbed

perichondrium – the layer of fibrous tissue covering cartilage

perinatal – around the time of birth, usually from a few days before to a few days after birth

periorbital – around the orbit

periosteal – referring to the layer of connective tissue that covers the surface of a bone

peritoneal – referring to the lining of the abdominal cavity

pertussis – whooping cough

petechial rash – small, round, flat spots caused by bleeding into the skin; *see* purpura

phlebitis – inflammation of the wall of a vein

phototherapy – treatment with bright light

pia – the innermost of the three meningeal layers covering the brain and spinal cord

pinna – the part of the ear that projects from the head

pituitary gland – the major hormone-secreting gland at the base of the brain

plasmin – an enzyme that dissolves blood clots

plasminogen – a substance present in the blood that can be activated to form plasmin

platelet – blood cells that help to stop bleeding

pleural cavity – the space between the coverings of the lungs and the inner surface of the chest wall

pneumocephalus – the presence of air within the skull, usually due to injury or surgery

pneumothorax – air in the pleural cavity

polymorph – another word for neutrophil

pons – the part of the brainstem that links the medulla oblongata and the midbrain

pontine – appertaining to the pons

porencephalic cyst – a cyst that forms in the brain at the site of damaged or injured brain tissue, most frequently in a cerebral hemisphere

posterior – towards the back

posterior fontanelle – the skin-covered opening towards the back of the skull of a baby where the sagittal and lambdoid sutures have not yet closed together

post-mortem examination (autopsy) – examination of the body after death to determine the cause of death or the presence of disease

postnatal – the time after birth

postpartum – the period of a few days after the birth of a baby

pre-eclampsia – high blood pressure during pregnancy in a woman whose blood pressure was normal before pregnancy

premature – *see* preterm

preretinal haemorrhage – bleeding into the eye in front of the retina

preterm – born before term, but often used to imply born at 36 weeks or earlier

prone – lying face downwards

prophylactic – a substance that prevents the development of a disease or condition, e.g. antibiotics given after an operation to prevent infection of the wound

prostaglandin – a hormone present in many tissues of the body

proteolysis – the process whereby protein molecules are broken down

prothrombin (PT) – a substance present in the blood plasma that helps with blood clotting

proximal – close to the origin or point of attachment, or close to the middle of the body, e.g. a nerve fibre that is close to the central nervous system, or the part of a limb that is close to the body

psychopath – a person who behaves in an antisocial way and displays no guilt or capacity to form emotional relationships; due to an abnormality, or failure of development, of his/her personality

psychotic – denotes loss of contact with reality, as in schizophrenia

PT – *see* prothrombin

PTT – *see* partial thromboplastin time

puerperal depression – the state of sadness that can affect a woman within the first few days after giving birth

pulse oximeter – a machine to measure oxygen saturation in the blood

purpura – a skin rash caused by bleeding into the skin from small blood vessels; *see* petechial rash

pyloric stenosis – narrowing of the outlet of the stomach that delays the passage of food and leads to food being vomited

pyrexia – fever, high temperature

radiograph – an image recorded onto a sheet of special photographic film, produced by variable absorption of X-rays by the different tissues in a part or parts of the body; used synonymously with X-ray

radiographic skeletal survey – X-ray pictures of the whole skeleton to check for old and new fractures or diseases of bones

radiologist – a doctor who specializes in the interpretation of imaging (ultrasound, X-ray, CT and MRI) in order to diagnose disorders

rehydration – giving fluids in order to correct an imbalance in the body

respiratory distress syndrome – a condition found in some newborn, especially preterm, babies where the lungs cannot expand sufficiently, causing rapid, laboured breathing

respiratory rate – number of breaths taken (usually per minute)

resuscitation – reviving respiratory and cardiac function in a person who appears to be dead

RETCAM – a camera used by ophthalmologists to take photographs of the retina

retina – the light sensitive layer that lines the interior of the eye

retinal haemorrhage – bleeding within the retina

retinopathy – a disease of the retina resulting in impairment or loss of vision

retinoschisis – a cleft or split in the retina

retraction bulbs (balls) – the microscopic finding in brain tissue of separation of nerve cell bodies from nerve cell fibres

rhinorrhoea – watery discharge from the nose

rickets – a disease of childhood caused by lack of vitamin D; it causes bones to become soft and malformed

sagittal – through the body, as to divide it into right and left halves

sagittal suture – the joint between the two parietal bones of the skull

schisis – a cleft or a split

schizophrenia – a mental disorder that is characterized by the breakdown of normal thinking, emotional responsiveness and contact with reality; can also involve delusions and hallucinations

sclera – the white outer layer of the eyeball

sclerosis – hardening of tissue, usually due to scarring after inflammation, or to ageing

scurvy – a disease caused by lack of vitamin C in the diet; it causes bleeding in gums and under the skin

seizure – a fit or convulsion; *see also* epilepsy, tonic, and tonic–clonic

sepsis – bacterial infection

septicaemia – 'blood poisoning' due to the presence of bacterial products in the bloodstream

sequela (*plural* sequelae) – a disorder or condition that results from an illness or an accident

serum biochemistry – the study of substances in the fluid that has separated from clotted blood, or blood plasma that has been allowed to stand

shunt – a length of tubing that diverts excess cerebrospinal fluid from the ventricles of the brain to another part of the body (usually the abdominal cavity), where it can be harmlessly absorbed

sinusoid – a small blood vessel found in some organs, such as the liver

skeletal survey – *see* radiographic skeletal survey

skull base – the bones at the base of the skull. These include the bones running from just above the eyes, lying behind the face, around the ears, and the back of the head

Sotos syndrome – a disorder of brain development associated with macrocephaly and some ventricular enlargement

special care baby unit – an intensive care unit for newborn babies who need extra nursing and medical care after birth, or who need to be closely observed for a time; often called a neonatal unit

sphenoid wing – bones forming part of the orbits

spina bifida – *see* myelomeningocele

splenium – the thickest part of the corpus callosum

squamous bone – part of the temporal bone at the side of the skull

squint – *see* strabismus

status epilepticus – repeated epileptic seizures without any intervening recovery of consciousness

strabismus – when the two eyes are not in alignment; they can be horizontally or vertically out of line with each other

subacute – of a disease, progressing more rapidly than a chronic one; implies of relatively recent origin

subarachnoid – the space between the arachnoid (the middle) and the pia (the innermost) meningeal layers, normally filled with cerebrospinal fluid

subconjunctival – beneath the conjunctiva, the clear covering of the eye

subdural – between the dura (the outermost) and the arachnoid (the middle) meningeal layers. In health, there is no space between the two

subdural effusion – a liquid collection in the subdural space, most commonly the result of bleeding or infection

subdural haematoma – blood that has accumulated or has clotted to form a semi-solid or liquid collection in the subdural space

subdural tap – the insertion of a hollow needle between the dura and the arachnoid layers in order to drain fluid from the subdural space

subgaleal – beneath the galea, a sheet of fibrous tissue that forms one of the layers of the scalp

subhyaloid – beneath the hyaloid membrane; this membrane surrounds the vitreous humour in the eye, separating it from the retina

subluxation – partial separation of a joint, whereby the ends of the bones are still in contact but are not aligned

suboccipital – below the occipital region of the skull

subpial – between the pia (the innermost meningeal layer) and the brain

subtemporal – underneath the temporal region of the scalp or the skull or the brain

sulcus (*plural* sulci) – a cleft, or infolding, on the surface of the brain

superior sagittal sinus – a major venous channel in the dura draining blood from the upper half of each cerebral hemisphere

supernatant – the fluid that lies uppermost when a specimen has been left to separate into liquid and solid components

supine – lying face upwards

supra – *prefix* meaning over or above

supratentorial – over or above the tentorium

sutural diastasis – separation of the cranial sutures

sutures – the joins between the skull bones

sylvian fissure – the deep groove on the surface of the brain that marks the border between the frontal and parietal lobes (above the fissure) and the temporal lobe (below the fissure)

syndrome – a combination of signs/symptoms that, taken together, point to a particular disorder

systolic – referring to the measurement of blood pressure; systolic pressure is the higher of the two measurements, when the ventricles are contracting; cf. diastolic

tachycardia – an increase in the heart rate to above the normal for age etc.

tachypnoea – rapid breathing

tap – *see* subdural tap

tegmentum – a region of the midbrain

temporal bones – bones in the part of the skull that encloses the brain

temporal horn – part of the lateral ventricle

temporal lobe – the part of the cerebral cortex that lies to the side, in front of the occipital lobe, and that is concerned with hearing and language, and also with memory

tentorium – an inward fold of the dura that separates the cerebellum below from the occipital lobes of the cerebral hemispheres above

Terson syndrome – vitreous haemorrhage secondary to non-traumatic intracranial haemorrhage

thalamus (*plural* thalami) – either of two masses of grey matter lying deep in the cerebral hemispheres; they relay sensory messages to the cortex

thrombin – the substance, derived from prothrombin, that aids in the final stages of blood coagulation (clotting)

tonic – in epilepsy, the continuous contraction of muscles

tonic–clonic – the combination of the contraction of muscles and rhythmical limb movements during epileptic seizures

transfontanelle – through the fontanelle, e.g. for ultrasound scanning or draining subdural effusions

transtentorial herniation – part of the cerebral hemisphere being pushed through the tentorium under pressure

trauma – physical wound or injury, or emotionally painful event

traumatic lumbar puncture – bleeding caused unintentionally during lumbar puncture; blood from injury to blood vessels in the surrounding tissues can enter the hollow needle used for the lumbar puncture, and it can therefore appear that there is blood in the cerebrospinal fluid due to disease or injury

triage nurse – a nurse, usually in an Accident and Emergency Department, who assesses the seriousness of an illness or injury when a patient arrives at a hospital

trigone – part of the lateral ventricles

ultrasound scan – a way of examining structures inside the body using sound waves; the echoes of reflected sound then form an electronic picture; ultrasound scanning is often used to examine a baby who is still inside the mother's uterus (womb)

uncal – referring to the uncus, which is a projection of the lower surface of the temporal lobes

unilateral – relating to one side of the body or of an organ; cf. bilateral

uraemia – the presence in the blood of excess waste compounds of protein breakdown that would normally be excreted by the kidneys

Valsalva manoeuvre – an attempt to breathe out against a closed airway

vasodilator – a drug used to dilate blood vessels and therefore increase blood flow

vein of Galen – a major vein that drains blood from deep structures within the brain

venepuncture site – the place where a vein has been punctured, e.g. where a blood sample has been taken

ventilated – placed on a ventilator

ventilator – a machine that maintains a flow of air into and out of the lungs of a patient who is not able to breathe normally

ventricles (cerebral) – cavities in the brain filled with cerebrospinal fluid; the lateral (the first and second) ventricles, one in each cerebral hemisphere, join up with the third ventricle, which in turn connects through a narrow channel with the fourth ventricle; this is located in the back part of the brain, and connects with the spinal canal

ventriculitis – inflammation in the ventricles of the brain

ventriculomegaly – enlargement of the cerebral ventricles

vertebra (*plural* vertebrae) – the individual bones that make up the spinal column

vertex – top part

visual acuity – sharpness of vision; the main requirements are a healthy retina and the ability of the eye to focus light onto the retina to form a sharp image, and for that image to be conveyed by the optic nerves to the brain

vitamin K – a vitamin that is important in blood clotting; *see* haemorrhagic disease of the newborn

vitreous haemorrhage – bleeding in the jelly-like substance that fills the space behind the lens and in front of the retina of the eye

vitreous humour – jelly-like material in the chamber behind the lens of the eye

white blood cell (leukocyte) – blood cells that are involved in protecting the body against foreign substances and are involved with antibody production and response to injury and/or disease

white matter – the lighter coloured tissue of the central nervous system containing the nerve fibres; cf. grey matter

xanthochromia – yellow discolouration; when this term is used to describe the cerebrospinal fluid, it indicates that red blood cells have been present in the fluid, and the breakdown products of these cells have left the cerebrospinal fluid yellow in colour

X-ray – radiation of very short wavelength that can penetrate any matter that is opaque to light; X-rays are used to produce radiographs

zygoma – one of the facial bones between the cheeks and the ear

INDEX

(Page numbers in *italics* refer to figures/tables.)

503

504

impact
  bridging vein stretch ratio, 141, 142
  hard, 141, 142
  minor, 298
  soft, 141, 142
  stress distribution, *144*
  tolerance limits, 119
impact injuries, 29, 47–9
  pathophysiology, 52–6
  shaking, 59
impulse, 129
indomethacin, intracranial pressure reduction, 325
infection
  subdural, 308
  treatment, 316–8
inflicted injury algorithm, *19*, 20
injuries
  acceleration, 48–9
  accidental, 40–1, 181
    falls, 49–52, *53*, *54*
  causes other than NAHI, *1*/*1*–*2*
  coexisting, 446–7
  compression, 43–7
    brain, 55
  dating, 286–7
  deceleration, 35, 49, 60–1
  disciplinary, 25–7
  dural, 218
  explanations, 475
  frustration, 25–7
  hanging, 91
  hyperextension, 92
  impact, 29, 47–9
    pathophysiology, 52–6
    shaking, 59
    subdural haemorrhage, 294–5
  laceration, 53–5
    cerebral, *236*, 238
  malicious, 24–5
  mechanisms, 43–56
    offered by parents/caregiver, 28–30
  penetrating, 43
    subdural haematoma, 67
  pre-existing, 400
  re-injury rate, 404–6
  rotational, 30, 48–9, 56
  skull, 214–8
  timing, 93, *93–4*, 95
  treatment, 475
  twisting, 37, 38, 39
  vulnerability to future, 430
  see also brain injury; contusional injuries; intra-
        ocular injuries; ocular injuries; scalp injury;
        shaking; shearing injury; skeletal injuries
intensive care admission for raised intracranial pres-
        sure, 11–2

intention, 453, 454–5
  not proved, 456
intentional acts, 454–5
intracerebral injury, direct, 266–7, *268*, 269
intracranial damage mechanisms, 43–56
intracranial haemorrhage, 114, 117
  retinal haemorrhage secondary to, 200
intracranial homeostasis, *86*
intracranial pressure
  normal, 86
  outcome in NAHI, 116
intracranial pressure, raised
  autoregulation, 88
  brain compression, 55
  brain swelling, 357
  cerebral oedema, 81, 82
  cerebrovascular autoregulation, 36
  cervico-medullary syndrome, 11–2
  glucose tolerance profile, 338, *339*
  incidence, 350
  monitoring, 82
  retinal haemorrhage, 15, *197*, 198
  treatment, 318–25
intracranial vessel compression by shifts/cones, 90–1
intradural bleeding, 62–3, 256, 258
intraocular injuries
  ageing, 194
  haemorrhage differential diagnosis, 195–200
  retinal haemorrhage pathology, 199
intraparenchymal haemorrhage, 12–3
intraretinal haemorrhage, 191–2
intrascleral haemorrhage, *193*, 194
intraventricular haemorrhage, 238
Investigator's Guide to Shaken Baby Syndrome (Wheeler),
        431
iron–oxygen complexes, 90
ischaemia, *see* hypoxic–ischaemic damage

J
jaundice, physiological, 96

K
KOSCHI score, 365

L
labetalol, 335
labour, compression injuries, 44–5
laceration injuries, 53–5
  cerebral, *236*, 238
language clarity, 470
laryngospasm, 256
learning disability, 27
  global, 398–9
legal aspects of shaken baby syndrome, 445–60
  clinical decision to refer, 449
  criminal offences, 453–5

505

507

509

shear–strain forces, 221
shunt catheter, non-valved silastic, 307
siblings
  decisions for, 470
  protection, 475
  vulnerability to injury, 430
sickle cell disease, 43
skeletal injuries, 5, 32–43, 271–88
  dating, 286–7
  differential diagnosis, 287–8
  imaging, 271–3
  incidence, 346
  see also fractures
skeletal survey, 285, 438
  guidelines, 272
skin lesions
  causes other than NAHI, 172, 173, 179–80
  see also scalp injury
skull
  added mass coefficients, 137–8
  compressibility, 35
  copper-beaten, 66
  CSF interface, 136
  deformity, 253
  elasticity, 34
  finite element modelling, 135
  impact area, 34–5
  injuries, 214–18
  protection, 34
  rigid body motion, 136
  vascular markings, 43
skull fractures, 32–7, 116, 283
  biomechanics, 33–5
  causes other than NAHI, 171, 173, 179
  characteristics of non-accidental, 35
  depressed, 67
  domestic accidents, 298
  force, 33–4
  growing, 36, 252–3, 254
  healing, 33
  imaging, 217–8
  impact site/time, 35
  importance, 36–7
  incidence, 148
  pathology, 351–2, 354
  pattern, 147
  prevalence, 147
  spreading, 354
social circumstances of family, 467
social pathology, 20–1
social work
  assessment, 465–6
  decision-making for children, 466–73
  early phases of work with family, 468–70
  implications of outcome of NAHI, 471
  interventions, 463, 465–6

investigations, 421
perspectives, 462–76
research, 466–8
role determination, 463
supportive culture, 466
sustaining intervention after hospital discharge, 470–1
time scales, 472–3
social workers, specialized knowledge, 463–4
sodium valproate, intravenous, 329
soft tissue injuries, scalp, 214–8
special needs of children, 476
spectrophotometry, 95–6
spinal cord
  axonal injury, 355
  pathology of injuries, 354–6
spine
  crush fractures, 285
  injuries, 285, 355
    cervical, 91–3
  post-mortem examination, 439
splintering, skull fracture, 32
Staphylococcus aureus, methicillin-resistant, 317
Staphylococcus epidermidis ventriculitis, 317
status epilepticus, 326, 327–8
  convulsive, 330
  treatment pathway, 331, 332
sternum fracture, 40, 285–6
steroids, intracranial pressure reduction, 323
strabismus, 204
subacute non-encephalopathic presentation, 15–16
subarachnoid haemorrhage, 73
  acute, 231
  imaging, 229–31
  pathology, 352
  subdural haematoma coexistence, 230
subcortical hyperintensity, 266, 269
subcortical laminar necrosis, 248
subcortical tears, shearing contusional, 233–4
subcortical white matter, cerebral infarction, 245–7
subdural collections, 251–2, 294
subdural effusion, 294
  differential diagnosis, 228, 229
  non-accidental injury, 152
subdural haematoma, 62, 106–13, 294
  acute, 66–7, 107, 221–2, 223–4, 228, 229, 263
    low-density, 225–6
  ageing, 222–3
  anterior, 222, 223
  arachnoid cyst complication, 301
  associated conditions, 68
  biomechanics, 114–5
  birth trauma, 300, 358
  bleeding continuation, 72–3
  causes, 63, 67, 68, 255–6, 346
  cerebral swelling, 229

510